GENERAL GYNECOLOGY

The Requisites in Obstetrics and Gynecology

Series Editor:

Mark Evans, MD

Director, Institute for Genetics and Fetal Medicine
St. Luke's-Roosevelt Hospital
New York, New York

Coming Soon in

The Requisites in Obstetrics and Gynecology Series

GYNECOLOGIC ONCOLOGY
HIGH-RISK OBSTETRICS
REPRODUCTIVE ENDOCRINOLOGY AND GYNECOLOGY

GENERAL GYNECOLOGY

The Requisites in Obstetrics and Gynecology

Andrew I. Sokol, MD

Associate Director, Section on Minimally Invasive Surgery
Division of Female Pelvic Medicine and Reconstructive Surgery
Washington Hospital Center
Adjunct Assistant Professor of Obstetrics and Gynecology, U.S.U.H.S.
Assistant Professor of Clinical Urology and Obstetrics and Gynecology,
    Georgetown University
Washington, DC

Eric R. Sokol, MD

Assistant Professor of Obstetrics and Gynecology
Co-Director, Urogynecology and Pelvic Reconstructive Surgery
Director of Gynecology Clinics
Stanford University School of Medicine
Stanford, California

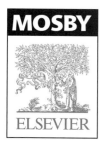

MOSBY

ELSEVIER

1600 John F. Kennedy Blvd.
Suite 1800
Philadelphia, PA 19103-2899

GENERAL GYNECOLOGY:
THE REQUISITES IN OBSTETRICS AND GYNECOLOGY

ISBN-13: 978-0-323-03247-6
ISBN-10: 0-323-03247-8

Notice

Medicine is an ever-changing field. Standard safety procedures must be followed, but as new research and clinical experience broaden our knowledge, changes in treatment and drug therapy may become necessary or appropriate. Readers are advised to check the most current product information provided by the manufacturer of each drug to be administered to verify the recommended dose, the method and duration of administration, and the contraindications. It is the responsibility of the treating physician, relying on experience and knowledge of the patient, to determine dosages and the best treatment for the patient. Neither the publisher nor the editors assume any liability for any injury and/or damage to persons or property arising from this publication.

The Publisher

Library of Congress Cataloging-in-Publication Data

General gynecology: the requisites in obstertics & gynecology / [edited by] Andrew I.
Sokol, Eric R. Sokol. – 1st ed.
    p. ; cm. – (Requisites in obstetrics & gynecology)
ISBN 0-323-03247-8
    1. Gynecology. I. Sokol, Andrew I.   II. Sokol, Eric R.   III. Series.
    [DNLM: 1. Genital Diseases, Female.   2. Pregnancy Complications. WP 140 G326 2007]
RG101.G4622 2007
48.1—dc26   2006046717

Acquisitions Editor: Rebecca Gaertner
Project Manager: Bryan Hayward
Designer: Steven Stave

Printed in the United States of America

Last digit is the print number: 9   8   7   6   5   4   3   2   1

This book is dedicated to my wife,
Alicia,
Whom I admire more than anyone else in the world;

To my son,
Matthew,
For making me see what is most important in life;

And to my parents,
Robert and Roberta,
For always steering me in the right direction.

Andrew I. Sokol

This book is dedicated to my wife,
Nikki,
Who is my best friend and my source of inspiration;

To my daughter,
Aria,
Who brings so much joy into our lives;

And to my parents,
Robert and Roberta,
Whose energy and enthusiasm set an example for us all.

Eric R. Sokol

CONTRIBUTORS

Marjan Attaran, MD
Department of Obstetrics and Gynecology, Cleveland Clinic, Cleveland, Ohio

Matthew D. Barber, MD, MHS
Associate Professor, Cleveland Clinic Lerner College of Medicine, Case Western Reserve University; Director of Clinical Research, Section of Urogynecology and Reconstructive Pelvic Surgery, Cleveland Clinic, Cleveland, Ohio

Mohammed A. Bedaiwy, MD, PhD
Department of Obstetrics and Gynecology, Cleveland Clinic, Cleveland, Ohio

Paul Blumenthal, MD
Professor, Department of Obstetrics and Gynecology, Johns Hopkins Bayview Medical Center, Baltimore, Maryland

Lori A. Boardman, MD, ScM
Associate Professor, Department of Obstetrics and Gynecology; Director, Colposcopy and Vulvar Clinics, Women and Infants Hospital of Rhode Island/Brown Medical School, Providence, Rhode Island

Linda D. Bradley, MD
Director, Center for Menstrual Disorders, Fibroids, and Hysteroscopic Services, Department of Obstetrics and Gynecology, Cleveland Clinic, Cleveland, Ohio

Mikael N. Brisinger, MD
Department of Obstetrics and Gynecology, Kaiser Permanente West Los Angeles Medical Center, Los Angeles, California

Jeffrey L. Clemons, MD, FACOG, LTC, MC
Chief, Division of Urogynecology and Pelvic Reconstructive Surgery, Department of Obstetrics and Gynecology, Madigan Army Medical Center, Tacoma; Clinical Assistant Professor, University of Washington, Seattle, Washington

Andres Chiesa-Vottero, MD
Department of Anatomic Pathology, Cleveland Clinic, Cleveland, Ohio

Amy S. Cooper, WHNP, MSN
Research Nurse Practitioner, Women and Infants Hospital of Rhode Island, Providence, Rhode Island

Allison A. Cowett, MD, MPH
Director, Center for Reproductive Health; Assistant Director, Fellowship in Family Planning; Clinical Assistant Professor, Department of Obstetrics and Gynecology, University of Illinois at Chicago, Chicago, Illinois

Lee Epstein, MD
Fellow, Department of Urogynecology, University of Louisville, Louisville, Kentucky

Pedro F. Escobar, MD
Department of Obstetrics and Gynecology, Florida Gynecologic Oncology, Fort Myers, Florida

Tommaso Falcone, MD, FRCSC, FACOG
Professor, Cleveland Clinic Lerner College of Medicine, Case Western Reserve University; Chairman, Department of Obstetrics and Gynecology, Cleveland Clinic, Cleveland, Ohio

Stephen S. Falkenberry, MD
Clinical Assistant Professor, Brown University School of Medicine, Providence, Rhode Island

Gita P. Gidwani, MD
Department of Obstetrics and Gynecology, Cleveland Clinic, Cleveland, Ohio

Jeffrey M. Goldberg, MD
Head, Section of Reproductive Endocrinology and Infertility, Department of Obstetrics and Gynecology, Cleveland Clinic, Cleveland, Ohio

Eric M. Heinberg, MD, MPH
Department of General Surgery, Swedish Medical Center, Seattle, Washington

Roxanne Jamshidi, MD, MPH
Assistant Professor, Department of Obstetrics and Gynecology, Johns Hopkins Bayview Medical Center, Baltimore, Maryland

David L. Keefe, MD
Professor and Chairman, Department of Obstetrics and Gynecology, University of South Florida College of Medicine, Tampa, Florida

Steven D. Kleeman, MD
Assistant Professor; Head, Section of Urogynecology, Department of Obstetrics and Gynecology, University of Cincinnati, Cincinnati, Ohio

Adam A. Klipfel, MD
Colorectal Surgeon and Program Coordinator, Colorectal Residency Program; Clinical Instructor, Department of Surgery, Brown Medical School, Providence; RI Colorectal Clinic, LLC, Pawtucket, Rhode Island

Jorge A. Lagares-Garcia, MD, FACS, FASCRS
Colon and Rectal Surgeon, Assistant Program Director, Colorectal Residency Program, Clinical Assistant Professor of Surgery, Brown University, Providence; RI Colorectal Clinic, LLC, Pawtucket, Rhode Island

Susan H. Lee, MD
Assistant Professor of Surgery in Clinical Obstetrics and Gynecology, Weill Medical College of Cornell University, New York; Breast Surgeon, Department of Surgery, New York Hospital Queens, Flushing, New York

Robert D. Legare, MD
Assistant Professor and Medical Director, Cancer Risk Assessment and Prevention Program, Department of Obstetrics and Gynecology, Women and Infants Hospital of Rhode Island/Brown Medical School, Providence, Rhode Island

E. Steve Lichtenberg, MD, MPH
Assistant Professor of Clinical Obstetrics and Gynecology, Feinberg School of Medicine at Northwestern University; Medical Director, Family Planning Associates Medical Group, Ltd., Chicago, Illinois

Lawrence Lurvey, MD, JD
Physician Director, Quality and Risk Management, Department of Obstetrics and Gynecology, Kaiser Permanente West Los Angeles Medical Center, Los Angeles, California

S. Gene McNeeley, MD
Professor of Obstetrics, Gynecology, and Urology, Wayne State University School of Medicine, Detroit, Michigan

Chad M. Michener, MD
Division of Gynecologic Oncology, Department of Obstetrics and Gynecology, Cleveland Clinic, Cleveland, Ohio

Magdy Milad, MD, MS
Professor, Department of Obstetrics and Gynecology, Feinberg School of Medicine at Northwestern University; Residency Program Director and Director of Gynecologic Endoscopy, Northwestern Memorial Hospital, Chicago, Illinois

Margaret A. Miller, MD
Assistant Professor, Department of Internal Medicine, Women and Infants Hospital of Rhode Island/Brown Medical School, Providence, Rhode Island

Deborah L. Myers, MD
Associate Professor, Department of Obstetrics and Gynecology, Director, Division of Urogynecology and Reconstructive Pelvic Surgery, Women and Infants Hospital of Rhode Island/Brown Medical School, Providence, Rhode Island

Renee T. Page, MD
Assistant Professor, Division of Gynecology, Wayne State University School of Medicine, Detroit, Michigan

Elizabeth H. W. Ricanati, MD
North American Menopause Society Certified Menopause Practitioner, Department of General Internal Medicine, Cleveland Clinic, Cleveland, Ohio

Adam A. Rojan
Brown Medical School, Providence, Rhode Island

Joseph S. Sanfilippo, MD, MBA
Professor, Department of Obstetrics, Gynecology, and Reproductive Sciences, The University of Pittsburgh School of Medicine, Magee-Womens Hospital, Pittsburgh, Pennsylvania

Jennifer Scalia Wilbur, MS
Clinical Program Manager, Cancer Risk Assessment and Prevention Program, Program in Women's Oncology, Women and Infants Hospital, Providence, Rhode Island

Steven Schechter, MD
Clinical Assistant Professor, Department of Surgery, Brown University; RI Colorectal Clinic, LLC, Pawtucket, Rhode Island

Megan O. Schimpf, MD
Department of Obstetrics and Gynecology, Division of Urogynecology, Hartford Hospital, Hartford, Connecticut

Andrea L. Sikon, MD, FACP
North American Menopause Society Certified Menopause Practitioner, International Society for Clinical Densitometry: Certified Densitometrist, Cleveland Clinic, Cleveland, Ohio

William Andre Silva, MD
Pacific Northwest Urogynecology, PLLC, Federal Way, Washington

Andrew I. Sokol, MD
Associate Director, Section on Minimally Invasive Surgery, Division of Female Pelvic Medicine and Reconstructive Surgery, Washington Hospital Center, Adjunct Assistant Professor of Obstetrics and Gynecology, U.S.U.H.S., Assistant Professor of Clinical Urology and Obstetrics and Gynecology, Georgetown University, Washington, DC

Eric R. Sokol, MD
Assistant Professor of Obstetrics and Gynecology, Co-Director, Urogynecology and Pelvic Reconstructive Surgery, Director of Gynecology Clinics, Stanford University School of Medicine, Stanford, California

Vivian W. Sung, MD, MPH
Assistant Professor, Department of Obstetrics and Gynecology, Division of Urogynecology and Reconstructive Pelvic Surgery,

Women and Infants Hospital/Brown Medical School, Providence, Rhode Island

Claire Templeman, MD
Assistant Professor, Department of Clinical Obstetrics and Gynecology, University of Southern California Women's and Children's Hospital, Los Angeles, California

Holly L. Thacker, MD, FACP, CCD
Director, Women's Health Center, Women's Health and Breast Pavilion, The Cleveland Clinic; Associate Professor of Surgery, The Cleveland Clinic Lerner College of Medicine, Case Western Reserve University, Cleveland, Ohio

Frank Tu, MD
Division Director, Endoscopic Surgery and Chronic Pelvic Pain; Assistant Professor of Obstetrics and Gynecology and Physical Medicine and Rehabilitation, Feinberg School of Medicine at Northwestern University, Chicago, Illinois

Paul K. Tulikangas, MD
Assistant Professor, Division of Urogynecology and Reconstructive Pelvic Surgery, Department of Obstetrics and Gynecology, University of Connecticut (Hartford Hospital), Hartford, Connecticut

Mark D. Walters, MD
Head, Section of Urogynecology and Reconstructive Pelvic Surgery, Department of Obstetrics and Gynecology, Cleveland Clinic, Cleveland, Ohio

James L. Whiteside, MD
Assistant Professor, Department of Obstetrics and Gynecology, Division of Urogynecology and Reconstructive Pelvic Surgery, Dartmouth Medical School, Lebanon, New Hampshire

John W. Whiteside, MD
Assistant Professor, Department of Family Medicine, Mayo Clinic, Scottsdale, Arizona

Nurit Winkler, MD
Department of Obstetrics and Gynecology, Division of Reproductive Endocrinology and Infertility, University of Texas Southwestern Medical Center, Dallas, Texas

Kyle J. Wohlrab, MD
Department of Obstetrics and Gynecology, Women and Infants Hospital of Rhode Island, Providence, Rhode Island

Kristen Page Wright, MD
Fellow, Reproductive Endocrinology and Infertility, Department of Obstetrics and Gynecology, University of Vermont, College of Medicine; Fletcher Allen Health Care, Burlington, Vermont

The Requisites in Obstetrics and Gynecology

FOREWORD

We are living in an era of rapidly changing technologies—an era in which technical and now many medical services can be performed remotely and often impersonally. At the same time, the cultures of medical practice and training have been radically transformed as resident work rules, the use of new procedures and equipment, and changing perspectives on the practice of medicine have evolved quite significantly over the past two decades. As a consequence, the overall approach to medical education, the slower rate of increasing responsibilities given to residents during their training, and the tolerance for nonstandardized approaches to patient care have likewise changed, with both positive and negative consequences. Thus, the basics, the "requisites," needed to operate in the current environment likewise have evolved. In this series, the editors and chapter authors crystalize the foundations needed for independent practitioners to survive and, in fact, thrive in the current medical climate. We hope readers will view the materials as the basis for evolving sophistication in the practice of obstetrics and gynecology.

Mark I. Evans, MD

PREFACE

General Gynecology: The Requisites in Obstetrics and Gynecology is written for the busy resident, fellow, and practicing physician. It is meant to be a comprehensive yet manageable textbook that can serve as both a primary reference text and a quick clinical guide. We believe this book fills a void left by other gynecology textbooks, which are too daunting or too brief in their coverage of important clinical topics in gynecology. Chapters in this textbook are meant to stand alone and can be read easily in one sitting. Similarly, although *General Gynecology: The Requisites in Obstetrics and Gynecology* is part of the *Requisites in Obstetrics and Gynecology* series, it is written as a freestanding textbook.

As editors, we have chosen to format *General Gynecology: The Requisites in Obstetrics and Gynecology* as a problem-based text. Readers should be able to quickly and easily locate pertinent information about specific gynecologic conditions. Each chapter is written in a practical, straightforward manner and is comprehensive but concise. Important information is summarized in easy-to-read tables and figures. Suggested readings are given at the end of each chapter for readers seeking more in-depth information.

General Gynecology: The Requisites in Obstetrics and Gynecology also differs from other general gynecology textbooks in two important respects. First, it devotes considerable space to disorders of the pelvic floor, including urinary incontinence, fecal incontinence, and pelvic organ prolapse. This depth of coverage is rare for a general gynecology textbook, but reflects the increasing importance of these disorders in gynecology. Second, minimally invasive therapies are covered in detail, as these technologies have become common in modern gynecology practice and are now considered the gold standard of care for many gynecologic conditions.

The contributors to this book are authorities in their respective fields, and we are greatly indebted to them for their collaboration in the creation of this unique volume. Our book would not have been possible without the help and support of many special people. Dr. Mark Evans invited our participation, and we are thankful for his continued support of our academic careers. We are also indebted to Dr. Mark Walters and Dr. Deborah Myers for their support of this significant project during our busy Female Pelvic Medicine/Reconstructive Surgery fellowships.

It is our hope that *General Gynecology: The Requisites in Obstetrics and Gynecology* will serve as a clinically useful reference in gynecology that can be read either chapter by chapter or cover to cover. We look forward to hearing your comments and ideas about how to improve this textbook for future generations of physicians.

Andrew I. Sokol, MD
Eric R. Sokol, MD

TABLE OF CONTENTS

Chapter 1   **EMBRYOLOGY**   1
David L. Keefe and Nurit Winkler

Chapter 2   **REPRODUCTIVE PHYSIOLOGY**   21
David L. Keefe and Kristen Page Wright

Chapter 3   **THE GENETICS OF BREAST AND GYNECOLOGIC CANCERS**   43
Jennifer Scalia Wilbur, Adam A. Rojan, and Robert D. Legare

Chapter 4   **GYNECOLOGIC ANATOMY**   73
Steven D. Kleeman and William Andre Silva

Chapter 5   **EVALUATION OF THE FEMALE PATIENT**   99
John W. Whiteside, Elizabeth H.W. Ricanati, and James L. Whiteside

Chapter 6   **PREVENTIVE HEALTH CARE FOR WOMEN**   125
Margaret A. Miller

Chapter 7   **FAMILY PLANNING**   157
Roxanne Jamshidi and Paul Blumenthal

Chapter 8   **PEDIATRIC AND ADOLESCENT GYNECOLOGY**   187
Claire Templeman and Joseph S. Sanfilippo

Chapter 9   **CONGENITAL AND DEVELOPMENTAL ANOMALIES**   205
Marjan Attaran and Gita P. Gidwani

Chapter 10   **PREGNANCY LOSS AND TERMINATION**   225
Allison A. Cowett and E. Steve Lichtenberg

Chapter 11   **ECTOPIC PREGNANCY**   257
Eric M. Heinberg

Chapter 12   **INFERTILITY: EVALUATION AND TREATMENT**   287
Jeffrey M. Goldberg

Chapter 13   ENDOMETRIOSIS AND ADENOMYOSIS   321
              Mohammed A. Bedaiwy and Tommaso Falcone

Chapter 14   ABNORMAL UTERINE BLEEDING   347
              Linda D. Bradley

Chapter 15   MENSTRUAL DISORDERS   367
              Eric R. Sokol, Lawrence Lurvey, and Mikael N. Brisinger

Chapter 16   MENOPAUSE   383
              Andrea L. Sikon and Holly L. Thacker

Chapter 17   VULVAR EPITHELIAL DISORDERS AND OTHER VULVAR
              CONDITIONS   409
              Lori A. Boardman and Amy S. Cooper

Chapter 18   DIAGNOSIS, WORKUP, AND MANAGEMENT OF PREINVASIVE
              LESIONS OF THE CERVIX   429
              Pedro F. Escobar, Andres Chiesa-Vottero, and Chad M. Michener

Chapter 19   LEIOMYOMAS   459
              Linda D. Bradley

Chapter 20   DISORDERS OF THE FALLOPIAN TUBE AND OVARY   481
              Renee T. Page and S. Gene McNeeley

Chapter 21   CONDITIONS OF THE FEMALE BREAST   497
              Susan H. Lee and Stephen S. Falkenberry

Chapter 22   GENITAL AND URINARY TRACT INFECTIONS   523
              Paul K. Tulikangas and Megan O. Schimpf

Chapter 23   PELVIC ORGAN PROLAPSE AND PELVIC FLOOR
              DYSFUNCTION   543
              Andrew I. Sokol and Mark D. Walters

Chapter 24   URINARY INCONTINENCE   583
              Eric R. Sokol

Chapter 25   BOWEL DISORDERS   609
              Jorge A. Lagares-Garcia, Adam A. Klipfel, and Steven Schechter

Chapter 26   URINARY TRACT INJURY AND GENITAL TRACT FISTULAS   639
              Vivian W. Sung, and Kyle J. Wohlrab

Chapter 27   INTERSTITIAL CYSTITIS AND CHRONIC PELVIC PAIN   663
              Deborah L. Myers

Chapter 28   **EVALUATION AND MANAGEMENT OF THE GYNECOLOGIC SURGICAL PATIENT**   687
Jeffrey L. Clemons

Chapter 29   **HYSTERECTOMY**   707
Matthew D. Barber

Chapter 30   **ENDOSCOPIC APPROACHES TO GYNECOLOGIC DISEASE**   755
Magdy Milad, Frank Tu, Lee Epstein, and Linda D. Bradley

INDEX   785

xix

EMBRYOLOGY
David L. Keefe and Nurit Winkler

INTRODUCTION

Understanding the earliest stage of development provides the clinician insight into the mechanisms underlying reproductive failure, congenital anomalies, preeclampsia, abnormal placentation, miscarriage, germ cell and trophoblastic neoplasms, and stem cell treatments. Development begins with *fertilization*, the process by which the sperm and oocyte unite to give rise to the *zygote*. A critical precursor to fertilization is cell *meiosis*, the two cell divisions that result in the formation of daughter cells known as *gametes*. Each gamete contains half the number of chromosomes and half the number of chromatids. Meiosis requires two consecutive cell divisions: *meiosis I*, in which homologous chromosome pairs exchange genetic material and then separate, and *meiosis II*, in which chromatids separate. Each cell is thus provided with a haploid number of chromosomes and half the amount of DNA of a normal somatic cell (Fig. 1-1).

GAMETOGENESIS

In females, the process of maturation from primitive germ cells to mature gametes begins before birth and is completed years later with the fertilization of the egg. At 4 weeks of development, primordial germ cells originate from the endoderm of the wall of the yolk sac and begin to migrate to the genital ridge (the indifferent gonad). Upon arriving at the genital ridge, the germ cells undergo a period of intense mitotic activity, increasing their number to 6 to 7 million. The number continues to rise until 20 weeks' gestation and then rapidly falls through an accelerated process of atresia. At birth, only about 2 to 4 million germ cells remain, and only about 40,000 persist until menarche. Fewer than 500 eventually will reach complete maturation and be ready to fertilize.

Once primordial germ cells arrive at the gonad of the female, they differentiate into *oogonia*. Although the majority of oogonia will continue to divide by mitosis, some oogonia differentiate into *primary oocytes* that enter the *prophase of the first meiosis division*. By 28 weeks of gestation, all primary oocytes have started the prophase of the first meiosis division where they are arrested at the *diplotene stage*, a resting stage of prophase

Figure 1-1

A, Mitosis.
B, Meiosis. (From Larsen WJ: Human Embryology, 3rd ed. New York, Churchill Livingstone, 2001.)

Mitosis

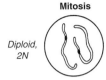

Diploid, 2N

Preparatory phase: DNA doubles

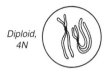

Diploid, 4N

Prophase: chromosomes condense

Metaphase: chromosomes line up on mitotic spindle; centromeres replicate

Anaphase: single-stranded chromosomes pull apart

Cell divides: each daughter cell contains two chromosomes of each type

Diploid, 2N

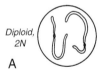

A

Meiosis

Diploid, 2N — Chromosomes each contain one chromatid

Preparatory phase: DNA doubles

Diploid, 4N — Chromosomes each contain two chromatids

Prophase 1: chromosomes condense

Chiasmata form; crossing over can occur

Metaphase I—anaphase I: double-stranded chromosomes pull apart

Telophase I: cell division

Haploid, 2N

Anaphase II: centromeres replicate and each double-stranded chromosome pulls apart to form two single-stranded chromosomes

Cell division yields four gametes

Haploid, 1N

B

characterized by a lacy network of chromatin. Primary oocytes remain in prophase until puberty.

At puberty, 5 to 15 *primary oocytes* begin to mature with each ovarian cycle. Usually only one reaches full maturity each month. The first meiotic division resumes shortly before ovulation, and the primary oocyte completes division with the formation of two daughter cells of unequal size: *secondary oocyte* receives most of the cytoplasm, whereas the first *polar body* receives practically no cytoplasm. Each daughter cell contains 23 double-stranded chromosomes. The secondary oocyte advances immediately to metaphase II of the second meiotic division around the time of ovulation. Meiosis II is completed only if the oocyte is fertilized. The maturation process from oogonium to secondary oocyte thus takes from about 12 to 50 years.

FERTILIZATION

Fertilization usually occurs in the widest part of the fallopian tube, the ampullary region. With each ejaculation, an average of 500 million sperm are deposited in the female tract. The flagellar activity of the spermatozoa, together with the contractions of the uterus and fallopian tubes, advances the spermatozoa to the ampullary region. Only about 300 to 500 spermatozoa reach the site of fertilization, and only one will fertilize the egg. The fertilization process includes two preliminary steps: *capacitation* and *acrosome reaction.* Both induce morphologic and biochemical changes in the acrosomal region of the spermatozoa. These modifications enable the spermatozoa to penetrate the oocyte's corona radiata and the zona pellucida. Once the spermatozoa have penetrated the oocyte's cytoplasm, the head of the spermatozoa separates from the tail, leaving the tail behind. The head of the spermatozoa progressively swells and forms the *male pronucleus.* Soon after the penetration of the spermatozoa, the oocyte undergoes two major processes: modification of the cortical area and zona pellucida to prevent other spermatozoa from penetrating the oocyte, and resumption of the second meiotic division with extrusion of the second polar body and formation of the *definitive oocyte.* The definitive oocyte then forms the *female pronucleus.*

After both pronuclei have replicated their DNA (from both paternal and maternal chromosomes), they undergo their first mitotic division, giving rise to the two-cell stage called the *zygote* or *one-cell embryo* (Fig. 1-2). The first division takes about 20 hours to complete. The ultimate results of fertilization are restoration of the diploid number of chromosomes, determination of the chromosomal sex, and initiation of embryo cleavage.

Five to six days after fertilization, the blastocyst differentiates into the inner cell mass, which is destined to form the embryo proper, and the *trophectoderm*, which is destined to form the placenta and membranes as well as a fluid-filled cavity called the *blastocele.*

Early Differentiation: Morula and Blastula

While the zygote is passing through the fallopian tube, it undergoes *cleavage*, a process of rapid mitotic divisions that result in the formation of progressively smaller cells. These smaller cells, called *blastomeres*, are totipotent (capable of forming a complete embryo). The first mitotic division of the zygote occurs about 30 hours after fertilization. Approximately 3 days after fertilization, the original zygote enters the uterine cavity. The zygote already is composed of 16 blastomeres, forming the *morula.* Upon entering the uterine cavity, fluid begins to penetrate through the zona pellucida and cell membrane of the morula, giving rise to a single cavity, the blastocele. The morula becomes the *blastocyst* (see Fig. 1-2). As the fluid gradually increases

3

Figure 1-2

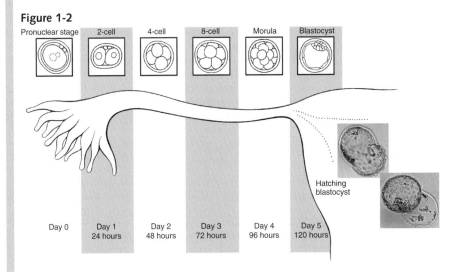

Fertilization occurs in the ampullary region of the fallopian tube. During the first few days, the zygote undergoes cleavage as it travels down the fallopian tube and enters the uterus. The blastocyst hatches from the zona pellucida and is then able to implant into the uterine endometrium. (From Larsen WJ: Human Embryology, 3rd ed. New York, Churchill Livingstone, 2001.)

within the cavity, it separates the blastocyst into two parts: the *trophoblast*, which is the mass of outer cells that lines the epithelial wall of the blastocyst, and the *embryoblast*, which is the inner pole that projects into the blastocyst cavity.

Implantation

Implantation involves the attachment, penetration, and embedding of the blastocyst within the endometrium. This process begins 6 days after fertilization, on the twentieth to twenty-second day of the cycle, and takes approximately 1 week. Implantation is an unusual process in that it resembles invasion by malignant neoplasm, and it involves tolerance of the antigenically foreign cells by the maternal host. At the time of implantation, the mucosa of the uterus is in the secretory phase, containing active glands, large amounts of nutrients, and tortuous arteries. It is composed of three layers: the superficial compact, intermediate spongy, and thin basal layers. Soon after the initiation of implantation, the endometrium undergoes a series of morphologic and biochemical changes known as the *Arias-Stella reaction*. This is followed by gradual decidualization of the endometrium, visualized between the fifth and sixth menstrual week as a bright echogenic ring within the uterus, providing the first sonographic evidence of pregnancy.

The blastocyst, arriving in the uterine cavity, hatches from the zona pellucida and differentiates into the trophoblast (outer cell mass) and embryoblast (inner cell mass). The trophoblast invades the endometrial epithelium and differentiates into the *cytotrophoblast* and *syncytiotrophoblast*. The cytotrophoblast, or inner cell layer, is mitotically active. New cells that originate from the cytotrophoblast join the increasing mass of the syncytiotrophoblast. The syncytiotrophoblast, or outer cell layer, is responsible for invasion of the endometrium and production of human chorionic gonadotropin. Human chorionic gonadotropin can be detected in the mother's peripheral blood as early as 6 days after ovulation, and always by the twelfth day (Table 1-1).

4

Table 1-1

Event	Days After Ovulation
Zona pellucida disappears	4–5
Blastocyst attaches to the epithelial surface of endometrium	6
Trophoblast erodes into endometrial stroma	7
Trophoblast differentiates into cytotrophoblast and syncytiotrophoblast	7–8
Lacunae appear around trophoblast	8–9
Blastocyst burrows beneath endometrial surface	9–10
Lacunar network forms	10–11
Trophoblast invades endometrial sinusoids, establishing uteroplacental circulation	11–12
Endometrial epithelium completely covers blastocyst	12–13
Strong decidual reaction occurs in stroma	13–14

5

SECOND WEEK OF DEVELOPMENT: BILAMINAR GERM DISC

The second week of development is characterized by formation of the *bilaminar germ disc* and associated structures including the amnion, chorion, and uteroplacental circulation. The blastocyst at this stage consists of trophoblast on the outside and embryoblast on the inside, as well as the blastocyst cavity.

Trophoblast

During this stage, the trophoblast already has differentiated into cytotrophoblast and syncytiotrophoblast (Fig. 1-3). The syncytiotrophoblast, which is a solid structure at the beginning of implantation, develops vacuoles that fuse together and form large lacunae. Concurrently, cells of the syncytiotrophoblast penetrate deeper into the stroma, until they reach the maternal sinuses. The syncytiotrophoblast erodes into the endothelium of the maternal sinuses, allowing maternal blood to enter the lacunar system. In this way, the syncytiotrophoblast establishes the first contact between maternal and fetal blood, creating the base for the uteroplacental circulation. Meanwhile, cells of the cytotrophoblast proliferate and penetrate into the syncytiotrophoblast, where they form cellular columns known as the *primary villi*.

Embryoblast

The embryoblast differentiates into two compact layers: the *hypoblast*, adjacent to the blastocyst cavity, and the *epiblast*, adjacent to the cytotrophoblast (see Fig. 1-3). These two layers together are known as the *bilaminar germ disc*. Soon after the formation of the bilaminar germ disc, a small cavity appears within the epiblast and gradually increases in size, giving rise to the *amniotic cavity* (see Fig. 1-3). Cells originated from the hypoblast proliferate and line the inner surface of the blastocyst cavity, forming the *primitive yolk sac*. With additional proliferation of these cells, the primitive yolk sac develops into the *secondary yolk sac*, which is also called the

Figure 1-3

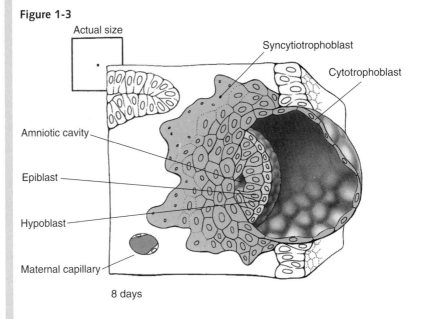

The blastocyst arriving at the uterine cavity differentiates into the trophoblast and embryoblast. The trophoblast invades the endometrial epithelium and differentiates into the cytotrophoblast, an inner cell layer, and the syncytiotrophoblast, an outer cell layer. The syncytiotrophoblast erodes into the endothelium, creating the base for the uteroplacental circulation. The embryoblast differentiates into the hypoblast, adjacent to the blastocyst cavity, and the epiblast. (From Larsen WJ: Human Embryology, 3rd ed. New York, Churchill Livingstone, 2001.)

definitive yolk sac. The definitive yolk sac is a much smaller structure than the original yolk sac (Fig. 1-4).

In the meantime, cells that originated from the yolk sac proliferate in the space between the cytotrophoblast and yolk sac cavity to form a loose connective tissue known as the *chorion.* Large cavities develop within the chorion and eventually become confluent, forming a new space called the *chorionic cavity.* The chorionic cavity surrounds the yolk sac and amniotic cavity, except where the bilaminar germ disc is connected to the trophoblast by the connecting stalk. The connecting stalk will become the umbilical cord (see Fig. 1-4).

THIRD WEEK OF DEVELOPMENT: FORMATION OF THE TRILAMINAR EMBRYO

The third week of gestation coincides with the first missed menstrual period. During this period, all three germ layers develop: the *ectoderm,* the *mesoderm,* and the *endoderm.*

Once the formation of the three germ layers is complete, organogenesis begins.

All three germ layers originate from the epiblast, with formation of a thickening of the epithelium on the surface of the epiblast known as the *primitive streak* (Fig. 1-5). Cells that originate at the primitive streak begin to proliferate in different directions:

Figure 1-4

The primitive yolk sac develops into the secondary yolk sac. The chorionic cavity surrounds the yolk sac and amniotic cavity, except where the bilaminar germ disc is connected to the trophoblast by the connecting stalk. The connecting stalk will become the umbilical cord. (From Larsen WJ: Human Embryology, 3rd ed. New York, Churchill Livingstone, 2001.)

Actual size

Syncytiotrophoblast

Connecting stalk

Cytotrophoblast

Extraembryonic mesoderm

Trophoblastic lacuna

14–15 days

Remnants of primary yolk sac (exocoelomic cysts)

7

Figure 1-5

Trilaminar embryo: all three germ layers originate from the epiblast, with formation of the primitive streak. Cells that originate at the primitive streak proliferate in different directions, giving rise to the endoderm (A), mesoderm (B), and ectoderm. (From Larsen WJ: Human Embryology, 3rd ed. New York, Churchill Livingstone, 2001.)

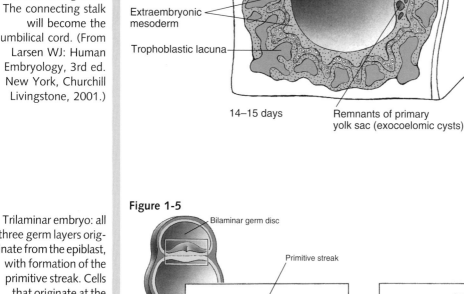

Bilaminar germ disc

Primitive streak

Epiblast

Hypoblast

14–15 days

Endoderm

A

16 days

Mesoderm   Definitive endoderm

B

1. Cranially, where they give rise to the *primitive node*
2. Between the epiblast and hypoblast, giving rise to the *endoderm* (see Fig. 1-5A)
3. Between the epiblast and the endoderm, giving rise to the *mesoderm* (see Fig. 1-5B)
4. Superiorly, where they give rise to the *ectoderm* and eventually become the developing nervous system

The embryonic disc, initially flat and round, gradually acquires a more elongated form with a broad cephalic and a narrow caudal end. Completing the formation of the three germ layers, cells that originated at the primitive node migrate cranially to form a midline cord, the *notochordal process*. The notochordal process will form the midline axis and the basis of the axial skeleton. Meanwhile, mesenchymal cells that originated in the primitive streak migrate cephalad and unite cranially to the notochordal process, giving rise to the *cardiogenic area*. At the cardiogenic area, they begin to proliferate and form two endothelial tubes that fuse together to form the *primitive heart tubes*. The primitive heart tubes are the origin of the cardiovascular system, which is the first system to reach a functional state.

NEURAL TUBE FORMATION

The nervous system originates primarily from the ectoderm. Ectodermal cells that originate at the notochord and cells from the adjacent mesoderm proliferate to form the *neural plate*. Invagination of the neural plate gives rise to the *neural groove* medially and to two *neural folds* laterally. Fusion of the neural folds gives origin to the primitive *neural tube*. The neural tube cranially will differentiate into the various compartments of the *brain*, whereas the remainder of the neural tube will give rise to the *spinal cord*. Defects of closure of the neural tube are the most frequent malformation of the central nervous system.

MUSCULAR AND SKELETAL SYSTEM

Mesenchymal cells originating from the mesoderm on each side of the notochords and the neural tube proliferate to form the *paraxial mesoderm*. on, the paraxial mesoderm begins to divide, giving rise to 42 to 44 pairs of linear bodies known as *somites*. The somites flank the notochord from the occipital region to the embryonic tail. The somites give rise to most of the axial skeleton, the voluntary musculature, and to part of the dermis of the neck and trunk.

FETAL-MATERNAL CIRCULATION

At the beginning of the third week of gestation, during the formation of the trilaminar embryo, establishment of the fetal-maternal circulation begins with the formation of the *primary villi*. The primary villi consist of a cytotrophoblast core covered by an external syncytial layer. Soon after formation of the primary villi, mesodermal cells penetrate the villi, transforming the primary villi to *secondary villi*. Within the secondary villi, mesodermal cells differentiate into blood cells and small vessels, giving rise to the *tertiary villi* or *definitive placental villous* (Fig. 1-6). The definitive villous communicates with the fetal circulation, establishing the final fetal-maternal circulation.

Figure 1-6

Fetal-maternal circulation: longitudinal section through a villus at the end of the third week of development. **A,** Primary stem villus (11–13 days). **B,** Secondary stem villus (16 days). **C,** Tertiary stem villus (21 days). Maternal vessels penetrate the cytotrophoblastic shell to enter intervillous spaces, which surround the villi. The capillaries in the villi are in contact with vessels in the chorionic plate and in the connecting stalk, which in turn are connected to intraembryonic vessels. (From Larsen WJ: Human Embryology, 3rd ed. New York, Churchill Livingstone, 2001.)

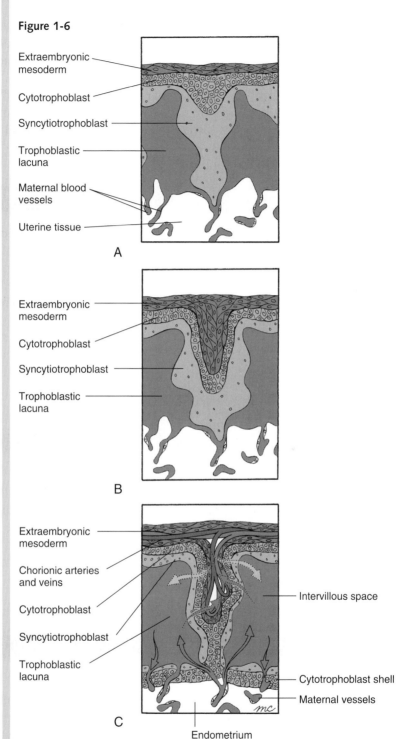

A

Extraembryonic mesoderm
Cytotrophoblast
Syncytiotrophoblast
Trophoblastic lacuna
Maternal blood vessels
Uterine tissue

B

Extraembryonic mesoderm
Cytotrophoblast
Syncytiotrophoblast
Trophoblastic lacuna

C

Extraembryonic mesoderm
Chorionic arteries and veins
Cytotrophoblast
Syncytiotrophoblast
Trophoblastic lacuna
Intervillous space
Cytotrophoblast shell
Maternal vessels
Endometrium

Morphologically, two types of villi can be distinguished: *anchoring villi*, which extend from the chorionic plate to reach the decidua basalis, and *free* or *terminal villi*, which branch from the anchoring villi and are responsible for the exchange of nutrients.

The embryonic circulatory system with blood vessels, plasma, and blood cells originates from the mesoderm in the yolk sac. Fetal hematopoiesis begins in the liver around the eighth week of gestation. Later, hematopoiesis takes place in the spleen, bone marrow, and lymph nodes.

By the end of the eighth week of gestation, the three primary germ layers have completed most of their differentiation, giving rise to the various tissues and organs.

The *ectoderm* germ layer gives rise to the following:

1. Central nervous system
2. Peripheral nervous system
3. Sensory epithelium of the ear, nose, and eye
4. Skin, including hair and nails
5. Pituitary gland, mammary glands, sweat organs, and enamel of the teeth

The *mesoderm* germ layer gives rise to the supporting tissues of the body, including the following:

1. Muscles
2. Cartilage and bone
3. Subcutaneous tissue

The *endodermal* germ layer gives rise to the following:

1. Epithelial lining of gastrointestinal tract
2. Epithelial lining of respiratory tract
3. Epithelial lining of urinary bladder
4. Parenchyma of the thyroid and parathyroid glands
5. Parenchyma of the liver and pancreas
6. Epithelial lining of the tympanic cavity and auditory tube

This period is considered to be the most critical for the developing fetus and is highly sensitive to teratogenic insult. Uncontrolled diabetes during this early stage of development can cause insufficient mesoderm formation at the caudal region of the embryo, resulting in a condition known as caudal dysgenesis or sirenomelia (Fig. 1-7A). Ethanol abuse during this stage can destroy cells in the anterior midline of the germ disc, producing holoprosencephaly (Fig. 1-7B).

UROGENITAL SYSTEM

The urinary and genital systems have a common embryologic origin, the mesodermal ridge (intermediate mesoderm), located along the posterior wall of the abdominal cavity. The common embryologic origin of the urinary and genital systems explains why malformations involving both systems appear so commonly.

Genital System

The genital system goes through an indifferent stage, from which development can proceed toward male or female genitalia, based on genetics and hormonal influences.

Sexual differentiation can be divided into the following categories:

1. Genetic sex—determined by the presence of the sex chromosomes (XX or XY)
2. Gonadal sex—determined by differentiation of the gonad into testis or ovary
3. Phenotypical sex—determined by differentiation of the external genitalia and secondary sexual characteristics into a phenotypic female or male

Genetic sex is determined at the time of conception by the presence of XX or XY chromosomes. Male sexual differentiation is an "active" process, requiring the presence of the SRY gene (sex-determining region), located on the short arm of the Y chromosome. In the absence of the Y chromosome, female development occurs.

11

Figure 1-7

A, Sirenomelia. Severe reduction of the caudal structures has resulted in fusion of the lower extremity limb buds.

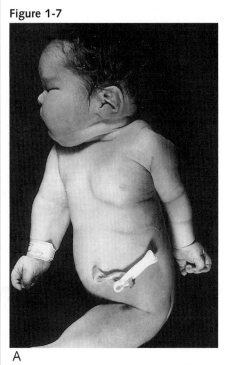

A

(continued)

Figure 1-7 Cont'd

B, Examples of holo-prosencephaly. This spectrum of malformations, which may occur as a manifestation of fetal alcohol syndrome, range in severity from minor midfacial defects to extremely devastating malformations. (From Larsen WJ: Human Embryology, 3rd ed. New York, Churchill Livingstone, 2001.)

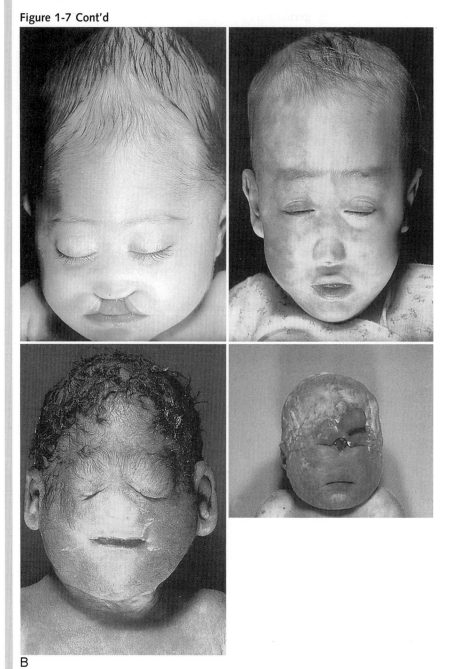

B

Gonads

The gonads do not acquire male or female morphologic characteristics until the seventh week of development. During the fifth week of gestation, at the medial side of each mesonephron, the coelomic epithelium and underlying mesenchyme proliferate to produce a thickened area known as the *genital ridge*. Primordial germ cells originating from the yolk sac migrate along the dorsal mesentery of the hindgut and reach the genital ridge at the sixth week of gestation. The germinal cells, upon arriving at the genital ridge, begin to proliferate, forming the *primitive sex cords*. These cells will determine the differentiation of the gonads into testis or ovary.

In the presence of the Y chromosome (Fig. 1-8A), the primitive sex cords proliferate in the medullary zone, giving rise to the *rete testis*. The sex cords, initially composed solely of germinal cells, later acquire *Sertoli cells*, which produce antimüllerian hormone. The production of antimüllerian hormone by Sertoli cells and of testosterone by Leydig cells induces male differentiation of the genital ducts and of the external genitalia. Production of testosterone takes place as early as the eighth week of gestation.

In the absence of a Y chromosome, the primitive sex cords regress and a second generation of sex cords develops. The second generation of sex cords in females does not develop in the medullary area as it does in males, but rather in the cortical area, and in females the cords are known as the

Figure 1-8

Primitive gonads: in the presence of the Y chromosome (A), the primitive sex cords proliferate in the medullary zone, giving rise to the rete testis. In females (B), primitive sex cords develop in the cortical area, called *cortical cords*. (From Larsen WJ: Human Embryology, 3rd ed. New York, Churchill Livingstone, 2001.)

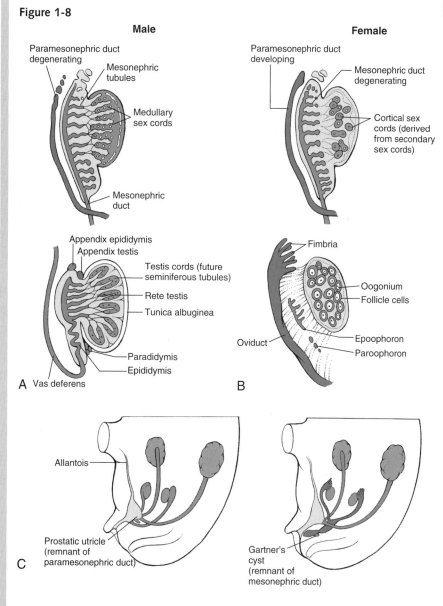

cortical cords (see Figs. 1-8B and 1-9). The cortical cords split into clusters of cells at the sixteenth week of gestation, and each cluster surrounds one or more primordial germ cell. The surrounding epithelial cells give rise to the *follicular cells*, and the germ cells become *oogonia* (see Fig. 1-9).

Genital Ducts

The genital ducts originate from the *mesonephric* ("wolffian") and the *paramesonephric* ("müllerian") ducts, both of which develop lateral to the urogenital ridge. The first to develop are the mesonephric ducts, followed by the paramesonephric ducts on either side of the mesonephric ducts.

Female

By the end of the fourth week of gestation, the paramesonephric ducts originate as a solid cord lateral to the mesonephric ducts. The mesonephric ducts regress in the absence of the Y chromosome. The paramesonephric ducts at the cranial end open into the abdominal cavity, giving rise to the *fallopian tubes* and *fimbria* (see Fig. 1-8). Distally, the paramesonephric ducts cross the mesonephric duct ventrally and unite, where they both open into the posterior wall of the urogenital sinus. At the point of entrance of the paramesonephric ducts into the urogenital sinus, the urogenital sinus proliferates, giving rise to the *müllerian tubercle*. Soon after, the two paramesonephric ducts begin to fuse together to form the *uterine canal*, the origin of the *uterus, cervix,* and *upper vagina*. The uterine canals complete their fusion by the tenth week of gestation. Meanwhile, along the border between the müllerian tubercle and the urogenital sinus, a solid cord of cells called the *vaginal plate* proliferates and elongates, increasing the distance between the uterus and the urogenital sinus. The vaginal plate canalizes at the sixteenth week of gestation, giving rise to the lumen of the *vagina*. The lumen of the vagina remains separated from that of the urogenital sinus by a thin tissue plate, the *hymen*. Perforation of the hymen usually occurs shortly before or after birth. The vagina has a dual origin: the upper portion of the vagina and the fornices originate from the paramesonephric ducts, whereas the lower portion of the vagina originates from the urogenital sinus.

Small remnants of the wolffian ducts, which can develop into cysts, can be found in the following locations:

Figure 1-9

Sex differentiation. (From Moore KL: The Developing Human: Clinically Oriented Embryology, 7th ed. Philadelphia, W.B. Saunders, 2003.)

Indifferent gonad

44 + XY	44 + XX
⇓	⇓
Testis	Ovary
1. Medullary cords develops	1. Medullary cords degenerate
2. No cortical cords	2. Cortical cords develop
3. Thick tunica albuginea	3. No tunica albuginea

1. Ovarian hilus and paravaginally, known as *Gartner cysts* (see Fig. 1-8C).
2. Broad ligament, known as *epoophoron*. Cysts of the epoophoron are known as *paraovarian cysts.*
3. Adjacent to the uterus, known as *paroophoron.*

Remnants of the paramesonephric ducts can be seen at the end of the fallopian tube and are known as *hydatid cysts of Morgagni.*

Failure of development of the paramesonephric ducts leads to agenesis of the cervix, uterus, and upper vagina, a condition known as *Rokitansky syndrome.*

Incomplete fusion of the paramesonephric tubes can give rise to a spectrum of uterine and vaginal abnormalities (Fig. 1-10). Since renal development occurs simultaneously, such uterine abnormalities often are combined with renal or ureteral anomalies, or both.

Male   In the presence of a Y chromosome and the SRY gene, müllerian-inhibiting substance produced by Sertoli cells causes regression of the paramesonephric ducts. Meanwhile, testosterone produced by the Leydig cells induces differentiation of the mesonephric ducts into the *efferent ducts* that communicate with the rete testis, followed cephalocaudally by the *epididymis, ductus deferens, seminal vesicle,* and *ejaculatory duct.* Remnants of the paramesonephric ducts can be found in the testis and prostate and are known as the *appendix of the testis* and the *prostatic utricle,* respectively (see Fig. 1-8C).

External Genitalia

Until about 9 weeks' gestation, the external genitalia are still in an indifferent stage. The definitive form can be seen at approximately 12 weeks of gestation. The origin of the external genitalia in both sexes begins at the cloacal membrane, where cells of mesenchymal origin proliferate on each side of the cloacal membrane, giving rise to the *urogenital fold.* The cloacal folds unite cranially to form the *genital tubercle.* Caudally they give rise to the *urethral groove* anteriorly, and *anal membrane* posteriorly. Soon after, two sets of lateral folds develop on either side of the urethral folds, becoming the *labioscrotal swelling* (Fig. 1-11).

Male   Under the influence of androgens, the genital tubercle elongates, giving rise to the *phallus* (see Fig. 1-11). Meanwhile, the urogenital fold closes over the urethral groove, forming the *penile urethra.* The labioscrotal swellings in the male grow toward each other and fuse in the midline, giving rise to the *scrotum* (see Fig. 1-11). Testicular descent into the inguinal canal begins at the twenty-eighth week of gestation, and at about the thirty-second week of gestation, the testes enter the scrotum. An incomplete fusion of the urethral folds will give rise to hypospadias (Fig. 1-12), in which an abnormal opening of the urethra occurs along the inferior aspect of the penis. In epispadias, the urethral meatus is therefore found on the dorsum of the penis.

Female   In females, the genital tubercle will give rise to the *clitoris.* The urogenital folds do not close as they do in males, and instead they give rise to the *labia minora.* The labioscrotal folds fuse posteriorly in the area of the

Uterine and vaginal abnormalities, results of incomplete fusion of the paramesonephric tubes. **A,** Normal uterus. **B,** Double uterus (uterus didelphys) and double vagina. **C,** Double uterus with single vagina. **D,** Bicornuate uterus. **E,** Bicornuate uterus with rudimentary horn. **F,** Septate uterus. **G,** Unicornuate uterus. (From Moore KL: The Developing Human: Clinically Oriented Embryology, 7th ed. Philadelphia, W.B. Saunders, 2003.)

16

Figure 1-10

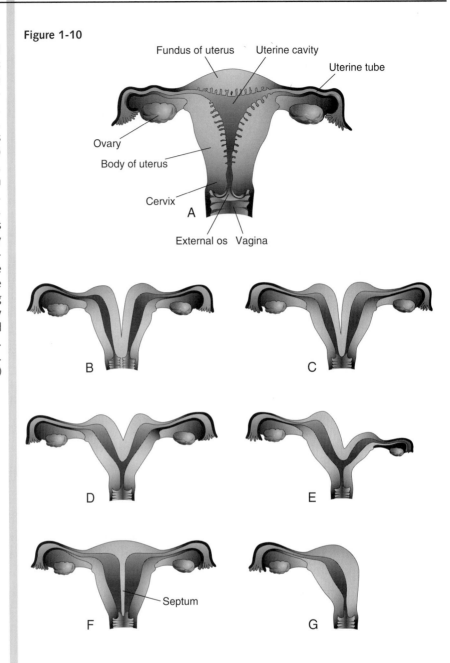

perineal body but laterally remain open to give rise to the *labia majora.* Anteriorly, the labioscrotal folds fuse together to form the *mons pubis* (Fig. 1-11 and Table 1-2).

Urinary System

The urinary system develops from three different systems that form in a cranial-caudal sequence during intrauterine life: the *pronephros, mesonephros,* and *metanephros.* The pronephros originates at the beginning of the fourth week of gestation in the cervical region of the embryo. It is a nonfunctional system that regresses completely by the end of the fourth week.

Figure 1-11

Development of the female and male external genitalia. **A** and **B,** Diagrams illustrating development of the genitalia during the indifferent stage (4 to 7 weeks). **C, E,** and **G,** Stages in the development of male external genitalia at 9, 11, and 12 weeks, respectively. To the left are schematic transverse sections of the developing penis illustrating formation of the spongy urethra. **D, F,** and **H,** Stages in the development of female external genitalia at 9, 11, and 12 weeks, respectively. (From Moore KL: The Developing Human: Clinically Oriented Embryology, 7th ed. Philadelphia, W.B. Saunders, 2003.)

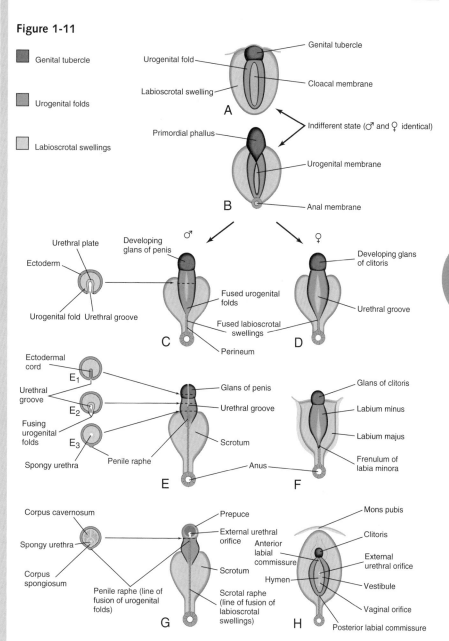

17

Soon after, more caudally along the upper thoracic to upper lumbar region, a new system develops from the intermediate mesoderm—the mesonephros with the *mesonephric duct.* The mesonephros functions only for a short period of time, producing urine for about 2 to 3 weeks, then regresses completely in females. In males, the mesonephros participates in the formation of the genital system. The definitive kidney develops from the *metanephric* mesoderm, which appears in the fifth week of gestation. The definitive kidney is composed of a collecting system and an excretory system. These two systems have different origins. The collecting system originates from the *ureteric buds* (Fig. 1-13). The ureteric buds are two

Figure 1-12

Infant with penoscrotal hypospadias. (From Larsen WJ: Human Embryology, 3rd ed. New York, Churchill Livingstone, 2001).

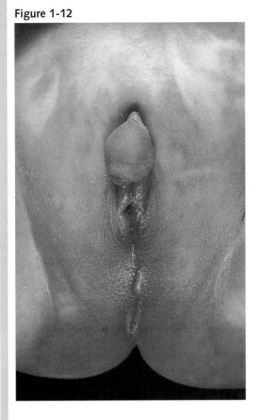

Table 1-2

Male and Female Derivatives of Embryonic Urogenital Structures

Embryonic Structure	Male Derivatives	Female Derivatives
Labioscrotal swelling	Scrotum	Labia majora
Urogenital folds	Ventral portion of penis	Labia minora
Genital tubercle	Phallus (penis)	Clitoris
Urogenital sinus	Urinary bladder	Urinary bladder
	Prostate gland	Urethral and paraurethral glands
	Prostate utricle	Vagina
		Hymen
Paramesonephric duct	Appendix of testes	Hydatid of Morgagni
		Uterus and cervix
		Fallopian tubes
		Upper vagina
Mesonephric duct	Appendix of epididymis	Duct of epoophoron
	Duct deferens	Gartner's duct
	Ejaculatory duct and seminal vesicle	
Metanephric duct	Ureter, renal pelvis, calyces, and collecting system	Ureter, renal pelvis, calyces, and collecting system
Mesonephric tubules	Ductuli efferents	Epoophoron
		Paroophoron

Development of the urinary system in the male and female. Diagram showing division of the cloaca into urogenital sinus and rectum, absorption of the mesonephric ducts, development of the urinary bladder, urethra, and urachus, and changes in the location of the ureters. **A,** Lateral view of the caudal half of the 5-week embryo; **B, D,** and **F,** dorsal views; **C, E, G,** and **H,** lateral views. The stages shown in **G** and **H** are reached at about 12 weeks' gestation. (From Moore KL: The Developing Human: Clinically Oriented Embryology, 7th ed. Philadelphia, W.B. Saunders, 2003.)

Figure 1-13

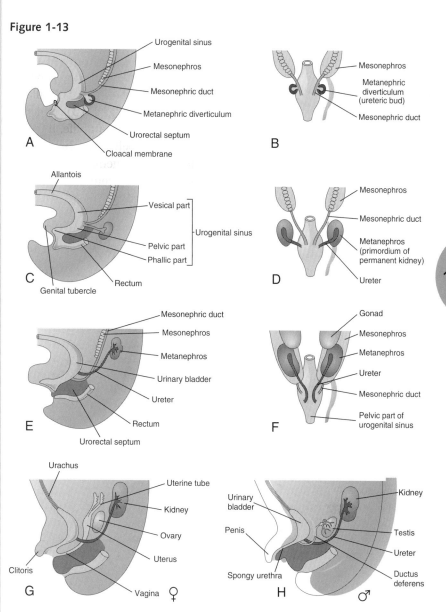

outgrowths of the mesonephric duct that originate just before its entrance into the cloaca. Once the ureteric buds are formed, they begin to penetrate into the metanephric tissue, where they continue to proliferate and subdivide. This process gives rise to the *renal pelvis,* the *major and minor calyces,* and about 1 to 3 million *collecting tubules.* Each tubule is covered by metanephric tissue that proliferates and differentiates, giving rise to the excretory units of the definitive kidney, the *nephrons.* The kidney initially develops in the pelvic region and later ascends to the lumbar region. The definitive kidneys become functional in the late seventh to early eighth week of gestation.

The bladder originates from the ventral part of the cloaca. During the seventh week of gestation, the cloaca divides anteriorly into the *urogenital sinus* and posteriorly into the *anal canal*. The primitive urogenital sinus is continuous superiorly with the *allantois* (see Fig. 1-13). The uppermost and largest part of the urogenital sinus gives rise to the *urinary bladder*, followed by a narrow neck that becomes the pelvic *urethra*. The urinary bladder is continuous with the allantois. The allantois later obliterates and gives rise to the *urachus* (see Fig. 1-13), which connects the apex of the bladder to the umbilicus; in postnatal life, it is known as the *median umbilical ligament*. In males, the pelvic urethra becomes the *membranous* and *prostatic urethra,* and the urogenital sinus becomes the *penile urethra.* In females, the pelvic urethra becomes the *membranous urethra* and the definitive urogenital sinus becomes the *vestibule of the vagina.* The caudal portions of the mesonephric ducts are absorbed into the wall of the urinary bladder. The *ureter,* which initially originated from the mesonephric duct, enters the bladder separately (see Fig. 1-13). As a result of the ascent of the kidneys to the lumbar region, the ureters are pulled cranially and the mesonephric ducts are pulled medially, until they enter the prostatic urethra and, in the male, become the *ejaculatory ducts.*

SUGGESTED READING

Copeland LJ: Textbook of Gynecology, 2nd ed. Philadelphia, W.B. Saunders, 1993.

Larsen WJ: Human Embryology, 3rd ed. New York, Churchill Livingstone, 2001.

Moore KL: The Developing Human: Clinically Oriented Embryology, 7th ed. Philadelphia, W.B. Saunders, 2003.

O'Rahilly R, Muller F: Human Embryology and Teratology. New York, Wiley-Liss, 1992.

Sadler TW: Langman's Medical Embryology, 8th ed, vol. 3. Philadelphia, Lippincott Williams & Wilkins, 2000.

Stenchever MA: Comprehensive Gynecology. St. Louis, Mosby, 1997.

2

REPRODUCTIVE PHYSIOLOGY

David L. Keefe and Kristen Page Wright

Coordination of the reproductive cycle is orchestrated by the elaborate interplay of hormonal signals affecting cyclic follicle development, steroid biosynthesis, and ovulation. The cycle is regulated by sex hormones that are at low levels during childhood, increase tremendously during the reproductive years, and decline again after menopause.

Ovulation and subsequent conception or menstruation during the reproductive years is determined by pulsatile gonadotropin-releasing hormone (GnRH) secreted from the hypothalamus, causing episodic release of follicle-stimulating hormone (FSH) and luteinizing hormone (LH) from the anterior pituitary gland. FSH stimulates dominant follicular growth, granulosa cell production, and increased estrogen biosynthesis. The FSH-induced rise in estrogen stimulates a midcycle surge in LH, triggering ovulation of the dominant follicle and subsequent formation of the corpus luteum. If conception occurs, the corpus luteum secretes the progesterone necessary to maintain the pregnancy through the first 10 weeks of gestation. If conception does not occur, the corpus luteum regresses and LH withdrawal causes a reduction in steroid hormone production and subsequent menstruation (Fig. 2-1). This chapter will examine the neuro-endocrinology of the hypothalamic-pituitary-ovarian axis and its intricate regulation of the menstrual cycle.

HYPOTHALAMUS

Gonadotropin-Releasing Hormone

The hypothalamus forms the lateral walls of the ventral aspect of the third ventricle at the base of the brain just above the junction of the optic nerves. During embryogenesis, the cells that produce GnRH originate in the medial olfactory placode and migrate along cranial nerves connecting the nose and the forebrain to their primary location. Failure of this migratory system results in a clinical entity known as Kallmann syndrome, characterized by hyposmia and hypogonadotropism. By mid-gestation, GnRH neurons are located predominantly in the arcuate nucleus of the medial basal hypothalamus, but also in the preoptic area of the anterior hypothalamus and the tuberal hypothalamus, all with neural projections

Figure 2-1

Coordinated events in the hypothalamus, pituitary gland, ovary, and endometrium. FSH, Follicle-stimulating hormone; LH, luteinizing hormone. (Couchman G, Hammond C: Physiology of reproduction. In Scott J, Disaia P, Hammond C, et al (eds): Danforth's Obstetrics and Gynecology. Philadelphia, Lippincott Williams and Wilkins, 1999, pp 47–64.)

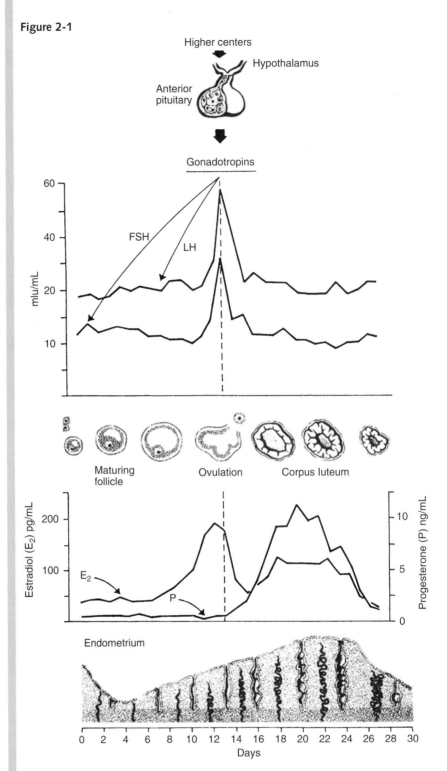

to the median eminence. The median eminence has a dense network of capillaries, formed by the superior hypophyseal arteries draining into the portal vessels, which descend along the pituitary stalk to the anterior pituitary gland (Fig. 2-2). This hypophyseal portal circulation has capillaries designed with a fenestrated endothelial lining, permitting the passage of large molecules such as GnRH. Secretion of hormones by the anterior pituitary gland is therefore controlled by neurohormones secreted by the hypothalamus and released into the portal circulation.

Regulation of the Hypothalamic Axis

Reproductive physiology is primarily orchestrated by pulsatile secretion of GnRH. GnRH is a decapeptide whose 92–amino acid precursor prohormone is encoded for on the short arm of chromosome 8. The prohormone is cleaved to yield GnRH and a 56–amino acid peptide, GnRH-associated peptide, during axonal transport to the median eminence. The function of GnRH-associated peptide is unknown. Episodic release of GnRH from the hypothalamus occurs every 60 to 90 minutes and causes episodic release of LH and, to a lesser extent, FSH. The circulatory half-life of GnRH is 2 to 4 minutes with rapid degradation, ensuring that biologically active amounts of GnRH do not escape the portal circulation. Normal gonadotropin secretion requires pulsatile GnRH secretion within a narrow range of frequency and amplitude.

Gonadotropins are secreted in a pulsatile pattern that reflects the pulsatile GnRH pattern. The follicular phase of the cycle is characterized by

23

Figure 2-2

The hypothalamus and the hypophyseal portal circulation. (Melmed S: Disorders of the anterior pituitary and hypothalamus. In Braunwald E, Fauci AS, Kasper DL, et al (eds): Harrison's Principles of Internal Medicine, 15th ed. New York, McGraw-Hill, 2001, pp 2029–2052.)

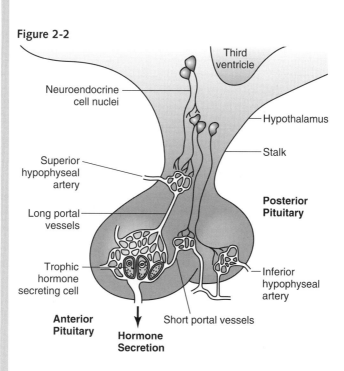

high-frequency, low-amplitude pulses and the luteal phase consists of low-frequency, high-amplitude pulses. Infrequent GnRH pulsation results in low levels of gonadotropin secretion and subsequent anovulation and amenorrhea. Higher than normal pulse frequency of GnRH down-regulates the GnRH receptors and causes a refractory response of FSH and LH. GnRH agonists used in the treatment of endometriosis, precocious puberty, and fibroids effectively downregulate the gonadotropin-gonadal axis, resulting in low levels of gonadotropins and sex steroids. These agonists have internal amino acid substitutions that increase their binding affinity to GnRH receptors and resist enzymatic degradation within the hypothalamus and pituitary gland.

Catecholamines modulate the frequency of GnRH pulsatile release, with norepinephrine causing stimulatory effects on GnRH and dopamine and serotonin exerting inhibitory effects. Estrogen and progesterone produced by the ovaries negatively feed back to the hypothalamus and pituitary, decreasing GnRH and consequent gonadotropin release. However, the pituitary—not the hypothalamus—is the major site of gonadal negative feedback in humans. Pituitary hormones also may directly inhibit hypothalamic GnRH secretion in a short feedback loop by retrograde portal blood flow from the pituitary to the hypothalamus.

Other Hypothalamic Hormones

There are other hypothalamic hormones influencing successful reproduction including corticotropin-releasing hormone (CRH), growth hormone–releasing factor (GHRF), somatostatin, and thyrotropin-releasing hormone (TRH).

CRH controls pituitary secretion of adrenocorticotropic hormone (ACTH) and subsequent cortisol, which mediates the body's stress response. Both the CRH and GnRH neuronal systems terminate in the median eminence, and experimental evidence suggests that CRH also may directly inhibit hypothalamic GnRH secretion. ACTH excess, in the form of both Cushing's syndrome and hypercortisolism, results in reproductive dysfunction. Hypothalamic amenorrhea and anorexia nervosa both produce states of hypercortisolism, suggesting that direct inhibition of GnRH by CRH is the mechanism for reproductive dysfunction in these patients.

GHRF localized in the medial basal hypothalamus triggers pulsatile growth hormone (GH) synthesis and release from the anterior pituitary. GH is a polypeptide involved in many aspects of growth, including regulation of lipolysis and skeletal and muscle development. GH is under tonic inhibition by the hypothalamic neuropeptide somatostatin. At the onset of puberty, the dynamics of GH secretion become critically dependent on the gonadal sex steroid hormones. Small doses of estrogen in early puberty stimulate GH secretion, resulting in long-bone cortical growth and the subsequent peak height velocity observed early in puberty.

Hypothalamic TRH release stimulates thyroid-stimulating hormone (TSH) release from the pituitary, which controls thyroid hormone regulation. TRH neurons are located in the paraventricular nucleus and project to the median eminence. The TSH response to TRH is predominantly influenced by negative feedback through thyroid hormone; however, more subtle effects are present. Estrogen, for example, increases the number of TRH receptors in the pituitary, resulting in a greater TSH response to TRH in women compared with men, and in particular, in women taking combined oral contraceptive pills. Both hypothyroidism and hyperthyroidism cause reproductive dysfunction. Hypothyroidism commonly results in menstrual irregularities and amenorrhea with or without hyperprolactinemia. Menstrual changes associated with hyperthyroidism are unpredictable, ranging from amenorrhea to oligomenorrhea to normal cycles.

PITUITARY

Gonadotropins

The pituitary gland is located at the base of the brain in the sella turcica and contains gonadotroph cells in its lateral portions that synthesize and secrete the gonadotropins LH and FSH.

FSH and LH are both heterodimeric glycoproteins consisting of two dissimilar noncovalently linked α- and β-chains. The α-subunit is essentially identical in both hormones and also in TSH and human chorionic gonadotropin (hCG). It consists of 92 amino acids and contains five disulfide bonds contributing to its tertiary structure. The β-subunit of each hormone contains differing amino acid sequences and carbohydrate side chains that are specific for either FSH or LH. The specific biologic activity of each hormone is therefore determined by the β-subunit. The α- and β-subunits are tightly attached noncovalently by a loop formed by the β-subunit, which wraps around the α-subunit.

FSH receptors are located on the granulosa cells of the ovary and the Sertoli cells of the testicle, where FSH binding promotes gamete production in the gonads. FSH stimulates the aromatization process by which androgens are converted to estrogen in the granulosa cell, and FSH may also stimulate granulosa cell division. FSH acts synergistically with LH, androstenedione, and estradiol to stimulate follicle maturation. During the menstrual cycle, FSH secretion peaks during the midcycle LH surge. The initial half-life of FSH is 3 to 4 hours.

The primary function of LH is to stimulate the theca cells of the ovary to produce androgens, mainly androstenedione, which can then be aromatized by the granulosa cells to estrogen. LH also stimulates ovarian maturation, resumption of the meiotic division of the ovum that was arrested in fetal life, ovulation, progesterone production, and corpus luteum formation. The initial half-life of LH is 20 minutes.

Regulation of Gonadotropins

Pulsatile GnRH binding the high-affinity receptors on the pituitary gonadotrophs causes pulsatile release of FSH and LH. This release of gonadotropins is mediated by calcium-dependent mechanisms via G protein coupling.

Estradiol has a biphasic inhibitory and stimulatory feedback effect on secretion of gonadotropins. At low levels, estrogen exerts an exquisitely sensitive negative feedback effect on the release of pituitary gonadotropins. At high levels, however, estrogen is capable of exerting a positive feedback effect on LH and FSH release. This positive stimulus initiates the preovulatory surge of gonadotropins in the follicular stage of the menstrual cycle. Progesterone levels, which rise midcycle, enhance the positive feedback of estradiol and amplify the duration of the LH surge. Loss of estrogen due to a postmenopausal or oophorectomized state results in chronically high levels of gonadotropins.

The secretion of gonadotropins also is influenced by the ovarian factors inhibin and activin. Inhibin is a nonsteroidal peptide synthesized by the granulosa cells and secreted into the follicular fluid and ovarian venous effluent. It exerts a potent inhibitory effect on FSH release and may contribute to ovarian follicular development. Activin is a potent stimulator of FSH release. Inhibin and activin are both members of the transforming growth factor β (TGF-β) family. Inhibin is composed of one α- and one β-subunit, whereas activin is a dimer composed of two inhibin β-subunits. The exact role of these factors in the control of gonadotropin secretion has yet to be elucidated.

Prolactin

The primary function of prolactin is lactogenesis, including mammary gland development as well as initiation and stimulation of milk secretion. Prolactin is secreted by lactotrophs in the anterior pituitary gland, which become more abundant during pregnancy and lactation. Prolactin is a single polypeptide of 198 amino acids and shares homology with human GH and human placental lactogen. Pituitary secretion of prolactin is under the tonic inhibitory control of dopamine released by the hypothalamus into the portal circulation. There are numerous medications that interfere with the metabolism, synthesis, or receptor binding of dopamine that can cause subsequent hyperprolactinemia. TRH exerts a modest stimulatory effect on prolactin secretion, and hypothyroidism can therefore cause hyperprolactinemia due to high circulating levels of TRH. Pituitary adenomas are another common cause of hyperprolactinemia. Clinical manifestations of hyperprolactinemia include galactorrhea and decreased gonadotropin secretion, which may lead to secondary amenorrhea, menstrual irregularity, and primary infertility.

Posterior Pituitary Hormones

Oxytocin and vasopressin or antidiuretic hormone (ADH) are synthesized as prohormones in the cell bodies of the supraoptic and paraventricular hypothalamic nuclei and are then transported to the neurohypophysis or posterior pituitary. ADH controls water diuresis by the kidney and is responsible for regulating plasma volume and osmolality. Oxytocin stimulates myometrial contractions during labor and also activates milk letdown. The increase in myometrial oxytocin receptors during pregnancy is mediated by estrogen and reaches peak levels near term. Stimulation of milk letdown relies on a complex neurogenic reflex arc beginning with the act of suckling stimulating nerve endings in the nipple. This stimulus travels to the hypothalamus via the spinal cord, where oxytocin release is stimulated from the neurohypophysis. Oxytocin causes contractions of the myoepithelial cells of the mammary gland and subsequent milk letdown. Acetylcholine and α-adrenergic neurons stimulate secretion of oxytocin and ADH while β-adrenergic neurons are suppressive.

OVARY

Steroid Hormone Biosynthesis

The ovary synthesizes estrogens, androgens, and progestins, which are all derived from the parent compound, cholesterol, containing 27 carbons. All three steroid hormone families are lipophilic and share a common carbon ring structure called *cyclopentanophenanthrene*, composed of four fused rings (Fig. 2-3). Progestins have 21 carbon backbones, androgens have 19, and estrogens have 18. The formation of the steroid sex hormones is summarized in Figure 2-4.

27

Progestins

Cholesterol is converted to pregnenolone and then to progesterone in two enzyme-requiring reactions. The major sites of progesterone biosynthesis are the granulosa-lutein cells of the corpus luteum, the syncytiotrophoblast of the placenta, and, to a lesser extent, the zona fasciculata and zona reticularis of the adrenal cortex. The primary function of progesterone is the preparation of the female reproductive tract for conception and implantation and the maintenance of the uterine environment during gestation until parturition.

Free, biologically active progesterone composes 3% to 5% of total progesterone, with the remainder being protein bound and therefore inactive. Circulating progesterone is 95% to 98% protein bound to either albumin (79.3%), cortisol-binding globulin (17.7%), or sex hormone–binding

Figure 2-3

Cyclopentano-phenanthrene ring system. (Couchman G, Hammond C: Physiology of reproduction. In Scott J, Disaia P, Hammond C, et al (eds): Danforth's Obstetrics and Gynecology. Philadelphia, Lippincott Williams and Wilkins, 1999, pp 47–64.)

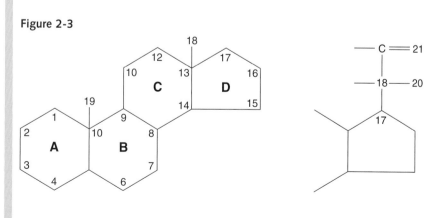

Figure 2-4

Formation of the steroid sex hormones. The synthesis of steroid hormones from cholesterol. (Speroff L, Glass R, Kase N: Clinical Gynecologic Endocrinology and Infertility, 6th ed. Baltimore, Lippincott Williams and Wilkins, 1999.)

28

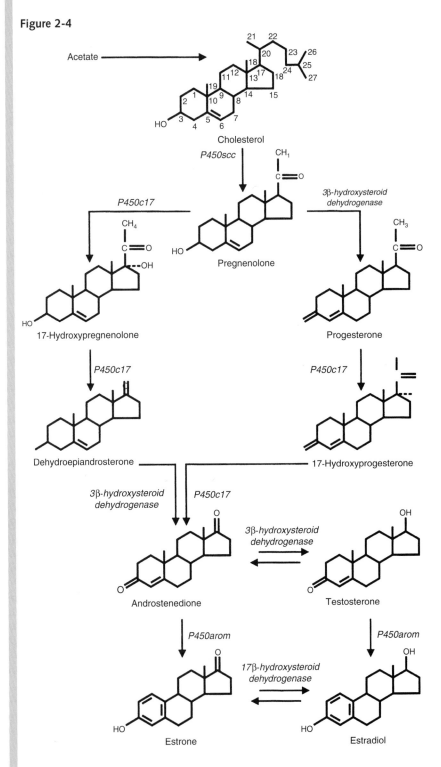

globulin (SHBG) (0.6%). Pregnancy causes an increase in the amount of progesterone bound to cortisol-binding globulin (37.7%) and a decrease in the fraction bound to albumin (54.7%), with virtually no change in the amount of free progesterone or progesterone bound to SHBG (Table 2-1).

Androgens

Ovarian interstitial cells located in the stroma and hilus of the ovary secrete testosterone and androstenedione. The major pathway for androstenedione synthesis from cholesterol is through dehydroepiandrosterone, produced predominantly by the adrenal gland. 17-Hydroxyprogesterone can also act as a precursor for androstenedione, especially when this precursor is produced in excess as in the case of 21-hydroxylase deficiency, the most common form of congenital adrenal hyperplasia. Androgen secretion is dependent on LH stimulation, peaks during the menstrual cycle around the time of the LH surge, and then gradually declines. Androgen secretion begins during puberty and continues but does not increase after menopause despite the increase in LH associated with menopause. Between 1% and 2% of testosterone is unbound, with the remainder bound equally to albumin and SHBG.

Estrogens

The principal sites of estrogen production in humans are the ovarian granulosa cells in premenopausal women, the stromal cells of adipose tissue in postmenopausal women, and the placental syncytiotrophoblast in pregnant women. Estrogen biosynthesis also occurs in a number of tissue sites, including the hypothalamus and amygdala regions of the brain, as well as the genital skin regions. Each tissue produces a different form of estrogen with the ovary synthesizing primarily estradiol, the placenta synthesizing estriol, and adipose synthesizing estrone. This tissue-specific biosynthesis reflects the available 19-carbon androgen substrate available to the aromatase enzyme in the different tissues. Estradiol is synthesized from dehydroisoandrosterone produced by the theca cells, estriol is synthesized from 16α-hydroxydehydroisoandrosterone sulfate produced by the fetal adrenal gland and the fetal liver, and estrone is synthesized from circulating androstenedione produced from the adrenal cortex (Table 2-2).

Free, biologically active estradiol represents 2% to 3% of total estradiol, with the remaining 60% bound to albumin and 38% bound to SHBG.

Table 2-1

Proportion of Protein-Bound Steroid Hormones

	Unbound	Albumin	SHBG	CBG
Estradiol	1% to 2%	60%	38%	
Testosterone	1% to 2%	49%	49%	
Progesterone (nonpregnant)	3% to 5%	79.3%	0.6%	17.7%
Progesterone (pregnant)	3% to 5%	54.7%	0.6%	37.7%

CBG, cortisol-binding globulin; SHBG, sex hormone–binding globulin.

Table 2-2

Tissue	Estrogen	Substrate	Source of Substrate
Ovary	Estradiol	Dehydroisoandrosterone	Theca cells
Adipose	Estrone	Androstenedione	Adrenal cortex
Placenta	Estriol	16α-hydroxydehydro- isoandrosterone sulfate	Fetal adrenal gland and fetal liver

Estradiol has one third the affinity for SHBG as dihydrotestosterone, and women have twice the concentration of SHBG as men. Levels of SHBG are increased by estrogens and thyroid hormones and decreased by androgens.

THE MENSTRUAL CYCLE

The menstrual cycle is driven by pulsatile GnRH release from the hypothalamus and, in the absence of this pulse generator, the pituitary-ovarian axis remains dormant. Coordination of the hypothalamic-pituitary-ovarian axis is via blood-borne signals, and the ovaries synchronize ovulation and the stimulatory and inhibitory feedback loops to the hypothalamus and pituitary. The duration of the menstrual cycle and the timing of ovulation appear to be determined by the ovary itself.

By convention, menstruation marks day 1 of the typical 25- to 30-day menstrual cycle. The significant variation in cycle length among women is largely due to variation in the length of the follicular phase; the luteal phase is consistently close to 14 days. There is a tendency toward longer menstrual cycles at the extremes of reproductive age because these times are characterized by less frequent ovulation. Dysfunctional uterine bleeding is also more common in these age groups as a consequence of oligo-ovulation.

Follicular Phase

Primordial germ cells begin development at 5 to 6 weeks' gestation and rapidly multiply, reaching a maximum of 6 to 7 million oocytes by 16 to 20 weeks' gestation. Depletion of this nongrowing pool occurs steadily due to constant recruitment for follicular growth and atresia. The rate of decrease is proportional to the total number of oocytes present. At birth, there are approximately 2 million primordial follicles in the human ovaries, each containing one oocyte arrested in prophase of meiosis I and surrounded by a single layer of spindle-shaped granulosa cells. By puberty, the number of primordial follicles has fallen to less than 300,000 and continues to decline steadily until the fourth decade of life, at which time there is a marked acceleration in the rate of depletion. Only about 400 follicles will ovulate during a woman's reproductive lifetime.

The 10- to 14-day follicular phase of the menstrual cycle involves an orderly sequence of events during which one surviving mature follicle is produced for ovulation. During each menstrual cycle, a cohort of many follicles begin their developmental course; however, typically all but one will undergo atresia via apoptotic programmed cell death. The number of follicles that begin growing in each cohort appears to be dependent on the size of the residual pool of inactive primordial follicles. Follicular development is characterized by an increase in the size of the oocyte, which becomes surrounded by a membrane called the *zona pellucida*. The granulosa cells surrounding the oocyte also proliferate and transition from squamous to cuboidal shaped. Initiation of follicular growth in each cohort of follicles occurs continuously at all phases of the cycle and is thought to be at least partially gonadotropin independent. However, in the early antral phase, each cohort will undergo atresia in the absence of FSH. The time required for early follicles to achieve the preantral stage is unknown and may occur over several months.

FSH rise in the early follicular phase provides the signal for recruitment of each cohort of antral follicles. Several follicles are initially recruited; however, by day 5 to 6 of the cycle, the dominant follicle has been irreversibly selected (Fig. 2-5). Experimental destruction of any of the follicles before day 5 to 6 of the cycle will not delay ovulation. However, experimental destruction of the largest follicle after day 7 will result in a delay to ovulation by approximately the length of a normal follicular phase because a new cohort of follicles must be recruited. The process of selection of the dominant follicle is incompletely understood and may represent

Figure 2-5

Recruitment and selection of the dominant follicle. (Adashi E, Rock JA, Rosenwalks Z: Reproductive Endocrinology, Surgery, and Technology. Philadelphia, Lippincott-Raven, 1996.)

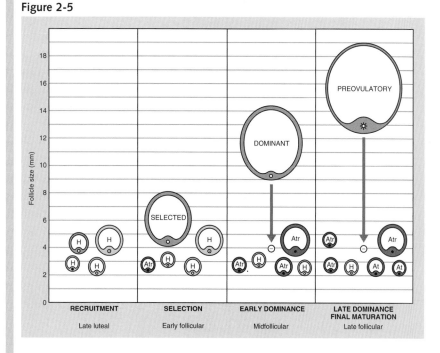

a competitive advantage of the selected follicle in producing estradiol. After selection of the dominant follicle, all other follicles in the cohort become destined for atresia.

The developing dominant follicle is the primary source of rising estradiol concentrations observed during the follicular phase. FSH receptors are noted to appear on the proliferating granulosa cells of the preantral follicle. The presence of FSH is necessary for granulosa cells to use aromatase to convert androgens to estrogens. The survival of the dominant follicle may be accomplished via its ability to elevate peripheral estradiol concentrations, thereby activating the negative feedback loop and inhibiting FSH. Thus, FSH secretion may be suppressed to a concentration insufficient to support the growth of the nondominant follicles in the cohort. The dominant follicle also likely exerts a paracrine mediated inhibition of other follicles.

Increasing estradiol concentrations during the follicular phase cause endometrial proliferation and enlargement of the endometrial glands via mitosis. Estradiol also mediates increased cervical mucus production, which becomes increasingly alkaline and elastic. The ferning capacity of the cervical mucus also increases and develops a positive fern test result.

As FSH is stimulating granulosa cells to produce estrogen, LH is stimulating theca cells to produce androstenedione, the estrogen precursor. Androstenedione diffuses across the lamina basalis and is converted into estrogens by the aromatase enzyme in the granulosa cells (Fig. 2-6). The granulosa and theca cells are so closely coupled during steroid estrogen biosynthesis that this interaction is known as the two-cell, two-gonadotropin theory of ovarian steroidogenesis. This system is delicately balanced because while low levels of androstenedione promote aromatase action, high levels of this androgen cause follicular atresia. The dominant follicle is distinguished by having increased estrogen production, whereas the follicles destined for atresia are characterized by a higher androgen-estrogen ratio.

Pharmacologic ovulation induction uses supraphysiologic concentrations of gonadotropins, resulting in a larger number of follicles recruited into each cohort. The endogenous gonadotropin supply also opposes the negative feedback effect of estradiol, interfering with the process of dominance by one follicle. Thus, multiple maturing graafian follicles are able to develop with ovulation induction.

Androgen production in the late follicular phase increases as theca cells of the lesser follicles return to their origin in the stromal tissue. These theca cells retain their ability to produce steroids, and a midcycle increase in stromal tissue is thus responsible for the increased production of androgens. Androgen production at this stage may facilitate the process of granulosa cell death and follicular atresia. Androgens also enhance midcycle libido as evidenced by a peak in female-initiated sexual activity observed during the ovulatory phase of the cycle. Thus, the midcycle increase in androgens results in increased sexual activity during the time when the female is most likely to conceive.

Figure 2-6

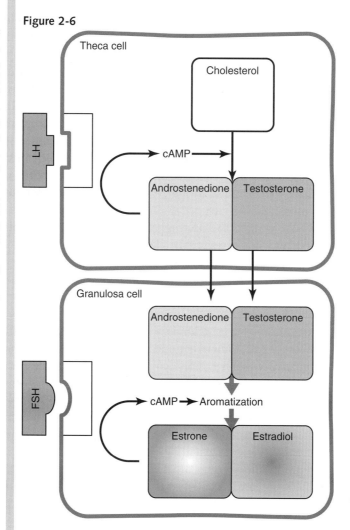

Formation of androgens by luteinizing hormone (LH) in the theca cell and formation of estrogens by follicle-stimulating hormone (FSH) in the granulosa cell. cAMP, Cyclic adenosine monophosphate. (Speroff L, Glass R, Kase N: Clinical Gynecologic Endocrinology and Infertility, 6th ed. Baltimore, Lippincott Williams and Wilkins, 1999.)

Ovulation

Estrogen concentrations increase slowly, then rapidly, during the follicular phase, and the midcycle LH surge is provoked when peak estrogen concentration is reached 24 to 36 hours before ovulation. LH promotes luteinization of the granulosa cells, causing production of progesterone from the dominant follicle around the time of ovulation. Progesterone facilitates positive feedback on the pituitary gland, initiating the LH surge when introduced in low doses after adequate estrogen priming. Progesterone administered before estrogen priming or given in high doses will block the LH surge. Midcycle progesterone also contributes to the estrogen-induced FSH surge. Although progesterone appears to enhance the effect of both the LH and FSH surge, it may not be obligatory. The mechanism that terminates the LH surge is unknown.

Ovulation typically occurs within 34 to 36 hours after the onset of the midcycle LH surge. Ovulation is preceded by rapid follicular enlargement and maturation of the nucleus and zona pellucida in preparation for fertilization. The LH surge stimulates the resumption of meiosis I within the preovulatory follicle and the first polar body is extruded in the metaphase II stage. The second meiotic arrest occurs at ovulation. Extrusion of the second polar body and completion of meiosis is not accomplished until fertilization occurs.

The LH surge arrests granulosa cell proliferation, decreasing both estradiol and androgen production. Levels of progesterone within the follicle continue to rise from the initiation of the LH surge until ovulation. Progesterone also increases the distensibility of the follicle wall, accommodating the rapid increase in follicular fluid volume without increasing intrafollicular pressure.

The gonadotropins and progesterone stimulate proteolytic enzymes such as plasminogen activator, which cause degenerative changes in the collagen of the follicular wall. These degenerative changes allow the oocyte-cumulus complex to be gently extruded from the ovary. Prostaglandin synthesis increases markedly at the time of ovulation, and prostaglandins appear to play a central role in follicle rupture. Pharmacologic inhibition of the synthesis of prostaglandins blocks follicle rupture and patients receiving infertility treatment should thus be advised to avoid drugs that inhibit prostaglandin synthesis around the time of ovulation.

Luteal Phase

Rapid vascularization and luteinization of the granulosa cell layer characterize development of the corpus luteum. The granulosa cells enlarge rapidly, become vacuolated, and acquire cellular organelles associated with steroidogenesis during their transition to luteal cells. Dissolution of the basal lamina between the granulosa and theca cell layers of the follicle also occurs, and the theca cells may differentiate to become part of the luteal cell population. There are at least two distinct sizes of luteal cells, and the larger luteal cells secrete 10 to 20 times more progesterone than the smaller luteal cells. It is unclear whether these subpopulations of luteal cells represent differing origins from granulosa or theca cells. In addition to luteal cells, the corpus luteum is also composed of vascular endothelial cells, leukocytes, and fibroblasts. By 4 to 6 days after ovulation the corpus luteum has become well organized.

The primary product of the corpus luteum is progesterone, and the corpus luteum secretes as much as 40 mg/day of this hormone. Neovascularization supplies the luteal cells with low-density lipoprotein cholesterol, the substrate for progesterone synthesis. Progesterone acts both locally and centrally to suppress new follicular growth. The corpus luteum also synthesizes estrogen, relaxin, and inhibin, all of which may play a role in early pregnancy initiation or maintenance. Secretion of progesterone and estradiol is episodic and correlates closely with LH pulses, which begin to decline in the late luteal phase.

Low levels of circulating LH are required for normal function of the corpus luteum. Luteal cells contain LH receptors that bind LH and activate an adenylate cyclase-cAMP–mediated increase in progesterone production. However, the exact mechanism by which the structure and function of the corpus luteum are maintained has yet to be elucidated.

Demise of the corpus luteum occurs 9 to 11 days after ovulation in the absence of fertilization. The process of luteolysis involves proteolytic enzymes; however, it is unclear which factor(s) signal the demise of the corpus luteum. Prostaglandin $F_{2\alpha}$ has been implicated in non-primate species as a luteolytic agent, but the role of this prostaglandin in primates remains unsubstantiated. Luteolysis is also not the result of declining LH support because artificially maintaining the frequency of LH pulses does not affect the lifetime of the corpus luteum in primates.

If pregnancy ensues, the demise of the corpus luteum is rescued by the emergence of hCG. hCG production by the conceptus emerges 9 to 13 days after ovulation and stimulates the luteal cells to continue the production of steroids. The production of progesterone will be maintained by hCG until approximately the ninth or tenth week of gestation, at which time placental steroidogenesis becomes well established.

PHYSIOLOGY OF THE ENDOMETRIUM

The endometrium is a complex tissue designed to provide the appropriate anatomic and hormonal environment for the growing conceptus. In the absence of implantation, the endometrium is shed in the late secretory phase.

Anatomy

The endometrium is composed of two tissue compartments: the upper transient functionalis is formed and shed during each menstrual cycle, whereas the deep germinal basalis persists from cycle to cycle. The blood supply to the basal portion of the endometrium is via the straight basal arteries, and the spiral arterioles supply the functionalis layer. Both the straight basal arteries and the spiral arterioles arise from the radial arteries at the myometrial-endometrial junction. The radial arteries arise from the arcuate arteries within the myometrium. The endometrium is composed of luminal and glandular epithelia, stromal fibroblasts, and vascular smooth muscle cells.

Proliferative Phase

The proliferative phase is characterized by the estrogen-dependent proliferation of endometrial glands and stroma. The endometrial height increases from 0.5 to 5.0 mm during this time, and mitoses are evident as nuclear DNA synthesis is increased. The endometrial glands are straight and tubular in shape at the beginning of the proliferative phase, and low columnar epithelium lines the glands in a pseudostratified configuration (Fig. 2-7). The endometrial glands become progressively more voluminous and tortuous during the late preovulatory period. Ciliated and microvillous

Figure 2-7

Proliferative phase of the endometrium. (Courtesy of J. Sung, MD, Division of Pathology, Women and Infant's Hospital of Rhode Island.)

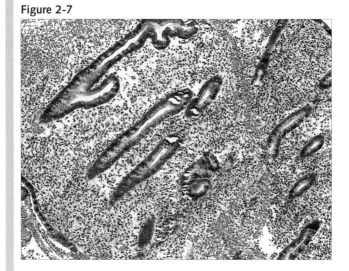

cells appear around days 7 to 8 of the cycle. Intracellular vacuoles and luminal secretions are not evident at this stage. The stromal cells are tightly packed and uniform and become slightly edematous as ovulation approaches.

Secretory Phase

The glands of the endometrium begin to demonstrate secretory activity in response to progesterone in the periovulatory period, marking the beginning of the secretory phase. Glycogen-rich secretory vacuoles appear within the cytoplasm of glandular cells and luminal secretion becomes evident throughout the secretory phase. The endometrial height remains fixed at 5 to 6 mm and mitosis and DNA synthesis declines as a result of increased progesterone. The stroma becomes edematous in response to high levels of estradiol and progesterone, resulting in coiling and compaction of the endometrial glands and spiral arteries (Fig. 2-8). The perivascular stromal cells begin to accumulate eosinophilic cytoplasm late in the secretory phase.

Thirteen days after ovulation, the endometrium has differentiated into three distinct zones. The basalis layer remains unchanged at the deepest portion of the endometrium and composes 25% of the total endometrial thickness. The middle 50% of the endometrium is termed the *stratum spongiosum* and is composed of loose edematous stroma with tightly coiled spiral vessels and dilated glands. The superficial portion overlying the stratum spongiosum is termed the *stratum compactum* and composes the remaining 25% of the total endometrial height. Large polyhedral stromal cells with less prominent glandular tissue characterize this layer.

If implantation occurs, the stromal cells become decidualized, and this decidua becomes an important structural and biochemical tissue for the developing pregnancy. Decidual cells are characterized by cytonuclear enlargement, increased mitotic activity, and the formation of a basement

Figure 2-8

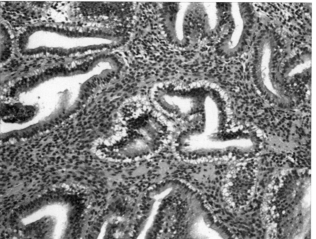

membrane. Decidual cells modulate the invasion of the trophoblast, respond to hormonal signals, and synthesize substances such as prolactin, relaxin, renin, insulin-like growth factors, and insulin-like growth factor–binding proteins. Kornchenzellen, or K, cells appear in the late secretory phase and increase in number throughout the first trimester of pregnancy. These cells are under hormonal control and are believed to have an immunoprotective role in implantation and placentation.

Endometrial Breakdown

In the absence of fertilization, resolution of the corpus luteum and subsequent withdrawal of estrogen and progesterone initiates menstruation. The rapid process of involution—the necrosis and shedding of the functionalis layer of the endometrium—is mediated by lysosomal enzymes, vasoconstriction, and myometrial contractions.

The integrity of the lysosomal membrane is disrupted with loss of hormonal support, and lysosomal enzymes are subsequently released. These lysosomal enzymes degrade the glandular and stromal cells as well as the vascular endothelium. Digestion of cellular material leads to the release of prostaglandins, extravasation of red blood cells, and tissue necrosis. Injury to the vascular surface promotes platelet deposits, resulting in minute foci of tissue necrosis.

Rhythmic vasoconstriction of the spiral arterioles mediated by prostaglandin $F_{2\alpha}$ and endothelin-1 leads to endometrial blanching and endometrial ischemia followed by necrosis. Swelling of the necrotic endothelial cells ultimately results in obliteration of the lumen. The spiral arteries are then shed with menstruation. Hemostasis during menstruation is accomplished by vasoconstriction of the ruptured basal arteries at the denuded basal layer of the endometrium.

The functionalis gradually detaches from the underlying basalis layer on days 2 to 4 of menstruation. The degenerated endometrium is expelled by prostaglandin-mediated myometrial contractions. The menstrual fluid is composed of autolyzed tissue with an inflammatory exudate, red blood cells, and proteolytic enzymes. Some of the proteolytic enzymes, particularly plasmin, have high fibrinolytic activity, which promotes liquefaction of the tissue and prevents clots. Approximately 50% of the menstrual component will be shed in the first 24 hours of menses. The usual duration of menstrual flow is 4 to 6 days, and the normal volume of fluid is 30 mL. More than 80 mL of menstrual fluid is considered abnormal.

PUBERTY

Puberty is a process of physiologic changes associated with activation of the hypothalamic-pituitary-gonadal axis that leads to adult reproductive functioning. Puberty is marked by the acceleration of linear growth, bone maturation, and the development of secondary sexual characteristics such as breast growth and pubic hair development. Puberty is initiated by two processes: adrenarche, the increased secretion of androgens from the adrenal gland; and gonadarche, the activation of steroidogenesis and gametogenesis in the gonads. Adrenarche typically precedes gonadarche; however, the two are independent endocrine events, and one may occur without the other.

Adrenarche

The increase in adrenal androgen production begins around 4 to 7 years of age and is one of the earliest endocrine changes associated with puberty. The activation in adrenal androgen secretion results in production of androstenedione, dehydroepiandrosterone, and androstenedione sulfate from the zona reticularis. The mechanism responsible for increased androgen production is not well understood and is independent of gonadarche initiation by pulsatile GnRH. Thus, patients with premature adrenarche will enter puberty at a normal age because acceleration of adrenal androgen production does not affect the GnRH activation of gonadarche. Additionally, children with Addison's disease who have adrenal insufficiency will also enter puberty at a normal age when supplied with appropriate mineralocorticoid and glucocorticoid replacement.

Gonadarche

Gonadarche results from activation of the hypothalamic-pituitary-gonadal axis and is initiated by a hypothalamic increase in pulsatile GnRH. Pulsatile GnRH secretion is detectable after 20 weeks' gestation and throughout the first year of life, after which time it gradually declines and becomes quiescent. Levels of gonadotropins and estradiol also remain low after the first year of life until the initiation of puberty. The initiation of puberty appears to be a centrally driven process because prepubertal girls will demonstrate a blunted pituitary and ovarian response to exogenous GnRH. The exact mechanism for the increase in GnRH pulsatility is not well understood, and it is not clear whether the hypothalamus is under tonic inhibition or lacks the appropriate excitatory stimulus before puberty.

The hypothalamic-pituitary-gonadal axis reactivates with the appearance of measurable sleep-induced LH pulses that correlate with nocturnal increases in GnRH pulsation. Before puberty, the hypothalamus and pituitary are extremely sensitive to the inhibitory effects of low levels of circulating steroids. The hypothalamus and pituitary become significantly less sensitive as GnRH pulsation increases, and production of gonadotropins and estradiol increases dramatically.

Physical Changes

The average age of puberty has decreased dramatically in the past two centuries, largely because of improved nutrition and access to health care. The average age of menarche in the United States is currently 12.8 years. Tanner systematically classified the orderly appearance of secondary sexual characteristics associated with puberty in the 1960s. The typical sequence of pubertal events in girls is thelarche (i.e., breast development), adrenarche (i.e., axillary and pubic hair development), peak height velocity, and menarche (i.e., development of menses). The processes of thelarche and adrenarche have discreet staging systems developed by Tanner (Table 2-3).

39

MENOPAUSE

The ovary becomes progressively less responsive to gonadotropins with advancing chronologic age until menses ultimately cease. The perimenopausal transition is marked by a 2- to 8-year period of menstrual irregularity preceding menopause. Cycle lengths increase and anovulation

Table 2-3

Stages of Pubertal Development in Girls as Defined by Tanner

Pubertal Stage	Breast	Pubic Hair
I	Infantile; areola not pigmented and only papilla is elevated	Prepubertal; no pubic hair
II	Subareolar tissue forms a breast bud—a mound of tissue limited to the areola; areola widens, papilla is erect	Coarser, curly, pigmented hair on each side of mons veneris or labia majora
III	Breast tissue enlarges beyond areola, but there is no separation of their contours	Coarse, curly hair spread across pubis
IV	Areola and papilla form a second mound above the plane of the enlarging breast tissue	Abundant adult pubic hair, limited to pubis
V	Adult breast; areola and breast tissue return to the same plane, papilla is erect	Pubic hair present on medial aspects of thighs

becomes more prevalent during this time, and ovarian follicles undergo an accelerated rate of loss until the supply of follicles is ultimately depleted. Elevated FSH levels, normal LH levels, slightly elevated estradiol levels, and decreased levels of inhibin mark these menstrual cycle changes. The elevation of FSH but not LH may be attributable to decreased levels of inhibin produced by the ovary. Estradiol levels remain slightly elevated, but in the normal range, until 6 months to 1 year before follicular growth and development cease. Menopause is defined by the permanent cessation of menstruation, indicating loss of ovarian activity. The average age of menopause is between 50 and 52 years in the United States. The age of menopause, unlike menarche, has changed little since early Greek times.

The postmenopausal ovary continues to produce significant amounts of testosterone and androstenedione but ceases the majority of its estrogen production. Estrogens in postmenopausal women are produced predominantly by aromatization of adrenal androgens outside of the ovary. The liver, kidney, and adipose tissue are predominantly responsible for estrogen production in the postmenopausal state, and the highest circulating form of estrogen is estrone. Obese women are therefore at higher risk for estrogenic stimulation due to aromatization of androgens by adipose tissue.

KEY POINTS

1. Hypothalamic pulsatile GnRH secretion within a narrow range of frequency and amplitude activates the monthly menstrual cycle by stimulating gonadotropin release from the pituitary and subsequent steroid biosynthesis in the ovary.

2. Coordination of the menstrual cycle relies on a complex interplay of blood-borne hormones using stimulatory and inhibitory feedback loops between the hypothalamus, pituitary gland, and ovary.

3. The two-cell, two-gonadotropin hypothesis for ovarian steroidogenesis stipulates that LH stimulates the theca cells of the ovary to produce androgens, and FSH stimulates the granulosa cells to aromatize androgens to produce estrogen.

4. The follicular phase is characterized by recruitment of a cohort of several developing follicles; however, typically only one dominant follicle will be selected to ovulate while the rest will undergo atresia.

5. The estradiol stimulatory feedback loop in the late follicular stage synchronizes the midcycle LH surge, which ensures maturation of the dominant follicle and subsequent ovulation.

6. The corpus luteum, formed from the ovarian remnant of the dominant follicle during the luteal phase, produces progesterone in response to LH or hCG stimulation and undergoes luteolysis after 12 to 15 days unless fertilization occurs.

Continued

KEY POINTS—CONT'D

7. The endometrium is a complex tissue designed to provide the appropriate anatomic and hormonal environment for the growing conceptus and has characteristic proliferative, secretory, and menstrual phases. The involution and necrosis that characterizes menstruation is initiated by lysosomal enzymes, vasoconstriction, and myometrial contractions.

8. The process of gonadarche in puberty is initiated by activation of hypothalamic pulsatile GnRH release, stimulating the hypothalamic-pituitary-gonadal axis. Adrenarche is a separate event marked by increased androgen production by the adrenal gland.

9. *Menopause* is defined as the cessation of menses and the termination of ovarian follicular maturation due to loss of the ability of the ovary to produce estrogen in significant quantities.

SUGGESTED READING

Adashi EY, Rock JA, and Rosenwaks Z (eds): Reproductive Endocrinology, Surgery, and Technology. Philadelphia, Lippincott-Raven, 1996.

Speroff L and Fritz MA (eds): Clinical Gynecologic Endocrinology and Infertility, 7th ed. Philadelphia, Lippincott Williams & Wilkins, 2005.

3

THE GENETICS OF BREAST AND GYNECOLOGIC CANCERS

Jennifer Scalia Wilbur, Adam A. Rojan, and Robert D. Legare

INTRODUCTION

Health care for women in their reproductive years is often governed by their obstetrician/gynecologist. Recognizing an increased risk of cancer can provide women, and possibly their family members, with important preventive and risk-reducing strategies. Since clinical and research testing has rapidly translated cancer gene discoveries into clinical practice, cancer genetics is slowly becoming part of routine patient care. With the exponential growth of the field of cancer genetics, it becomes continually more difficult to remain current in the literature as it relates to accurate risk assessment; the medical, legal, and social issues of genetic testing; and surveillance, chemoprevention, and surgical prophylaxis options. Internationally, there are approximately 450 health care professionals specializing in the area of cancer genetic counseling. Referring at-risk women to a cancer genetic specialist can provide patients with a personal cancer risk assessment, the option of genetic testing (if appropriate), and an individualized medical management strategy. Therefore, obtaining a deeper understanding of the role of the cancer genetic specialist may facilitate referrals, easing the anxiety most women face when asked to explore their personal risk of cancer.

This chapter describes the multiple components of a cancer genetics and risk assessment program, provides an overview of hereditary cancer syndromes associated with breast cancer and gynecologic tumors, and discusses the basic controls on the cell cycle as it relates to oncology.

CANCER GENETIC COUNSELING

In 1971, Sarah Lawrence College offered the first masters degree program in human genetics. This was the onset of a new medical field called *genetic counseling.* The profession's growth and development provided impetus for the establishment of a professional society that was named the National Society of Genetic Counselors. This society carries the mission to promote the genetic counseling profession as a recognized and integral part of health care delivery, education, research, and public policy. Initially, the field of genetics and genetic counseling primarily focused on prenatal and pediatric genetics. However, with exponential growth of this area of medicine, multiple subspecialties have quickly emerged with the most prominent being oncology.

Over the last several years, there has been a strong initiative to offer clinical cancer genetics services in major medical universities and comprehensive cancer centers in the United States. The development of these services has also been present in the private practice arena as well as health maintenance organizations. Genetic counseling for women concerned about their risk of cancer involves an individual risk assessment based on a comprehensive pedigree analysis and providing education regarding appropriate risk-reducing and screening strategies, which, at times, involves the option of cancer genetic testing. Ideally, this service is offered within the setting of a multidisciplinary team of specialists who are able to offer cancer risk–reducing strategies such as increased surveillance, chemoprevention, and surgical prophylaxis.

Medical specialties such as medical oncology and surgery have initiated educational programs to keep their members current as better risk-assessment tools and medical management options for breast, ovarian, endometrial, and colorectal cancer enter the clinical mainstream. However, this is not particularly true for obstetricians and gynecologists; studies have concluded that obstetricians/gynecologists should become familiar with the principles of assessing family history for specific familial and hereditary cancer syndromes given their primary role in the health care of women.

INDICATION FOR CANCER RISK ASSESSMENT

Family history remains the most critical tool when evaluating cancer risk. Multiple publications have suggested a combination of clinical features, epidemiologic factors, and the aggregation of cancers in a family that would warrant further investigation of familial or hereditary cancer risk (Box 3-1). The accepted family features that raise concern for an increased cancer risk are purposely broad to compensate for the inaccuracy documented when confirming verbally reported cancer family histories and to capitalize on the reported reassurance "low-risk" patients often gain after a cancer risk evaluation. When cancer is present in a family, patients

> **Box 3-1** Features of a Family History That Would Warrant Further Investigation or Referral
>
> Multiple cancers (either of the same or different primaries) within the same lineage of a family
>
> Multiple primary cancers within the same person (e.g., colon and endometrial cancer occurring in one family member)
>
> Ashkenazi Jewish heritage
>
> Bilateral cancer or multifocal cancer within the same organ
>
> Cancer in a person with congenital anomalies
>
> An unusual or rare cancer (e.g., male breast cancer)
>
> A previously identified genetic mutation in a family member

often overestimate their lifetime risk of developing cancer; undergoing a cancer evaluation may significantly reduce this high perceived risk. Therefore, the "worried well" may benefit from a cancer risk evaluation even though their family history may not appear overly concerning.

FAMILY HISTORY

As familial cancer history remains the backbone of risk analysis, algorithms have been devised to ensure an accurate compilation of information. Cancer genetics specialists generally obtain a three-generation pedigree, including all relatives with their current age or age of death, whether or not they have been diagnosed with cancer. This allows the clinician to evaluate the size of the family, particularly noting the number of male and female members, which could influence the assessment of familial and/or hereditary disease. The pedigree should document each person who has developed an invasive or preinvasive diagnosis of cancer, as well as the age of cancer diagnosis and primary site. Additional clinical features such as colorectal polyps, use of hormone replacement therapy, and bilateral oophorectomy procedures should also be obtained because these factors may influence or limit accurate risk analysis. Last, because most cancer syndromes carry an autosomal dominant inheritance pattern, it is important to document all first-degree relatives of affected persons, even if they fall beyond the three-generation pedigree parameters.

Models for the development of cancer genetics and risk assessment programs are similar among national and international cancer genetics services. With each new patient referral, most centers will request that the patient complete a family history questionnaire before their appointment. This allows the patient time to obtain medical records and contact affected relatives to most accurately report the requested medical family history. Unfortunately, inaccurate family history information is often still observed, particularly beyond first-generation relatives. Love et al. documented that accurate reporting of the cancer diagnoses in second-degree relatives was correct only two thirds of the time, with familial gynecologic malignancies being reported less accurately than breast and colon cancers. Familial ovarian cancer is also often mistakenly reported as uterine, stomach, or cervical cancer, which dramatically modifies risk analyses, recommended screenings, and cancer risk–reducing strategies. Clinical geneticists and genetic counselors therefore invest a great deal of time and effort in the collection of pathology reports and death certificates to verify diagnosis age and tumor types in affected family members. During the creation and assessment of a three-generation pedigree, inaccurate patient reporting must be taken into account when formulating medical recommendations.

Modes of Inheritance

There are five categories of single-gene or mendelian trait disorders: autosomal dominant, autosomal recessive, X-linked recessive, X-linked dominant, and mitochondrial inheritance. The different modes are based on where the gene for the disease is located and the number of mutant allele copies required to express the phenotype.

Mendelian Inheritance Patterns

Autosomal dominant inheritance is classically the most recognizable type of mendelian inheritance. Usually, only one inherited mutant allele is necessary for a person to be affected by an autosomal dominant disorder (i.e., Huntington's disease). When a person carries an autosomal dominant gene mutation, each offspring carries a 50% chance of inheriting that mutated allele. The most common hereditary cancer syndromes, hereditary breast and ovarian cancer (HBOC) syndrome and hereditary nonpolyposis colorectal cancer (HNPCC), are autosomal dominant in nature. Nevertheless, because persons with HBOC, HNPCC, and other dominantly inherited conditions do not carry a 100% disease risk, persons may present with pedigree patterns that are misleading. This phenomenon is called *reduced penetrance* and is seen only in autosomal dominant disorders. *Variable expressivity* refers to the degree to which a condition or disorder is expressed in a person. *Late phenotypic onset, sex-specific expression* and *high recurrent mutation rates* are other genetic occurrences seen in autosomal dominant disease that can alter the expected family disease patterns.

Autosomal recessive inheritance also presents with the locus on an autosomal chromosome, but both inherited alleles must be mutant to express the phenotype. Therefore, most persons affected by a recessive disorder have parents with normal phenotypes. Since parents of an affected child both carry a mutant allele, their risks for a second pregnancy are as follows: a 25% chance to have another affected child, a 50% chance to have an unaffected child who carries one mutant allele, and a 25% chance to have an unaffected child with two normal alleles. Other cancer predisposition syndromes inherited in an autosomal recessive pattern include Fanconi's anemia and Bloom syndrome.

X-linked dominant/recessive inheritance involves the locus on the X chromosome. An X-linked gene is said to express dominant inheritance when a single dose of the mutant allele affects the phenotype of a female. A recessive X-linked gene requires two doses of the mutant allele to affect the female phenotype. Cancer susceptibility syndromes are rarely inherited in an X-linked fashion, with X-linked lymphoproliferative disorder being one such example.

Mitochondrial inheritance involves the locus on the mitochondrial "chromosome." The DNA of mitochondria contains about 10 genes involved in oxidative phosphorylation as well as a few other genes. Since this DNA is capable of mutation, a few human diseases have been found to be associated with mitochondrial inheritance. Leber's optic atrophy is a classic example of a disease of mitochondrial DNA. The ovum, originating in the female, has about 100,000 copies of mitochondrial DNA; the sperm, originating in the male, has fewer than 100 copies, and these are probably lost at fertilization. Virtually all of a person's mitochondria come from his or her mother. Affected fathers produce no affected offspring, whereas the offspring of affected mothers are all affected.

Nonmendelian Inheritance Patterns

Multifactorial and chromosomal inheritance patterns account for the remaining nonmendelian disorders. Multifactorial diseases are caused by a combination of the effects of multiple genes or by interactions between genes and the environment. With the use of genetic microarray processes, there is hope for a deeper understanding and improved treatment options for diseases of this type. Such disorders are more difficult to analyze because their genetic causes are often unclear, and they do not follow distinct patterns of inheritance. Examples of conditions caused by multiple genes or gene-environment interactions include certain types of cancer, heart disease, diabetes, and schizophrenia. Chromosomal disorders also do not follow the mendelian patterns of inheritance and are caused by changes in the number or structure of chromosomes. Chromosomal conditions include sex chromosome abnormalities such as Turner's, XXX, and XYY syndromes.

CANCER GENETICS RISK ASSESSMENT PROCESS

Cancer genetics and risk assessment is an innovative approach to patient care that is multidimensional. This multistep counseling process incorporates varying degrees of medical, legal, social, and psychological concerns. Health professionals trained in cancer genetics will need to possess knowledge in each of these areas to assist patients in understanding their risks, making informed decisions, and appreciating the implications for cancer prevention and risks for other family members (Box 3-2).

Determining Cancer Risk

A woman's family history regarding cancer assists in categorizing the disease into a sporadic, familial, or inherited pattern (Fig. 3-1). Having one or two relatives diagnosed with cancer at an average age, possibly involving both the maternal and paternal lineages, typically would not increase a person's risk of cancer appreciably. This type of presentation generally

---

Box 3-2 Cancer Risk Assessment Process

1. Contracting—understanding the patient's reason for referral, perceived risks, and current medical and social situation
2. Discussing personal and family history (obtaining pathology reports for confirmation, if possible)
3. Translating risk analyses into language appropriate for the patient
4. Discussing the risks, limitations, and benefits of genetic testing (if appropriate); these include the medical, legal, social, psychological, and family issues related to a positive, negative, and uncertain test result
5. Discussing appropriate research opportunities that may be helpful to the patient, the patient's family, and/or the advancement of medicine
6. Disclosing and interpreting genetic test results as they relate to the patient's personal and medical history
7. Discussing an appropriate medical management strategy
8. Coordinating referrals for social/psychological support as well as with other health care specialists for cancer treatment/surveillance
9. Communicating, with the patient's consent, the counseling outcome and plan with the patient's treating physician team

---

denotes *sporadic* disease, which is the most common cause of cancer. Aside from age, most sporadic cancers are thought to be caused by a combination of environmental and polygenetic influences. A person's *familial* cancer risk, which is commonly influenced by an affected relative's age of cancer diagnosis and degree of relationship, is also likely caused by multiple interacting factors. An example of familial cancer risk would be breast cancer clustering in families where there is no suggestion of an autosomal dominant inheritance pattern. Familial multifactorial theories include the modifying effects of other genes, as well as possible interactions of the gene(s) with environmental factors. The majority of data determining familial cancer risk are derived from statistical modeling and epidemiologic studies. Epidemiologic publications studying women who have a first-degree relative diagnosed with ovarian cancer, at any age, propose a threefold to fourfold increased lifetime risk of developing ovarian cancer compared with

Figure 3-1

The majority of cancers can be subdivided into sporadic, familial, and hereditary causes.

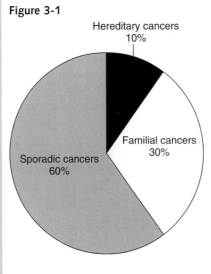

Hereditary cancers
10%

Familial cancers
30%

Sporadic cancers
60%

the general population. Based on the lack of effective screening methods available for early ovarian cancer detection, as well as emotional status, women may choose a different course of action once informed of this slightly increased ovarian cancer risk. With clinical suggestion of an autosomal dominant family cancer pattern, an *inherited* cancer syndrome should be investigated. Practitioners should be cautious of sex-specific expression, variable age of onset and expressivity, and reduced penetrance, which can easily disguise a dominant mutant allele. Additionally, limitations in family history (i.e., adoption) and inaccurate family history reporting can change the typical autosomal dominant pattern. Therefore, a comprehensive evaluation of family history is critical for the identification of an inherited cancer syndrome, which when identified, may have a major impact on a woman's medical, family, and social welfare.

Cancer Genetic Testing

The most common means for genetic testing is leukocyte DNA, a simple blood sample. However, buccal swab and tumor tissue are also viable options. Buccal swab, though only available for a limited number of genetic tests, is less invasive and is of particular benefit when the patient has difficulty with peripheral blood draws. When an affected relative is deceased or it is not feasible to obtain a blood sample, analyzing DNA extracted from paraffin-embedded tumor blocks acquired during surgery is yet another testing strategy. Specific tumor DNA studies are commercially available to help aid in the diagnosis of inherited susceptibility to cancer. In the case of HNPCC, microsatellite instability (MSI) analysis and gene expression assays performed on tumor tissue can facilitate the next phase in the genetic testing process. The presence of MSI within a tumor increases the probability for an HNPCC germline mutation, and similarly, immunohistochemistry expression assays may help identify which HNPCC gene to sequence. Screening for germline BRCA1 mutations using RNA expression assays is under investigation.

Algorithm for Genetic Testing

An overall basic schema (Box 3-3) has emerged and has been accepted in medical practice for patients undergoing cancer genetic counseling with the option of testing. The patient seeking counseling may be unaffected with a positive family history, affected with a suspected inherited cancer, or unaffected with a relative positive for a hereditary genetic mutation. Because current molecular testing cannot identify all of the genetic mutations associated with inherited cancer genetic syndromes, a negative test result in an unaffected person has limited clinical significance. Therefore,

---

Box 3-3 Hereditary Genetic Testing: A Multistep Process

1. Identify at-risk patient.
2. Provide pretest counseling.
3. Obtain informed consent.
4. Select and offer test.
5. Disclose results.
6. Provide post-test counseling and follow-up.

if a family has an increased probability of harboring a germline mutation, it is recommended to initially offer DNA analysis to an affected relative. Offering genetic testing to a patient's family member can be complex both logistically as well as psychologically. This will often require the patient to contact a relative he or she has not seen or heard from for many years. Even if the affected relative is a first-degree relative (i.e., siblings, offspring, or parents) and close relationships are established, this person may choose not to pursue a cancer genetics consultation or genetic testing for personal reasons. Although the person's test result may affect the medical care of other relatives, the decision for genetic testing is ultimately his or her own. This can cause complex emotions and disrupt family relationships. Lastly, there may not be a living affected relative available in a family to offer genetic testing. Under these circumstances, with the ability to obtain appropriate legal consent, paraffin-embedded tumor block analysis is at times an option (i.e., MSI analysis for HNPCC investigation or BRCA gene analysis for three common mutations recognized in the Ashkenazi Jewish population). Nevertheless, if the unaffected patient is unable to obtain the genetic carrier status of an affected relative, the complex interpretation of a negative test result must be explained during the pretesting consultation.

Pretest Counseling   After a comprehensive review of the family history with the determined suspicion for a possible hereditary genetic syndrome, time is invested with the patient to ensure he or she has sufficient information to make an informed decision regarding genetic testing. Most pretest counseling appointments last approximately 120 minutes and cover the following:

1. *The cancer genetic syndrome.* This step involves a discussion regarding the clinical description, cancer risks, and management of the suspected disease. In addition, the counselor addresses estimated chance for the presence of a germline mutation and the consequences of a positive, negative, and inconclusive test result, as well as predicted cancer risks, recommended screening, and risk-reduction guidelines for each possible test outcome.
2. *A testing strategy.* Next comes a discussion of which family member is the most appropriate person for testing to obtain the most medically meaningful results for the patient. If not the patient, what is the existing relationship with this person, and would providing contact information for a cancer genetic specialist close to where this relative lives assist in facilitating counseling with the option of genetic testing?
3. *Family members.* Although persons undergoing genetic testing should primarily base their decision for testing on personal medical management and psychological effects, recognizing its implication for the health of other relatives is a critical component. For example, once a person is found to carry an autosomal dominant mutation, a 50% risk for offspring, siblings, and each parent to also carry the same predisposition mutation can be recognized. Similarly, the genetic test result of a parent whose child carries a dominant gene mutation will yield the carrier status of his or her spouse (assuming the spouses are the biologic parents of that child). Therefore, genetic testing results can yield a

definitive carrier risk and possible carrier status of other relatives, which often hold serious implications for the person who was not even tested. Since studies have shown that the first family member who tests positive is more likely to experience difficulty and distress with sharing the test results with family members, special attention and support needs to be directed to this person. There have been few studies analyzing the communication among a hereditary cancer genetic family. Clase et al. (2003) report that the dissemination of information was largely focused on first-degree relatives due to the superficial and/or lack of relationships that existed with distant relatives.

4. *Experiences with cancer.* Past family and personal cancer experiences can have profound effects on actions related to medical screening, relationships with health professionals, morbidity and mortality, perceived disease risk, and stigmatization of cancer within the family. These experiences may be multigenerational, dividing those who were caretakers with those uninvolved because of physical distance, psychological reasons, or both. Reactions to a positive or negative test result may compound or confuse already complex relationships. Therefore, exploration of present and past cancer encounters often provides insight into a patient's perspective, which can prove to be critical when supporting patients during result disclosure.

5. *Perceived risk.* Understanding a patient's perceived risk can assist in adjusting the counseling approach to better serve patient needs and enhance the patient's understanding of his or her risks and compliance with the recommended screening and risk-reduction guidelines.

6. *Psychological issues.* Multiple studies have examined psychological distress among persons undergoing cancer genetic testing. The majority of studies focus on offering BRCA gene analysis to persons suspected of carrying a mutation causing HBOC syndrome. The overriding conclusion is that genetic testing and counseling can occur with little anxiety and stress. In fact, psychological benefit has been reported for persons receiving a negative test result. However, on the contrary, several studies have documented that the individual whose test results are negative (having a previously identified positive test result in the family) can be plagued with survivor guilt. Wagner et al. report that depression scores increased in women with negative test results and decreased in women with positive results. Wood et al. analyzed women with cancer discovered less than 1 year from their testing experience and found they expressed increased distress associated with genetic testing and counseling. Therefore, as more comprehensive analyses are performed, there may be specific subgroup populations identified that may require greater psychological support.

7. *Risk of genetic discrimination.* Persons who carry an increased disease risk due to a positive genetic test result fear the possibility of health insurance and employment discrimination. There has been heightened legislative attention given to medical privacy with the focus on protection from genetic discrimination. In 1996, the Health Insurance Portability and Accountability Act implemented policy recommendations on health insurance and provided some protection from discrimination; however,

51

many holes in this legislation remain, and genetic discrimination is still a possibility. Although there are many recent publications that have demonstrated that the fear of employment and health insurance discrimination in the United States far outweighs the reality, counseling and education of patients considering genetic testing remains critical.

Informed Consent

The decision to pursue genetic testing should be voluntary and made without coercion. Patients should possess a clear understanding of the consequences associated with positive, negative, and uncertain test results. Proper consenting is a complex and time-consuming process usually accounting for a large majority of the pretest appointment. A patient review and signature of a written document describing the risks, limitations, and benefits of the specific test being ordered is strongly recommended.

Post-Test Counseling

Receiving genetic test results can be an extremely emotional experience for the patient in the setting of both a negative and positive test result. For this reason, and to ensure accurate result interpretation, a face-to-face meeting with the patient is recommended. Since a negative genetic test result can indicate a broad spectrum of cancer risks (ranging from the risks observed in the general population to those associated with a hereditary cancer syndrome), it is critical that patients with negative results not be given false reassurance. The interpretation of uncertain genetic variants often leads to confusion about medical management recommendations and family genetic testing options. The discovery of a positive deleterious mutation carries dramatically higher cancer risks as well as important implications for family members. Follow-up visits are encouraged for patients with positive test results to further address personal medical screenings, chemopreventive and surgical strategies, and communication to at-risk family members. Follow-up visits are also useful for addressing anxiety and fears related to passing the mutation on to children, providing support, and coordinating referrals to other appropriate health care professionals, such as psychiatrists and endocrinologists. Last, it is also reasonable to follow those high-risk families wherein a hereditary mutation cannot be identified. As the field of cancer genetics continues to rapidly advance, additional genetic testing options may become available that could be important to the management of these families.

CELL CYCLE CONTROL

Acquired Versus Inherited Gene Mutations

Cancer is caused by the serial acquisition of inherited and/or acquired genetic mutations that ultimately result in the malignant phenotype. The root of cancer evolution rests in altered or perturbed cell cycle kinetics. Although acquired mutations are necessary for the development of most cancers, in 5% to 10% of cancers, inherited germline mutations confer greatly increased risks for specific tumor types. This is the case in cancer syndromes such as hereditary nonpolyposis colorectal carcinoma and HBOC syndrome. In other instances, clustering of similar cancers in a given family is seen even when no inherited mutations can be found. Cancer susceptibility in these families is clearly higher than for the general population, but it is less than in the hereditary cancer syndromes. For example, the lifetime risk of breast cancer in women with two affected first-degree family members diagnosed between the ages of 40 to 49 years is increased approximately threefold over that of the general population. The lifetime risk of colorectal carcinoma is increased by twofold to threefold in those with one affected first-degree relative. Modest levels of increased cancer susceptibility may be due in part to the inheritance of some single-nucleotide polymorphisms (SNPs). SNPs are single base-pair substitutions occurring relatively frequently (>1%) in a population. SNPs in genes involved in DNA repair, carcinogen metabolism, and hormone metabolism may affect cancer susceptibility and are an area of active investigation.

Types of DNA Alterations Seen in Cancer Cells

Cancer cells have DNA alterations at the level of the gene and the chromosome, and in some cancers, through the presence of exogenous viral DNA.

Genes
Mutations restricted to small regions or single genes include point mutations, substitutions, and small insertions, deletions, and duplications. These generally occur within the coding or regulatory regions of the gene. Members of the ras gene family, for instance, are activated by point mutations in many cancers.

Chromosomes
Cancers also demonstrate gross changes visible at the chromosomal level. These include the following: (1) changes in chromosome number, by loss or gain of chromosomes; (2) gross deletions of chromosomal segments; (3) inversion of segments; (4) translocation between two chromosomes, creating new sequences; (5) amplification of chromosome segments, which cytogenetically are visualized as homogenously staining regions within chromosomes or extrachromosomally as small fragments called *double minutes.*

For example, in ovarian carcinomas, highly complicated rearrangements and fusions are often seen. Deletions within the long arms of chromosomes 6 and 17 and the short arm of chromosome 11 are common. Other rearrangements, such as translocations between chromosome 6 and chromosome 14, have also been observed. Amplification of the myc and her2/neu oncogenes is also seen in approximately 20% of breast, cervical, and ovarian cancers. The clinical relevance of her2/neu amplification in breast cancer is well known.

Viruses
Although most cancers are not related to viruses, certain strains of human papilloma virus (particularly HPV-16 and HPV-18) can cause cervical, anal, and oropharyngeal carcinomas. Nearly all invasive cervical carcinomas and more than 70% of preinvasive cervical lesions contain HPV DNA.

Two viral gene products, E6 and E7, are required for malignant transformation. E6 and E7 bind and inhibit the tumor suppressors (discussed below) p53 and pRB, respectively, and promote accumulation of mutations in DNA by preventing cell cycle arrest after DNA damage. The key difference between low-risk and high-risk strains of HPV is binding affinity and activity of these two proteins.

Classes of Genes Mutated

Three classes of genes mutated in cancer can be identified: proto-oncogenes, tumor suppressors, and DNA repair genes.

Proto-Oncogenes

The normal function of proto-oncogenes is to promote cell division or inhibit cell death. These genes and their protein products are intricately regulated to prevent excess cellular proliferation. Oncogenes result from activating mutations of proto-oncogenes, causing overexpression of the gene or dysregulation of the gene product. Oncogenes act dominantly, in that mutation in only one of the two copies of the gene is necessary for cellular transformation. Members of the myc family of proto-oncogenes encode transcription factors necessary for cell division and are commonly mutated by amplification or by chromosomal translocations in cancers.

Among the most commonly mutated proto-oncogenes are members of the ras family, mutated in approximately 20% of all cancers, including 50% of colorectal, 95% of pancreatic, and up to 25% of endometrial and ovarian carcinomas. Ras mutations in ovarian carcinomas are seen more commonly in borderline and low-malignant-potential tumors of mucinous histology than in high-grade tumors. Ras is a small G protein that cycles between an active guanosine triphosphate (GTP)-bound form that promotes cell division and an inactive guanosine diphosphate (GDP)-bound form. Point mutations cause loss of the ability to cycle to the inactive form and result in dysregulated, constitutively active ras.

Tumor Suppressors

The role of tumor suppressors is opposite to that of proto-oncogenes. Tumor suppressors normally inhibit cell division or promote cell death. Mutations in tumor suppressors act recessively in that deletion or loss of function mutations in both copies of a tumor suppressor gene are necessary for tumorigenesis. The tumor suppressor p53, encoded by the TP53 gene, is the most commonly mutated gene in human cancer, present in 30% to 40% of ovarian carcinomas. p53 can cause cell cycle arrest as well as cell death after DNA damage. Another commonly mutated tumor suppressor, pRB, was named after its association with hereditary and sporadic retinoblastoma and is mutated in a wide variety of cancers. In its hypophosphorylated state, pRB is able to bind and inhibit members of the E2F family of transcription factors. This prevents transit of damaged cells from entering the S phase of the cell cycle and replicating their DNA. As previously discussed, pRB and p53 are inactivated in cervical carcinomas through the action of HPV proteins.

Most hereditary cancer syndromes are caused by the inheritance of a germline mutation in a tumor suppressor gene. The inheritance of a single recessive mutation can be responsible for an autosomal dominant cancer syndrome and is explained by Knudson's "two-hit" hypothesis (Fig. 3-2). In normal cells, two separate somatic mutations (two hits) are required to inactivate a tumor suppressor gene. Each mutation is a low-probability event, so it is relatively rare for one cell to have both of its alleles inactivated. In hereditary cancer syndromes, every cell inherits a germline mutation in one of the alleles (i.e., the first hit). In these cases, a second hit in at least one cell in the target organ is highly likely to occur. What causes this second hit to occur is unknown. However, the role of modifier genes is an active area of research. These are genetic changes that may influence the expression of the known inherited germline mutation (i.e., BRCA genes). Two examples specific to inherited BRCA gene mutations are as follows:

1. The *HRAS1 proto-oncogene* located on chromosome 11p15.5 has been identified to carry a polymorphism of variable number of tandem repeats (VNTR). Phelan et al. reported that the risk of ovarian cancer in BRCA1 carriers with one or two HRAS1 VNTR alleles was twice as great as that of carriers with the common HRAS1 alleles.
2. According to an abstract presented at the 1998 meeting of the American Society of Human Genetics, the CY1A1 gene was identified as a possible modifier gene in BRCA gene carriers with and without breast cancer.

Figure 3-2

Alfred Knudson's "two-hit" hypothesis.

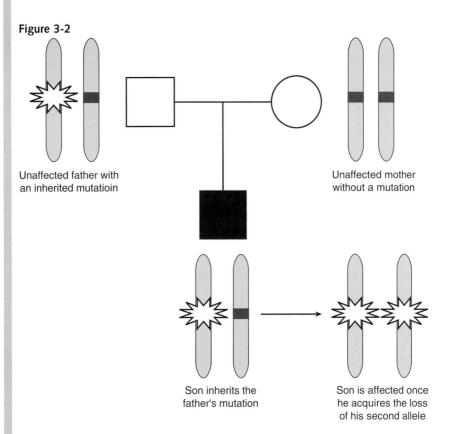

Unaffected father with an inherited mutatioin

Unaffected mother without a mutation

Son inherits the father's mutation

Son is affected once he acquires the loss of his second allele

CY1A1, in its wild-type form, encodes for an enzyme involved in estradiol hydroxylation and polyaromatic hydrocarbon metabolism. A specific gene variant was identified in affected and unaffected women carrying a BRCA gene mutation, yielding an approximate 40% breast cancer risk reduction.

With further studies examining gene-gene and gene-environment interactions, there is hope to further knowledge in the area of tumor genesis and the care of persons with both hereditary and noninherited carcinomas.

DNA Repair Genes

A third class of mutated genes in cancers is DNA repair genes. These genes are involved in DNA repair as well as maintenance of genomic stability and integrity. Loss of function in DNA repair genes increases mutation rates in the entire genome, including proto-oncogenes and tumor suppressors. Although these genes are not specifically involved in cell growth, they can be considered a subset of tumor suppressors because mutations in these genes act recessively. HNPCC is caused by mutations in the DNA mismatch repair system, resulting in elevated risks of colorectal and other cancers, including endometrial and ovarian cancers. Mutations in DNA mismatch repair genes, commonly MSH2 or MLH1, cause genetic instability, resulting in MSI. Mutation rates are elevated twofold to threefold with the identification of repetitive DNA sequences within the tumor called *microsatellites.* Mutations in tumor suppressors, such as transforming growth factor (TGF)-βRII, which encodes for a receptor responsible for the growth-inhibiting factor TGF-β, and Bax promoting cell death, are common in HNPCC.

Multistep Process for Carcinogenesis

Molecular and epidemiologic analysis suggests that cancers require at least 4 to 10 mutations for clinical expression. In most cases, this process occurs over decades. Each mutation confers some selective growth advantage or increase in mutational rate, until a cell has acquired enough mutations to become malignant. Although the precise order of mutations varies from cancer to cancer and is not well understood for most cancers, the process of carcinogenesis in colorectal cancer has been extensively studied and is currently well known as the Vogelstein hypothesis. It is thought that at least seven mutations involving four genes (inactivation of three tumor suppressor genes and activation of one proto-oncogene) are necessary for the development of colorectal cancer. Although the order of mutations is not always identical, the order of the sequence of events is significant. For instance, inactivation of both alleles of the tumor suppressor gene APC is one of the first events, whereas inactivation of p53 is generally one of the last events in colorectal carcinogenesis. As well, cells undergoing mutations in a different sequence are less likely to become malignant tumors.

Gene Expression Profiling

Gene expression profiling uses microarrays to simultaneously compare gene transcription in cancer cells versus normal tissues in thousands of genes. This allows for the identification of genes that are overexpressed or underexpressed in cancers. Although gene expression profiling currently is used primarily as a research tool, many potential clinical applications of the method are being developed. The expression profile may provide prognostic information addressing the aggressiveness of a tumor, including biomarkers tracing disease prognosis and its response to therapies. It may also give information about potential therapeutic targets, as well as sensitivity and resistance to different chemotherapies.

HEREDITARY CANCER SYNDROMES

Clinicians should make efforts to recognize genetic syndromes that predispose patients to the development of gynecologic cancers so that patients are afforded the opportunity to have genetic testing to assist them and their family members in making the most appropriate medical management decisions. Table 3-1 lists the recognized hereditary genetic syndromes associated

Table 3-1

Hereditary Genetic Syndromes Associated with Breast Cancer or Gynecologic Tumors

Hereditary Cancer Syndromes	Clinical Features	Identified Gene(s)	Inheritance Pattern
Breast and ovarian cancer syndrome	Breast, ovarian, and prostate cancers	BRCA1, BRCA2	Autosomal dominant
Hereditary nonpolyposis colorectal cancer syndrome	Colorectal, endometrial, ovarian, gastric, hepatobiliary, brain, and small bowel cancers	MLH1, MSH2, MSH6, PMS1, PMS2	Autosomal dominant
Li-Fraumeni syndrome	Soft tissue sarcomas, leukemia, breast, brain, ovarian, adrenocortical, prostate, melanoma, and pancreatic cancers	p53	Autosomal dominant
Cowden syndrome	Thyroid cancer, breast cancer, mucocutaneous lesions, and colonic neoplasms	PTEN	Autosomal dominant
Peutz-Jeghers syndrome	Abnormal melanin deposits, gastrointestinal tract polyposis and cancers, sex cord tumors with annular tubules (SCAT), breast cancer, cervical adenoma malignum, endometrial cancer, and endometrial cancer	STK11	Autosomal dominant
Ataxia-telangiectasia	Cerebellar ataxia, oculocutaneous telangiectasia, radiation hypersensitivity, leukemia, lymphoma, numerous other tumors, and breast cancer in carriers	ATM	Autosomal recessive

with breast cancer or gynecologic tumors. Because most are caused by autosomal dominant tumor suppressor or mismatch repair gene mutations, the respective types of cancers are usually seen in multiple generations and occur at young ages. HBOC and HNPCC are the most common disorders among inherited gynecologic cancer syndromes. Therefore, the remaining portion of this chapter focuses on a detailed description of HBOC and HNPCC and on reviewing the specific genes involved, genetic testing options, the associated cancer risks, and current medical management options.

Hereditary Breast and Ovarian Cancer

HBOC is largely accounted for by deleterious BRCA1 or BRCA2 gene mutations, discovered in 1994 and 1996, respectively. The BRCA1 and BRCA2 genes normally function as tumor suppressor genes; however, when a deleterious BRCA germline mutation is present, the risk of cancer is increased, causing HBOC. Approximately 16% of mutations in families with hereditary breast cancer are not found by standard BRCA1 and BRCA2 DNA sequencing/large BRCA1 genomic rearrangement analysis and are believed to be caused by either an undiscovered gene(s) or mutations within BRCA1 and BRCA2 that are being missed with current testing methods. Additionally, there are less common hereditary breast syndromes that can be recognized by associated clinical characteristics and confirmed with molecular testing, such as Cowden syndrome, Bloom syndrome, Peutz-Jeghers syndrome, xeroderma pigmentosum, ataxia-telangiectasia, and Li-Fraumeni syndrome. Similarly, there are other syndromes associated with hereditary epithelial ovarian cancer such as HNPCC as reviewed below in this chapter.

Guidelines updated and published by the American Society of Clinical Oncology (ASCO) recommend that genetic testing be offered when (1) the individual has personal or family history features suggestive of a genetic cancer susceptibility condition; (2) the test can be adequately interpreted; and (3) the result will aid in diagnosis or influence the medical or surgical management of the patient or family members at hereditary risk of cancer. These guidelines also state that testing should only be carried out in the setting of pre- and post-test counseling, which should include discussion of possible risks and benefits of cancer early detection and risk-reducing strategies.

BRCA1 and BRCA2 Cancer-Predisposing Mutation Probability

Overall, studies indicate that a BRCA1 or BRCA2 cancer-predisposing gene mutation is more likely to be present if the family history includes breast cancer diagnosed before age 50 years, bilateral breast cancer (with a premenopausal initial diagnosis), ovarian cancer, male breast cancer, Ashkenazi Jewish ancestry, or the occurrence of both breast cancer and ovarian cancer in the same woman (Fig. 3-3). Because each study evaluated BRCA carrier risk from a selected population, it is often best to determine an individual's/family's carrier probability according to the data set that is clinically most similar or applicable.

There are two popular models available to estimate the probability for the presence of a cancer-predisposing BRCA1 or BRCA2 mutation.

Figure 3-3

An example of a family with hereditary breast and ovarian cancer syndrome.

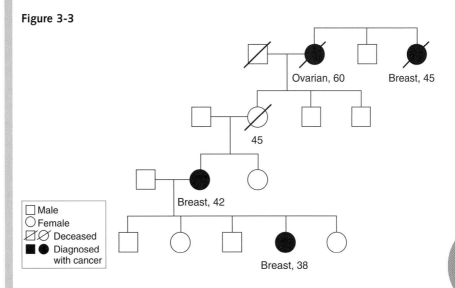

Male
Female
Deceased
Diagnosed with cancer

Ovarian, 60   Breast, 45

45

Breast, 42

Breast, 38

The first is a software model called BRCAPRO (http://astor.som.jhmi.edu/BayesMendel/brcapro.html). This calculation is based on observations in referral populations in which the majority of women tested were affected with breast or ovarian cancer. This model adjusts risk according to Bayesian theorem, but it may overestimate or underestimate carrier risk dependent on the family characteristics present. The second model is an empiric model derived by Myriad Genetic Laboratories, Inc. These data were obtained from a series of 238 women with a positive family history who developed breast cancer before the age of 50 years or ovarian cancer at any age. The development of ovarian cancer within such families significantly increased the chance of finding a BRCA1 or BRCA2 mutation. The Myriad model was later applied to 10,000 tested persons by the same group (observational data). Of importance, these risk estimates are calculated directly from the clinician's completed test request form, which is usually history that is obtained only from the patient's verbal report. Therefore, due to each model's limitations, it is recommended that hereditary cancer risk assessment be performed by experienced clinicians to ensure that the most accurate assessment is calculated.

Cancer Risks Associated with a BRCA Deleterious Mutation

The majority of HBOC families have been linked to gene mutations affecting the normal function of the BRCA1 or BRCA2 protein. Most studies report that women carrying a deleterious BRCA gene mutation have a 56% to 85% cumulative lifetime risk of developing breast cancer up to the age of 70 years and a 16% to 44% cumulative lifetime risk of developing ovarian cancer. Additionally, BRCA-positive women already diagnosed with breast cancer carry a higher risk of a second primary breast cancer, both in the ipsilateral and contralateral breasts. Several studies demonstrate a 30% to 40% 10-year risk of second primary breast cancer among BRCA1/2 carriers. There are recent data suggesting that cancer risks for BRCA2-positive women may be lower when compared with BRCA1 carriers. Antoniou et al. performed a meta-analysis of 22 studies reporting an approximate 45% breast cancer risk and an 11% ovarian cancer risk for BRCA2 carriers by the age of 70 years. Additionally, reports have shown the average age of ovarian cancer to be younger in BRCA1 carriers compared with BRCA2 carriers (52 and 62 years, respectively).

Male BRCA heterozygotes carry an approximate 6% male breast cancer risk by the age of 70 years and a threefold to fourfold increased relative risk of prostate cancer by the age of 80 years. Although low, the risk of pancreatic cancers in men and women carrying a BRCA2 mutation was estimated to be approximately 2% to 3% by age 80. Suggestive evidence remains of additional cancer risks influenced by an absent BRCA protein, such as pancreatic cancer and melanoma. However, further studies need to be conducted to substantiate these findings.

Retrospective analyses are also beginning to report a relationship between breast cancer histology and BRCA heterozygosity. Data thus far suggest that BRCA1 breast tumors more commonly have features suggestive of a poor prognosis, including aneuploidy; higher histologic grade; a high proliferative rate (S-phase fraction); and negative estrogen receptor (ER), progesterone receptor (PR), and Her-2/*neu* expression (triple negative). BRCA2 tumors are more often ER/PR positive and less likely to overexpress Her-2/*neu*. However, there is also evidence that medullary carcinoma (which has a histology associated with a more favorable prognosis) is more common among women with BRCA1 mutations.

Management of Risk in Carriers of BRCA Gene Mutations

Management of persons found to be positive for HBOC susceptibility syndrome includes discussion regarding cancer screening protocols, possible options for chemoprevention, as well as prophylactic surgery. The majority of these strategies are available through research protocols. Although a number of interventions have been postulated to reduce the morbidity and mortality from breast cancer in women confirmed to carry a BRCA1 or BRCA2 cancer-predisposing mutation, data are still evolving to substantiate these claims. Nevertheless, several strategies have been prospectively studied and proved to detect early-stage cancers or to decrease the risk of cancer development in BRCA heterozygotes. These strategies include cancer screening, prophylactic mastectomy and/or oophorectomy, and chemoprevention. As a result, management recommendations are most appropriately made based on recent publications along with expert opinion.

Cancer Screening

Recommendations for cancer screening of persons with a BRCA1 or BRCA2 cancer-predisposing mutation have been made by a task force convened by the Cancer Genetics Studies Consortium (CGSC), an National Institutes of Health–sponsored consortium of researchers assessing the ethical, legal, and social implications of genetic testing for cancer risk. The CGSC statement emphasizes that, at the time of publication, recommendations were based on presumed benefit and may change as new evidence becomes available. Patients must therefore be counseled regarding the limited knowledge about strategies to reduce risk in combination with patient preference regarding follow-up decisions. Recommendations similar to those of the CGSC are also practiced in 16 European family cancer centers.

Breast Cancer Screening

The three-pronged breast cancer screening regimen is based on data from families with cancer-predisposing BRCA1 or BRCA2 mutations, addressing the elevated breast cancer risk beginning in a woman's late 20s or early 30s. Persons predisposed to an inherited breast cancer risk are recommended to consider the following:

- Monthly breast self-examination beginning at the age of 18 years.
- Clinical breast examination two to four times annually beginning at the age of 25 years.
- Annual mammography beginning at the age of 25 years: There is evidence that BRCA1 and BRCA2 gene products may be necessary to assist with DNA damage repair caused by radiation. Despite concerns expressed regarding the repeated low doses of radiation exposure caused by mammography in BRCA-positive women, the Human Genome Research Institute's (NHGRI) task force states that this hypothetical risk would likely be outweighed by mammography's benefit for early cancer detection.
- Annual magnetic resonance imaging (MRI) screening: Although the sensitivity of MRI appears to be superior to that of mammography and breast ultrasound for the detection of invasive cancers in high-risk women, the specificity is debated and appears to be directly related to the clinical experience of the radiologist. There have been several studies supporting the use of MRI in women having an increased breast cancer risk. The detection of small foci of breast disease in BRCA gene–positive women (which were undetectable with mammography) has supported the integration of screening MRI in germline carriers. There is great need for further studies to enable health practitioners to recommend the most effective use of MRI screening for women at high risk for breast cancer.

Men with BRCA mutations may also be at increased risk for breast cancer, and evaluation of any breast mass or change is advisable; however, there are insufficient data to recommend a formal surveillance program at this time.

Ovarian Cancer Screening

The ovarian cancer screening measures available have limited sensitivity and specificity and have not been shown to reduce ovarian cancer mortality. Nevertheless, the CSGC and NHGRI task forces recommend the following for women carrying a deleterious BRCA1 or BRCA2 gene mutation:

- Annual or semiannual pelvic examination beginning at the age of 25 to 35 years.
- Annual or semiannual transvaginal ultrasound examination with color Doppler beginning at the age of 25 to 35 years.
- Annual or semiannual serum CA-125 concentration beginning at the age of 25 to 35 years: Serum screening can be associated with a high false-positive rate, especially in premenopausal women, and is often not practiced by physicians even in the setting of a germline carrier.

Promising data, reported from Memorial Sloan-Kettering Cancer Center, provide the first prospective evidence demonstrating that the above surveillance strategy used in BRCA-positive women may result in the diagnosis of early-stage ovarian tumors.

Prophylactic Surgery

Prophylactic Mastectomy

In a publication by Hartmann et al., of 6039 women found to carry a BRCA gene mutation and/or with a family history of breast cancer who underwent prophylactic mastectomy, there was an estimated 90% to 94% reduction in breast cancer risk and an 81% to 94% reduction in breast cancer–related deaths. Additional prospective data regarding 251 BRCA-positive persons followed up at Memorial Sloan-Kettering Cancer Center demonstrated the detection of two occult intraductal breast cancers within the 29 persons choosing risk-reducing mastectomy.

Although only a small percentage of women from high-risk families choose to undergo prophylactic bilateral mastectomy, and those who do generally feel content with their decision. In a follow-up study of high-risk women who pursued preventive surgery, approximately 74% reported a reduced emotional concern regarding breast cancer development and seemed to naturally sustain other psychological and social functioning.

Prophylactic Oophorectomy

Data presented at the 2001 American Society of Human Genetics 50th Annual Meeting indicate that prophylactic bilateral salpingo-oophorectomy (BSO) reduces the risk of ovarian cancer by 95% in women with BRCA deleterious mutations. The risk of primary peritoneal carcinomatosis does not appear to be effected by salpingo-oophorectomy. A study conducted by the National Cancer Institute found that women from families at high risk for ovarian cancer had an equal rate of primary peritoneal cancer after oophorectomy compared with the rate of primary peritoneal cancer in women who had not had the procedure. Further studies are necessary to investigate whether hysterectomy or any other strategy would further reduce the risk of ovarian cancer or primary peritoneal cancer after BSO.

Rebbeck et al. have also demonstrated that prophylactic oophorectomy reduces the risk of breast cancer by approximately 50% in BRCA carriers. Additionally, in 21 of 36 BRCA gene–positive women diagnosed with breast cancer who underwent BSO either before or within 6 months of their cancer diagnosis, only 1 of 15 (4.8%) relapsed versus the 7 of 15 (47%) women who retained their ovaries. Therefore, after comprehensive counseling, study results now advocate for BRCA-heterozygous persons to consider risk-reducing prophylactic salpingo-oophorectomy to reduce the risk of *both* ovarian and breast cancers at the appropriate time.

As preventive oophorectomy is becoming more common secondary to the identification of an inheritable mutation, specific recommendations are emerging related to this surgical procedure, as well as regarding the pathologic examination of the tissue removed. Unexpected gynecologic neoplasms were discovered in five high-risk breast/ovarian cancer patients (four of the five patients had a documented deleterious BRCA mutation) who underwent prophylactic salpingo-oophorectomy with hysterectomy. Therefore, more rigorous tissue examination, as well as specified surgical interventions, should be considered for the detection of early neoplastic changes when BRCA carriers choose preventive BSO as a risk-reducing strategy.

After comprehensive cancer genetic counseling, the majority of women are pleased with their decision to pursue surgical interventions for ovarian cancer prevention. Although approximately 93% of high-risk women who underwent prophylactic oophorectomy expressed no regret about their decision, 50% preferred more information about the risk and benefits of hormone replacement therapy (HRT) before making decisions about surgery. Armstrong et al. studied the use of HRT after BSO in premenopausal BRCA gene carriers. Consistent with previous publications, they found that short-term HRT use is reasonable for women experiencing a compromise in quality of life; however most recommend discontinuing use before or at the time of expected menopause. Women in this situation must assume at least a theoretical increase in breast cancer risk.

63

Chemoprevention

Breast Cancer Risk Reduction

The national surgical adjuvant breast and bowel project (NSABP) P-1 prevention trial assessed the use of tamoxifen (a partial estrogen receptor antagonist) in women identified by the Gail model to have an increased breast cancer risk. This study reported a 49% reduction in breast cancer in the 5-year group treated with tamoxifen. It was concluded that tamoxifen prophylaxis was most beneficial in women with an elevated risk of breast cancer who were younger than 50 years of age because premenopausal women did not seem to be at increased risk for venous thrombosis or uterine cancer compared with their postmenopausal counterparts. However, tamoxifen reduced the incidence of breast cancers that were estrogen-receptor positive, but not estrogen-receptor negative. Since breast cancers occurring in women with BRCA1 mutations are more likely to be estrogen-receptor negative, it is difficult to estimate the benefit of tamoxifen prophylaxis without specifically testing the effect in women with BRCA1 or BRCA2 cancer-predisposing mutations.

To assess the effect of tamoxifen in BRCA carriers, complete BRCA sequencing analysis was performed on 288 of the 315 women who developed invasive breast carcinoma within the NSABP-P1 tamoxifen trial. However, only 19 women (6.6%) were found to be heterozygous for BRCA mutations. Due to the small number of cases and wide confidence intervals, conclusions could not be drawn from these data. However, encouraging results from Narod et al. demonstrated an estimated 75% reduction for a contralateral breast cancer in those carrying BRCA1 and BRCA2 mutations. Nevertheless, because there are significant adverse consequences of tamoxifen treatment, including a higher rate of endometrial cancer and thromboembolic episodes such as pulmonary embolism, each patient should be counseled appropriately, enabling him or her to make the best personal decision.

Ovarian Cancer Risk Reduction

One case-controlled study has found a substantial decreased risk of ovarian cancer in women with BRCA1 or BRCA2 cancer-predisposing mutations who took oral contraceptives for more than 3 years. These data remain consistent with general population studies, which indicate a reduced risk of somatic ovarian carcinoma with oral contraceptive use. However, the study is currently debated primarily because it did not assess other outcomes, such as the effect of oral contraceptives on breast cancer risk, and thus, should be interpreted cautiously.

Hereditary Nonpolyposis Colorectal Cancer

This disorder was first described by Dr. Henry Lynch and colleagues upon the discovery of two families having multiple relatives diagnosed with colorectal, endometrial, and stomach cancers. Initially called Lynch syndrome, this disorder was later termed *hereditary nonpolyposis colorectal cancer* and is believed to be responsible for an estimated 3% to 5% of colorectal cancers. Because endometrial cancer is not generally recognized as an inherited tumor type, HNPCC is reviewed with emphasis on the related extracolonic gynecologic malignancies.

Clinical Manifestations

The colorectal cancers seen in HNPCC families usually occur at an average age of 44 years, develop primarily in the right side of the colon (proximal to the splenic flexure), and progress more rapidly. Persons with an HNPCC gene mutation have a lifetime risk of colorectal cancer of approximately 80%. In addition to colorectal cancer, patients and family members are more susceptible to a wide variety of extracolonic malignancies. Women heterozygous for an HNPCC mutation also have an approximate 39% risk for endometrial cancer and a 9% risk for an ovarian malignancy by the age of 70 years. However, mutation-specific studies have documented endometrial risks as high as 71% by the age of 70 years. Other increased HNPCC cancer risks that have been well documented include transitional cell carcinoma of the ureter and renal pelvis and adenocarcinomas of the stomach, small bowel, and biliary system. Also, an excess of pancreas, larynx, brain, and hematopoietic malignancies has also been described. Figure 3-4 illustrates a typical pedigree for a family with HNPCC.

Families meeting the established "Amsterdam criteria" are most likely to hold an inherited HNPCC genetic mutation as the primary cause of the associated cancers in the family. The Amsterdam criteria (Box 3-4) requires the presence of at least three family members with colorectal cancer, extending over at least two generations, with at least one person diagnosed before the age of 50 years, and one affected person a first-degree relative of the other two. Up to 70% of families meeting this criteria link to one of the known HNPCC genes. Nevertheless, because families not meeting this criteria have been found to harbor an HNPCC mutation, less restrictive guidelines called the Amsterdam II criteria (see Box 3-4) were established and include the characteristic clinicopathologic features of HNPCC. Last, the Bethesda and Revised Bethesda criteria (see Box 3-4) are primarily focused on a specific patient rather then the entire family.

Genetic Testing

HNPCC is an autosomal-dominant condition that is caused by one of several DNA mismatch repair gene mutations. These genes normally function

Figure 3-4

An example of a family with hereditary nonpolyposis colorectal cancer syndrome.

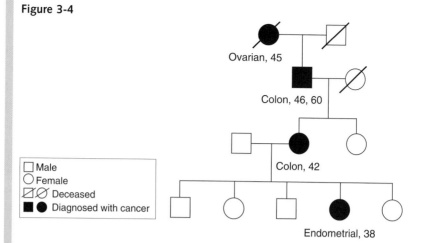

Ovarian, 45

Colon, 46, 60

□ Male
○ Female
⊠∅ Deceased
■● Diagnosed with cancer

Colon, 42

Endometrial, 38

Box 3-4 Hereditary Nonpolyposis Colorectal Cancer (HNPCC): Clinical Characteristics That Increase the Probability of an HNPCC Germline Mutation

65

Amsterdam criteria

Three relatives with colorectal cancer (CRC):
  With one relative being the first-degree relative (FDR) of the other two
  Within two successive generations
  With one CRC diagnosed before the age of 50 years

Modified Amsterdam criteria

Two CRC cases younger than 55 years of age in small families
Two FDR with CRC, plus a relative with endometrial cancer or unusual neoplasm
  (gastrointestinal, brain, kidney, ureter; diagnosed before the age of 55 years)

Bethesda criteria

Families that meet either set of Amsterdam criteria
Any CRC or endometrial cancer diagnosed before the age of 45 years
Two HNPCC-associated cancers (includes synchronous, metachronous CRC) or
  associated extracolonic tumors—endometrial, ovarian, gastric, hepatobiliary,
  small bowel or TCC of the renal pelvis or ureter
CRC plus an FDR with: CRC and/or HNPCC extracolonic cancer and/or
  colorectal adenoma, with one cancer diagnosed before the age of 45 years,
  and adenoma diagnosed before the age of 40 years
CRC or endometrial cancer diagnosed before the age of 45 years
Right-sided CRC with an undifferentiated pattern (solid or cribriform) of histology
  diagnosed before the age of 45 years, defined as poorly differentiated or
  undifferentiated carcinoma composed of irregular, solid sheets of large
  eosinophilic cells, and containing small gland-like spaces
Signet-ring-cell–type CRC diagnosed before the age of 45 years
Adenomas diagnosed before the age of 40 years

Revised Bethesda criteria

Diagnosed with colorectal cancer before the age of 50 years
Synchronous or metachronous colorectal or other HNPCC-related tumors (which include
  stomach, bladder, ureter, renal pelvis, biliary tract, brain (glioblastoma), sebaceous
  gland adenomas, keratoacanthomas and carcinoma of the small bowel), regardless of age
Colorectal cancer with a high-microsatellite instability morphology that was
  diagnosed before the age of 60 years
Colorectal cancer with one or more first-degree relatives with colorectal cancer or other
  HNPCC-related tumors—one of the cancers must have been diagnosed before the age
  of 50 years (this includes adenoma, which must have been diagnosed before the
  age of 40 years)
Colorectal cancer with one or more relatives with colorectal cancer or other
  HNPCC-related tumors, regardless of age

to correct DNA errors during cellular replication. The identified mismatch repair genes that mutate in HNPCC include *hMLH1, hMSH2, hPMS1, hPMS2,* and *hMSH6.* Because these five genes do not account for the entire HNPCC syndrome, there still remain undiscovered genes, as well as possible mutations within the known inherited genes, missed with current testing methods. Nevertheless, *hMLH1* and *hMSH2* are thought to account for an estimated 70% of HNPCC families, and all five genes are currently available for clinical testing. Full gene sequencing was thought to be the "gold standard" when searching for a family mutation; however, Southern blot analysis has recently become commercially available and is believed to identify up to 32% of HNPCC mutations (specifically large rearrangements of MLH1 and MSH2) not detectable by sequencing technology.

In accordance with published studies, the American Gastroenterological Association recommends the consideration of MSI testing when a person meets any of the first three Bethesda criteria or any of the revised criteria points (see Box 3-4). MSI testing is an evaluation of repeating DNA sequences in the colorectal tumor. Colorectal cancers testing positive for MSI indicates an increased probability of an HNPCC gene mutation. Approximately 80% of HNPCC colon cancers will be MSI positive, compared with only 10% to 15% of noninherited tumors. Therefore, because the sensitivity of MSI in HNPCC-related tumors is not 100%, HNPCC mutation analysis should still be pursued in compelling colorectal/endometrial cancer families found to be MSI negative. However, because immunohistochemistry of the HNPCC gene products with MSI analysis has been reported to enhance mutation detection rate, this also is a reasonable strategy to better specify the defective HNPCC gene before direct DNA analysis.

HNPCC Management

Surveillance Recommendations for colorectal cancer screening in HNPCC have been published by several authors on the basis of expert and consensus opinion. Persons with germline mutations are recommended to start colonoscopy at the age of 25 years or 5 years before the youngest colorectal cancer diagnosed in the family, whichever comes first, and to continue this practice annually. Jarvinen et al. showed that colorectal screening decreases morbidity and mortality from colorectal cancer for the children of patients with HNPCC.

Annual screening for endometrial cancer is recommended by expert opinion beginning at the age of 25 to 35 years. There is no consensus on the optimal method of screening, but choices include endometrial aspiration and transvaginal ultrasonography. The efficacy of these tools remains uncertain. Some experts have recommended screening for ovarian and genitourinary cancers when these tumors have been observed in the family, although insufficient data exist to recommend a specific regimen. Proposed methods of screening for ovarian cancer include transvaginal ultrasonography and serum CA-125, and urine analysis for genitourinary tumors. However, these screening tests have not been proven to detect ovarian and genitourinary tumors at their early curable stages.

Chemoprevention

Currently, there are no chemopreventive therapies available for HNPCC carriers outside of clinical research trials. Nevertheless, once studies complete the evaluation of the use of cyclo-oxygenase–2 inhibitors and aspirin in this high-risk group, additional risk-reducing options may become available.

Surgical Strategies

For patients with HNPCC who have been previously diagnosed and treated for colon cancer, prophylactic colectomy is a reasonable option to consider because of the high risk of metachronous colon malignancies. This surgical prophylaxis is also a reasonable strategy in heterozygotes diagnosed with adenomas at a young age or in those who are unwilling or unable to undergo routine colonoscopy. A consensus panel found insufficient evidence to recommend for or against prophylactic hysterectomy and oophorectomy as a measure for reducing cancer risk and advised that women who are carriers of an HNPCC germline mutation be counseled appropriately. However, preventive total abdominal hysterectomy and BSO should be considered at the time of surgery for an HNPCC-associated colorectal cancer.

KEY POINTS

1. Cancer risk assessment is an evolving critical component of cancer risk reduction and prevention. Cancer risk assessment of persons at high risk is best achieved through referrals to a high-risk program.

2. Genetic counseling programs have defined curricula regarding cancer genetics. Genetic counselors trained in cancer genetics are best suited to convey risk assessment and contribute in a multidisciplinary fashion to risk reduction and prevention.

3. Cancer develops because of the serial acquisition of genetic mutations. Cancer genetic syndromes are associated with an inheritable genetic risk that increases the probability of cancer development in a person's lifetime.

4. Most cancers are sporadic. Approximately 5% to 10% of cancers are caused by an autosomal-dominant inherited cancer risk.

5. Understanding cancer risk can lead to effective risk-reduction strategies (e.g., oral contraceptive and tamoxifen use) and prevention (e.g., prophylactic oophorectomy/mastectomy/colectomy).

6. The understanding of environmental and polygenic influences on cancer development is in its infancy. Understanding the relative contributions of each will give insight and hopefully effective treatment and prevention strategies for the 90% to 95% of cancers that are not associated with an autosomal dominant syndrome.

WEBSITES

Genetic Testing Site Listing and Education Resource:
http://www.genetests.org/
National Cancer Institute: http://www.nci.nih.gov/
National Institutes of Health: http://www.nih.gov/

SUGGESTED READING

Agoff SN, Mendelin JE, Grieco VS, et al: Unexpected gynecologic neoplasms in patients with proven or suspected BRCA-1 or -2 mutations: Implications for gross examination, cytology, and clinical follow-up. Am J Surg Pathol 26:171–178, 2002.

American Society of Clinical Oncology: Resource document for curriculum development in cancer genetics education. J Clin Oncol 15:2157–2169, 1997.

American Society of Clinical Oncology policy statement update: Genetic testing for cancer susceptibility. J Clin Oncol 21(12):2397–2406, 2003.

Antoniou A, Pharoah PD, Narod S, et al: Average risks of breast and ovarian cancer associated with BRCA1 or BRCA2 mutations detected in case series unselected for family history: A combined analysis of 22 studies. Am J Hum Genet 73(3):1117–1130, 2003.

Bane AL, Beck JC, Bleiweiss I, et al: BRCA2 mutation-associated breast cancers exhibit a distinguishing phenotype based on morphology and molecular profiles from tissue microarrays. Am J Surg Path 31(1):121–128, 2007.

Bast RC, Urban N, Shridhar V, et al: Early detection of ovarian cancer: Promise and reality. Cancer Treatment and Research 107:61–97, 2002.

Bernhardt BA, Tambor ES, Fraser G, et al: Parents' and children's attitudes toward the enrollment of minors in genetic susceptibility research: Implications for informed consent. Am J Med Genet A (United States) 116(4):315–323, 2003.

Berry DA, Parmigiani G, Sanchez J, et al: Probability of carrying a mutation of breast-ovarian cancer gene BRCA1 based on family history. J Natl Cancer Inst 89:227–238, 1997.

Biesecker BB, Ishibe N, Hadley DW, et al: Psychosocial factors predicting BRCA1/BRCA2 testing decisions in members of hereditary breast and ovarian cancer families. Am J Med Genet 93:257–263, 2000.

Boland CR, Thibodeau SN, Hamilton SR, et al: A National Cancer Institute workshop on microsatellite instability for cancer detection and familial predisposition: development of international criteria for the determination of microsatellite instability in colorectal cancer. Cancer Res 58:5248–5257, 1998.

Brain K, Norman P, Gray J, et al: A randomized trial of specialist genetic assessment: psychological impact on women at different levels of familial breast cancer risk. Br J Cancer 86:233–238, 2002.

Brunet JS, Vesprini D, Abrahamson J, et al: Breast cancer risk in BRCA1/BRCA2 carriers is modified by the CYP1A1 gene (Abstract). Am J Hum Genet 63:A247, 1998.

Burke W, Daly M, Garber J, et al: Recommendations for follow-up care of individuals with an inherited predisposition to cancer II. BRCA1 and BRCA2. JAMA 277:997–1003, 1997.

Burke W, Petersen G, Lynch P, et al: Recommendations for follow-up care of individuals with inherited predisposition to cancer. I. Hereditary nonpolyposis colon cancer. JAMA 277:915–919, 1997.

Chang-Claude J, Dong J, Schmidt S, et al: Using gene carrier probability to select high risk families for identifying germline mutations in breast cancer susceptibility genes. J Med Genet 35:116–121, 1998.

Claes E, Evers-Kiebooms G, Boogaerts A, et al: Diagnostic genetic testing for hereditary breast and ovarian cancer in cancer patients: women looking back on the pre-test period and a psychological evaluation. Genet Test 8:13–21, 2004.

Claes E, Evers-Kiebooms G, Boogaerts A, et al: Communication with close and distant relatives in the context of genetic testing for hereditary breast and ovarian cancer in cancer patients. Am J Med Genet 116A:11–19, 2003.

Couch FJ, DeShano ML, Blackwood MA, et al: BRCA1 mutations in women attending clinics that evaluate the risk of breast cancer. N Engl J Med 336:1409–1415, 1997.

Cummings S: The genetic testing process: How much counseling is needed? J Clinc Oncol 18:60S–64S, 2000.

David YB, Modan B, and the National Israeli Study of Ovarian Cancer: Effect of BRCA mutations on the length of survival in epithelial ovarian tumors. J Clin Oncol 20(2):463–466, 2002.

DePasquale SE, Giordano A, Donnenfeld AE: The genetics of ovarian cancer: molecular biology and clinical application. Obstet Gynecol Surv 53:248–256, 1998.

Easton DF, Ford D, Bishop DT: Breast Cancer Linkage Consortium: Breast and ovarian cancer incidence in BRCA1-mutation carriers. Am J Human Genetics 56:265–271, 1995.

Ford D, Easton DF, Bishop DT, et al: Risks of cancer in BRCA1-mutation carriers. Lancet 343:692–695, 1994.

Frank TS, Critchfield GC: Hereditary risk of women's cancers. Best Pract Res Clin Obstet Gynaecol 16:703–713, 2002.

Frank TS, Deffenbaugh AM, Reid JE, et al: Clinical characteristics of individuals with germline mutations in BRCA1 and BRCA2: Analysis of 10,000 individuals. J Clin Oncol 20:1480–1490, 2002.

Frank TS, Manley SA, Olopade OI, et al: Sequence analysis of BRCA1 and BRCA2: correlation of mutations with family history and ovarian cancer risk. J Clin Oncol 16:2417–2425, 1998.

Frank T, Deffenbaugh A, Reid J, et al: Clinical characteristics of individuals with germline mutations in BRCA1 and BRCA2: Analysis of 10,000 individuals. J Clin Oncol 20(6):1480–1490, 2002.

Friedenson B: Is mammography indicated for women with defective BRCA genes? Implications of recent scientific advances for the diagnosis, treatment, and prevention of hereditary breast cancer. Med Gen Med 9:E9, 2000.

Friedman L, Kramer R: Reproductive issues for women with BRCA mutations. J Nat Cancer Inst Monogr 34:83–86, 2005.

Frost MH, Schaid DJ, Sellers TA, et al: Long-term satisfaction and psychological and social function following bilateral prophylactic mastectomy. JAMA 284:319–324, 2000.

Garber J, Offit K: Hereditary cancer predisposition syndromes. J Clin Oncol 23:276–292, 2005.

Geller G, Botkin JR, Green MJ, et al: Genetic testing for susceptibility to adult-onset cancer. The process and content of informed consent. JAMA 277:1467–1474, 1997.

Grabrick DM, Hartmann LC, Cerhan JR, et al: Risk of breast cancer with oral contraceptive use in women with a family history of breast cancer. JAMA 284:1791–1798, 2000.

Grann V, Jacobson J, Thomason D, et al: Outcomes of tamoxifen chemoprevention for breast cancer in high-risk women: A cost-effectiveness analysis. J Clin Oncol 20(10):2520–2529, 2002.

Halford SE, Rowan AJ, Lipton L, et al: Germline mutations but no somatic changes at the MYH locus contribute to the pathogenesis of unselected colorectal cancers. Am J Pathol 162:1545–1548, 2003.

Hall MA, Rich SS: Laws restricting health insurers' use of genetic information: Impact on genetic discrimination. Am J Human Genet 66:293–307, 2000.

Hanahan D and Weinberg RA: The hallmarks of cancer. Cell 100:57–70, 2000.

Hartmann LC, Schaid DJ, Woods JE, et al: Efficacy of bilateral prophylactic mastectomy in women with a family history of breast cancer. N Engl J Med 340:77–84, 1999.

Hendriks YM, Wagner A, Morreau H, et al: Cancer risk in hereditary nonpolyposis colorectal cancer due to MSH6 mutations: impact on counseling and surveillance. Gastroenterology 127:17–25, 2004.

Holtzman NA, Watson MS: Promoting safe and effective genetic testing in the United States. Final report of the Task Force on Genetic Testing. J Child Fam Nurs 2:388–390, 1999.

Hopwood P, Wonderling D, Watson M, et al: A randomized comparison of UK genetic risk counseling services for familial cancer: psychosocial outcomes. Br J Cancer 91:884–892, 2004.

Jarvinen H, Aarnio M, Mustonen H, et al: Controlled 15-year trial on screening for colorectal cancer in families with hereditary nonpolyposis colorectal cancer. Gastroenterology 118:829–834, 2000.

Johannsson OT, Idvall I, Anderson C, et al: Tumour biological features of BRCA1-induced breast and ovarian cancer. Eur J Cancer 33:362–371, 1997.

Kainu T, Kononen J, Johansson O, et al: Detection of germline BRCA1 mutations in breast cancer patients by quantitative messenger RNA in situ hybridization Cancer Res 56:2912–2915, 1996.

King MC, Wieand S, Hale K, et al: Tamoxifen and breast cancer incidence among women with inherited mutations in BRCA1 and BRCA2: National Surgical Adjuvant Breast and Bowel Project (NSABP-P1) Breast Cancer Prevention Trial. JAMA 286:2251–2256, 2001.

Kmet LM, Cook LS, Magliocco AM: A review of p53 expression and mutation in human benign, low malignant potential, and invasive epithelial ovarian tumors. Cancer 97(2):389–404, 2003.

Kriege M, Brekelmans CT, Boetes C, et al: Efficacy of MRI and mammography on breast-cancer screening in women with familial or genetic predisposition. N Engl J Med 351(5):427–437, 2004.

Lakhani SR, Van De, Vijver MJ, et al: The pathology of familial breast cancer: predictive value of immunohistochemical markers estrogen receptor, progesterone receptor, HER-2, and p53 in patients with mutations in BRCA1 and BRCA2. J Clin Oncol 20:2310–2318, 2002.

Lerman C, Schwartz M, Peshkin B, et al: Impact of BRCA1/BRCA2 mutation testing on psychological distress in a clinic-based sample. J Clin Oncol 20(2):514–520, 2002.

Legare RD: Screening and management of hereditary breast cancer. Med Health R I 82:172–175, 1999.

Lerman C and Shields AE: Genetic testing for cancer susceptibility: The promise and the pitfalls. Nat Rev Cancer 4:235, 2004.

Love RR, Evans AM, Josten DM: The accuracy of patient reports of a family history of cancer. J Chronic Dis 38:289–293, 1985.

Lynch HT, Fitzsimmons ML, Lynch J, et al: A hereditary cancer consultation clinic. Nebr Med J 74:351–359, 1989.

Lynch E, Doherty R, Gaff C, et al: Cancer in the family and genetic testing: Implications for life insurance. Med J Australia 179:480–483, 2003.

Lynch H, de la Chapelle A: Hereditary colorectal cancer. N Engl J Med 348:919–932, 2003.

Marcus JN, Watson P, Page DL, et al: Hereditary breast cancer: Pathobiology, prognosis, and BRCA1 and BRCA2 gene linkage. Cancer 77:697–709, 1996.

Meijers-Heijboer H, van Geel B, van Putten WL, et al: Breast cancer after prophylactic bilateral mastectomy in women with a BRCA1 or BRCA2 mutation. N Engl J Med 345:159–164, 2001.

Meiser B, Halliday JL: What is the impact of genetic counselling in women at increased risk of developing hereditary breast cancer? A meta-analytic review. Soc Sci Med 54:1463–1470, 2002.

Moller P, Borg A, Evans DG, et al: Survival in prospectively ascertained familial breast cancer: analysis of a series stratified by tumour characteristics. BRCA mutations and oophorectomy. Int J Cancer 101:555–559, 2002.

Narod SA, Risch H, Moslehi R, et al: Oral contraceptives and the risk of hereditary ovarian cancer. N Engl J Med 339:424–428, 1998.

Narod S, Brunet JS, and the Hereditary Breast Cancer Clinical Study Group: Tamoxifen and risk of contralateral breast cancer in BRCA1 and BRCA2 mutation carriers: A case-control study. Lancet 356:1876–1881, 2000.

Narod S, Liede A, Karlan B, et al: Cancer incidence in a population of Jewish women at risk of ovarian cancer. J Clin Oncol 20(6):1570–1577, 2002.

Narod S, Offit K: Prevention and management of hereditary breast cancer. J Clin Oncol 23:1656–1663, 2005.

National Comprehensive Cancer Network: NCCN colorectal cancer screening practice guidelines. Oncology 13:152–179, 1999.

Noller KL: Estrogen replacement therapy and risk of ovarian cancer. JAMA 288:368–369, 2002.

Offit K: Clinical Cancer Genetics: Risk Counseling and Management. New York, Wiley-Liss, Inc, 1998.

Parent ME, Ghadirian P, Lacroix A, et al: The reliability of recollections of family history: implications for the medical provider. J Cancer Educ 12:114–1120, 1997.

Parmigiani G, Berry DA, Aguilar O: Determining carrier probabilities for breast cancer susceptibility genes BRCA1 and BRCA2. Am J Hum Genet 62:145–158, 1998.

Petricoin E, Ardekani A, Liotta L, et al: Use of proteomic patterns in serum to identify ovarian cancer. Lancet 359:572–577, 2002.

Phelan CM, Rebbeck TR, Weber BL, et al: Ovarian cancer risk in BRCA1 carriers is modified by the HRAS1 variable number of tandem repeat (VNTR) locus. Nat Genet 12:309–311, 1996.

Pierce LJ, Strawderman M, Narod SA, et al: Effect of radiotherapy after breast-conserving treatment in women with breast cancer and germline BRCA1/2 mutations. J Clin Oncol 18:3360–3369, 2000.

Powell SM, Petersen GM, Krush AJ, et al: Molecular diagnosis of familial adenomatous polyposis. N Engl J Med 329:1982–1987, 1993.

Rebbeck TR, Levin AM, Eisen A, et al: Breast cancer risk after bilateral prophylactic oophorectomy in BRCA1 mutation carriers. J Natl Cancer Inst 91:1475–1479, 1999.

Rebbeck T, Weber B, Lynch H, and the Prevention and Observation of Surgical End Points Study Group: Prophylactic oophorectomy in carriers of BRCA1 or BRCA2 mutations. N Engl J Med 346(21):1616–1622, 2002.

Ries LAG, Eisner MP, Kosary CL, et al: SEER Cancer Statistic Review, 1973–1998. National Cancer Institute Bethesda MD, 2001.

Robson M, Gilewski T, Haas B, et al: BRCA-associated breast cancer in young women. J Clin Oncol 16:1642–1649, 1998.

Robson M: Breast cancer surveillance in women with hereditary risk due to BRCA1 or BRCA2 mutations. Clin Breast Cancer 5(4):260–268; discussion 269–271, 2004.

Rodriguez-Bigas MA, Bosland CR, Hamilton SR, et al: A National Cancer Institute workshop on hereditary nonpolyposis colorectal cancer syndrome: Meeting highlights and Bethesda Guidelines. J Natl Cancer Inst 89:1758–1762, 1997.

Russell SE, McCluggage WG: A multistep model for ovarian tumorigenesis: the value of mutation analysis in the KRAS and BRAF genes. J Pathol 203(2):617–9, 2004.

Russo G, Zegar C, Giordano A: Advantages and limitation of microarray technology in human cancer. Oncogene 22:6497–6507, 2003.

Scartozzi M, Bianchi F, Porfiri E, et al: Mutations of hMLH1 and hMLSH2 in patients with suspected hereditary nonpolyposis colorectal cancer: Correlation with microsatellite instability and abnormalities of mismatch repair protein expression. J Clin Oncol 20(5):1203–1208, 2002.

Schneider K: Counseling About Cancer: Strategies for Genetic Counseling. New York, Wiley-Liss, Inc, 2002.

Scheuer L, Kauff N, Robson M, et al: Outcome of preventive surgery and screening for breast and ovarian cancer in BRCA mutation carriers. J Clin Oncol 20(5):1164–1166, 2002.

Shattuck-Eidens D, Oliphant A, McClure M, et al: BRCA1 sequence analysis in women at high risk for susceptibility mutations. JAMA 278:1242–1250, 1997.

Sherr CJ: Principles of tumor suppression. Cell 116(2):235–246, 2004.

Smith RA, Saslow D, Sawyer KA, et al: American Cancer Society guidelines for breast cancer screening: update 2003. CA Cancer J Clin 53:141–169, 2003.

Statement of the American Society of Clinical Oncology: Genetic testing for cancer susceptibility. J Clin Oncol 14:1730–1736, 1996.

Struewing JP, Brody LC, Erdos MR, et al: Detection of eight BRCA1 mutations in 10 breast/ovarian cancer families, including one family with male breast cancer. Am J Hum Genet 57:1–7, 1995.

Struewing JP, Hartge P, Wacholder S, et al: The risk of cancer associated with specific mutations of BRCA1 and BRCA2 among Ashkenzi Jews. N Engl J Med 336:1401–1408, 1997.

Swisher EM, Babb S, Whelan A, et al: Prophylactic oophorectomy and ovarian cancer surveillance. Patient perceptions and satisfaction. J Reprod Med 46:87–94, 2001.

The Breast Cancer Linkage Consortium: Cancer risks in BRCA2. J Natl Cancer Inst 61:1310–1316, 1999.

Thibodeau SN, French AJ, Cunningham JM, et al: Microsatellite instability in colorectal cancer: different mutator phenotypes and the principal involvement of hMLH1. Cancer Res 58:1713–1718, 1998.

Tilanus-Linthorst MM, Obdeijn IM, Bartels KC, et al: First experiences in screening women at high risk for breast cancer with MR imaging. Breast Cancer Res Treat 63:53–60, 2000.

Vasen HF, Haites NE, Evans DG, et al: Current policies for surveillance and management in women at risk of breast and ovarian cancer: a survey among 16 European family cancer clinics. European Familial Breast Cancer Collaborative Group. Eur J Cancer 34(12):1922–1926, 1998.

Verhoog LC, Brekelmans CT, Seynaeve C, et al: Survival and tumour characteristics of breast-cancer patients with germline mutations of BRCA1. Lancet 351:316–321, 1998.

Vogelstein B, Kinzler K: The Genetic Basis of Human Cancer, 2nd ed. New York, McGraw-Hill, 2002.

Wagner CJ, Itzen M, Malick J, et al: Communication of BRCA1 and BRCA2 results to at-risk relatives: a cancer risk assessment program's experience. Am J Med Genet 119C:11–18, 2003.

Wagner TM, Moslinger R, Langbauer G, et al: Attitude towards prophylactic surgery and effects of genetic counseling in families with BRCA mutations. Austrian Hereditary Breast and Ovarian Cancer Group. Br J Cancer 82:1249–1253, 2000.

Warren R: Screening women at high risk of breast cancer on the basis of evidence. Eur J Radiol 39:50–59, 2001.

Webb MJ: Symposium: Genetic testing and management of the cancer patient and cancer families. J Am Coll Surg 187:449–456, 1998.

Whittemore AS, Gong G, Itnyre J: Prevelance and contribution of BRCA1 mutations in breast cancer and ovarian cancer: results from three U.S. population-based case-control studies of ovarian cancer. Am J Human Genetics 60:496–504, 1997.

Winawer SJ, Fletcher RH, Miller L, et al: Colorectal cancer screening and surveillance: clinical guidelines, evidence, and rationale. Gastroenterology 112: 594–642, 1997.

Wood MD, Mullineax L, Rahm AK, et al: Impact of BRCA1 testing on women with cancer: A pill study. Genet Test 4:265–272, 2000.

4

GYNECOLOGIC ANATOMY

Steven D. Kleeman and William Andre Silva

INTRODUCTION

Understanding the anatomy of the pelvis and perineum is a difficult task; the relationships of bones, muscles, ligaments, and organs are complex. This chapter will give the reader a good basis for an understanding of the anatomic relationships in and around the pelvis. However, the reader must further this understanding with time in the cadaver laboratory and observation in the operating room. Only then will the reader be able to think of the pelvis in global terms. Similar to the process of looking at fine art, one will gain increased appreciation by observing anatomy from several different vantage points.

This chapter will review the anatomy in sections: first, the bony pelvis and ligaments; then muscles, nerves, and arteries; and finally, organs including the external genitalia and perineum. The final section regarding the anatomy of the pelvic floor will incorporate all of these components.

BONY PELVIS AND LIGAMENTS

The bony pelvis forms the foundation to which all of the pelvic structures are attached. Five bones make up the bony pelvis. The ilium, ischium, and pubis fuse together at the acetabulum to form the coxal bones (Fig. 4-1). It is these bones that form the lateral and anterior part of the pelvis. The sacrum and coccyx complete the pelvis posteriorly and form the posterior border of the pelvic outlet.

Several important bony anatomic landmarks are important to the gynecologist (Figs. 4-1 and 4-2), including the anterior superior iliac spine, which is readily felt in most patients, and the posterior superior iliac spine, which can be followed from the superior edge of the ilium. In the standing position, the anterior superior iliac spine and symphysis pubis are in the same vertical plane and pressure is directed down onto these bony structures, diverting pressure away from the muscles of the pelvic floor.

Figure 4-1

The bony pelvis and ligaments. (From Hinman F Jr: Atlas of Urosurgical Anatomy. Philadelphia, W.B. Saunders, 1993.)

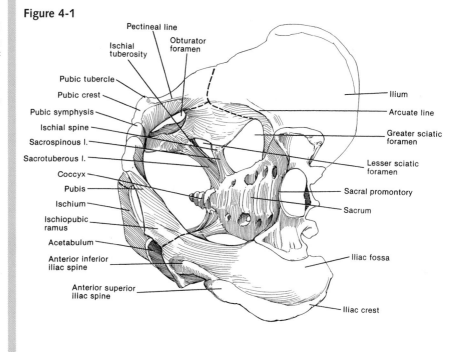

Figure 4-2

A posterior view of the bony female pelvis. (Reprinted from Gabbe SG, Niebyl JR, Simpson JL: Obstetrics: Normal and Problem Pregnancies, 4th ed. New York, Churchill Livingstone, 2002.)

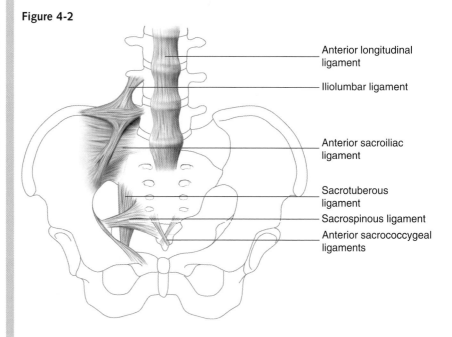

Other important bony landmarks are seen in Figure 4-1, including the ischial spine, ischial tuberosity, pectineal and arcuate lines, and pubic tubercle. These are important gynecologic surgical landmarks. The inguinal ligament runs between the anterior superior iliac spine and the pubic tubercle. The area between the ligament and superior pubic ramus forms the space where arteries, nerves, and muscles have access to the anterior part of the thigh (femoral canal). The pectineal and lacunar ligaments run along the arcuate line from the pubic tubercle. More inferiorly, the sacrospinous ligament runs between the ischial spine and the lateral edge of the sacrum and coccyx (see Figs. 4-1 and 4-2). The sacrotuberous ligament runs between the ischial tuberosity and the lateral margin of the sacrum and coccyx. These two ligaments define the greater and lesser sciatic foramina. These foramina give access to the posterior thigh and buttocks.

Clinical Relevance

The bony and ligamentous landmarks used regularly in obstetrics and gynecology include the ischial spine, anterior superior iliac spine, pectineal ligament (Cooper's ligament), and sacrospinous ligament. During labor and delivery, the ischial spine is palpated to determine the station of the presenting fetal part. Additionally, it is used as a landmark and serves as a point of fixation for many structures important for vaginal support. The pectineal ligament is used as a point of attachment during incontinence surgery (i.e., Burch colposuspension). Similarly, the sacrospinous ligament is used to help support the vaginal apex in cases of vaginal vault prolapse. Finally, the anterior superior iliac spine is palpated before laparoscopic surgery to determine placement of laparoscopic ports.

75

MUSCLES OF THE PELVIS

The muscles of the pelvic floor can be divided into the lateral rotators of the thigh and the pelvic diaphragm. The pelvic diaphragm is made up of the levator ani muscles (e.g., puborectalis, pubococcygeus, iliococcygeus) and the coccygeus muscles (Figs. 4-3 and 4-4). These muscles collectively

Figure 4-3

A superior view of the muscles of the pelvic diaphragm. (Reprinted from Gabbe SG, Niebyl JR, Simpson JL: Obstetrics: Normal and Problem Pregnancies, 4th ed. New York, Churchill Livingstone, 2002.)

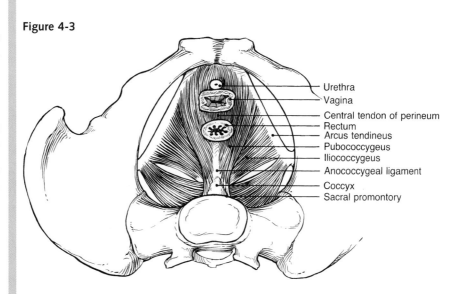

Urethra
Vagina
Central tendon of perineum
Rectum
Arcus tendineus
Pubococcygeus
Iliococcygeus
Anococcygeal ligament
Coccyx
Sacral promontory

Figure 4-4

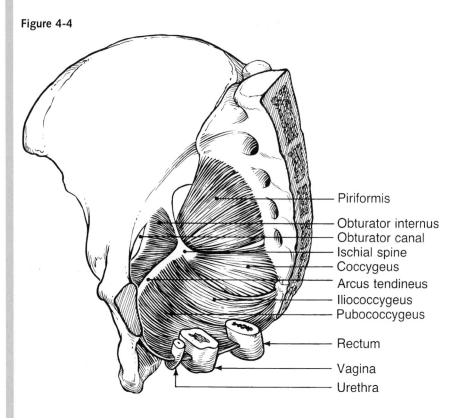

An oblique view of the muscles of the pelvic diaphragm. (Reprinted from Gabbe SG, Niebyl JR, Simpson JL: Obstetrics: Normal and Problem Pregnancies, 4th ed. New York, Churchill Livingstone, 2002.)

Piriformis

Obturator internus
Obturator canal
Ischial spine
Coccygeus
Arcus tendineus
Iliococcygeus
Pubococcygeus

Rectum

Vagina
Urethra

form the diaphragm of the pelvis. Their role in pelvic organ support will be discussed later.

The lateral rotators of the thigh include the obturator internus, obturator externus, and piriformis muscles (see Fig. 4-4). The obturator internus muscle lies on the intrapelvic side of the obturator membrane, a fibrous membrane that covers the obturator foramen. The tendon of the obturator internus muscle traverses the lesser sciatic foramen to insert on the greater trochanter of the femur, facilitating lateral thigh rotation. A thickening of the obturator fascia, called the *arcus tendineus levator ani*, serves as a point of attachment of the levator ani muscles to the pelvic sidewall. It is visible as a white line extending from the ischial spine to the superior pubic ramus.

The piriformis muscle extends from the anterolateral sacrum, through the greater sciatic foramen, to the greater trochanter.

Clinical Relevance

A strong and properly coordinated pelvic floor is essential for normal bladder, bowel, and sexual function (see below). Additionally, the pelvic floor muscles maintain constant tone and react to increases in abdominopelvic pressure, maintaining visceral structures in their proper anatomic positions and promoting continence of urine and feces. The role of the pelvic floor muscles is discussed in detail in Chapter 23, Pelvic Organ Prolapse and Pelvic Floor Dysfunction.

ARTERIES OF THE PELVIS

The abdominal aorta is a direct continuation of the thoracic aorta. It passes along the anterior surface of the vertebral column and divides at approximately the fourth lumbar vertebra, dividing into two common iliac arteries. Before this, the aorta gives off several branches (Fig. 4-5).

After dividing into the right and left common iliac arteries, each common iliac artery divides into the internal (hypogastric) and external iliac arteries. The inferior epigastric arteries are the terminal branches of the right and left external iliac arteries. Each courses superiorly and medially forming the lateral boundary of the inguinal triangle. They continue on the posterior aspect of the rectus abdominis muscles and eventually anastomose with the superior epigastric branch of the internal thoracic artery. The deep circumflex iliac artery courses along the inguinal ligament laterally, continuing along the inner aspect of the crest of the ileum, and eventually enters the abdominal musculature.

The internal iliac arteries further divide into anterior and posterior divisions. Branches of the posterior division include the iliolumbar, lateral sacral, and superior gluteal arteries (Fig. 4-6). The posterior division of the hypogastric artery terminates as a large superior gluteal artery that exits through the greater ischiatic foramen, superior to the piriformis muscle. The lateral sacral arteries course inferiorly and medially and enter the four anterior sacral foramina supplying the structures in the sacral canal. The iliolumbar artery courses superiorly and laterally between the obturator

77

Figure 4-5

The arterial vessels derived from the abdominal aorta. (Reprinted from Walsh PC, Retik AB, Vaughan ED, et al: Campbell's Urology, 8th ed. Philadelphia, W.B. Saunders, 2002.)

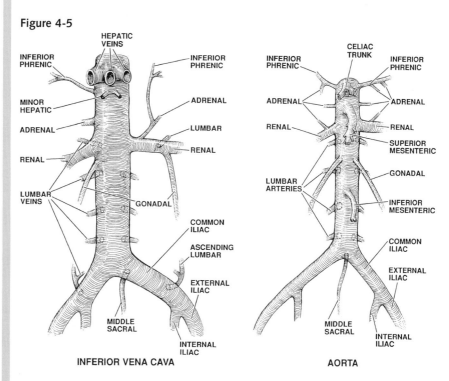

Figure 4-6

A lateral view of the pelvis and its major arterial systems. (Reprinted from Gabbe SG, Niebyl JR, Simpson JL: Obstetrics: Normal and Problem Pregnancies, 4th ed. New York, Churchill Livingstone, 2002.)

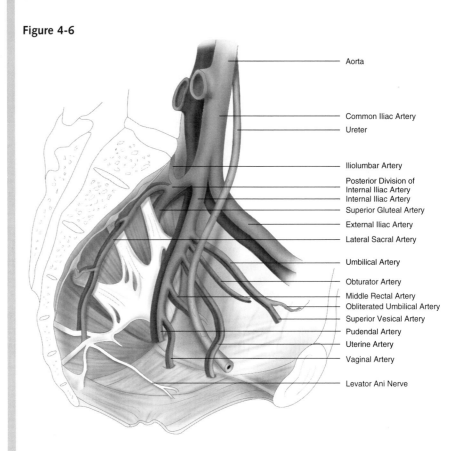

- Aorta
- Common Iliac Artery
- Ureter
- Iliolumbar Artery
- Posterior Division of Internal Iliac Artery
- Internal Iliac Artery
- Superior Gluteal Artery
- External Iliac Artery
- Lateral Sacral Artery
- Umbilical Artery
- Obturator Artery
- Middle Rectal Artery
- Obliterated Umbilical Artery
- Superior Vesical Artery
- Pudendal Artery
- Uterine Artery
- Vaginal Artery
- Levator Ani Nerve

nerve and the lumbosacral trunk. It is posterior to the common iliac artery, and it divides into an iliac branch that ramifies the iliac fossa and a lumbar branch, which ascends superior in a position posterior to the psoas muscle.

The anterior division of the internal iliac artery branches into a number of arteries important to the gynecologic surgeon, including the superior vesical, uterine, middle rectal, obturator, internal pudendal, and inferior gluteal arteries (see Fig. 4-6). The umbilical artery and superior vesical artery continue along the side wall of the pelvis, posterior to the obturator nerve and lateral to the ureter and round ligament. After giving off the superior vesical artery, this artery continues on as the medial umbilical ligament.

The uterine artery courses anteriorly on the levator ani muscle at the base of the broad ligament, then turns medially between the layers of the broad ligament superior to the ureter and on the lateral fornix of the vagina (Fig. 4-7). It yields branches to the vagina and lateral side of the uterus (Fig. 4-8). The middle rectal artery courses medially on the lateral pelvic side wall and supplies the rectum. The obturator artery courses inferiorly and laterally along the sidewall of the pelvis, along with the obturator nerve (see Fig. 4-6). In 35% to 45% of patients, the obturator artery may arise from the inferior epigastric branch of the external iliac, also

Figure 4-7

The arterial supply to the uterus and adnexal structures. The vessels anastomose near the cornual region at the lateral uterus. a., Artery; br., branch. (Reprinted from Gabbe SG, Niebyl JR, Simpson JL: Obstetrics: Normal and Problem Pregnancies, 4th ed. New York, Churchill Livingstone, 2002.)

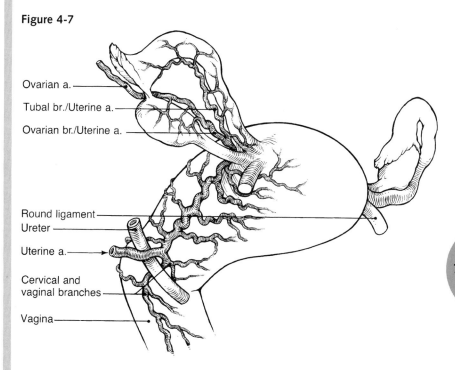

Ovarian a.
Tubal br./Uterine a.
Ovarian br./Uterine a.
Round ligament
Ureter
Uterine a.
Cervical and vaginal branches
Vagina

Figure 4-8

The arterial supply to the vagina. a., Artery; br., branch; U-G, urogenital. (Reprinted from Gabbe SG, Niebyl JR, Simpson JL: Obstetrics: Normal and Problem Pregnancies, 4th ed. New York, Churchill Livingstone, 2002.)

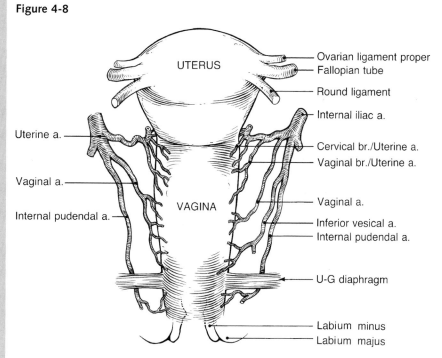

UTERUS
Ovarian ligament proper
Fallopian tube
Round ligament
Internal iliac a.
Uterine a.
Cervical br./Uterine a.
Vaginal br./Uterine a.
VAGINA
Vaginal a.
Vaginal a.
Internal pudendal a.
Inferior vesical a.
Internal pudendal a.
U-G diaphragm
Labium minus
Labium majus

called an *anomalous obturator artery*. The internal pudendal artery courses inferiorly and exits the pelvic cavity into the gluteal region through the greater ischiatic foramen. It then loops around the ischial spine and enters the perineum by crossing through the lesser ischiatic foramen.

NERVES

The following nerves are involved with innervation of the anterior abdominal wall (Fig. 4-9): the 7th to 11th intercostal nerves and the subcostal, iliohypogastric, and ilioinguinal nerves. The 7th to 11th intercostal nerves travel between the transversus abdominis and internal abdominis oblique muscles to the lateral edge of the rectus sheath. These nerves pierce the rectus sheath, course posterior to the rectus muscles, and then pierce it in the anterior wall of the rectus sheath to become the anterior cutaneous nerves. The subcostal nerve (T12) follows the plane between the transversus abdominis and internal abdominis oblique muscles to enter the rectus sheath as described above. The iliohypogastric nerve is a branch of the lumbar plexus (L1) and transverses between the transversus abdominis and internal abdominis oblique. It pierces the internal abdominis oblique muscle approximately 1 cm superior to the anterior superior iliac spine and becomes cutaneous about 1 inch superior to the superficial inguinal ring. It gives off a lateral cutaneous branch to the gluteal region. The

Figure 4-9

The arterial and nervous supply of the abdominal wall. m., Muscle; n., nerve; a., artery; v., vein. (Reprinted from McVay C: Anson and McVay's Surgical Anatomy, 6th ed. Philadelphia, W.B. Saunders, 1984.)

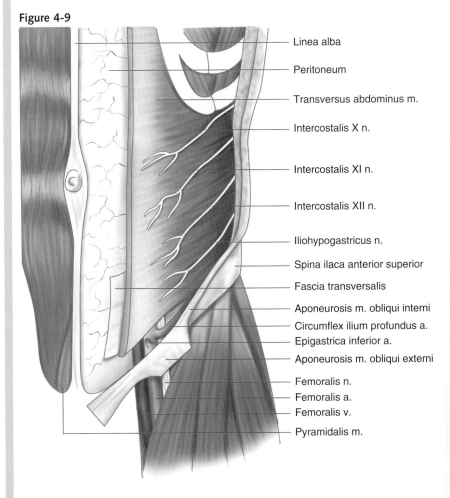

- Linea alba
- Peritoneum
- Transversus abdominus m.
- Intercostalis X n.
- Intercostalis XI n.
- Intercostalis XII n.
- Iliohypogastricus n.
- Spina ilaca anterior superior
- Fascia transversalis
- Aponeurosis m. obliqui interni
- Circumflex ilium profundus a.
- Epigastrica inferior a.
- Aponeurosis m. obliqui externi
- Femoralis n.
- Femoralis a.
- Femoralis v.
- Pyramidalis m.

ilioinguinal nerve arises from the lumbar plexus (L1) and follows a course similar to the iliohypogastric but is more inferior in its course. This nerve pierces the internal abdominis muscle and travels between the internal and external abdominis muscles, enters the inguinal canal, and leaves through the superficial inguinal ring. It sends cutaneous branches to the skin over the pubis and anterior labia majora and a cutaneous branch to the thigh (Fig. 4-10).

The following nerves arise from the lumbar plexus (Fig. 4-11): the iliohypogastric, ilioinguinal, genitofemoral, lateral femoral cutaneous, femoral, and obturator nerves. The ilioinguinal and iliohypogastric nerves have been previously discussed. The genitofemoral nerve comes from the first and second lumbar segments. It pierces the psoas major muscle and descends over its anterior surface, giving off genital and femoral branches. The genital branch courses inferiorly, passes through the deep inguinal ring of the inguinal canal, innervates the round ligament, and terminates in the skin of the labia majus and thigh. The femoral branch descends on the lateral side of the external iliac and femoral artery and supplies the anterior surface of the thigh.

The femoral nerve arises from the second, third, and fourth lumbar segments of the spinal cord. It courses within the psoas major muscle, emerging from the lateral surface of the psoas near the inguinal ligament. It gives branches to the psoas and iliacus muscles; after entry into the lower limb posterior and distal to the inguinal ligament, it breaks up into several branches. The branches of the femoral nerve include the medial cutaneous, intermediate cutaneous, and saphenous nerves, as well as muscular

Figure 4-10

The cutaneous nervous supply to the perineum. m., Muscle. (Reprinted from Gabbe SG, Niebyl JR, Simpson JL: Obstetrics: Normal and Problem Pregnancies, 4th ed. New York, Churchill Livingstone, 2002.)

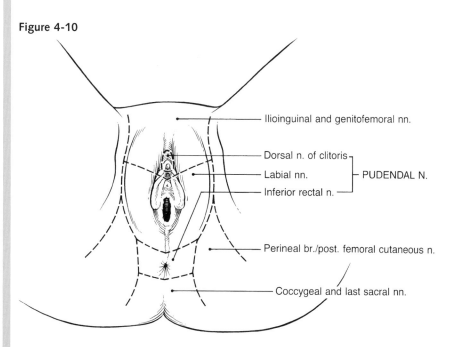

Ilioinguinal and genitofemoral nn.

Dorsal n. of clitoris

Labial nn. — PUDENDAL N.

Inferior rectal n.

Perineal br./post. femoral cutaneous n.

Coccygeal and last sacral nn.

Figure 4-11

The lumbar plexus. n., Nerve; m., muscle. (Reprinted from Miller RD: Miller's Anesthesia, 6th ed. New York, Churchill Livingstone, 2005.)

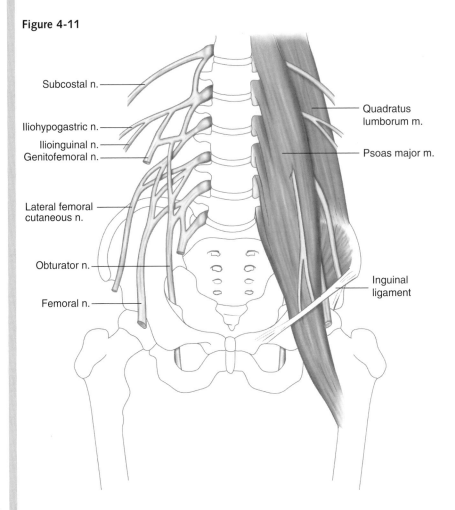

Subcostal n.

Iliohypogastric n.

Ilioinguinal n.

Genitofemoral n.

Lateral femoral cutaneous n.

Obturator n.

Femoral n.

Quadratus lumborum m.

Psoas major m.

Inguinal ligament

branches. The medial cutaneous nerve courses inferiorly and slightly medially, crossing anterior to the femoral vessels. The intermediate cutaneous nerve divides into medial and lateral branches and supplies the skin of the distal two thirds of the anterior surface of the thigh (Fig. 4-12). The saphenous nerve runs inferior, pierces the deep fascia on the medial side of the knee, and accompanies the long saphenous vein. Muscular branches include nerves to the psoas and iliacus muscles.

The lateral femoral cutaneous nerve arises from the second and third lumbar segments and courses in the substance of the psoas muscle. It appears at the lateral border at the level of the iliac crest. The nerve courses anterior to the iliacus muscle. It enters the thigh deep to the inguinal ligament and courses on the anterior surface of the sartorius muscle.

The obturator nerve arises from the second, third, and fourth lumbar segment. It courses in the substance of the psoas muscle and escapes from the psoas muscle on the medial side rather than the lateral. It courses

Figure 4-12

Lumbosacral dermatomes (A) and cutaneous distribution (B) of peripheral nerves. (Reprinted from Miller RD: Miller's Anesthesia, 6th ed. New York, Churchill Livingstone, 2005.)

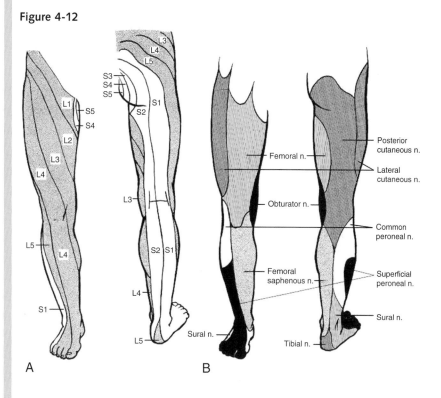

along the lateral pelvic sidewall, lateral to the internal iliac vessels, ureter, ovary, and broad ligament but anterior to the obturator vessels. It then enters the obturator canal and leaves the pelvic cavity to enter the thigh, where it divides immediately into an anterior branch and courses inferiorly deep to the pectineus and adductor long muscles and anterior to the adductor breves muscle. The posterior branch of the obturator nerve innervates the obturator externus muscle, pierces it, courses inferiorly between the adductor brevis and anteriorly to the adductor magnus posteriorly. It then splits into branches that are distributed to the upper (adductor) part of the adductor magnus and sometimes to the adductor brevis.

EXTERNAL GENITALIA

The external genitalia comprise the mons veneris, labia (majora and minora), clitoris, vestibule, urethral meatus, and the ostia of the accessory glands (Fig. 4-13). Superiorly, the perineum is bounded by the pelvic diaphragm, whereas inferiorly it is bounded by the skin covering the external genitalia, anus, and neighboring structures. The perineum is bounded laterally by the inferior pubic rami, the obturator internus, the coccygeus

Figure 4-13

The external genitalia. (A) Mons pubis; (B) prepuce; (C) clitoris; (D) labia majora; (E) labia minora; (F) urethral meatus; (G) Skene's ducts; (H) vagina; (I) hymen; (J) Bartholin's glands; (K) posterior fourchette; (L) perineal body. (Reprinted from Townsend CM, Beauchamp RD, Evers BM, Mattox KL: Sabiston Textbook of Surgery, 17th ed. Philadelphia, W.B. Saunders, 2004.)

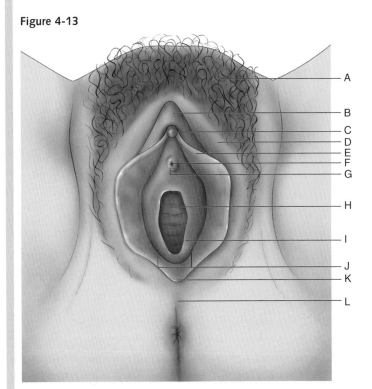

muscle, the sacrotuberous ligaments, and the gluteus maximus. The pelvic outlet can be divided into two triangles separated by a line drawn between the ischial tuberosities (Figs. 4-14 and 4-15). The urogenital triangle has its apex anteriorly at the symphysis pubis, and the anal triangle has its apex at the coccyx.

The urogenital triangle contains the perineal membrane, a fibrous connective tissue layer extending between the pubic rami and penetrated by the urethra and vagina and the external genitalia (i.e., mons pubis, labia majora and minora, clitoris, and vestibule). The mons pubis is a suprapubic fat pad covered by dense skin appendages. The labia majora form the lateral borders of the vulva. The labia minora and interlabial grooves are found medial to the labia majora and do not contain hair follicles. Found at the lower edge of the pubic symphysis is the glans, formed by the fusion of the paired roots of the clitoris in the midline. The labia minora fuse over the clitoris to form the hood clitoral frenulum. The vulvar vestibule extends to the hymeneal sulcus medially and is contiguous to the medial aspect of the labia minora laterally, demarcated by Hart's line. Bartholin's glands (situated at 5 and 7 o'clock), the paraurethral Skene's glands, and minor vestibular glands (positioned around the lateral vestibule) are found under the vestibular bulb, which has ostia that pass through the vestibular mucosa.

The muscles of the external genitalia include the transverse perineal muscles (deep and superficial), the ischiocavernosus muscles that cover the crura of the clitoris, and the bulbocavernosus muscles that overlie the vestibular bulbs (Figs. 4-14 and 4-15).

The anal triangle consists of the anal canal with its internal and external sphincters, the ischiorectal fossa, the median raphe, and skin.

Figure 4-14

The muscles of the superficial perineal space as demonstrated in the dorsal lithotomy position. (Reprinted from Gabbe SG, Niebyl JR, Simpson JL: Obstetrics: Normal and Problem Pregnancies, 4th ed. New York, Churchill Livingstone, 2002.)

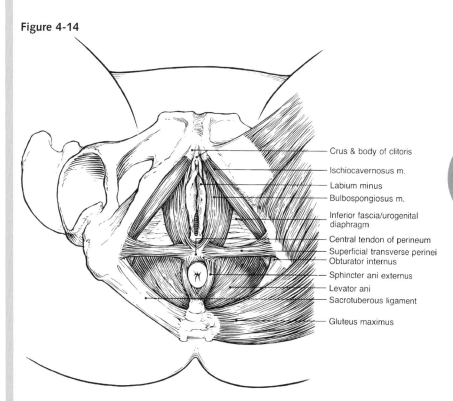

Crus & body of clitoris
Ischiocavernosus m.
Labium minus
Bulbospongiosus m.
Inferior fascia/urogenital diaphragm
Central tendon of perineum
Superficial transverse perinei
Obturator internus
Sphincter ani externus
Levator ani
Sacrotuberous ligament
Gluteus maximus

Figure 4-15

An inferior view of the muscles of the deep perineal space. The inset shows the boundaries of the urogenital triangle and anal triangle. (Reprinted from Gabbe SG, Niebyl JR, Simpson JL: Obstetrics: Normal and Problem Pregnancies, 4th ed. New York, Churchill Livingstone, 2002.)

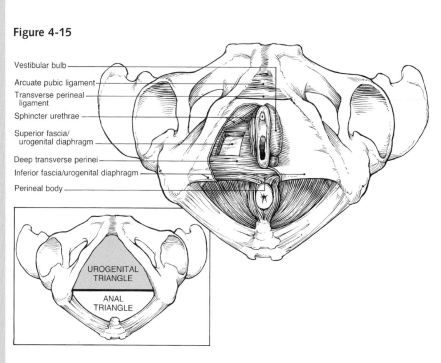

Vestibular bulb
Arcuate pubic ligament
Transverse perineal ligament
Sphincter urethrae
Superior fascia/urogenital diaphragm
Deep transverse perinei
Inferior fascia/urogenital diaphragm
Perineal body

UROGENITAL TRIANGLE
ANAL TRIANGLE

The blood supply to the perineum is predominantly derived from the internal pudendal artery (Fig. 4-16). This artery arises from the internal iliac artery and passes through Alcock's (pudendal) canal, a fascial tunnel along the obturator internus muscle below the origin of the levator ani muscle. On emerging from Alcock's canal, the internal pudendal artery sends branches to the urogenital triangle and anal triangle. Blood supply to the mons pubis arises from the inferior epigastric artery, a branch of the external iliac artery. Blood supply to the lateral aspect of the vulva is derived from the external pudendal artery which arises from the femoral artery. Venous return from the perineum drains into the internal iliac and femoral veins.

The major nerve supply to the perineum originates from the internal pudendal nerve (S2–S4), which travels through Alcock's canal with the internal pudendal artery and vein. The anterior branches supply the perineal membrane and external genitalia, whereas the posterior branch, the inferior rectal nerve, supplies the anus, ischiorectal fossa, and neighboring skin. The ilioinguinal and genitofemoral nerves from the lumbar plexus travel through the inguinal canal and exit through the superficial inguinal ring, supplying the mons pubis and anterior labia (see Fig. 4-10). The visceral efferent nerves responsible for clitoral erection arise from the pelvic splanchnic nerves.

Figure 4-16

The arterial and nervous supply of the perineum. n., Nerve; a., artery; v., vein; inf., inferior; int., internal; ext., external. (Reprinted from Doherty MG: Clinical anatomy of the pelvis. In Copeland LJ [ed]: Textbook of Gynecology. Philadelphia, W.B. Saunders, 1993, pp 17–58.)

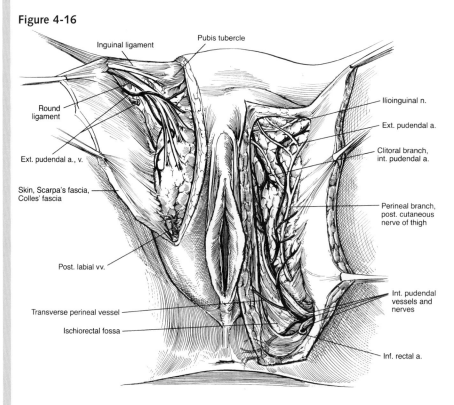

Inguinal ligament · Pubis tubercle · Ilioinguinal n. · Ext. pudendal a. · Round ligament · Clitoral branch, int. pudendal a. · Ext. pudendal a., v. · Skin, Scarpa's fascia, Colles' fascia · Perineal branch, post. cutaneous nerve of thigh · Post. labial vv. · Int. pudendal vessels and nerves · Transverse perineal vessel · Ischiorectal fossa · Inf. rectal a.

INTERNAL GENITAL ORGANS

The reproductive organs include the ovaries, fallopian tubes, uterus, cervix, and vagina and their associated blood supply and innervation (Fig. 4-17).

Ovary

The glistening white, oval-shaped ovaries are suspended from the lateral pelvic sidewall inferior to the pelvic brim by the infundibulopelvic ligaments and attach to the superolateral aspect of the uterine fundus with the utero-ovarian ligaments. The ovaries vary in size depending on the age of the person and the status of the ovulatory cycle. A nonovulating ovary will characteristically measure about $3 \times 2 \times 1$ cm.

The ovaries contain approximately 1 to 2 million oocytes at birth. On average, women release up to 300 ova during their lifetimes. Histologically, the ovary is divided into the outer cortex and inner medulla. The cortex consists of a very cellular connective tissue stroma in which the ovarian follicles are embedded. The medulla is composed of loose connective tissue, which contains blood vessels and nerves. The cortex is surrounded by a single layer of cuboidal epithelium called the *germinal epithelium.*

Each ovary is supplied by an ovarian artery that arises directly from the aorta and courses with the vein through the infundibulopelvic ligament into the ovarian medulla. The right ovarian vein drains to the inferior vena cava, and the left drains to the left renal vein. An anastomotic arterial complex originating from the uterine artery spreads across the broad ligament and mesosalpinx. Autonomic fibers from the lumbar sympathetic and the sacral parasympathetic plexus innervate the ovaries.

87

Figure 4-17

A posterior view of the pelvis and its organs. The ureter and its relationship to the uterine artery is noted at the window through the posterior leaf of the broad ligament (lig.). The ureter is also seen crossing the bifurcation of the iliac vessels. (Reprinted from Gabbe SG, Niebyl JR, Simpson JL: Obstetrics: Normal and Problem Pregnancies, 4th ed. New York, Churchill Livingstone, 2002.)

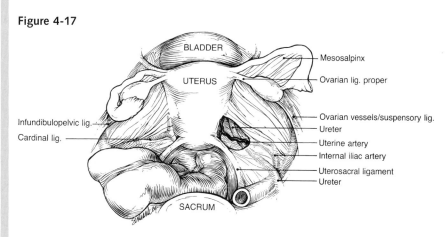

Clinical Relevance

The infundibulopelvic ligament, with the ovarian blood supply, crosses over the ureter as it descends into the pelvis. Identifying this relationship is critical to avoid transecting, ligating, or kinking the ureter during surgical procedures. By dividing the broad ligament, the peritoneum lateral to the bifurcation of the common iliac artery is opened and reflected to expose the ureter. Thus, even a distorted ovarian pedicle can be safely clamped after the ureter has been exposed.

Fallopian Tubes

The main function of the fallopian tubes is the transport of the egg and sperm in opposite directions, followed by transport of the developing embryo into the uterus. A fallopian tube is able to generate a variety of contractile patterns due to the arrangement of circular and longitudinal muscle fibers. Ciliary activity is also of major importance in ovum transport. Tubal epithelium is mainly composed of ciliated and secretory cells. A ciliated cell contains 250 to 300 elongated kinocilia at its apex and predominates at the fimbria. Cilia contract in an organized and synchronized fashion in which a propulsive power stroke is followed by a nonpropulsive retracting stroke.

The cylindrical fallopian tubes, approximately 8 cm long, originate at the uterine cavity in the uterine cornua. They consist of a 1- to 2-cm intramural segment and a narrow 4- to 5-cm isthmic segment. The tubes flare over 2 to 3 cm to the funnel of the infundibular segment and terminate at the fimbria. The branches of the uterine artery and vessels in the mesosalpinx supply the tube, with a secondary supply from the anastomosis with the ovarian vessels (see Fig. 4-7).

Uterus and Cervix

The uterus is a pear-shaped organ suspended in the midline by the cardinal and uterosacral ligaments (see Fig. 4-17). Dense fibrous condensations arising from the fascial covering of the levator ani muscles form the cardinal ligaments and insert into the lateral portions of the uterocervical junction. The uterosacral ligaments arise posterolaterally from the uterocervical junction and course posterolaterally to insert into the parietal fascia at the sacroiliac joint. The round ligaments of the uterus arise from the superior aspect of the uterus, course through the internal inguinal ring, and insert into the labia majora. The broad ligaments are composed of visceral peritoneum.

The uterine cavity is lined by the endometrium, a complex epithelial tissue. Its arterial supply is derived from branches of the uterine artery that perforate the myometrium to the basalis layer. The uterine cervix is the small cylindrical neck that leads from the uterus into the vagina.

The blood supply for the uterus and cervix are the paired uterine arteries, which originate from the anterior division of the internal iliac artery, course through the broad ligament and tortuously up the side of the uterus, and give off multiple concentrically arranged anterior and posterior arcuate arteries. The arcuate arteries travel from lateral to medial along the anterior and posterior aspects of the uterus and anastomose in

Figure 4-18

A lateral view of the anatomic relationships of the uterus. Note that the ureter crosses underneath the uterine artery at this level. lig., Ligament. (Reprinted from Gabbe SG, Niebyl JR, Simpson JL: Obstetrics: Normal and Problem Pregnancies, 4th ed. New York, Churchill Livingstone, 2002.)

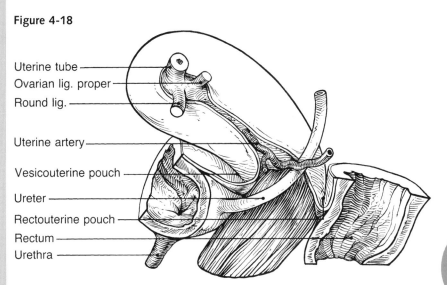

Uterine tube
Ovarian lig. proper
Round lig.

Uterine artery

Vesicouterine pouch

Ureter

Rectouterine pouch

Rectum

Urethra

the midline, giving off numerous radial arteries that supply the deep myometrium and endometrium. Additional blood flow comes from anastomoses with the ovarian and vaginal arteries. Venous return from the uterus empties into the internal iliac veins (see Fig. 4-7). Innervation of the uterus and cervix is derived from the autonomic plexus.

Clinical Relevance

The primary surgical consideration for managing the uterine vessels is the close proximity of the ureter, which courses approximately 1 cm below the uterine artery and 1 cm lateral to the cervix (Fig. 4-18). If the surgeon loses control of one of the branches of the vessel, it is important to use techniques that avoid clamping or kinking the ureter.

Vagina

The vagina extends from the vestibule to the cervix. The anterior and posterior walls of the upper two thirds of the vagina are normally apposed to each other to create a transverse potential space. The lower third of the vagina is relatively vertically oriented.

The blood supply to the vagina courses along its lateral walls and is provided by descending branches of the uterine artery and ascending branches of the internal pudendal artery (see Fig. 4-8). Innervation is derived from the autonomic plexus and the pudendal nerve.

ANATOMY OF THE PELVIC FLOOR

Normal pelvic floor function is paramount to the maintenance of urinary and fecal continence and pelvic support. Damage to anatomic support structures may lead to derangements in urethral and bladder function, defecatory dysfunction, and pelvic organ prolapse. In addition, disorders related to physiologic and neurologic function of the lower urinary tract can result in abnormalities in the storage and evacuation of urine.

Bladder

The bladder is composed of three layers of smooth muscle and serves as a low-pressure reservoir. It is located dorsal to the pubic bone and is bounded by the symphysis anteriorly and the uterovesical peritoneum dorsally. The bladder neck is located at the junction of the bladder base and the urethra. The thickened detrusor musculature at this area contributes to sphincteric closure. The bladder base lies directly on the endopelvic fascia of the anterior vaginal wall. The trigone is triangular and bounded by the internal urethral opening and the ureteric orifices. At its superior border is a raised area called the *interureteric ridge.* The superior vesical, inferior vesical, and hemorrhoidal arteries branch off from the internal iliac artery and supply the bladder. Bladder innervation is supplied by parasympathetic and sympathetic autonomic fibers.

Ureter

Near the bladder, the ureter contains three muscular layers: the inner longitudinal, middle circular, and outer longitudinal layers. However, these layers are indistinct and only roughly organized into layers. The small outer longitudinal layer is surrounded by adventitia. The ureters course through the retroperitoneum into the pelvis over the psoas muscle, lateral to the inferior vena cava. They cross over the common iliac arteries as they enter the pelvis, follow the posterolateral pelvic sidewalls, run parallel to the uterine arteries for 2.5 to 3 cm, and then continue under the uterine arteries, which cross over them as they course toward the uterus. The ureters lie 1 to 2 cm lateral to the cervix at the level of the internal cervical os, then travel upward and medially to enter the bladder obliquely. The anatomic relationship of the ureter to the adjacent pelvic structures can be seen in Figure 4-17.

Surgical compromise of the ureters may occur during clamping or ligating of the infundibulopelvic vessels, clamping or ligating of the cardinal ligaments, or wide suturing in the endopelvic fascia during an anterior repair.

Urethra

The female urethra is approximately 3.8 cm in length and extends from the bladder neck to the vestibule, opening approximately 2.5 cm below the clitoris. The lower portion of the urethra is fused to the adjacent vagina. It is directed obliquely downward and forward and is slightly curved with the concavity directed forward. Its epithelium is composed of stratified squamous cells and variably becomes transitional as it approaches the bladder.

Both intrinsic and extrinsic factors in the urethra promote continence. Intrinsic factors include the striated urethral sphincter, submucosal venous congestion, circular and longitudinal smooth muscles, coaptation of the urethral epithelium, urethral elasticity, and α-adrenergic–mediated urethral tone. Extrinsic factors include the components of the urethral hammock including the levator muscles, the endopelvic fascia, and their attachments. This extrinsic function will be discussed below. Intrinsic and extrinsic factors play equally important roles for urinary continence.

The smooth muscle portion of the urethra consists of an outer circular and an inner longitudinal layer. The circular layer is a thin, poorly formed entity. Contraction of the circular muscle leads to constriction; however, little is known about the role of the longitudinal muscle layer (Fig. 4-19).

The striated urogenital sphincter (or external urethral sphincter) (Fig. 4-20) is composed of the sphincter urethrae, the compressor urethrae, and the urethrovaginal sphincter, the latter two being part of the deep transverse peroneus muscle. The circularly oriented sphincter ure-

Figure 4-19

A cross-sectional view of the mid-urethra. m., Muscle. (Reprinted from Strohbehn K, DeLancey JOL: The anatomy of stress incontinence. Oper Techn Gynecol Surg 2:5–16, 1997.)

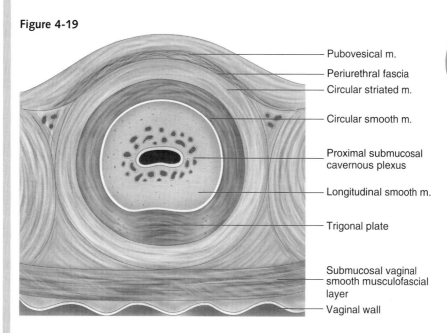

- Pubovesical m.
- Periurethral fascia
- Circular striated m.
- Circular smooth m.
- Proximal submucosal cavernous plexus
- Longitudinal smooth m.
- Trigonal plate
- Submucosal vaginal smooth musculofascial layer
- Vaginal wall

Figure 4-20

The internal and external urethral sphincter. (From DeLancey JO: Anatomy of the female bladder and urethra. In Bent AE, Ostergard DR, Cundiff GW, Swift SE: Ostergard's Urogynecology and Pelvic Floor Dysfunction, 5th ed. Philadelphia, Lippincott, Williams and Wilkins, 2003, pp 3–18.)

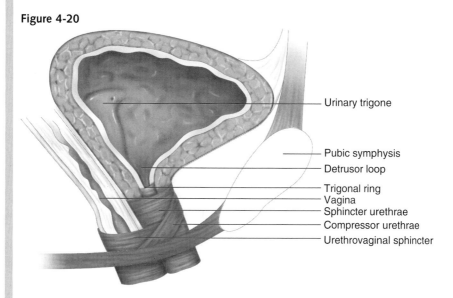

- Urinary trigone
- Pubic symphysis
- Detrusor loop
- Trigonal ring
- Vagina
- Sphincter urethrae
- Compressor urethrae
- Urethrovaginal sphincter

thrae is found innermost and is prominent in the proximal two thirds of the urethra. Previous authors have termed this the *rhabdosphincter*. More distally, the compressor urethrae and urethrovaginal sphincter are present. These two muscles emanate from the anterolateral aspect of the distal half to one third of the urethra. Thus, their formation is not circular but, instead, arches over the anterior or ventral urethral surface to surround the vagina (urethrovaginal sphincter) or traverse the inferior pubic rami (compressor urethrae). The three-muscle complex functions as a unit. The rich content of type I fibers enable urethral tone to be maintained. The muscles also contribute to voluntary and reflex urethral closure during times of increased intra-abdominal pressure. In half of continent women with a bladder neck that is incompetent, the striated urogenital sphincter provides this secondary continence mechanism.

Pelvic Organ Support

Support of the pelvic organs is achieved by the interaction of the anatomic attachments of the bony, muscular, and connective tissue elements with nervous system control. The *pelvic floor* refers to all the components that support the pelvic cavity, in addition to the levator ani muscles.

Endopelvic Fascia

Controversy exists surrounding the use of the term *fascia* as it applies to the pelvis. Histologic studies reveal that the lining of the levator ani, piriformis, and obturator internus are genuine examples of pelvic fascia. One example in which the term *fascia* has been incorrectly used is in reference to the tissue that is plicated in an anterior colporrhaphy. Histologically, it is the muscular lining of the vagina that is plicated. There are no discrete capsules of fascia that separate the bladder and vagina from one another.

The endopelvic fascia is a sheet of fibroareolar tissue following the blood supply to the visceral organs that acts as a retroperitoneal mesentery. The fascia divides the retroperitoneal space into avascular planes. The endopelvic or pubocervical fascia attaches the cervix and vagina to the lateral pelvic sidewall. It is composed to two parts: the parametrium, which is the part connected to the uterus (i.e., the uterosacral and cardinal ligaments), and the paracolpium, which is the part connected to the vagina. The parametrium and cardinal ligaments continue to the vaginal introitus and fuse directly to the supporting tissues associated with the vagina. The uterine and vaginal arteries travel in these structures. The uterosacral ligaments are the posterior components of the cardinal ligaments, extending from the cervix and upper vagina to the lateral sacrum. Lateral pelvic support is provided by linear condensations of obturator and levator ani fascia termed the *arcus tendineus fascia pelvis* and the *arcus tendineus levator ani*, respectively (Figs. 4-21 and 4-22). The arcus tendineus levator ani serves as a point of attachment for the pubococcygeus and iliococcygeus muscles and lies on the fascia of the obturator internus. It runs from the posterolateral pubic ramus to the ischial spine. The arcus tendineus fascia pelvis runs from the anterior pubis to the ischial spine as it joins with the arcus tendineus levator ani. It provides lateral (paravaginal) support to the anterior vagina.

Figure 4-21

Space of Retzius. The vaginal attaches laterally to the arcus tendineus fascia pelvis. a., Artery; v., vein; m., muscle. (Reprinted from Baggish MS, Karram MM: Atlas of Pelvic Anatomy and Gynecologic Surgery. Singapore, W.B. Saunders, 2001.)

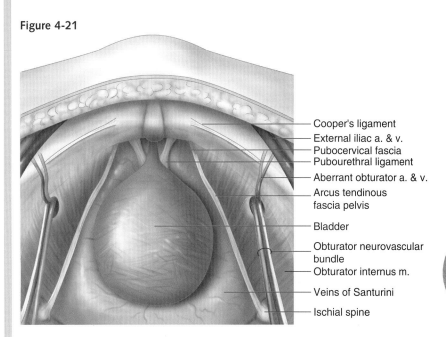

Cooper's ligament
External iliac a. & v.
Pubocervical fascia
Pubourethral ligament
Aberrant obturator a. & v.
Arcus tendinous fascia pelvis
Bladder
Obturator neurovascular bundle
Obturator internus m.
Veins of Santurini
Ischial spine

93

There are three levels of vaginal support as described by DeLancey (1992) (see Fig. 4-22). Level I support consists of paracolpium that suspends the apical portion of the vagina and is composed of the cardinal-uterosacral ligament complex. Level II support comprises the paracolpium that is attached to the vagina laterally via the arcus tendineus fasciae pelvis and superior fascia of the levator ani. Level III support consists of the distal vaginal attachments: anteriorly, via fusion of the urethra to the vagina; laterally, to the levators; and posteriorly, with the perineal body.

Clinical Relevance
Disruption of level I support may lead to prolapse of the uterus or vaginal vault, whereas damage to level II and III supports predispose to anterior and posterior vaginal prolapse. All levels of defective support should be repaired during reconstructive surgery.

Pelvic Diaphragm

A muscular diaphragm bounds the abdominopelvic cavity on its inferior end and sweeps from side to side and anteroposteriorly. The pelvic diaphragm arises from the posterior pubic bone on both sides and from the fascia of the obturator internus (i.e., arcus tendineus levator ani) and ischial spine. The levator ani consists of two parts: the pubovisceral and diaphragmatic parts. The pubovisceral portion consists of the pubococcygeus and the puborectalis muscles. These two muscles arise from the posterior pubic bone and converge on a tendon called the *anococcygeal raphe*, which is a narrow fibrous band extending from the coccyx to the posterior margin of the anus. The puborectalis muscle and its tendinous insertion form the puborectal sling, whose role is to pull the anal canal forward and stop fecal matter from passing from the superior to the anal portion of the rectum. It plays a role in fecal continence.

Figure 4-22

Three levels of vaginal support. **A,** Removal of the bladder exposes the vagina with its supporting structures. **B,** Level I support suspends the vaginal apex from the lateral pelvic walls via the paracolpium. Level II support consists of the paracolpium that attaches the vagina laterally to the arcus tendineus fascia pelvis. Level III support consists of distal vaginal attachments. (Reprinted from DeLancey JO: Anatomic aspects of vaginal eversion after hysterectomy. Am J Obstet Gynecol 166:1717–1724, 1992.)

94

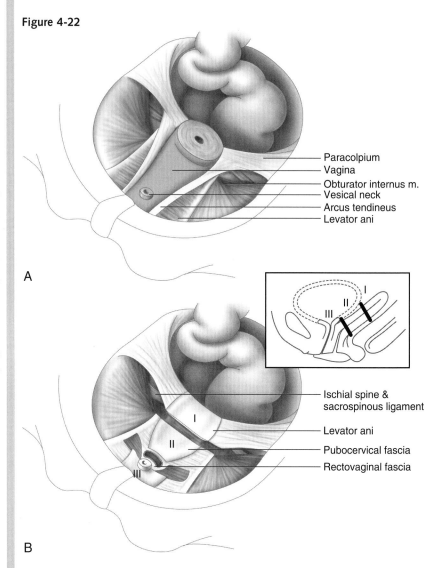

A

Paracolpium
Vagina
Obturator internus m.
Vesical neck
Arcus tendineus
Levator ani

Ischial spine & sacrospinous ligament

Levator ani

Pubocervical fascia

Rectovaginal fascia

B

The diaphragmatic portion of the levator ani consists of the iliococcygeus and coccygeus muscles. The iliococcygeus muscle arises from the ischial spine and arcus tendineus levator ani and inserts onto the coccyx and anococcygeal raphe. It composes the largest part of the levator complex. The coccygeus (or ischiococcygeus) is situated just posterior to the iliococcygeus. It arises from the ischial spine ligament and inserts into the lateral coccyx and sacrum. The sacrospinous ligament forms the tendineus part of the coccygeus muscle. The genital hiatus allows passage of the anus, urethra, and vagina through the muscles of the pelvic diaphragm.

Type I and type II muscle fibers are present in the levator ani muscle to allow, respectively, a baseline tone and voluntary contraction. Type II fibers are fast-twitch fibers, and they contract forcefully for a shorter duration of time. Type I fibers are slow-twitch and contract slowly to provide a sustained tone. Thus, in the pelvis, type I fibers support the viscera during normal activity whereas type II fibers reflexively contract during sudden increases in intra-abdominal pressure. By tonic contraction of the pubococcygeus muscle, the genital hiatus coapts. This closure of the pelvic floor contributes to a stable structure on which the pelvic organs are supported. In addition, type II fiber contraction leads to the elevation of the visceral organs and vaginal closure. The vagina and rectum rotate posteriorly over the anococcygeal raphe, elevating that structure and narrowing the genital hiatus.

Clinical Relevance

Defects in any of the musculofascial components of the pelvic floor can result in pelvic organ prolapse and increase the risk of incontinence. For instance, damage to the pelvic floor muscles resulting from childbirth can lead to a widening of the genital hiatus, resulting in a vagina further exposed to the effects of intra-abdominal pressure. The vagina may be adequately supported as long as the endopelvic fascia is intact. However, defects in the endopelvic fascia may result in prolapse. Pelvic organ prolapse is discussed in detail in Chapter 23, Pelvic Organ Prolapse and Pelvic Floor Dysfuntion.

Urethral and Vesical Neck Support

The urethra is maintained in a retropubic position by the sling-like anterior vaginal wall, which attaches bilaterally to the levator ani and obturator muscles. The distal urethra is fixed in position through its fusion to the vagina, whereas the proximal portion and bladder neck are usually mobile. Older schools of thought have attributed most of the urethral support to the pubourethral ligaments that run from the mid-urethra to the intrapelvic inferior pubis. These ligaments cover the proximal urethra and are derived from condensations of the endopelvic fascia surrounding the obturator internus, floor of the retropubic space, and posterior pubis. Various authors have refuted the importance of the pubourethral ligaments in urethral stabilization and continence. Intact support of the bladder neck and proximal urethra are important for the maintenance of urinary continence. Various theories exist regarding the maintenance of urinary continence.

Richardson et al. reintroduced the concepts of White describing lateral paravaginal attachment between the arcus tendineus fascia pelvis and the periurethral tissues and anterior vaginal wall. The muscular attachment of the periurethral fascia to the medial levator ani allows the bladder neck to rotate downward during micturition and maintain its resting position at end-micturition. Separation of the pericervical fascia from the arcus tendineus fascia pelvis can lead to stress incontinence and anterior vaginal wall prolapse. DeLancey proposed "hammock hypothesis," which states that the underlying stability of the suburethral layer is more important for urethral closure and the maintenance of continence than the position of the urethra relative to the pelvis (Fig. 4-23). Increases in intra-abdominal pressure compress the urethra against the vaginal wall on which it lies, maintaining continence.

Figure 4-23

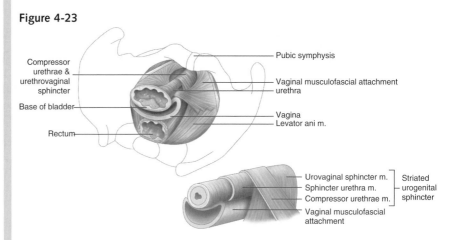

The hammock hypothesis. Increases in intra-abdominal pressure compress the urethra against the vaginal wall on which it lies, which acts as a hammock of support. (Reprinted from Walters MD, Karram MM: Urogynecology and Reconstructive Pelvic Surgery, 2nd ed. St. Louis, Mosby, 1992.)

96

Clinical Relevance

Damage to the underlying supporting structures of the bladder base and proximal urethra may lead to stress incontinence because the urethra cannot be adequately compressed against a stable suburethral layer. Additionally, detachment of the vagina from its lateral support (i.e., paravaginal defect) may lead to prolapse of the anterior vaginal wall.

CONCLUSION

The anatomy of the pelvic floor has been classically divided into the external and the internal genitalia. The external genital organs include the mons pubis, clitoris, urinary meatus, labia majora, labia minora, vestibule, Bartholin's glands, and periurethral glands. The internal genital organs are located in the true pelvis and include the vagina, uterus, cervix, oviducts, ovaries, and surrounding supporting structures. Pelvic organ support and continence are maintained by a complex interplay between the bony structures of the pelvis, pelvic diaphragm muscles, nerves that innervate the pelvic floor, and endopelvic fascia.

KEY POINTS

1. Five bones make up the pelvis. The ilium, ischium, and pubis fuse together at the acetabulum to form the coxal bones. The sacrum and coccyx complete the pelvis posteriorly.
2. The levator ani, the major supporting structure for the pelvic viscera, is composed of the iliococcygeus, coccygeus, pubococcygeus, and puborectalis muscles; the iliococcygeus is the broadest and most posterior portion.
3. The arterial supply of the pelvis is paired and bilateral and has multiple collaterals and numerous anastomoses.

Continued

KEY POINTS—CONT'D

4. The pelvic outlet can be divided into the urogenital and anal triangles by a line drawn between the ischial tuberosities.

5. The cardinal ligaments are located at the base of the broad ligament, are continuous with the connective tissue of the parametrium, and are attached to the pelvic diaphragm through continuity with the superficial superior fascia of the levator ani.

6. The ureter lies in the retroperitoneal space and crosses over the common or internal iliac artery at the pelvic brim.

7. The distal ureter enters into the cardinal ligament, where it is approximately 1 to 2 cm lateral to the uterine cervix and surrounded by a plexus of veins.

8. Surgical compromise of the ureters may occur during clamping or ligating of the infundibulopelvic vessels, clamping or ligating of the cardinal ligaments, or wide suturing in the endopelvic fascia during an anterior repair.

9. Disruption of level I support may lead to prolapse of the uterus or vaginal vault, whereas damage to level II and III supports predispose to anterior and posterior vaginal prolapse.

10. The suburethral vaginal wall acts as a hammock of support; the urethra is compressed against it during increases in intra-abdominal pressure.

SUGGESTED READING

Aronson MP: Atlas of pelvic anatomy and gynecologic surgery. J Pelvic Med Surg 9(4):195, 2003.

Baggish MS, Karram MM: Atlas of Pelvic Anatomy and Gynecologic Surgery. Singapore, W.B. Saunders, 2001.

Brooks J: Anatomy of the lower urinary tract and male genitalia. In Walsh PC, Retik AB, Vaughan ED Jr, Vein AJ (eds): Campbell's Urology, 7th ed. Philadelphia, Elsevier, 1997, pp 89–128.

Buller JL, Thompson JR, Cundiff GW, et al: Uterosacral ligament: Description of anatomic relationships to optimize surgical safety. Obstet Gynecol 97(6): 873–879, 2001.

Clemente CD: Gray's Anatomy, 30th ed. Philadelphia, Lea & Febiger, 1985.

DeLancey JO: Anatomic aspects of vaginal eversion after hysterectomy. Am J Obstet Gynecol 166(6 Pt 1): 1717–1724, 1992.

DeLancey JOL: Anatomy and biomechanics of genital prolapse. Clin Obstet Gynecol 36:897–909, 1993.

Grant JCB: An Atlas of Anatomy, 9th ed. Baltimore, Williams & Wilkins, 1991.

Netter FH: Atlas of Human Anatomy. East Hanover, NJ, Novartis, 1997.

Reiffenstuhl G: Practical pelvic anatomy for the gynecologic surgeon. In Nichols DH (ed): Gynecologic and Obstetric Surgery. St Louis, Mosby, 1993, pp 26–71.

Strohbehn K: Normal pelvic floor anatomy. Obstet Gynecol Clin North Am 25:683–705, 1998.

Strohbehn K, DeLancey JOL: The anatomy of stress incontinence. Oper Techn Gynecol Surg 2:5–16, 1997.

Walters M, Weber A: Anatomy of the lower urinary tract, rectum, and pelvic floor. In Walters M, Karram MM (eds): Urogynecology and Reconstructive Pelvic Surgery, 2nd ed. Philadelphia, Elsevier, 1999, pp 3–14.

Weber AM, Walters MD: Anterior vaginal prolapse: Review of anatomy and techniques of surgical repair. Obstet Gynecol 89:311–318, 1997.

5

EVALUATION OF THE FEMALE PATIENT

John W. Whiteside, Elizabeth H.W. Ricanati, and James L. Whiteside

INTRODUCTION

Medical evaluation begins with a thorough history and physical examination; the methodic gathering of historical and physical examination findings is indispensable to administering good patient care. In evaluating a patient, a physician relies on innate or learned skills of perception, communication, and physical examination. No single chapter could successfully detail the lessons required in becoming proficient in these skills. Furthermore, these skills are not static; each physician should become progressively more capable in them with time. The reader of this chapter is assumed to possess knowledge of the basic elements of a medical history and familiarity with performing a physical examination. This chapter will focus on common diseases and the historical and physical examination elements that are unique or required to thoroughly evaluate female patients. Our focus will be further limited to the well-woman evaluation, since subsequent chapters in this textbook discuss gynecologic disease presentations and diagnostic workup.

NONGYNECOLOGIC WELL-WOMAN HISTORY AND ORGAN-BASED ASSESSMENT

Screening and Prevention

The annual physical examination of a gynecologic patient is a tailored periodic health visit based on an individual's particular risk of disease. When screening for disease, the aim is prevention of morbidity and mortality. Although recommended screening tests are discussed elsewhere in this textbook, we briefly mention some in the context of a well-woman evaluation. These include measurement of blood pressure at every visit and at least every 2 years in all patients regardless of age. Chapter 6, Preventive Health Care for Women, will detail the currently recommended screening tests and strategies in women. Other health maintenance issues include counseling on smoking cessation, alcohol and drug use, seatbelt use, adequate nutrition (including calcium) and exercise, injury prevention, daily dental hygiene, and functional assessment (e.g., elicitation of marital and sexual problems). Convincing data are now available that all women of childbearing age should take 400 µg of folic acid to prevent fetal neural tube defects.

Annual influenza vaccination should be offered to all female persons older than 6 months, particularly those who are pregnant or immunocompromised. Tetanus vaccination should be administered every 10 years to those who have completed their primary series as children; for those who have not received their primary series, this should be done first. The Centers for Disease Control and Prevention recommends that women receive a single administration of the pneumococcal vaccine at the age of 65 years. In addition, other vaccinations are advised for women at higher risk such as travelers or residents in areas of endemic disease.

History

A thorough history is the single best element of the evaluation to render diagnostic insight. Obtaining a history for a well-woman visit is similar in structure to the standardized history format (see Box 5–1), with a few notable exceptions. Past obstetric and gynecologic history are important additions, and these will be considered separately later. A sexual history and abuse history should also be obtained because sexual health affects overall well-being; many sexual problems reflect underlying disease processes or psychological morbidity (e.g., anger, anxiety, and depression). Obtaining a sexual history also facilitates dialogue about topics such as sexually transmitted diseases and pregnancy. The practitioner must maintain a nonjudgmental approach as she or he inquires about sexual orientation, contacts, practices, and problems. Physical and sexual violence are common, often affecting women more than men. Intimate partners or relatives with a normally protective role may also perpetrate violence against women. It is imperative to inquire about all forms of abuse, including emotional, physical, and sexual abuse as part of a good history.

Box 5-1 Outline of Historical Information Obtained During Well-Woman Evaluation

Chief complaint
History of present illness
Past medical history
Past surgical history
Past obstetric and gynecologic history
Allergies/medications: Prescription, over-the-counter, herbal, and alternative medicine preparations and vitamins
Social history
Sexual and abuse history
Family history (e.g., breast cancer, ovarian cancer, colon cancer, thyroid disease, and coronary artery disease)
Health maintenance: Diet, exercise, calcium intake, tetanus status, seatbelt use, smoke detectors
Review of systems

Nongynecologic Organ System Assessments

Cardiovascular System

Heart disease is the leading cause of death of women in the United States, accounting for more than 50% of female mortality. The risk of cardiovascular disease increases dramatically after menopause. Nonetheless, heart disease is both underdiagnosed and undertreated in women. Women are twice as likely as men to die from a myocardial infarction after controlling for age and comorbidities, and they have a higher mortality rate after coronary bypass surgery and angioplasty. Ultrasensitive C-reactive protein testing has recently been shown to be useful in stratifying a woman's risk of heart disease and should be offered to high-risk women in addition to routine lipid and fasting-glucose testing.

The risk factors that contribute to ischemic cardiac disease in women are similar to those found in men and are listed in Box 5-2. Any well-woman office assessment should include consideration of these risk factors and should trigger a discussion regarding the patient's individual risk of coronary event. Multiple prediction models exist to aid this discussion (such as the Framingham Prediction Score). These models contribute to the patient's understanding of risk and assist the physician in choosing targets for the treatment of cholesterol, blood pressure, and other cardiac risk factors. Since smoking cessation reduces the risk of heart attack by approximately 50%, all women should be counseled to discontinue smoking.

Elevated blood pressure is an independent risk factor for heart attack, heart failure, stroke, and renal disease. The risk of these disorders rises

---

Box 5-2 Cardiovascular Risk Factors for Myocardial Infarction

Hypercholesterolemia
Goals:
  Total cholesterol < 200
  Low-density lipoprotein cholesterol < 130
  High-density lipoprotein cholesterol > 50
  Triglycerides < 150

Menopause

Smoking

Diabetes mellitus

Hypertension
Goal < 120/80
Prehypertension 120–140/80–90
Hypertension > 140/90

Family history of heart disease

Metabolic syndrome
Defined as meeting three or more of the following criteria:
  Blood pressure > 185/85 or already receiving antihypertensive medication
  Blood glucose levels > 110
  High-density lipoprotein < 50
  Triglycerides > 150
  Waist circumference > 35 inches

exponentially across the entire blood pressure range, from 115/75 to 185/115 mm Hg. The diagnosis of hypertension is made when blood pressure measurements are elevated during three separate office visits. The initial workup should focus on identifying potential causes of "secondary hypertension" such as oral contraceptive use, Cushing's disease, obstructive sleep apnea, pheochromocytoma, and renal disease. Secondary hypertension accounts for less than 5% of hypertension cases, but identification of these disorders is important because intervention may be curative.

Treatment of primary hypertension begins with lifestyle modification. However, to achieve the goal office blood pressure of less than 140/90, most persons with hypertension will require two or more medications. For patients with greater risk of heart disease, diabetes or chronic renal disease, the goal office blood pressure is lower, less than 130/80. A thiazide-type diuretic agent should be considered as initial therapy in most patients. Alternative or additional medications may be chosen based on the presence of comorbid disease states such as coronary artery disease, heart failure, diabetes, or renal disease.

Beyond myocardial ischemia and its risk factors, other common cardiac disorders include arrhythmias, valvular disease, and congestive heart failure. Most of these disorders are equally prevalent among men and women and are treated similarly between the sexes.

Pulmonary System

The diagnosis of pulmonary disease often depends on specific symptoms that the patient experiences. However, unlike other disease systems, pulmonary diseases often have a long latency period, thus requiring a high index of suspicion on the part of the physician.

The symptoms of dyspnea and cough correspond to many pathologic pulmonary processes. Normally, breathing is an unconscious behavior. The sensation of breathlessness, therefore, is often an early complaint of pulmonary disease. Cough may be a result of the need to rid the lung of excess mucus or the result of an irritation of the airways. Although an acute cough usually has an infectious etiology, the three most common causes of chronic cough are asthma, postnasal drip, and gastroesophageal reflux disease (GERD). A carefully taken history is crucial for better characterizing these symptoms (i.e., association with exercise, lying flat, chronicity).

Obstructive lung diseases such as asthma and chronic obstructive pulmonary disease are common in women. Asthma may occur in the absence of tobacco exposure and is characterized by episodic, reversible inflammation of the airways in response to internal or external stimuli. In contrast, chronic obstructive pulmonary disease is characterized by chronic non-reversible inflammatory and architectural changes in the lungs that usually result from persistent tobacco smoke exposure. Patients with both diseases may present with wheezing, cough, and shortness of breath (a result of widespread bronchospasm and inflammation). Patients with moderate to severe obstructive disease may require inhaled or systemic steroids in addition to bronchodilating therapies. The physician should consider prophylactic treatment for osteoporosis in patients requiring long-term steroid use. During pregnancy, patients with asthma must be carefully monitored; one third of these patients will have worsening symptoms, one third will stay the same, and one third will have improvement. In addition, pregnant women already have some compromised breathing due to the pressure of the growing uterus on the thoracic cavity.

Sleep disorders may present alone or as a consequence of other respiratory illnesses such as those already mentioned. Women with these disorders complain of interrupted sleep, restless sleep, morning headaches, poor concentration, memory difficulties, and daytime sleepiness. Box 5-3 lists respiratory conditions associated with disordered sleep. Obstructive sleep apnea is the leading cause of daytime sleepiness and is a risk factor of cardiovascular morbidity. Patients develop symptoms when the pharyngeal airway is temporarily occluded during sleep. Obstructive sleep apnea is more common in obese, postmenopausal women. Significantly, a small percentage of these patients may develop pulmonary hypertension with resultant cor pulmonale.

Lung cancer is currently the leading cause of cancer death in women in the United States, having surpassed all other cancers as a result of increasing tobacco usage among women in recent decades. Although there are other risk factors for this disease, such as occupational and environmental exposures, tobacco use is the most common and modifiable risk factor (Box 5-4). Currently, no consensus guidelines for lung cancer screening exist; routine chest x-rays are not recommended.

Gastrointestinal System

Absorption of nutrients in the gastrointestinal (GI) system is dependent on a complex interplay of neurologic reflexes, smooth muscle contraction, and the action of multiple specialized cells. Complaints related to the GI system may result from a failure in any of these cellular actions. Specifically, GI

Box 5-3 Respiratory Conditions Associated With Disordered Sleep
Obstructive sleep apnea
Central sleep apnea
Periodic breathing
Hypoventilation resulting from neuromuscular or pulmonary disease

---

Box 5-4 Risk Factors for Lung Cancer
Tobacco
Occupational exposures
Asbestos
Radon
Environmental
Diet

symptoms may result from altered motility, compromise of a mucosal surface, or distension of the bowel lumen.

Dyspepsia refers to chronic or recurrent pain in the upper abdomen and may be caused by gastroduodenal ulcer, GERD, *Helicobacter pylori*–induced gastritis, or gastric cancer. For patients presenting with dyspepsia, management options include empiric acid-lowering therapy, *H. pylori* testing (serology vs. breath test), or diagnostic testing such as endoscopy. Because the incidence of gastric cancer increases with age, upper endoscopy is recommended for patients older than 45 years who present with new dyspepsia. Patients younger than 45 years should be tested for *H. pylori* exposure and treated with antibiotics if results are positive or an antisecretory agent if they are negative. Patients younger than 45 years who fail to respond to antibiotic or antisecretory therapy should be referred for upper endoscopy. Approximately 60% of patients with dyspepsia have no identified cause for pain and are classified as having functional dyspepsia.

GERD is one of the most prevalent GI disorders among women. Approximately 60% of patients report experiencing heartburn intermittently, and the incidence of GERD in pregnant women exceeds 80%. Beyond heartburn, other symptoms include sour or acid taste, food regurgitation, chronic cough, belching, and chest pain. Surgical and endoscopic treatments exist for GERD, but most patients respond well to lifestyle changes and antisecretory medications.

Chronic reflux of stomach acid into the esophagus can lead to esophagitis and Barrett's esophagus, a condition associated with increased risk of developing esophageal adenocarcinoma. Indications for endoscopic evaluation of GERD symptoms are outlined above. In addition, the diagnosis of Barrett's esophagus mandates repeated endoscopy. The frequency of this monitoring depends on the presence and degree of cellular dysplasia.

Irritable bowel syndrome (IBS) is a functional bowel disorder that occurs in the absence of a structural or biochemical explanation of the patient's symptoms. Approximately 15% to 20% of adults have experienced this disorder, but fewer than half seek medical attention. Women are affected more often than men. Symptoms include diarrhea, constipation, pain, and bloating. The specific criteria ("Rome II criteria") for the diagnosis of IBS are listed in Box 5-5. Note that although psychosocial stressors and disease may contribute to the presentation of IBS, they are not considered when making the diagnosis. IBS is a diagnosis of exclusion; as such, some level of evaluation and testing is warranted for all patients. Depending on age and symptoms, blood and stool studies may be indicated. Routine lower endoscopy is recommended for patients older than 50 years. However, endoscopy is only indicated for younger patients with evidence of significant disease (e.g., weight loss, anemia). Treatment of IBS is based on predominant symptoms and may include medication, counseling, and dietary/lifestyle modifications.

Abdominal pain is one of the most common presenting complaints among women in the ambulatory setting. Multiple organ systems can contribute to this complaint, and the complete differential diagnosis is beyond the scope of this chapter. The physician should attempt to elicit details about the onset,

---

> **Box 5-5** Rome II Criteria for the Diagnosis of Irritable Bowel Syndrome
>
> During at least 12 weeks (need not be consecutive) in the preceding 12 months, the patient must have experienced abdominal discomfort or pain having two of the following three features:
>
> 1. Relieved with defecation; and/or
> 2. Onset associated with a change in frequency of stool; and/or
> 3. Onset associated with a change in form (appearance) of stool
>
> Symptoms that cumulatively support the diagnosis of IBS include the following:
>
> 1. Abnormal stool frequency (i.e., >3 bowel movements per day or <3 per week)
> 2. Abnormal stool form (i.e., lumpy/hard or loose/watery)
> 3. Abnormal stool passage (e.g., straining, urgency, or feeling of incomplete evacuation)
> 4. Passage of mucus
> 5. Bloating or feeling of abdominal distension
>
> *The Rome II diagnostic criteria of IBS presume the absence of a structural or biochemical explanation for the symptoms.*

severity, quality, timing, location, and aggravating or alleviating factors associated with the pain. Usually, a thorough history and focused physical examination can considerably narrow the differential diagnosis for the pain. A list of common causes of abdominal pain is provided in Box 5-6.

Widespread availability of chemistry testing and increased public interest in lipid monitoring has resulted in a dramatic increase in the number of abnormal liver test results that must be interpreted by physicians. When liver enzyme levels are elevated, the evaluation should include a detailed review of the patient's alcohol use, medications, and supplements. Further investigation should include a check of serologies for viral hepatitis as well as iron studies to rule out hemochromatosis. Nonalcoholic steatohepatitis or "fatty infiltration" of the liver is the most common cause of mild elevations in transaminase levels. Therefore, a hepatic ultrasound should be considered before ordering tests for more rare disorders.

The diagnosis of hematochezia or GI bleeding may result from a screening stool study or from the patient's complaint of frankly bloody or melanotic stools. When stools are overtly bloody, patients are generally hospitalized and evaluated expeditiously under the presumption that the bleed is active. When occult bleeding is detected or suspected based on iron deficiency or anemia, investigation is done in the outpatient setting. Upper and lower endoscopies are the primary investigative tests done for occult GI blood loss. Other diagnostic modalities include radioisotope bleeding scans, barium studies, and capsule enteroscopy.

The differential diagnosis of hematochezia includes malignancy of the colon. Colorectal cancer is the third leading cause of cancer-related death among American women and accounts for approximately 14% of all annual cancer deaths. Survival is directly related to the stage of cancer at the time of diagnosis. As a result, screening for colorectal cancer is recommended for all persons. Most women begin screening at the age of 50 years;

Box 5-6 Common Causes of Abdominal Pain

Gastrointestinal
Gastric or duodenal ulcer
Small or large bowel obstruction
Intussusception
Appendicitis
Pancreatitis
Cholecystitis, cholangitis
Biliary colic
Diverticulitis
Inflammatory bowel disease (ulcerative colitis, Crohn's disease)
Inguinal, umbilical, ventral, or femoral hernia
Volvulus
Meckel's diverticulum
Mesenteric lymphadenitis
Abscess

Vascular
Dissecting abdominal aortic aneurysm
Mesenteric ischemia or infarction

Genitourinary
Urinary tract infection, pyelonephritis
Ovarian cyst or torsion
Mittelschmerz
Ectopic pregnancy, threatened abortion
Pelvic inflammatory disease

Musculoskeletal
Muscular pain
Ilioinguinal or iliohypogastric nerve entrapment

Neurologic
Shingles, postherpetic neuralgia
Radiculopathy

those with higher risk of disease, such as those with hereditary or inflammatory bowel disorders, are offered earlier screening through fecal occult blood testing, flexible sigmoidoscopy, colonography, or colonoscopy.

Endocrine System

Beyond reproductive hormonal disorders, the most common endocrine diseases in women are thyroid disease, diabetes, obesity, and osteoporosis. The thyroid gland may either underproduce or overproduce thyroid hormone, resulting in hypothyroidism or hyperthyroidism, respectively.

Box 5-7 lists common thyroid disorders. Hypothyroidism, common in women, is treated with chronic supplementation of levothyroxine with the goal of restoring serum thyrotropin levels to normal. It often takes several weeks for an elevated thyroid-stimulating hormone to correct in response to an appropriate levothyroxine dose. Weight reduction and increases in pulse rate and blood pressure occur early with thyroxine supplementation. However, hoarseness, anemia, and changes in skin and hair

Box 5-7 Common Thyroid Disorders
Hypothyroidism
Overt hypothyroidism
Subclinical hypothyroidism
Transient hypothyroidism
Pregnancy-related disorder
Postablative hypothyroidism
Hyperthyroidism
Graves' disease
Toxic adenoma or toxic nodular goiter
Thyroiditis
Pregnancy-related disorder
Thyrotoxic crisis (thyroid storm)

may take longer to resolve. Thyroid levels need to be closely monitored over time. Over-replacement increases the risk of arrhythmia, anxiety, and osteoporotic fractures; under-replacement increases the risks of hypercholesterolemia and ischemic heart disease.

As opposed to hypothyroidism, hyperthyroidism is a result of an overactive thyroid gland. However, like hypothyroidism, this condition is common and affects women more than men. Graves' disease is the most common cause of hyperthyroidism (80% to 90% of all cases) and may be easily diagnosed if a patient's presenting signs include a diffuse goiter and ophthalmopathy. Other causes of hyperthyroidism include toxic adenoma, toxic nodular goiter, and thyroiditis. Treatment options include antithyroid medications, radioactive iodine, and surgery. Hyperthyroidism may also occur during pregnancy. In this case, the preferred treatment is an antithyroid medication at the lowest possible dose since radioactive iodine is known to harm the developing fetus.

Diabetes is an increasing epidemic in the United States and results in significant morbidity and mortality in women. The disease affects almost 16 million Americans, though many are unaware that they have the disease. There are three main types of diabetes: type I, type II, and gestational diabetes. Type I diabetes results from diminished insulin levels produced by the pancreas, whereas type II diabetes results from decreased sensitivity to insulin among other cells in the body. Type II diabetes is the most common form and usually presents in adults older than 40 years, particularly among persons with obesity. Further, women with gestational diabetes have a 50% chance of developing type II diabetes later in life. Despite differences in pathophysiology, all types of diabetes share a common list of complications, including pathologic changes in the cardiovascular, renal, ocular, and neurologic systems.

Risk factors for diabetes are listed in Box 5-8. Treatment may consist of dietary restrictions, weight loss, oral medication, or insulin, depending on the type and severity of disease. Patients are advised regarding recommended lifestyle changes and are instructed to monitor their glucose levels. In addition, physicians regularly follow up with the patient, checking for

Box 5-8	Risk Factors for Diabetes
Family history	
Obesity	
Race	
African American	
Hispanic	
Native American	

changes in sensation, proteinuria, skin condition, and hemoglobin Alc. The American Diabetes Association advises annual eye examinations for changes in the retina. Given the high morbidity and mortality rates associated with diabetes, physicians now recognize the importance of primary preventions identifying women at risk and encouraging weight loss and exercise.

Obesity, a chronic disease with complications such as hypertension, diabetes, and hypercholesterolemia, is increasing in prevalence in the United States and worldwide. Bariatric diseases are defined using body mass index (BMI), which is the patient's weight in kilograms divided by height in meters squared. *Overweight* is defined as a BMI of 25 to 29.9 kg/m,^{2} *obesity* is a BMI higher than 30 kg/m,^{2} and *severe* or *morbid obesity* is defined as a BMI higher than 40 kg/m^2 (or >35 kg/m^2 in the presence of comorbid disease). It should be noted that the use of BMI as a measure of obesity has some significant shortcomings; bodybuilders, who have a greater amount of muscle, would often be classified as obese despite their low body fat percentage.

Most cases of obesity are related to nonmedical disorders such as a sedentary lifestyle and excessive caloric intake. However, smoking cessation may be a cause of weight gain, as are some medicines, such as insulin, sulfonylureas, and steroids. At any one time, more than two thirds of adults in the United States report either trying to lose weight or to maintain weight. Significantly, only 20% are both eating less and engaging in more than 150 minutes of physical activity per week. Despite the U.S. Preventive Services Task Force recommendation that clinicians screen all adult patients for obesity and offer intensive counseling and behavioral interventions to promote sustained weight loss for obese adults, fewer than half of obese adults report being advised to lose weight by a health professional. In examining an overweight or obese patient during a well-woman evaluation, it is a physician's duty to identify this health risk and to offer meaningful strategies to correct the disorder.

Osteoporosis is characterized as low bone mass and microarchitectural bone tissue deterioration. The World Health Organization defines *osteoporosis* as bone mineral density two and half or more standard deviations below that of a "young normal adult." The nonmodifiable and modifiable risk factors for osteoporotic fractures are listed in Box 5-9. Fifty percent of all white women will experience an osteoporotic fracture at some point in their lifetime. The goals of treating decreased bone mass include reducing

---

Box 5-9 Risk Factors for Osteoporotic Fractures

Nonmodifiable
History of adult fractures
First-degree family history of fracture
Caucasian race
Advancing age
Female gender
Dementia

Comorbid disease
Chronic obstructive pulmonary disease
Hyperparathyroidism
Type I diabetes
Pernicious anemia
Multiple sclerosis
Rheumatoid arthritis
Sarcoidosis
Cirrhosis

Modifiable
Low body weight
Cigarette smoking
Estrogen deficiency
Sedentary lifestyle
Alcoholism
Low calcium intake
Impaired eyesight
Medications
Anticonvulsants
Levothyroxine
Glucocorticosteroids
Heparin
Lithium

Box 5-10 Bone Mineral Density Testing Recommendations

Bone mineral density testing is recommended in the following populations:
All postmenopausal women younger than 65 years with one or more risk factors for osteoporosis
All women older than 65 years, regardless of additional risk factors
Postmenopausal women presenting with fractures
Women who are weighing benefits of therapy for osteoporosis and want to use bone mineral density to aid in decision making
Women considering the cessation of prolonged hormone replacement therapy

---

the risk of fracture through risk modification and stemming further bone loss through medications such as bisphosphonates and calcium supplementation. The diagnosis of osteoporosis is based on the bone mineral density testing results. Guidelines regarding use of this test are listed in Box 5-10.

Renal System

Advanced azotemia (the presence of nitrogenous wastes in the blood) and electrolyte disturbances can arise from numerous causes, and the symptoms associated with renal failure are often vague and nonspecific. These disorders can and should be screened for in any woman presenting with somatic complaints without clear cause. The testing of blood urea nitrogen, creatinine, sodium, potassium, chloride, and total carbon dioxide is an effective first step in assessing a woman with possible renal disease. Other renal disorders to consider in assessing a patient in the course of a well-woman evaluation include tumors and infections of the urinary tract. Risk factors associated with genitourinary tumors should be identified (see further discussion) and high-risk lifestyles should be discouraged.

Benign or malignant tumors of the genitourinary tract can cause hematuria. Genitourinary cancer is found in 20% to 40% of cases of gross hematuria and 5.1% of microscopic hematuria. Isolated hematuria is the sole presenting symptom in 60% of all renal cell carcinomas, whereas the classic triad of hematuria, flank pain, and a palpable mass occurs in only 10% to 15% of cases. The most important modifiable risk factor for renal cancer is tobacco exposure, conferring a two-fold greater risk of the disease. Bladder cancer should also be suspected in the workup of hematuria; approximately 85% to 90% of cases present with this finding. Here again, the most important modifiable risk factor for bladder cancer is tobacco exposure, accounting for approximately 30% of cases. If a urinary tract tumor is suspected during the evaluation of hematuria, the patient should be referred to a urologist.

Dipstick urinalysis is commonly performed in the evaluation of urinary complaints. Although reagent strip results can be diagnostic in symptomatic patients, more than 20% of unselected persons screened with reagent strips will have an abnormality. False-positive findings can precipitate unnecessary and possibly harmful treatments or diagnostic tests. The reagent strip renders information on urine pH, protein, hemosiderin pigment, nitrite, specific gravity, and leukocyte esterase. Despite its relatively good sensitivity, positive results from a reagent strip should be confirmed with more specific tests. The diagnoses of bacteriuria, hematuria, and proteinuria all require additional testing. Boxes 5-11 and 5-12 review the basic evaluation and differential diagnosis of hematuria and proteinuria.

Although urinary frequency, urgency, and incontinence are considerably bothersome to the patient, these conditions are often overlooked by their physician. Subsequent chapters will discuss in detail the problem of female bladder dysfunction, but it should be emphasized these symptoms are a major source of morbidity among women. Queries regarding a woman's voiding frequency (should generally be fewer than 8 times in a 24-hour period), presence of nocturia (normally fewer than two times per night), urgency with voids, and urinary incontinence should be included in any comprehensive well-woman evaluation.

Musculoskeletal System

Inquiry and diagnosis of musculoskeletal disease is usually triggered by a specific patient complaint. In general, a patient first complains of pain in a

---

Box 5-11 Basic Evaluation and Differential Diagnosis of Hematuria

Evaluation
Most cost-effective approach unclear; historical standard has been intravenous
pyelogram, cystoscopy, and cytology.

Differential
Congenital
  Cystic renal disease
  Benign familial hematuria
  Hematologic abnormalities (e.g., bleeding disorders, sickling disorders)
  Anatomic (e.g., diverticula, posterior urethral valves, vesicoureteric reflux)
Trauma (degree of hematuria does not correlate with the extent of injury)
  Exercise-induced hematuria ("athletic hematuria")
  Foreign body (urethral catheters, ureteral stents)
Inflammatory
  Infection
  Glomerulonephritis
Metabolic
  Urinary calculi
Neoplastic
  Benign or malignant tumors of the genitourinary tract
Other
  Drugs
  Endometriosis
  Postoperative

joint, muscle, or limb. This pain may result from trauma, overuse, pain syndromes, or other disease such as inflammatory and crystalline arthritides as well as tumors of the skeletal system.

Persistent overuse of the musculoskeletal system can result in injury to tendons, ligaments, bones, and cartilage. However, most cases of osteoarthritis are not related to the patient's history of athleticism. Indeed, less than 20% of the American public reports exercising regularly, but the prevalence of osteoarthritis exceeds 80% in those older than 75 years. The treatment of osteoarthritis usually includes activity modification, weight loss, stretching, strengthening exercises, and analgesics.

In addition to trauma and overuse, the etiology of joint pain can be infectious or crystal induced (e.g., gout, pseudogout), or it may present as a symptom of a systemic inflammatory disorder. Causes of inflammatory arthritis include systemic lupus erythematosus, rheumatoid arthritis, psoriatic arthritis, and gonococcal tenosynovitis (septic arthritis). These inflammatory diseases are more common in women than in men. In contrast, 95% of gouty arthropathy occurs in men. Inflammatory arthritis usually involves more than one joint, whereas gout and infection usually involve a single joint. The clinician should consider the presence of a septic joint in any woman presenting with fever and monoarthropathy. Treatment of gout involves rest and use of nonsteroidal anti-inflammatory medications, whereas inflammatory arthritides are treated with systemic immunologic agents. A septic joint presents a clinical emergency, and treatment requires urgent parenteral antibiotics.

Box 5-12   Basic Evaluation and Differential Diagnosis of Proteinuria

Evaluation
Quantitative protein measurement with 24-hour urinalysis for all qualitative findings
Protein electrophoresis for proteinuria of 300 to 2000 mg/24 hours
Fasting glucose for patients with evidence of renal insufficiency
Renal ultrasound or intravenous pyelogram depending on renal function
Management based on suspected cause:
  If suspected to be exercise induced, hydration, rest, and repeat analysis are recommended.
  Renal consultation is recommended in cases of persistent proteinuria.

Differential
Glomerular proteinuria (increased glomerular capillary permeability)
  Immunoglobulin A nephropathy
  Diabetic nephropathy
  Drug induced (e.g., heroin, captopril, lithium, nonsteroidal anti-inflammatory drugs)
  Minimal change disease
  Autoimmune (e.g., systemic lupus erythematosus, Henoch-Schönlein purpura)
  Congestive heart failure
  Other (e.g., exercise-induced, orthostasis, fever)
Tubular proteinuria (failed resorption of low-molecular-weight proteins)
  Obstructive uropathy
  Glucosuria
  Toxins and drugs
  Aminoaciduria
  Phosphaturia
Overflow (i.e., overflow of excess or abnormally accumulating immunoglobulins and low-molecular-weight proteins)
  Multiple myeloma
  Leukemia
  Hemoglobinuria/myoglobinuria
Tissue proteinuria (associated with inflammation)
  Acute inflammation of urinary tract: cystitis, urothelial tumors

---

Fibromyalgia is a common condition that is characterized by fatigue as well as widespread aching and stiffness in muscles and soft tissues. It is more prevalent in women than in men. Diagnosis is based on the patient's description of chronic widespread pain for at least 3 months and the finding of multiple areas of muscle tenderness on examination. There are no tissue or laboratory abnormalities in fibromyalgia, and abnormal laboratory findings may suggest another etiology for the pain. Treatment of this condition includes reassurance and assistance in self-management.

Excluding bone marrow malignancies such as leukemia and lymphoma, tumors of the musculoskeletal system are rare. Most patients with these malignancies present with the complaint of pain. Other findings may include weight loss, presence of a mass, or focal tenderness on examination. Treatment is specific to the tissue pathology of the tumor, and prognosis for the patient varies considerably depending on the malignancy type and size. The evaluation and treatment is complicated and requires the involvement of an orthopedic cancer specialist as well as an oncologist.

Breast Assessment

Fibrocystic Changes

Fibrocystic changes are the most common of all benign breast conditions and are present in up to half of all premenopausal women. Among those affected, half are symptomatic. They are thought to be associated with an exaggerated response to estrogen and progesterone and are more prevalent during a woman's reproductive years. The most common presentation involves cyclic, bilateral breast pain, and engorgement. Breast tenderness and nodules on examination are most prominent in the days just before menstruation.

Fibroadenoma

After fibrocystic changes, fibroadenomas are the most common form of benign breast disease. Unlike fibrocystic changes, fibroadenomas remain constant throughout the menstrual cycle. They are generally slow-growing, firm, painless, and freely mobile masses comprising a mixture of proliferating epithelial and supporting fibrous tissue. Generally, they are small in size, approximately two to three centimeters. As with other breast masses, they are often biopsied and/or excised to definitively rule out malignancy.

Breast Cancer

Breast cancer ranks second to lung cancer as the leading cause of cancer-related death in the United States. In 1997, approximately 182,000 new cases of breast cancer were diagnosed, and 44,000 women died of the disease. The most important risk factor for developing breast cancer is a positive family history. Other risk factors include increasing age, early menarche, late menopause, nulliparity, early exposure to ionizing radiation, long-term postmenopausal hormone replacement therapy, and alcohol ingestion.

Screening mammography and clinical examination by a trained practitioner have resulted in early diagnosis and a 25% to 30% reduction in mortality in women older than 50 years of age. The utility of screening women younger than 50 years is controversial. This has led to discrepancies in guideline recommendations regarding when to initiate screening in patients with a standard risk of developing breast cancer. The decision to screen women before the age of 50 years should be individualized after discussion of the risks and benefits of the screening test. Most guidelines recommend screening every 1 to 3 years between ages 40 and 50 years. Women from high-risk families, especially those who have the BRCA-1 or BRCA-2 mutations, should begin annual screening 10 years prior to the earliest age at which breast cancer was detected in a relative, or at age 40, whichever comes first.

Skin Assessment

The integument is the largest organ in the body. Likewise, this organ is the most likely to develop malignancy—the bulk of these being related to sun exposure. Although most skin lesions that initiate physician visits are benign, some are malignant, and others are signs of underlying systemic disease. Identifying skin lesions and knowing which require biopsy or referral is essential to the physician's care of a patient during a well-woman evaluation. Inappropriate trivialization of asymptomatic skin lesions may lead to disfigurement, systemic spread of the disorder, or death. Although a thorough listing of skin lesions and their management is beyond the scope of this chapter, the reader should learn the characteristics of worrisome lesions and should be able to perform a complete skin examination of patients presenting for a well-woman examination. Likewise, it is the physician's role to advise the patient regarding the dangers of excessive sun exposure.

Psychosocial Assessment

Eating Disorders

These biopsychosocial syndromes encompass anorexia nervosa, bulimia, binge-eating disorders, and their variants. The morbidity and mortality of these illnesses are very high and are frequently potentiated by delay between the onset of symptoms and initiation of treatment. Eating disorders of all kinds are more common among white, adolescent to young-adult women who are typically in the upper to upper-middle classes of an industrialized society. Approximately half of affected persons recover, with an additional 30% obtaining partial recovery. The disorders tend to fluctuate between periods of illness and remission.

The complications of anorexia are primarily related to starvation, whereas those of bulimia are more related to the sequelae of the binge-purge cycle. Altered nutritional status can cause many physical problems, and careful history and physical examination is required. The examiner must inquire not only about dietary habits and weight fluctuations, but also about exercise habits and purging. The use of laxatives, enemas, and other medications must be addressed. On examination, height, weight, and BMI should be evaluated. Signs and symptoms of eating disorders are listed in Box 5-13. Diagnostic criteria for both anorexia and bulimia are listed in Box 5-14. Overall, the clinical picture of anorexia suggests hypothyroidism or hypopituitarism, whereas that of bulimia depends on whether it is primarily a binge illness or a purge illness.

Psychological assessment is paramount to the evaluation of eating disorders since they are usually accompanied by other comorbid psychiatric illnesses, such as depression.

Anxiety Disorders

Many people are affected by anxiety disorders such as generalized anxiety disorder, panic attack, and social phobias. Differentiation between the various disorders is often difficult, particularly since the disorders may coexist and overlap. Symptoms may be cardiac (e.g., chest pain, hyperventilation, tachycardia, and palpitations), neurologic (e.g., tremulousness, dizziness,

---

Box 5-13 Signs and Symptoms of Eating Disorders

Orofacial: Dental caries, enlargement of the parotid glands
Cardiovascular: Hypotension, prolonged QT interval, arrhythmias
Gastrointestinal: Decreased intestinal motility, constipation
Endocrine and metabolic: Amenorrhea, electrolyte abnormalities, and osteoporosis
Renal: Calculi
Integument: Dry skin and hair, hair loss, lanugo

Box 5-14 Diagnostic Criteria for Anorexia Nervosa and Bulimia
Anorexia (All four criteria required for diagnosis.) Body weight less than 85% of expected weight Intense fear of weight gain Inaccurate perception of own body, size, or shape Amenorrhea **Bulimia** (All four criteria required for diagnosis.) Recurrent binge eating (two or more times a week for 3 months) Recurrent purging Excessive exercise or fasting (two or more times a week for 3 months) Absence of anorexia

lightheadedness, faintness, and headache), or gastrointestinal (e.g., nausea, vomiting, diarrhea, and abdominal pain). Anxiety disorders are often chronic and require long-term treatment. Symptoms commonly flare up during times of stress or depression. Optimal treatment requires a combination of pharmacotherapy and psychotherapy. Pharmacologic intervention includes benzodiazepines, β-blockers, tricyclic antidepressants, and selective serotonin reuptake inhibitors. Psychotherapeutic methods include brief interventions (supportive and cognitive approaches) and behavioral therapies, such as biofeedback and systematic desensitization.

Violence Against Women

Approximately 4.5 million women in the United States between the ages of 18 and 65 are victims of domestic violence each year. More than 90% of domestic violence involves women abused by men, and approximately one in four women using the emergency department has a history of partner violence within the past year. During pregnancy, one in six women is abused every year in the United States, and more than 3 million children between ages 3 and 17 years witness parental abuse. Violence cuts across all age, race, educational, and socioeconomic lines. In 1994, the U.S. federal government enacted the Violence Against Women Act that provides measures for preventing violence against women and includes a national toll-free hotline for information and referrals (National Domestic Violence Hotline, 1–800–799-SAFE).

Although domestic violence is widely prevalent, most medical professionals fail to recognize it in clinical practice due to their discomfort in discussing the topic. Diagnosing domestic violence may also be difficult due to its varied presentations. Findings range from specific physical signs (e.g., dental trauma, head, and neck injuries) to more general complaints (e.g., chronic abdominal, pelvic, or chest pain; somatic disorders; IBS; sexually transmitted diseases; or HIV exposure). Psychological symptoms such as depression, anxiety and panic disorders, eating disorders, substance abuse, or post-traumatic stress disorder may be the first manifestations of domestic violence. Other clinical indicators of abuse include delaying treatment for or poor explanation of injuries, repeat emergency room or clinic visits, and an overly attentive or verbally abusive partner. Simple, but important, screening questions include: "Do you ever feel unsafe at home?" and "Has anyone at home hit you or tried to injure you in any way?"

Once abuse is admitted, providers must carefully document as precisely as possible evidence of abuse because the information may be needed for future medical practitioners and potential legal proceedings. It is imperative not to include the patient's address or phone number in the medical record because the abuser may inadvertently be given access to the patient's chart and may seek retaliation. Providers should inform patients of resources that are available, such as the National Domestic Violence Hotline.

GYNECOLOGIC ASSESSMENT: HISTORY, PHYSICAL EXAMINATION, AND DIAGNOSTIC TESTING

Gynecologic History

The following is an outline of a detailed gynecologic history that, depending on the chief complaint, could be elicited. An in-depth gynecologic history may be obtained to investigate a specific gynecologic complaint. The questions asked are directed at eliciting the necessary information to diagnose and treat the patient's complaint. Preceding any history gathering, a physician is first presented with an observed impression and chief complaint. Such information will, to the experienced physician, form the basis of a "sick" versus "not sick" determination and a decision about how best to triage the patient and her problem or problems.

I. Primary Compliant (in patients presenting for a well-woman visit, this section may not be appropriate)
   a. Onset
   b. Duration
   c. Severity
   d. Precipitating or relieving factors
   e. Associations (e.g., relationship to eating, coital activity, voiding)
   f. Previous occurrences and outcome

II. Menstrual History
   a. Age at menarche
   b. Length of cycle
   c. Regularity of cycle
   d. Date of last menstrual period and previous menstrual period (if the patient is presenting with an "abnormal" menses, then the date of the patients last "normal" menses)
   e. Premenstrual molimina (e.g., skin changes, headaches, weight gain, mood swings)
   f. Duration of flow
   g. Amount of flow (i.e., number of sanitary pads, presence of clots, size of clots)
   h. Dysmenorrhea, primary or secondary (i.e., kind of pain, location, onset, precipitating and relieving factors)
   i. Prior therapy for menstrual disorders

      j. If postmenopausal, then age of menopause, associated menopausal symptoms, and use of hormone replacement therapy

III. Sexual History

Obtaining a sexual history can be a particularly intrusive exercise for an older patient and should be tempered by the patient's problem and value of the information gained. In many instances, knowing a patient is not a victim of sexual abuse, her sexual activity and her satisfaction with this activity will suffice. Among younger women, particularly teenagers, a more thorough sexual history can help identify high-risk behaviors that can be the basis of health instruction and disease-prevalence determinations. Young age, greater coital frequency, and lack of contraception (either barrier or hormonal) are associated with upper genital tract disease.

    a. Age at first sexual intercourse

    b. Frequency of sexual intercourse and most recent activity

    c. Satisfaction with sexual activity and dyspareunia

    d. Contraception use and type

IV. Obstetric History

    a. Number of pregnancies and dates (i.e., gravidity)

    b. Number of deliveries and dates (i.e., parity)

    c. Type of delivery (i.e., vaginal or cesarean, spontaneous or forceps/vacuum assisted, full or pre-term, complications including perineal lacerations)

    Numerous studies have made an association between vaginal delivery and development of urinary incontinence and pelvic organ prolapse. The association is even stronger among those women having sustained a forceps- or vacuum-assisted vaginal delivery.

    d. Birth weights of offspring

    e. Postpartum complications

    f. Number of spontaneous abortions and gestational age

    g. History of ectopic pregnancies

    The common nomenclature of gravida x, parity f-p-a-l, specifies the number of pregnancies x, births after gestation longer than 37 weeks f, births after gestation shorter than 37 weeks p, abortions (spontaneous or induced) a, and living children l. Thus a G 5, P 4-3-0-6 would designate a woman who had five pregnancies, two of which were twin gestations, 3 pregnancies delivered after 37 weeks' gestation, 2 pregnancies were preterm, 1 child died, and there are 6 remaining live children.

V. Past Medical History (including medical problems not already elicited, allergies, medication use, and hospitalizations)

VI. Past Surgical History (including type, approach, reason, and outcome of previous surgeries)

Complications of surgery can give insight into undiscovered medical problems such as factor V Leiden deficiency, the most commonly inherited bleeding disorder. In patients with surgically correctable gynecologic conditions, a careful past surgical history can greatly aid the surgeon.

VII. Social History

Social history with ascertainment of exposures to tobacco, alcohol, and illegal substances can be important in assessing a patient risk profile for some gynecologic diseases. Marital and employment status also can be useful in risk assessment.

Specific gynecologic disease presentations are the focus of subsequent chapters; pertinent components of the history and physical examination will be presented in the appropriate chapters.

Examination and Diagnostic Testing

To optimize the clinical information gained from a female pelvic examination, a thorough understanding of female pelvic anatomy is necessary. For instance, lack of familiarity with the location and orientation of the levator ani muscles limits an examiner's assessment of pelvic organ support or sources of pelvic pain. As pelvic anatomy is discussed elsewhere in this volume, the reader is encouraged to begin there when seeking to learn or improve the pelvic examination technique. Beyond this, assessment of the pelvis is tailored to the patient's presenting issue(s).

Assessment of the Breast

The breast examination is included as a routine part of the gynecologic examination. If the patient has complaints about discomfort or pain in a breast, the health care professional should begin by examining the nonaffected breast and axilla. Inspect the breasts with the patient in the supine and sitting positions, with her hands above her head and then on her hips. Care should be taken to observe the contour, symmetry, and vascular pattern of the breasts for signs of skin retraction, edema, or erythema. Then, the examiner should systematically palpate each breast, the axillae, and the supraclavicular areas using the pads of the fingers to feel for masses. This can be accomplished by going in a circle, dividing the breast into segments, or by going up and down. Regardless, care must be taken to examine the breast in its entirety. Finally, the nipple should be evaluated for discharge, crusting, or ulceration.

Assessment of the External Genitalia

Pelvic examination begins with visual inspection of the vulva, clitoris, urethra, vaginal introitus, perineal body, and anus. Care should be taken to expose all these structures for adequate visualization. The location and appearance of any abnormal vaginal discharge should be noted. Swelling or tenderness at the lateral base of the introitus could suggest a Bartholin's gland abscess. Palpation of a problematic Bartholin's gland between the examiner's thumb and forefinger should elicit tenderness. It should be confirmed that the swelling is oriented at the location of Bartholin's gland and not in association with the anus or ischiorectal fossa. Swelling along the anterior vagina wall together with a patient complaint of pelvic pain should prompt palpation of the urethra. Purulent urethral discharge and tenderness in association with a urethral swelling is strongly suggestive of a urethral diverticulum. Other possible vaginal swellings include

Gartner's duct cysts. These cysts are usually painless and can occur virtually anywhere in the vagina; they usually arise on the lateral vaginal walls. On occasion, they are associated with the ipsilateral ureter, and caution should be exercised in any attempt at removal.

Vulvar Examination

Disorders of the vulva are poorly understood. This lack of understanding begins with etiology and extends to assessment and treatment. For a patient undergoing a well-woman evaluation who denies any vulvar complaints, examination begins by visually inspecting the vulvar skin for any surface or color irregularities. Early vulvar cancer is easily overlooked by both the patient and the physician, and punch biopsy is recommended if the diagnosis of a vulvar condition is uncertain. The value of vulvar colposcopy is controversial. Vulvar pain disorders such as vestibulitis may have associated erythema at the vestibule (the boat-shaped fossa inside the labia minora), but it is often diagnostically helpful to use a cotton swab to reveal tenderness along Hart's line. The clinician should take care to appreciate normal vulvar architecture, since this may be distorted with vulvar dystrophies such as lichen sclerosis and lichen planus. It should be noted that, though not specifically documented in the literature, there is some normal loss of vulvar architecture with age.

119

Urethral Examination

Examination of the urethra begins with visual inspection. Any evidence of urethral discharge, prolapse, or the presence of a caruncle should be noted. In patients who complain of continuous urinary incontinence or leakage of urine from the vagina, the urethra and anterior vaginal wall should be carefully inspected for urethrovaginal fistulae with the help of the posterior blade of the speculum or Sims' retractor. The urethra is palpated for masses or tenderness, which could indicate a urethral diverticulum or urethritis, respectively.

Measurement of urethral mobility can be done using the end of a lubricated cotton swab inserted through the urethra into the bladder. Once in place, the woman is asked to perform a Valsalva maneuver or cough, and the angle of arc movement of the cotton swab is measured. Movement of the swab more than 30 degrees between the resting and straining angles indicates urethral hypermobility. In the past, emphasis was placed on the mobility of the urethra in determining the type of urinary incontinence. A hypermobile urethra was thought to be causative of anatomic urinary incontinence, and surgical correction of this incontinence was aimed at limiting urethral movement. Since any significant anterior vaginal wall prolapse will lead to urethral hypermobility, the cotton swab test is usually not needed when significant anterior vaginal wall prolapse is present. Recently, improvements in treatment modalities for urinary incontinence and a continued lack of understanding of the mechanisms of urinary incontinence have brought into question the need to assess urethral mobility.

Anus and Perineal Body

Examination of the anus and perineal body begins with careful inspection for evidence of hemorrhoids, anal fissures, rectal prolapse, or fecal soiling. Close examination of the perineal body can also be instructive. In a young, nulliparous female the perineal body is approximately 2-cm long, firm, and at an approximately 45-degree angle from the orientation of the anus with the patient in the lithotomy position. The angulation of the anus relative to the plane of the vagina is due to the pull of the puborectalis muscle against the distal portion of the anal canal. Obstetric injury can cause tissue or nerve injury with resultant loss of this normal anatomy. A "dovetail" sign can be noted in those women who have sustained disruption of the external anal sphincter. In this case, the normal radial rugations of the anus are diminished or lost atop the scarred external anal sphincter. Bulging of the perineal body or lost angulation of the anus relative to the vaginal plane suggest pelvic floor dysfunction.

Beyond visual inspection of the anus, digital examination of the anus can sample for occult GI tract bleeding and can render further insight into the integrity of the external anal sphincter. In recent years, endoanal ultrasonography has been found to be very good at identifying internal and external anal sphincter disruptions. Other tests of the anal canal include manometry and pudendal nerve terminal motor latency. Both tests are used in the evaluation of the woman with defecatory dysfunction.

Assessment of the Vagina and Cervix

An important but often overlooked part of any pelvic assessment is the wet mount. Consideration for collecting a wet mount specimen must be made before proceeding with any other portion of the pelvic examination to avoid contamination. The basic tools for wet mount assessment include litmus paper, a cotton swab, a test tube filled with a small amount of saline, a slide, coverslip, and a microscope. Collection of the specimen includes dragging the cotton swab along the full length of the vagina that is exposed with aid of a speculum. The swab is placed on the litmus paper to determine the vaginal pH and then put in the saline filled test tube. The cotton swab and test tube can then be taken to the microscope, where the vaginal smear can be suspended in a small amount of saline on the slide and then covered with the coverslip. The slide should be viewed at both low (10×) and high (40×) magnification to assess: (1) vaginal cell appearance and relative number, (2) bacterial appearance and load, and (3) presence of infectious organisms. Vaginal cells covered with bacteria are called *clue cells*, and normally up to 10% of a low-magnification view can include these cells. Greater than 20% clue cells, a pH higher than 4.5, a fishy odor when the sample is suspended in potassium hydroxide (positive "whiff test"), and a grey adherent discharge are known as Amsel's criteria for the diagnosis of bacterial vaginosis. Other findings on wet mount examination include motile trichomonads (trichomoniasis), parabasilar cells (atrophic vaginitis), and hyphae (candidiasis).

Cervical cytology screening should be performed on all sexually active women every 1 to 3 years, beginning at the age of first intercourse. Details of how to triage cervical cytology are covered elsewhere in this text. The technique of collecting cervical cytology is relatively well known. The advent of human papilloma virus subtyping has changed the media used to collect the sampled cells. Colposcopy, always an alternative to Papanicolaou smear assessment but limited by availability, time, and cost, will remain an essential skill for the obstetrician/gynecologist. The basic techniques for colposcopic assessment of the cervix are covered elsewhere and are beyond the scope of this chapter.

Assessment of the Upper Genital Tract

The upper genital tract can be assessed using the bimanual examination as well as diagnosis-directed procedures. Such procedures include the endometrial biopsy and pelvic ultrasound, which are essential to the workup of abnormal vaginal bleeding. Infusion of saline into the uterine cavity during pelvic ultrasound (i.e., saline infusion sonography) can also be helpful in the workup of abnormal uterine bleeding. A variety of methods are available to sample the endometrium. In recent years, the endometrial Pipelle has become more widely used, with improvements in both its ease of use and patient comfort. The technique involves swabbing the cervix with a cleaning solution (e.g., Betadine or Hibiclens) and slowly inserting the Pipelle through the cervical os. It may be necessary to either slightly bend the tip to account for uterine flexion or grasp the cervix with a single-tooth tenaculum. Grasping the cervix with the tenaculum and applying slight downward traction straightens the cervical canal to allow the Pipelle access to the uterine cavity. Use of the tenaculum, however, results in patient discomfort and with practice should become a rare event.

Assessing the uterus and adnexa is challenging, especially in obese women, in whom the bimanual is often suboptimal. This challenge is highlighted by the fact that there is no commonly accepted means to screen for ovarian cancer. Imaging techniques such as abdominal or transvaginal ultrasound, magnetic resonance imaging, and computed tomography scanning may be useful in the evaluation of uterine or adnexal masses, or when the bimanual examination is suboptimal because of body habitus. Imaging techniques and the evaluation of adnexal masses will be covered in detail in Chapter 20, Disorders of the Fallopian Tube and Ovary.

Assessment of Pelvic Organ Prolapse

Standardized assessment of the vagina has been and continues to be a source of active research. Before 1996, there were a variety of methods to assess prolapse. These methods included the Baden-Walker half-way and Beecham systems, but they also included nonobjective descriptive methods such as using words like *massive* to describe prolapsed segments of the vagina. In 1996, an international multidisciplinary committee adopted the Pelvic Organ Prolapse Quantification (POPQ) system. This system offers a standardized method of measuring the vagina that is invaluable in objectifying treatment outcomes. Although it is unnecessary to perform POPQ on all patients presenting with prolapse, the test can offer a way to objectify the patient's management outcomes. Furthermore, familiarity with the system will aid in the generalist's understanding of forthcoming research on the topic. Performance of the POPQ system is covered in depth in Chapter 23, Pelvic Organ Prolapse and Pelvic Floor Dysfunction; readers are encouraged to familiarize themselves with the technique.

CONCLUSION

The well-woman gynecology visit often serves as a woman's most consistent health care contact. For this reason, the general obstetrician/gynecologist or other women's health care professional should be familiar with common health problems in addition to the gynecologic conditions faced by women in different age groups. Careful history taking and physical examination may identify risky behaviors or disease processes early in their course, decreasing patient morbidity. Healthy lifestyle choices and reproductive health should be reinforced at each visit. Understanding the unique risks of women is paramount to tailoring the well-woman examination and, ultimately, to promoting the improved health of our female patients.

KEY POINTS

1. The well-woman examination should focus on disease prevention and health promotion. In addition to gynecologic care, routine health maintenance should include blood pressure monitoring, cholesterol measurement, breast and colon cancer screening, vaccination maintenance, and healthy lifestyle counseling.

2. Heart disease is the leading cause of death in women in the United States. Control of hypertension, hypercholesterolemia, diabetes, tobacco use, and obesity can greatly reduce the morbidity and mortality of heart disease.

3. Lung cancer is the leading cause of cancer death in women in the United States. Tobacco use is the most important modifiable risk factor.

4. Irritable bowel syndrome is a diagnosis of exclusion and is made according to the Rome II criteria.

5. Serum transaminase levels are often incidentally found to be elevated. Initial workup includes testing for fatty infiltration of the liver, viral hepatitis, and hemochromatosis.

6. All women should begin screening for colorectal cancer by the age of 50 years except those with higher risk as a result of familial or inflammatory disease, who should begin screening at an earlier age.

7. Skin cancer has a higher incidence than all other forms of malignancy; every well-woman examination should include a thorough inspection of the skin.

8. Well-woman examinations should include screening for eating disorders, sexual abuse, and physical abuse.

9. Knowledge of pelvic anatomy greatly improves the diagnostic yield of pelvic examination. Pelvic organ prolapse and urinary incontinence are important causes of morbidity in women, and assessment for these disorders should be done as part of the routine well-woman evaluation. Physical examination tools such as the Pelvic Organ Prolapse Quantification system will aid in the standardization of prolapse measurement and in the assessment of management outcomes.

10. Wet mount of vaginal secretions with determination of vaginal pH should be performed for all patients with symptomatic vaginal discharge. Determination of vaginal pH can be a useful tool in screening for vaginal atrophy.

SUGGESTED READING

Anderson MR, Klink K, Cohrssen A: Evaluation of vaginal complaints. JAMA 291:1368–1379, 2004.

Bump RC, Mattiasson A, Bo K, et al: The standardization of terminology of female pelvic organ prolapse and pelvic floor dysfunction. Am J Obstet Gynecol 175:10–17, 1996.

Drossman DA, Camilleri M, Mayer EA, Whitehead WE: AGA technical review on irritable bowel syndrome. Gastroenterology 123:2108–2131, 2002.

Eisenstat WE, Bancroft SA: Domestic violence. N Engl J Med 341:886–892, 1999.

Grady D, Herrington D, Bittner V, et al: Cardiovascular disease outcomes during 6.8 years of hormone therapy: Heart and estrogen/progesterone replacement follow up [HERS II]. JAMA 288:49, 2002.

Grossfeld GD, Wolf JS Jr, Litwan MS, et al: Asymptomatic microscopic hematuria in adults: Summary of the AUA best practice policy recommendations. Am Fam Physician 63:1145–1154, 2001.

National Institutes of Health: The Seventh Report of the Joint National Committee on Prevention, Detection, Evaluation and Treatment of High Blood Pressure. NIH Publication No. 03–5233, 2003.

North American Menopause Society: Management of Postmenopausal Osteoporosis: Position Statement of NAMS. Menopause 9:84–101, 2002.

Pearce EN, Farwell EN, Braverman LE: Current concepts: Thyroiditis. N Engl J Med 348:2646–2655, 2003.

Preventive Services Resource Links: U. S. Preventive Services Task Force. Agency for Healthcare Research and Quality, Rockville, MD. Septermber 2003. http://www.ahrq.gov/clinic/uspstf/resource.htm

Rome ES, Ammerman S: Medical complications of eating disorders: An update. J Adolesc Health 33: 418–426, 2003.

Seltzer VL, Pearse WH: Women's Primary Health Care: Office Practice and Procedures. New York, McGraw-Hill, 2000.

Shivers SC, Wang X, Li W, et al: Molecular staging of malignant melanoma: Correlation with clinical outcome. JAMA 280:1410–1415, 1998.

Talley NJ, Silverstein MD, Agreus L, et al: AGA technical review: Evaluation of dyspepsia. Am Gastroenterological Association. Gastroenterology 114:582–595, 1998.

123

6

PREVENTIVE HEALTH CARE FOR WOMEN

Margaret A. Miller

PREVENTION AND SCREENING

It is estimated that nearly one half of deaths from the 10 leading causes of death in the United States are attributed to modifiable behavior. Early detection and treatment of many common diseases can lead to significant reductions in morbidity and mortality. The obstetrician/gynecologist plays a pivotal role in effective prevention and screening for women. Many women, especially during reproductive years, rely solely on their obstetrician/gynecologist for preventive care. This chapter is intended to provide the clinician with a framework for implementing good screening and preventive practices for women.

Screening refers to the detection of disease at an asymptomatic or preclinical stage. Screening may be done by history, physical examination, laboratory testing, or other procedure.

Primary prevention occurs before disease onset and is intended to prevent disease from occurring at all. Examples of primary prevention include immunization to prevent disease and folic acid to prevent neural tube defects. The goal of secondary prevention is to detect disease when it is asymptomatic and prevent progression of disease. Examples include Papanicolaou (Pap) smears and fecal occult blood testing to detect malignancies in their earliest stages. Tertiary prevention occurs after the onset of clinically apparent disease and is aimed at preventing further complications. An example of tertiary prevention is β-blockers to reduce recurrent myocardial infarction (MI).

Putting prevention and screening into practice can be difficult for busy clinicians. First, clinicians must be aware of and have access to the most updated guidelines for preventive services. Evidence-based practice guidelines for prevention and screening have been published by the American College of Physicians, the United States Preventive Services Task Force (USPSTF), and the Canadian Task Force on Preventive Health Care. A comprehensive database of evidence-based clinical practice guidelines is provided by the National Guideline Clearinghouse (NGC). The NGC is an initiative of the Agency for Healthcare Research and Quality, U.S. Department of Health and Human Services, and is available online (http://www.

guideline.gov). Many of the guidelines are available in a summary format ideal for posting, carrying in a pocket, or downloading to a portable computer. Second, a plan should be developed to implement these guidelines in the office. Helpful tools include a "Health Maintenance" flow sheet to be placed in the front of the chart. Nurses or medical assistants can be trained to review the flow sheet and to provide reminders for the physician and patient about preventive services that may be due. Computer-based programs are also very helpful in monitoring such services. Many providers also find it useful to include "health maintenance" as part of the problem list, which may serve as a prompt to review and update screening and preventive services at each yearly examination.

The components of prevention and screening that will be reviewed in this chapter include the following:

1. Assessment of cardiovascular risk including screening and detection of hypertension, hyperlipidemia, and diabetes as well as assessment of smoking status, level of physical activity, and weight management
2. Prevention and detection of osteoporosis
3. Screening and detection of thyroid disease
4. Adult immunizations
5. Cancer screening including screening for breast, ovarian, cervical, colorectal, lung, and skin cancer
6. Screening and detection of depression, dementia, substance abuse, and domestic violence

PREVENTION OF CARDIOVASCULAR DISEASE

Cardiovascular disease is the leading cause of death in women in the United States. Mortality from cardiovascular disease is greater than all other causes combined. It is estimated that nearly one in two women in the United States will die from heart disease or stroke. Women as well as health care providers often lack an understanding of their risk of cardiovascular disease. Recognizing this deficit in knowledge, the American Heart Association has recently identified education of women as a top priority in the fight to prevent cardiovascular disease.

Risk Factor Assessment

An important part of the preventive health examination for all women is identification of cardiovascular risk factors. Risk factors for cardiovascular disease have been well documented (Box 6-1) and should be reviewed with patients on a yearly basis. Many of these risk factors are modifiable and, if identified early, can lead to significant reduction in morbidity and mortality. Pregnancy offers an ideal opportunity to identify risk factors and to promote lifestyle changes to reduce future risk. Pregnant women are often highly motivated to make healthy lifestyle choices, and the regular prenatal office visits provide a unique opportunity to promote behavior change. In menopause, the risk of cardiovascular disease increases

---

Box 6-1 Cardiovascular Risk Factors

Primary risk factors
Personal history of coronary heart disease (CHD)
Age older than 55 years
Dyslipidemia (high levels of low-density lipoproteins or low levels of high-density lipoproteins)
Family history of CHD (first-degree male relative younger than 55 years, or female younger than 65 years)
Diabetes mellitus
Smoking
Hypertension
Peripheral vascular disease

Other risk factors
Sedentary lifestyle
High triglyceride levels
Obesity

127

---

substantially, so the yearly preventive health examination for postmenopausal women should emphasize assessment and modification of cardiovascular risk factors. For all women, the yearly examination should include screening for hypertension, hyperlipidemia, and diabetes when appropriate (see below); counseling about smoking cessation, weight management, healthy diet, and physical activity; and a discussion about pharmacologic interventions that may modify the risks of developing cardiovascular disease, such as aspirin and hormone replacement therapy (HRT).

Hypertension

It is estimated that 52% of women older than 45 years of age have elevated blood pressure. African American women have a significant increase in the incidence of hypertension as well as complications from hypertension and therefore warrant special attention. Blood pressure should be measured as part of a routine evaluation.

Accurate blood pressure measurement is essential to correct diagnosis. Proper blood pressure measurement requires the following conditions:

1. Patient should be seated quietly for 5 minutes in a chair with feet on the floor and arm held at the level of the heart.
2. An appropriately sized cuff should be used (cuff bladder should encircle 80% of the arm).
3. The bladder should be inflated to 20 mm Hg above the systolic pressure as estimated by loss of the radial pulse.
4. The bladder should be deflated slowly (no more than 3 mm Hg/sec).
5. The blood pressure should be taken in both arms, with the higher pressure documented.

A diagnosis of hypertension should only be made after two elevated readings over the course of separate visits. Table 6-1 provides the most recent classification of blood pressure with recommendations for initial

Table 6-1

Blood Pressure Classification	mm Hg	Lifestyle Changes	Medication
Normal	<120/80	Encourage	None
Prehypertension	120–139/80–89	Recommend	No drug indicated except in patients with compelling indications*
Hypertension			
Stage 1	140–159/90–99	Recommend	First choice is thiazide diuretic
Stage 2	>160/100	Recommend	Initiate two-drug therapy. Thiazide diuretic in combination with β-blocker, ACE-I, ARB, CCB

*Compelling indications include heart failure, post–myocardial infarction, diabetes, chronic kidney disease, cerebrovascular disease, or high coronary disease risk.
ACE-I, angiotensin-converting enzyme inhibitors; ARB, angiotensin-receptor blockers; CCB, calcium channel blocker.

therapy. Evaluation of newly diagnosed hypertension includes three objectives: to identify other cardiovascular risk factors, to assess for evidence of target-organ damage, and to identify reversible causes of hypertension.

Hypertension is categorized as either essential hypertension (idiopathic or primary) or secondary hypertension (due to a known cause). Between 90% and 95% of newly diagnosed hypertension is due to essential hypertension. Although a complete workup for secondary causes is not necessary, all patients should be screened for underlying disorders that may lead to hypertension (Table 6-2). Risk factors for essential hypertension include a family history of hypertension, increased salt intake, excess alcohol intake, obesity, African American race, and certain personality traits.

Primary target organs affected by hypertension include the heart, brain, kidney, and eyes. Patients should be screened for target-organ damage at initial diagnosis and yearly thereafter (Table 6-3). Assessment of cardiac risk factors should also be done at initial diagnosis as well as yearly in hypertensive patients.

Laboratory testing for newly diagnosed patients with hypertension should include an electrocardiogram, urinalysis, blood glucose, hematocrit, serum potassium, creatinine, calcium, and a lipid profile. More extensive testing should be pursued only if the history and/or physical examination results are suggestive of a secondary cause (see Table 6-2). The electrocardiogram, fasting blood glucose, and lipid panel as well as assessment of renal function with a urinalysis and creatinine should be repeated yearly in all patients with hypertension. Also, all hypertensive patients should be counseled about lifestyle changes that have been shown to lower blood pressure. These include weight reduction, healthy diet rich in fruits and vegetables and low in fat, reduced sodium intake, regular physical activity, and moderation of alcohol consumption (Table 6-4).

Table 6-2   Secondary Causes of Hypertension

Condition	Symptoms	Signs Other Than Hypertension	Screening Test
Primary renal disease Renal artery stenosis Glomerular disease	Usually none	Abdominal/flank bruit Hematuria, large palpable kidneys, edema	Urinalysis, creatinine
Drugs (OCP, NSAIDs, pseudoephedrine)	Usually asymptomatic	None	Medication history
Pheochromocytoma	"5 Ps": Palpitation Pallor Perspiration Pain (chest, head, abdomen) Pressure (HBP)	Tremor, weight loss, anxiety	Screen for signs and symptoms; if present, do plasma-free metanephrine level; if none, no lab evaluation necessary
Primary hyperaldosteronism	Usually asymptomatic	Abnormalities found during exam are rare	Electrolytes (may have low K+, high Na)
Hyperthyroidism	Anxiety, increased sweating, heat intolerance, palpitations, dyspnea, fatigue, weight loss	Tachycardia, weight loss, may have goiter, tremor, warm, moist skin, exophthalmos	Thyroid-stimulating hormone
Hyperparathyroidism	"Bones, stones, groans, moans"; that is, painful bones, renal stones, abdominal pain, and psychiatric symptoms	Nephrolithiasis, polyuria, weight loss, bone pain, muscle weakness, apathy	Calcium
Cushing's disease	Emotional lability, muscle weakness, easy bruising	Moon facies, central obesity, striae, osteoporosis, diabetes, hirsutism	Screen for signs and symptoms; if present, check 24-hour urinary free cortisol or consider dexamethasone suppression test; if none, no lab evaluation necessary
Sleep apnea	Excessive daytime sleepiness, snoring	Obesity, low-lying palate	Screen for signs and symptoms; if present, refer for sleep study
Coarctation of the aorta	Usually asymptomatic, may have headaches, exertional leg fatigue and pain, epistaxis	Prominent neck pulsations, delayed peripheral pulses bruit over back	Screen for signs and symptoms; if present, check CXR (may have rib notching, "3 sign"); if none, no lab evaluation necessary

OCP, Oral contraceptive pill; NSAIDs, nonsteroidal anti-inflammatory drug; HBP, high blood pressure; K+ = potassium; Na, sodium; CXR, chest x-ray.

129

Table 6-3

Evaluation for
End-Organ Damage

Heart	Check ECG to rule out LVH
Kidneys	Check urinalysis, creatinine. If abnormal, do 24-hour urine for protein and creatinine clearance
Eyes	Funduscopic examination to check for retinopathy
Brain	Check for signs and symptoms of brain injury/dementia

ECG, electrocardiogram; LVH, left ventricular hypertrophy.

Table 6-4

Lifestyle
Modifications to
Prevent and Manage
Hypertension

Modification	Recommendation	Approximate SBP Reduction
Weight reduction	Maintain healthy body weight (BMI < 25 kg/m^2)	5–20 mm Hg/10 kg
Adopt DASH eating plan	Diet rich in fruits, vegetables, and low-fat dairy products with a reduced content of saturated and total fat	8–14 mm Hg
Dietary sodium reduction	Reduce dietary sodium intake to no more than 100 mmol/day (2.4 g sodium or 6 g sodium chloride	2–8 mm Hg
Physical activity	Regular aerobic physical activity, such as brisk walking (at least 30 min/day most days of the week)	4–9 mm Hg
Moderation of alcohol consumption	Limit consumption to no more than one drink per day in women	2–4 mm Hg

Adapted from Chobanian AV, Bakris GL, Black HR, et al: The Seventh Report of the Joint National Committee on Prevention, Detection, Evaluation and Treatment of High Blood Pressure. The JNC 7 Report. JAMA 289:2560–2572, 2003.
SBP, Systolic blood pressure; BMI, body mass index; DASH, dietary approaches to stop hypertension.

Pharmacologic therapy should be initiated in patients with blood pressure higher than 140/90 mm Hg on two or more readings. Thiazide-type diuretics should be the initial drug of choice, either alone or in combination with another drug for most patients. Several classes of drugs have been shown to be effective in lowering blood pressure and reducing complications from hypertension, including angiotensin-converting enzyme inhibitors, angiotensin-receptor blockers, β-blockers, calcium channel blockers, and thiazide-type diuretic agents. Patients with diabetes or kidney, cardiac, or pulmonary disease may have compelling reasons to use or avoid specific medicines.

Dyslipidemia

Data from epidemiologic studies show a clear relationship between plasma cholesterol levels and risk of coronary heart disease (CHD). High concentrations of low-density lipoproteins (LDLs) are directly related to risk for coronary disease and cardiac mortality. Low concentrations of high-density lipoproteins (HDLs) are also predictive of CHD and appear to constitute a more potent risk factor in women than men. A meta-analysis of 38 studies found that for every 10% reduction in serum cholesterol, CHD mortality was reduced by 15% and total mortality risk by 11%. For these reasons, identifying and treating dyslipidemia is an important part of the preventive examination.

The most recent guidelines from the National Cholesterol Education Program recommend that all patients older than 20 years of age have an initial screening test for cholesterol. A fasting lipid profile is recommended. Subsequently, persons with no known coronary disease who have a desirable LDL level should be rescreened in 5 years. Patients who have borderline results and fewer than two cardiac risk factors should be rescreened in 2 years. Goals for cholesterol are based on LDL levels and should be individualized based on the patient's other cardiac risk factors. Determining the LDL goal and cutpoint for treatment requires the following four steps:

Step 1. Identify CHD or CHD equivalents. CHD equivalents include the following:

a. Diabetes
b. Symptomatic carotid stenosis
c. Peripheral vascular disease
d. Aortic abdominal aneurysm
e. Multiple risk factors that confer a 10-year risk of cardiac event of more than 20%

Step 2. Identify cardiac risk factors other than hyperlipidemia. These include the following:

a. Smoking
b. Hypertension
c. Low HDL (<40)
d. Family history of premature coronary artery disease (CAD; first-degree male relative with onset of CAD at an age younger than 55 years, first-degree female relative with onset of CAD at an age younger than 65 years)
e. Age (men older than 45 years, women older than 55 years)
f. If HDL is greater than 60, subtract 1 risk factor

Step 3. If more than two cardiac risk factors are present, determine the 10-year risk of a cardiac event using the Framingham scoring system (Table 6-5).

Step 4. Use the information to determine the risk category and the corresponding LDL goal.

Table 6-6 reviews the LDL cholesterol goals and cutpoints for treatment based on risk category. Therapeutic lifestyle changes are an important part of treatment for all patients with hyperlipidemia. Reduction in dietary saturated fat and cholesterol is recommended. The addition of plant stanols and sterols has also been shown to improve cholesterol. Referral to a nutritionist to help establish a diet plan is very helpful for most patients.

Table 6-5

Framingham Scoring System (Estimate of 10 Year Risk of CHD Event for Women)

Point Score by Age Group	
Age	Points
20–34	−7
35–39	−3
40–44	0
45–49	3
50–54	6
55–59	8
60–64	10
65–69	12
70–74	14
75–79	16

Point Scores by Age Group and Cholesterol					
Total Cholesterol	Age 20–39	Age 40–49	Age 50–59	Age 60–69	Age 70–79
<160	0	0	0	0	0
160–199	4	3	2	1	1
200–239	8	6	4	2	1
240–279	11	8	5	3	2
280+	13	10	7	4	2

Point Scores by Age Group and Smoking Status					
	Age 20–39	Age 40–49	Age 50–59	Age 60–69	Age 70–79
Nonsmoker	0	0	0	0	0
Smoker	9	7	4	2	1

Point Scores by HDL Level	
HDL	Points
60+	−1
50–59	0
40–49	1
<40	2

Point Scores by Systolic Blood Pressure (BP) and Treatment Status		
Systolic BP	If Untreated	If Treated
<120	0	0
120–129	1	3
130–139	2	4
140–159	3	5
160+	4	6

10-Year Risk of Cardiac Event by Total Point Scores	
Point Total	10-Year Risk
<9	<1%
9–12	1%
13–14	2%
15	3%
16	4%
17	5%

10-Year Risk of Cardiac Event by Total Point Scores—cont'd	
Point Total	**10-Year Risk**
18	6%
19	8%
20	11%
21	14%
22	17%
23	22%
24	27%
>25	>30%

HDL, high-density lipoprotein.

Table 6-6

LDL Cholesterol Goals and Cutpoints for Therapeutic Lifestyle Changes (TLCs) and Drug Therapy in Different Risk Categories

	LDL Goal	LDL Level at Which to Initiate TLC	LDL Level at Which to Initiate Medications
CHD or CHD equivalent (see text)	<100	>100	>130 100–129, drug optional
2+ CHD risk factors	<130		10-year risk 10% to 20% >130
		>130	10-year risk < 10% >160–190
0–1 CHD risk factors	<160	>160	160–190 drug optional

Adapted from Executive Summary of the Third Report of the National Cholesterol Education Program (NCEP) Expert Panel on Detection, Evaluation and Treatment of High Blood Cholesterol in Adults (Adult Treatment Panel III).
LDL, low-density lipoprotein; CHD, coronary heart disease.
Use Framingham Scoring System for estimate of 10-year risk for women.

In addition, patients should be encouraged to engage in moderate physical activity and maintain a healthy weight (body mass index [BMI] < 25). If the target LDL is not achieved after 6 to 12 weeks of therapeutic lifestyle changes, pharmacotherapy should be initiated.

Diabetes

Diabetes mellitus (DM) is a heterogeneous group of conditions with hyperglycemia as their most common clinical manifestation. Type I DM (previously referred to as insulin-dependent DM) accounts for 6% to 10% of all persons with DM and is an autoimmune disease associated with certain human leukocyte antigen genes. Type II DM (previously referred to as non–insulin dependent DM) accounts for 85% to 90% of all persons with DM in the United States and is not linked to human leukocyte antigen. However, evidence for a genetic predisposition to type II DM is overwhelming.

Diabetes is considered a powerful risk factor for cardiovascular disease, especially in women. The American Diabetes Association recommends screening for diabetes in all patients who have any of the following risk factors:

- Age older than 45 years
- Family history of diabetes in parents or sibling
- Obesity (BMI > 27 kg/m^2)
- Member of high-risk ethnic group (e.g., Native American, Asian American, Hispanic, African American, Pacific Islander)
- Previously identified impaired glucose tolerance or impaired fasting glucose
- Hypertension or hyperlipidemia
- History of gestational diabetes or baby weighing more than 4 kg (9 pounds) at birth

A fasting blood sugar test is the screening of choice. A diagnosis of diabetes is made if one or more of the following conditions are met:

1. Classic symptoms (e.g., polyuria, polydipsia, unexplained weight loss) and a random plasma blood sugar level of at least 200 mg/dL
2. Fasting blood sugar level of more than 126 mg/dL on two occasions
3. Two-hour postprandial blood sugar level of more than 200 mg/dL on two occasions

Glucose values for normal, impaired blood sugar and diabetes are shown in Table 6-7.

The initial evaluation of a patient with diabetes should include a thorough history and physical examination as well as laboratory evaluation (Box 6-2). The goal of therapy in all patients is euglycemia (HbA1c < 7%). It is well documented in randomized controlled trials that intensive control of both type I and type II diabetes will lead to a significant reduction in microvascular complications. Initial therapy for an asymptomatic patient with type II diabetes begins with diet, weight reduction, and exercise. Medications are often needed to achieve normal glucose levels and target HbA1c range (Table 6-8).

Obesity

In the United States, 64% of adults are either overweight (33%) or obese (31%). The rise in the prevalence of obesity in the United States has been marked and sudden, especially in children. Obesity is associated with a three-fold increased risk of hypertension, diabetes, hyperlipidemia, and death from cardiovascular disease. In addition, obesity increases the risk of a number of other conditions including obstructive sleep apnea,

Table 6-7

Glucose Values

	Normal	Impaired Fasting Glucose	Diabetes
Fasting plasma glucose	<100 mg/dL	100–126 mg/dL	>126 mg/dL
2-hour postload glucose	<140 mg/dL	140–200 mg/dL	>200 mg/dL

Box 6-2   Initial Evaluation for Type II Diabetes

History
Symptoms of hyper- or hypoglycemia
Medications (including current or previous use of insulin or oral hypoglycemics)
Glucose self-monitoring program (current or previous)
Dietary habits and nutritional education
Exercise and daily activity habits
Other cardiovascular risk factors
Reproductive status, contraceptive methods
Substance use, especially smoking status

Physical examination
Weight, height, BMI
Blood pressure
Funduscopic exam (with referral to ophthalmologist for ongoing care)
Periodontal exam
Cardiovascular exam (including peripheral pulses and bruits)
Foot and skin exam
Neurologic exam for peripheral sensation, loss of proprioception, autonomic
    dysfunction (lack of sweating, tachycardia)

Laboratory evaluation
Fasting blood sugar
HbA1C
Fasting lipid profile
Blood urea nitrogen/creatinine, potassium
Urine for microalbumin
ECG

thrombosis, osteoarthritis, and several types of cancer. The definitions of obesity can be found in Table 6-9. The patient's height and weight should be measured yearly and the BMI calculated. Weight loss strategies that promote gradual and sustained weight loss should be encouraged. Pharmacotherapy for the treatment of obesity has, in general, been associated with little benefit in sustained weight loss and is often limited by adverse effects. Surgical intervention may be considered in patients with morbid obesity (BMI > 40 or BMI > 35 with obesity-related morbidity) after a careful consideration of all options and risks of surgery.

Smoking

Screening for tobacco use should be considered an essential "vital sign," and all patients should be asked about smoking status at each visit. Smoking is the number one preventable cause of death in the United States. Patients should be asked about total years of exposure to cigarettes, and a pack-year history (number of packs multiplied by years smoked) should be documented. Counseling for smoking cessation should include the "5 A's":

1. **Ask:** Patients should be asked about smoking at each visit, and the answer should be documented in the chart.

Table 6-8 Oral Diabetes Medications

Drug	Mechanism	Side Effects	Cautions/Contraindications
Sulfonylurea	Increase insulin secretion	Weight gain and hypoglycemia	Diabetic ketoacidosis (DKA)
First generation			
Tolbutamide (Orinase)			
Chlorpropramide (Diabinase)			
Acetohexamide			
Second generation			
Glipizide (Glucotrol)			
Glyburide (Micronase, Diabeta)			
Glimerpride (Amaryl)			
Biguanides	Improve insulin sensitivity in peripheral tissues, inhibit hepatic glucose output and stimulate glucose uptake by peripheral tissues	Lactic acidosis, diarrhea, nausea, vomiting, flatulence, abdominal discomfort, hypoglycemia, myalgia, dizziness	Renal insufficiency because of lactic acidosis
Metformin (Glucophage)			Hold for iodinated contrast study Monitor creatinine
Thiazolidinediones	Decrease insulin resistance	Congestive Heart Failure (CHF) and liver abnormalities	Liver abnormalities, edema, CHF Monitor liver function tests every 2 months for 1 year
Rosiglitazone (Avandia)			
Pioglitazone (Actos)			
Glucosidase inhibitors	Inhibit enzymatic breakdown of starches in the small intestine, delay absorption of carbohydrates and reduce postprandial hyperglycemia	Diarrhea, bloating, cramping	Diarrhea, bloating, cramping Contraindicated in cirrhosis, irritable bowel syndrome, DKA, bowel obstruction Use caution in cases of impaired renal function
Acarbose (Precose)			
Miglitol (Glyset)			
Other	Stimulates pancreatic islet cells to release insulin	Hypoglycemia; rare cases of hepatic dysfunction, Stevens Johnson, hemolytic anemia, pancreatitis	Insulin-dependent diabetes mellitus, ketoacidosis Use caution with renal disease
Repaglinide (Prandin)			
Nateglinide (Starlix)			

Table 6-9

Overweight	BMI 25.0–29.9 kg/m^2
Obese	BMI >30 kg/m^2
Morbid obesity	BMI > 40 kg/m^2

BMI, body mass index.

2. **Assess:** Assess the patient's readiness to quit. If patient not ready to commit to quit date, address barriers to quitting.
3. **Advise:** Advise patients about the dangers on smoking with a clear, strong, and personalized message. The benefits of cessation should be stressed.
4. **Assist:** Assist the patient to set a quit date. Offer educational materials and referral for behavioral therapy or formal cessation program. Discuss pharmacologic options as indicated.
5. **Arrange:** Arrange a follow-up. Reinforce nonsmoking status.

Exercise

A recent report of the U.S. Surgeon General found that 25% of women report no sustained physical activity. Additionally, a national survey found that women were significantly less likely to enroll in cardiac rehabilitation after an MI than men. Providers should ask about physical activity including household work, leisure time, and occupational physical activity. All patients should be encouraged to engage in a minimum of 30 minutes of physical activity on most days of the week. This may be achieved with several shorter bouts of activity of at least 10 minutes. In addition to aerobic activity, strengthening exercises are important in the prevention of osteoporosis as well as maintaining adequate functional ability as a woman ages.

HRT and Aspirin for Primary Prevention

Although a number of observational studies have suggested that HRT protects against cardiovascular disease, a large multicenter randomized controlled trial (i.e., Women's Health Initiative) recently found that HRT had no benefit and even increased the rate of cardiovascular disease in the first year of its use. Despite known benefits in preventing osteoporotic fractures, HRT is associated with a number of risks including thrombosis, breast cancer, and cholecystitis. The weight of the evidence would suggest that the risks of HRT would exceed the benefit in most patients.

The benefit of aspirin in patients with known cardiovascular disease is well established. Whether aspirin may prevent cardiovascular disease in patients with no history of cardiovascular disease is controversial. A number of randomized controlled trials have not included women, but those studies that have included women have shown a reduction in the incidence of MI, yet with no effect on the incidence of ischemic stroke in the aspirin group. Aspirin also increases the risk of hemorrhagic stroke and gastrointestinal bleeding. These potential risks and benefits must be weighed in each individual patient. The balance of benefit and harm is

137

most favorable in patients at high risk for cardiovascular disease. Primary prevention with aspirin should not be recommended for patients with a history of gastrointestinal bleeding.

OSTEOPOROSIS

It is estimated that 50% of white women will experience an osteoporotic fracture at some time in her life. Most often these fractures occur in the spine, hip, or wrist; however, almost all fractures in older women are at least in part due to low bone mass. Fractures in older women are often followed by chronic pain, limitations in function, and even death. For example, 25% of women who sustain a hip fracture will require long-term nursing care, and only 40% fully regain their prior level of functioning. Hip fractures are also associated with a 10% to 20% excess mortality within 1 year.

Screening for osteoporosis should be performed in all postmenopausal women. Assessment of clinical risk factors should be done on a yearly basis (Box 6-3).

Bone mineral density (BMD) testing should be done on all women older than 65 years regardless of risk factors, younger postmenopausal women with one or more risk factor (other than being white, postmenopausal, and female), and postmenopausal women who present with a fracture. Dual-energy x-ray absorptiometry (DEXA) of the central hip and spine is the preferred technique for screening and diagnosis.

Interventions to reduce fracture risk should be discussed with all postmenopausal women. All women should be assessed for adequate intake of calcium (at least 1200 mg/day) and vitamin D (at least 400 to 800

Box 6-3   Risk Factors for Osteoporosis

Major risk factors
Personal history of fracture as an adult
History of fragility fracture in a first-degree relative
Low body weight
Current tobacco smoking
Use of oral corticosteroid therapy for longer than 3 months

Additional risk factors
Impaired vision
Estrogen deficiency at an early age (younger than 45 years)
Dementia
Poor health/frailty
Recent falls
Low calcium intake (lifelong)
Low physical activity
Alcohol intake of more than 2 drinks per day

IU/day). Women should be encouraged to participate in regular weight-bearing and strengthening exercise. Additionally, avoidance of tobacco or excess alcohol and treatment of any other risk factors such as vision impairment should be addressed. Pharmacologic therapy should be considered in women with a BMD T-score below -2 by hip DEXA with no other risk factors, a BMD T-score below -1.5 by hip DEXA with one or more risk factors, or a personal history of a prior vertebral or hip fracture.

Table 6-10 provides information on drugs approved by the U.S. Food and Drug Administration (FDA) for the prevention or treatment of osteoporosis. Repeat bone density testing should be done every 1 to 2 years to monitor progression of disease. There is some evidence that combination drug therapy (usually a bisphosphonate with nonbisphosphonate) may provide minor improvements in bone density compared with monotherapy. However, the effect of combination therapy on the incidence of fracture is unknown. This, along with potential side effects and costs, needs to be weighed against potential benefits in each individual patient.

139

THYROID DISEASE

The prevalence of thyroid dysfunction is increased in women, especially older women, compared with men. Although thyroid dysfunction encompasses hypothyroidism, hyperthyroidism, and goiter, hypothyroidism is by far the most common clinical entity. Hypothyroidism most often occurs in women between the ages of 40 and 60 years. The overall incidence is around 1% of the female population, but it can be as high as 6% in women older than 60 years of age. Subclinical hypothyroidism is reported to occur in 5% to 17% of the population. Symptoms of hypothyroidism are nonspecific and include weakness, fatigue, sleepiness, cold intolerance, constipation, dry skin, hair loss, hoarseness, muscle aches and stiffness, menstrual disturbances, decreased libido, and depression. Myxedema (i.e., nonpitting peripheral edema) occurs only in severe cases.

The thyroid-stimulating hormone (TSH) assay is a highly sensitive test that can detect subclinical disease in an asymptomatic patient. Data regarding the clinical benefit of screening for thyroid disease are inconsistent and therefore recommendations regarding screening of asymptomatic patients are varied. The American Thyroid Association recommends that all adults be screened for thyroid dysfunction with a TSH assay beginning at the age of 35 years and every 5 years thereafter. The USPSTF concludes that the evidence is insufficient to recommend for or against routine screening for thyroid disease. Clinicians should be alert to the sometimes subtle presentation of thyroid disease and should consider screening in all patients with symptoms. This is particularly important in pregnancy since even subclinical disease may have an impact on the cognitive functioning of the offspring.

Table 6-10

FDA-Approved Drugs
for the Prevention
and Treatment of
Osteoporosis

Drug	Dose	Side Effects	Comments
Bisphosphonates Alendronate (Fosamax)	Prevention: 5 mg/day or 35 mg/week Treatment: 10 mg/day or 70 mg/ week	Upper gastrointestinal disorders (e.g., dysphagia, esophagitis, esophageal or gastric ulcer)	Should be taken on an empty stomach, first thing in the morning with water only. Patients should be instructed to refrain from eating or drinking and remain upright for 30 minutes after taking the dose.
Risedronate (Actonel)	Prevention and treatment: 5 mg/day or 35 mg/week		
Calcitonin (Miacalcin)	200 IU single intranasal spray Also available by subcutaneous delivery	Rarely rhinitis and epistaxis	Approved for treatment of osteoporosis in women who are at least 5 years postmenopausal. Instruct patient to alternate nostrils each day.
Estrogen/HRT	Various preparations	May increase risk of cardiovascular disease, breast cancer, thrombosis, cholestasis	FDA recommends that non- estrogen treatments should be considered first for prevention of osteoporosis.
Parathyroid hormone (Forteo)	20 µg daily subcutaneous	Leg cramps, dizziness	Approved for treatment of osteoporosis for postmenopausal women at high risk of fracture. Contraindicated in women with a history of Paget's, prior radiation therapy of the skeleton, bone metastases, hypercalcemia, or skeletal malignancy.
Raloxifene (Evista)	60 mg/day po	May increase hot flashes, increases risk of thrombosis	Approved for prevention and treatment.

IMMUNIZATIONS

Routine immunizations continue to be an important part of preventive health for all women. Although most women are very aware of the importance of immunizations for children, they may be less knowledgeable about the need for ongoing immunizations in adulthood. Table 6-11 provides information about indications and dosing for adult immunizations as well as recommendations for immunization during pregnancy. Because of the theoretical risk of transmission to the fetus, live-virus vaccines are contraindicated during pregnancy. Most other vaccines are safe and should be offered to pregnant women when indicated.

CANCER SCREENING

Breast Cancer

Breast cancer is the second deadliest cancer in women. A large body of evidence exists to support screening for breast cancer. Screening strategies may include breast self-examination, clinical breast examination by a health care provider, and screening mammography. All expert groups agree on the benefit of screening mammography with or without clinical breast examination for all women older than 50 years on an annual basis. There is some controversy over the benefit of screening mammography for women aged 40 to 50 years. Most groups agree that routine screening should be recommended every 1 to 2 years for women at average risk for breast cancer. Forty- to 50-year-old women with risk factors for breast cancer—particularly a strong family history of breast cancer—should be screened every year. There is also no clear consensus about promoting breast self-examination. Studies are few and have not shown a clear benefit in reducing mortality from breast cancer. In addition, a few studies have shown an increase incidence of breast biopsies for benign disease in women who learn to perform breast self-examination.

A reasonable approach to breast cancer screening is to recommend mammography and clinical breast examination to all women older than 50 years of age. Screening for women aged 40 to 50 years must be individualized based on each patient's risk factors and the potential for a false-positive result. Women who wish to do breast self-examination should be advised about the limitations of this practice.

Yet another area of controversy is the age at which screening mammography may be discontinued. The role of screening mammography in women older than 70 years of age has never been adequately studied. Most experts agree that women with a life expectancy of more than 5 years are likely to benefit from continued screening.

In recent years, much attention has been focused on the development of pharmacologic agents to prevent breast cancer. Selective estrogen receptor modulators have been found to be an effective tertiary prevention strategy to prevent the recurrence of breast cancer. A large randomized controlled

Table 6-11 Adult Immunizations

Vaccine/Dose	Indications	Revaccinate	Pregnancy
Influenza, 1 dose	All adults older than 50 years All adults with chronic disease (e.g., heart, pulmonary, renal, metabolic, immunosuppression, sickle cell anemia) Residents of chronic care facilities Health care workers Pregnancy of more than 13 weeks' gestation during influenza season	Annually	All women who will be pregnant during influenza season should be vaccinated. Pregnant women may be vaccinated in any trimester. Vaccine should be given subcutaneously. Intranasal influenza vaccine is a live attenuated vaccine and should not be given in pregnancy
Pneumococcal, 1 dose	All adults older than 65 years Persons younger than 65 years with chronic disease (e.g., heart, pulmonary [excluding asthma], diabetes, renal, liver, alcoholism, immunosuppressed, sickle cell anemia, asplenia) Alaska natives and Native Americans	If initial dose given when a person is younger than 65 years, revaccinate once after age 65 years, at least 5 years after initial dose. In patients with chronic disease at highest risk of pneumococcus (e.g., asplenia, organ transplant, HIV, nephrotic syndrome, malignancy, chronic renal failure, immunosuppression), revaccinate once at least 5 years after initial dose	Indications for administration are not altered by pregnancy. Safety in first trimester has not been evaluated.
Tetanus, diphtheria, 1 dose	All adults	Booster every 10 years in all adults. For patients with wounds, revaccinate if last dose was given more than 5 years previously	No evidence of harmful fetal effects. Should be considered if otherwise indicated.

| Hepatitis B, 3 doses at 0, 1, and 6 months | All children younger than 18 years
Adults older than 18 years with risk factors (i.e., IV drug use, multiple sexual partners, recent STD, male homosexual sex, household contact or sex partners of persons with chronic hepatitis B, health care workers, staff of institutions for developmentally disabled or imprisoned, inmates of correctional institutions, persons receiving hemodialysis or who receive clotting factor concentrates, international travelers who will be in countries with high or intermediate prevalence of hepatitis B for more than 6 months) | None | Pregnant women with risk factors should be immunized. All neonates of women with acute or chronic hepatitis should be given hepatitis B immunoglobulin and hepatitis B vaccine. |
| Hepatitis A, 2 doses at 0 and 6 months | History of chronic liver disease
Clotting disorder
IV drug use
Men who have sex with men
Travelers to countries with high or intermediate prevalence of hepatitis A
Persons with occupational risk who work with hepatitis A virus-infected primates | None | Should be considered if otherwise indicated. |

continued

Table 6-11 Adult Immunizations—cont'd

Vaccine/Dose	Indications	Revaccinate	Pregnancy
Measles, mumps, rubella	No evidence of immunity to measles and are: Health care workers College students Travelers to foreign countries Asymptomatic persons infected with HIV who have CD4 counts less than 200 Persons recently exposed to measles	**One dose** in women of childbearing age with no evidence of immunity to rubella, health care workers with no evidence of immunity to rubella, college students and travelers if no evidence of immunity to rubella or mumps. Consider for persons previously vaccinated with killed mumps vaccine or before 1979 with an unknown mumps vaccine. **Two doses at 0 and at least 1 month subsequent** if previously vaccinated with killed measles vaccine or between 1963 and 1967 with unknown measles vaccine.	Contraindicated in pregnancy. Pregnancy should be avoided for at least 4 weeks after immunization.
Varicella, 2 doses at 0 and 4 to 8 weeks	Health care workers with no evidence of immunity and no reliable history of disease Susceptible family members and other close contacts of immunocompromised persons Consider for susceptible persons who have high risk of exposure (e.g., school teachers, college students, residents and staff of residential institutions, day care workers) and for women considering pregnancy	None	The effects of varicella vaccine on the fetus are unknown. Pregnant women should not be vaccinated. Pregnancy should be avoided for 1 month after each dose. VZIG should be given to pregnant women who have been exposed to varicella.

HIV, Human immunodeficiency virus; IV, intravenous; STD, sexually transmitted disease; VZIG, varicella zoster immunoglobulin.

trial also found the selective estrogen receptor modulator tamoxifen to be an effective primary prevention agent in women with an increased risk of breast cancer. The FDA has approved the use of tamoxifen for primary prevention of breast cancer in certain high-risk women. Tamoxifen should not, however, be routinely used for primary prevention of breast cancer in women carrying low or average risk. Breast cancer screening is discussed at length in Chapter 21, Conditions of the Female Breast.

Ovarian Cancer

In the United States, ovarian cancer remains the leading cause of death from gynecologic malignancies. Ovarian neoplasms can be broadly divided into three categories: epithelial tumors, sex cord stromal tumors, and germ cell tumors. Epithelial ovarian cancer is responsible for the preponderance of morbidity and mortality and has been the focus of multiple studies evaluating screening programs.

The incidence of ovarian cancer increases with age, with the highest incidence occurring between the ages of 50 and 60 years. The majority of women with ovarian cancer present only after the cancer has spread beyond the ovary. Early-stage disease rarely causes significant symptoms. Although early detection would certainly reduce mortality, there is currently no adequate screening strategy for average risk women. Studies of the marker for ovarian and endometrial carcinomas (CA-125) and ultrasound in this population have been associated with an unacceptably high rate of false-positive results, leading to increased morbidity and cost. Women with a family history of ovarian cancer may benefit from screening. Most of these women will have a sporadic case of ovarian cancer in the family. Such patients should be counseled about the possible benefit and limitations of screening and may be offered serial CA-125 and ultrasound screenings on a yearly basis. This may be particularly beneficial in postmenopausal women. It is likely that women with a suspected hereditary ovarian cancer syndrome will benefit the most from screening. Surveillance includes CA-125 and other tumor markers as well as transvaginal ultrasound every 6 months. Testing for BRCA gene mutations should be considered in this population. Prophylactic oophorectomy after childbearing years or by the age of 35 years is generally recommended for women with true hereditary ovarian cancer syndrome. Ovarian neoplasms are more thoroughly discussed in Chapter 20, Disorders of the Fallopian Tube and Ovary.

Cervical Cancer

Although there has never been a randomized controlled trial documenting the benefit of screening Papanicolaou (Pap) smears, it is clear that the incidence of cervical cancer and death from cervical cancer has significantly declined with the introduction of this simple test.

Pap smears to detect early cervical cancer are recommended in all women within 3 years of initiating vaginal intercourse or by the age of 21 years. Recommendations regarding appropriate interval of screening are varied. The American College of Obstetricians and Gynecologists and the Society of Gynecologic Oncologists agree with recent recommendations set forth by the American Cancer Society that all women younger than the age of 30 years be screened annually with conventional Pap smears or every 2 years with liquid-based Pap tests. After the age of 30 years, the interval may be extended to every 2 to 3 years if a woman is healthy and has had three normal Pap smears in a row. After the age of 70 years, Pap smears may be stopped if the patient has had three normal Pap smears and no abnormal results in the last 10 years. There is a general consensus that there is no clear benefit to screening in women who have had a hysterectomy for benign reasons and in whom the cervix has been removed. Older women should, however, continue to have an annual pelvic exam with visual inspection of the vulva and vagina and bimanual and rectovaginal examinations. The reader is referred to Chapter 18, Diagnosis, Workup, and Management of Preinvasive Lesions of the Cervix, for a more detailed discussion of cervical cancer screening protocols.

Colorectal Cancer

The approach to screening for colorectal cancer varies widely depending on the individual patient's risk. Risk stratification should include the following points:

1. A history of colon cancer or adenomatous polyp
2. Presence of disease that may increase the risk of colon cancer (e.g., inflammatory bowel disease)
3. A family history of colon cancer
4. A family history of a genetic syndrome such as familial adenomatous polyposis or hereditary nonpolyposis colorectal cancer

Patients with a history of colon cancer or adenomatous polyp should be followed up by a gastroenterologist or colorectal surgeon, who will determine the appropriate interval for surveillance. Table 6-12 outlines the appropriate timing of screening according to other risk factors. A number of screening strategies have been studied and are presented in Table 6-13. A detailed discussion of colon cancer can be found in Chapter 25, Bowel Disorders.

Lung Cancer

Lung cancer is the leading cause of cancer death in both men and women. No screening strategies have clearly demonstrated a reduction in mortality from lung cancer. Specifically, routine screening with chest x-ray and/or sputum samples has not been found to be effective. Preliminary data suggest the feasibility of computed tomography scan as a screening tool. Large trials are now underway. Currently, the most effective preventive measure is to strongly encourage smoking cessation.

Skin Cancer

Skin cancer is common, with more than 1 million cases diagnosed per year in the United States. The most common types are basal cell carcinoma, squamous cell carcinoma, and melanoma. Although basal cell carcinoma has the highest incidence, it is infrequently associated as a cause of mortality. Squamous cell carcinoma is the second most common form of skin cancer and tends to afflict people in their 60s and 70s in areas exposed to the sun. Actinic keratosis is a common precursor lesion.

Table 6-12

Risk Factor	Age to Initiate Screening	Interval of Screening
Average risk	At age of 50 years	FOBT yearly Sigmoidoscopy every 5 years Colonoscopy every 10 years
Family history of colon cancer (one second- or third-degree relative)	Screen as average risk	Interval as in average risk
Family history of colon cancer (one first-degree relative with colon cancer diagnosed before the age of 60 years or two first-degree relatives)	At age of 40 years or 10 years before patient reaches the age of the index case, whichever comes first	Colonoscopy every 5–10 years
Familial adenomatous polyposis	Age of 10–12 years	Yearly sigmoidoscopy If genetic test results are positive, colectomy recommended
Hereditary nonpolyposis colorectal cancer	At age of 20–25 years or 10 years before patient reaches the age of the youngest diagnosis of colon cancer in the family	Colonoscopy every 1–2 years
Inflammatory bowel disease	Begin screening after 8–10 years of disease	Yearly colonoscopy

FOBT, fecal occult blood testing.

Table 6-13

Test	Comments
Digital rectal examination	Only 10% of colorectal cancers are within reach of the examining finger. There is no evidence of reduced mortality and no adverse effect.
Fecal occult blood testing (FOBT)	Home FOBT with three consecutive stool samples is preferred over one office FOBT. Sensitivity is low and will miss 50% of cancers. This is not an adequate screening test alone.
Sigmoidoscopy	Fair evidence from case control studies exists to show that sigmoidoscopy reduces mortality. This test detects 68% to 78% of advanced neoplasia.
Colonoscopy	No studies have addressed the benefit of colonoscopy as a screening tool. This test is more sensitive than sigmoidoscopy and detects 90% of large adenomas. Sensitivity is probably higher for cancer.
Barium enema	No evidence on mortality rates exists. This test is less sensitive than colonoscopy. Barium enema is not an effective screening strategy.

Melanoma, on the other hand, tends to be diagnosed at a younger age and behaves more aggressively; therefore, early diagnosis is paramount. The incidence of malignant melanoma is on the rise. Risk factors for melanoma include a history of sunburns, fair skin, family history of melanoma, and precursor lesions such as congenital or dysplastic nevi. A thorough skin examination takes only a few minutes and can be life saving. Melanomas may occur anywhere on the skin, but they are frequently located on the back and other areas that are difficult to visualize on self-inspection. The "ABCDEs" of melanoma are used to remind both clinicians and patients about worrisome features of a skin lesion that should prompt further investigation. These are as follows:

- Asymmetry
- Border irregularities
- Color variegation (i.e., different colors within the same area)
- Diameter greater than 6 mm
- Enlargement

Preventive measures include reducing sun exposure and using adequate sunscreens because ultraviolet radiation is a major causative factor for basal cell carcinoma, squamous cell carcinoma, and melanoma. Any suspicion of skin cancer should prompt a rapid referral to a dermatologist.

DEPRESSION

The lifetime risk for developing major depression is 10% to 25% for women (compared with 4.5% to 9.3% for men). Although major depression may occur at any age, the typical age of onset is in the 20s or 30s. Some patients may experience only a single episode of depression, but for most it is a chronic disease with relapses and remissions. Depression that goes unidentified and untreated is more likely to become chronic. Not all patients will present with depressed mood and, in fact, most patients will present to the primary care provider with somatic complaints. Providers should be aware of the most common presentations of depression (Box 6-4). In addition, patients who have a history of major depression, substance abuse, or dysthymia are at increased risk for depression. A number of questionnaires have been developed to identify and diagnose depression. Useful initial questions for the primary care physicians include the following:

In the past month have you been bothered by:

- Little interest or pleasure in doing things?
- Feeling down, depressed, or hopeless?

Patients who answer "yes" to either of the above questions should be further assessed for *Diagnostic and Statistical Manual of Mental Disorders*, ed 4, criteria for major depression (Box 6-5). Those who meet criteria should be immediately screened for suicide risk. Additionally, secondary causes of depression should be considered. These include the following:

148

Box 6-4   Common Presentations of Depression

Multiple (more than five per year) medical visits
Multiple unexplained symptoms
Work or relationship dysfunction
Changes in interpersonal relationships
Dampened affect
Poor behavioral follow-through
Weight gain or loss
Sleep disturbance
Fatigue
Dementia
Irritable bowel syndrome
Volunteered complaints of stress or mood disturbance

Box 6-5   DSM Criteria for Diagnosis of Depression

Five or more of the following symptoms present concomitantly on most days for consecutive days for at least 2 weeks constitute depression. (At least one of the symptoms is either depressed mood or loss of interest or pleasure.)
Depressed mood
Markedly diminished interest or pleasure in all or almost all activities
Significant weight loss
Insomnia or hypersomnia
Psychomotor agitation or retardation
Fatigue or loss of energy, feelings of worthlessness, or excessive or inappropriate guilt
Diminished ability to think, concentrate, or make decisions
Recurrent thoughts of death

DSM, *Diagnostic and Statistical Manual of Mental Disorders.*

- Substance abuse
- Medication (e.g., opioids, β-blockers, methyldopa, benzodiazepines, steroids, Accutane)
  - Uncommon and when occurring, generally presents soon after starting medication
- General medical disorders (e.g., hypothyroidism, malignancy, Parkinson's disease, dementia)
- Grief reaction
  - Lasts 2 to 6 months and improves steadily without specific treatment
- Other psychiatric disorders

Depression is a treatable condition. Studies indicate that behavioral therapy and medication appear to be equally effective for mild to moderate depression, though coadministration of medication and psychotherapy is more effective than either treatment modality alone. Medications, behavioral therapy, and electroconvulsant therapy are indicated for persons with severe depression. Commonly used antidepressant medications include selective serotonin reuptake inhibitors such as fluoxetine, heterocyclic agents such as amitriptyline, dual-action medications such as venlafaxine, monoamine oxidase inhibitors such as phenelzine, and other medications such as trazodone and bupropion.

DEMENTIA

Dementia occurs in 8% to 10% of all patients older than 65 years and in 30% to 50% of patients older than 85 years. Alzheimer's dementia is by far the most common, causing 60% to 80% of cases. Delayed diagnosis is common because many signs of memory impairment may be inaccurately attributed to normal aging. Cognitive decline in normal aging may consist of mild memory impairment as well as delayed information processing; however, these symptoms are not progressive and do not interfere with daily functioning. In contrast, dementia is associated with a decline in cognitive function, particularly memory impairment, behavioral disturbance, and impairment in social and occupational functioning. Dementia differs from delirium in that sensorium (i.e., the patient's level of arousal or alertness) is not affected. Dementia from Alzheimer's disease is associated with a slow and gradual onset and progression. Most cases come to diagnosis only after 2 to 3 years of symptoms. A more rapid onset of dementia (less than 6 months of symptoms) should alert the clinician to other possible diagnoses such as Creutzfeldt-Jakob disease. With the introduction of medications to slow the progression of dementia, focus on early identification of cognitive impairment is important.

A new classification of memory impairment has emerged and is referred to as *mild cognitive impairment* (MCI). MCI includes the conditions of patients who have memory impairment but do not meet criteria for a diagnosis of dementia. Patients with MCI typically have good overall cognitive functioning and are independent in terms of activities of daily living. Approximately 6% to 25% of patients with MCI will progress to Alzheimer's-type dementia and should be screened annually for progression to dementia. The most useful screening tool for dementia is the mini-mental status examination (Box 6-6). A score of less than 24 is suspicious for a diagnosis of dementia, and these patients should be referred for further evaluation. All patients with a new diagnosis of MCI or dementia should be evaluated for possible reversible causes. Laboratory evaluation should include a complete blood count and measurements of electrolyte levels, blood urea nitrogen and creatinine concentrations, thyroid function, calcium, and vitamin B_{12} to rule out metabolic or hematologic causes. Brain imaging is recommended in the initial evaluation of all patients with dementia. Magnetic resonance imaging without contrast will provide the most clinically useful information. Screening for neurosyphilis, lumbar puncture, toxicology screen, and electroencephalogram should be considered only if clinically indicated.

DOMESTIC VIOLENCE

It is estimated that more than 1 million women in the United States are the victims of physical or sexual abuse by their partners each year. Abuse

---

Box 6-6   Mini-Mental Status Examination

Orientation
1. What is the (year)(season)(date)(day)(month)? Score 1 point for each.
2. Where are we (state)(county)(town)(hospital)(floor)? Score 1 point for each.

Registration
Name three objects. Ask the patient all three immediately after you have said them. Give 1 point for each correct answer.

Attention and Calculation
1. Serial 7s: Have the patient start from 100 and subtract 7, then repeat. Stop after five answers. (Award 1 point for each correct answer.) Alternatively, ask the patient to spell "world" backwards. (Give 5 points for correct answer.)
2. Ask the patient to name the three objects mentioned above. (Give one point for each correct answer.)
3. Point to a pencil and wristwatch and ask the patient to name each. (Award 1 point for each.)
4. Ask the patient to repeat "no ifs, ands, or buts." (Give 1 point.)
5. Follow a three-stage command: For example, "Take this paper in your right hand, fold it in half, and put it on the floor." (Give 3 points.)
6. Ask the patient to read and obey the following:
   Close your eyes. (Give 1 point.)
   Write a sentence. (Give 1 point.)
   Copy design. (1 point)

Adapted from Folstein MF, Folstein SE, McHugh PR: "Mini-mental state." A practical method for grading the cognitive state of patients for the clinician. J Psychiatr Res 12(3):189–198, 1975. Copyright 1975, 1998, MiniMental LLC.

may begin as emotional or verbal abuse but often escalates to physical violence. Although domestic violence occurs among women of all ages, races, and socioeconomic background, a number of factors have been associated with an increased risk of domestic violence (Box 6-7). Victims live with constant fear and shame and are often reluctant to report the abuse. For this reason, clinicians should be alert to clues in the history or physical examination that may lead one to suspect domestic violence (Box 6-8). Many groups have recommended screening of all women for domestic violence. Screening and assessment for domestic violence should be done in a private setting, and confidentiality should be ensured. A screening question may be asked during the social history taking; this question can be introduced, for example, as follows: "I have found that in my practice, many of my patients are involved in relationships that

---

Box 6-7   Risk Factors for Domestic Violence

Aged younger than 35 years
Having a marital status of single, divorced, or separated
Abusing alcohol or having a partner who does
Being pregnant or postpartum
Having low socioeconomic status
Having a history of childhood physical or sexual abuse

Box 6-8	Warning Signs of Domestic Violence

Any suspicious injury (e.g., injury in unusual location, multiple injuries in various stages of healing, pattern of injury inconsistent with history, repeated visits for minor injuries)

Chronic somatic complaints (e.g., headaches, abdominal pain, pelvic pain, fatigue, vague complaints)

Other medical conditions such as IBS, PID, STDs

Psychiatric illness or substance abuse

Pregnancy, especially if woman has injuries

Change in office visit pattern (e.g., late or missed appointments, frequent change of provider, sudden increase or decrease in visit frequency, increased use of emergency room)

Controlling behavior of partner

IBS, Irritable bowel syndrome; PID, pelvic inflammatory disease; STDs, sexually transmitted diseases.

can be violent, so I now routinely ask all of my patients about violence in their lives." This introductory statement may then be followed by one or more of the following questions:

- Have you ever been physically abused (e.g., kicked, hit, slapped, or punched)?
- Have you and your spouse/partner ever used physical force when you were arguing?
- Are you ever afraid of your partner?

If domestic violence is suspected, it is important that the clinician remain nonjudgmental and supportive. Patients should be offered educational material including phone numbers for the local resources for domestic violence victims. If domestic violence is confirmed, the patient's immediate safety status should be confirmed, and if there appears to be imminent danger, a referral to a local shelter should be arranged. Confronting the abuser or suggesting couples therapy is of no benefit and may even lead to an escalation of violence when the abuser is again alone with the victim.

SUBSTANCE ABUSE

It is estimated that 10% to 15% of all primary care patients have problems related to addiction. Screening for substance abuse should be part of the routine history for all patients. A simple screening tool called the *CAGE questionnaire* has been validated for the assessment of alcohol disorders (Box 6-9). One positive response warrants further investigation for the possibility of alcohol abuse. Two positive responses have a sensitivity of 85% and specificity of 90% for a diagnosis for alcohol abuse. The CAGE questionnaire has also been adapted for use in screening for drug use; the revised version is called *CAGE-AID* (Box 6-10). The CAGE-AID

Box 6-9 CAGE Questionnaire

C: Have you ever tried to *cut down* on your alcohol or drug use?
A: Do you get *annoyed* when people comment about your drinking or drug use?
G: Do you feel *guilty* about things you have done while drinking or using drugs?
E: Do you need an *eye-opener* to get started in the morning?

Box 6-10 CAGE-AID Questionnaire (Adapted to Include Drugs)

Since your eighteenth birthday, have you:
Had any fractures or dislocations of your bones or joints (excluding sports injuries)?
Been injured in a traffic accident?
Injured your head (excluding sports injuries)?
Been in a fight or been assaulted while intoxicated?
Been injured while intoxicated?

---

questionnaire screens for a history of trauma. A positive response to two or more of these questions indicates a high likelihood of addiction. Specific criteria for a diagnosis of substance abuse or substance dependence have been developed by the American Psychiatric Association. A diagnosis of *substance abuse* is made when one or more of the following occur in a 12-month period:

- Recurrent substance use resulting in failure to fulfill major role obligations
- Recurrent substance use in situations that are physically hazardous
- Legal problems related to substance use
- Continued substance use despite persistent or recurrent social or interpersonal problems

Substance dependence occurs when three or more of the following occur in a 12-month period:

- Evidence of tolerance, withdrawal, or use of a substance in larger amounts or over a longer period than intended
- Persistent desire or unsuccessful efforts to cut down
- Great deal of time spent in activities necessary to obtain the substance
- Reduction in social, occupational, or recreational activities because of substance use
- Continuation of substance use despite knowledge of problems

Once a substance abuse problem has been identified, a referral should be made to a community-based program, such as Alcoholics Anonymous or Narcotics Anonymous, or to a behavioral health specialist. Behavioral change is not easy for most patients, and the health care provider can use the following strategies to aid in a patient's recovery:

- Discuss the relationship between substance use and current medical concerns or psychosocial problems.
- Assess the patient's readiness to change.

- Negotiate goals and strategies for reducing consumption and instituting other changes.
- Involve family members as appropriate.
- Schedule a follow-up appointment to monitor status and changes.

SUMMARY

A physician's advice is often the most influential factor in a patient's decision to reduce the risk of disease in the future. The obstetrician/gynecologist has the unique opportunity to put prevention into practice at the annual gynecologic examination and during routine prenatal visits. Early detection of many common diseases will lead to significant reduction in morbidity and mortality. An organized, informed approach to prevention and screening is an integral part of high-quality comprehensive care for women.

KEY POINTS

1. Cardiovascular disease is the leading cause of death in women in the United States.
2. Cardiac risk factors should be reviewed with all patients on a yearly basis.
3. Modifiable cardiac risk factors include hypertension, hyperlipidemia, diabetes, smoking, obesity, and physical inactivity.
4. Hip fractures are a leading cause of morbidity in elderly woman, and osteoporosis prevention has been shown to reduce the incidence of hip fractures.
5. Lung cancer is the leading cause of cancer death in women in the United States.
6. Screening strategies for lung cancer are not effective, and smoking cessation is the most important intervention to reduce the risk for lung cancer.
7. Routine screening for breast, cervical, colorectal, and skin cancer have been shown to reduce mortality.
8. Regular and timely immunizations are an important part of the periodic health examination.
9. Lifestyle modifications have been shown to have a powerful effect on reducing the risk for cardiovascular disease, diabetes, and many forms of cancer.
10. Women have a high lifetime risk of depression and often initially present to a primary care provider.
11. Memory impairment in the elderly is not always part of the normal aging process and warrants screening for dementia.
12. The incidence of domestic violence and substance abuse in primary care practices is high, and caregivers must be alert for warning signs.

SUGGESTED READING

American Diabetes Association: Clinical Practice Recommendations 2005. Diabetes Care 28:S1–S2, 2005.

Anderson GL, Limacher M, Assaf AR, et al: Women's Health Initiative Steering Committee. Effects of conjugated equine estrogen in postmenopausal women with hysterectomy: The Women's Health Initiative randomized controlled trial. JAMA 291(14): 1701–1712, 2004.

Bach PB, Niewoehner DE, Black WC: Screening for lung cancer: The guidelines. Chest 123:83S–88S, 2003.

Canadian Task Force on the Periodic Health Examination: Canadian Guide to Clinical Preventive Health Care. Ottawa, Canada Communication Group, 1994.

Centers for Disease Control and Prevention: Recommended Adult Immunization Schedule. Summary of Recommendations Published by the Advisory Committee on Immunization Practices. October 2004–September 2005.

Chobanian AV, Bakris GL, Black H, et al: The Seventh Report of the Joint National Committee on Prevention, Detection, Evaluation, and Treatment of High Blood Pressure. The JNC 7 Report. JAMA 289(19): 2560–2572, 2003.

Clinical Guidelines on the Identification, Evaluation, and Treatment of Overweight and Obesity in Adults: National Institutes of Health, National Heart, Lung, and Blood Institute. NIH Publication No. 98–4083. Available from: http://www.nhlbi.nih.gov

Colorectal cancer screening and surveillance: Clinical guidelines and rationale—Update based on new evidence. Gastroenterology 124:544–560, 2003.

Fiore MC: US public health service clinical practice guideline: Treating tobacco use and dependence. Respir Care 45:1200–1262, 2000.

Humphrey LL, Helfand M, Chan BK, Woolf SH: Breast cancer screening: A summary of the evidence for the U.S. Preventive Services Task Force. Ann Intern Med 137:347–360, 2002.

Implications of recent clinical trials for the National Cholesterol Education Program Adult Treatment Panel III Guidelines. J Am Coll Cardiol 44(3): 720–732, 2004.

Institute for Clinical Systems Improvement: Major Depression in Adults in Primary Care. 8th ed. 2004. Available from: http://www.icsi.org

Karlawish JH, Clark CM: Diagnostic evaluation of elderly patients with mild memory problems. Ann Intern Med 138:411–419, 2003.

Ladenson PW, Singer PA, Ain BA: American Thyroid Association Guidelines for Detection of Thyroid Dysfunction. Arch Intern Med 160:1573–1575, 2000.

McLellan AT, Lewis DC, O'Brien CP, Kleber HD: Drug dependence, a chronic medical illness: Implications for treatment, insurance, and outcomes evaluation. JAMA 284:1689–1695, 2000.

Mosc L, Appel LJ, Benjamin EJ, et al: Evidence-based guidelines for cardiovascular disease prevention in women. Circulation 109:672–693, 2004.

National Osteoporosis Foundation Physician's guide to prevention and treatment of osteoporosis. Washington, DC, 2003. Available from: http://www.nof.org

Ovarian Cancer NIH Consensus Development Panel: Ovarian cancer screening, treatment and follow-up. JAMA 273:491–497, 1995.

Ramsay J, Richardson J, Carter YH, et al: Should health professionals screen women for domestic violence? Systematic review. BMJ 325:314, 2002.

Rex DK, Johnson DA, Lieberman DA, et al: Colorectal cancer prevention 2000: Screening recommendations of the American College of Gastroenterology. American College of Gastroenterology. Am J Gastroenterol 95:868–877, 2000.

Saslow D, Runowicz CD, Solomon D, et al: American Cancer Society guideline for the early detection of cervical neoplasia and cancer. CA Cancer J Clin 52:342–362, 2002.

Third Report of the National Cholesterol Education Program (NCEP) Expert Panel on Detection, Evaluation, and Treatment of High Blood Cholesterol in Adults (Adult Treatment Panel III) final report. Circulation 106(25):3143–3421, 2002.

United States Preventive Services Task Force: Guide to Clinical Preventive Services. 2nd ed. Baltimore, MD, Williams and Wilkins, 1996.

Weinstock MA: Early detection of melanoma. JAMA 284:886–889, 2000.

Winawer S, Fletcher R, Rex D, et al: Colorectal cancer screening and surveillance: Clinical guidelines and rationale. Update based on new evidence. Gastroenterology 2003 Feb 124 (2):544–560, 2003.

Wright TC, Schiffman M, Solomon D, et al: Interim guidance for the use of human papillomavirus DNA testing as an adjunct to cervical cytology for screening. Obstet Gynecol 103:304–309, 2004.

7

FAMILY PLANNING
Roxanne Jamshidi and Paul Blumenthal

CONTRACEPTIVE DEVELOPMENT: A HISTORICAL CONTEXT

Since the beginning of history, humans have employed a wide range of methods by which to avoid pregnancy. The oldest written document referring to contraception techniques, the Kahun papyrus, dates to over 4000 years ago, and describes a pessary made of crocodile dung and fermented dough that a woman would insert into the vagina before intercourse. Subsequent historical texts describe a variety of preparations thought to prevent pregnancy, including recipes for supposed sterilizing agents such as leaves of hawthorn, ivy, willow, and poplar, and barrier methods such as alum applied to the uterus or lemon halves placed over the cervix. In the Middle Ages, many women died from poisoning resulting from lead, arsenic, mercury, and strychnine, all agents believed to have contraceptive value.

The modern era of contraception was marked by the development of the condom in 1709 by a physician to King Charles II. In contrast to earlier times, this era is marked by the development of methods based on more accurate knowledge concerning the process of conception. By the early 1800s, a contraceptive sponge and a contraceptive syringe (for the injection of an aqueous solution of alum or zinc sulfate into the vagina immediately after ejaculation) were available. Over the next 100 years, various forms of vaginal suppositories, douches, pessaries, diaphragms, and cervical caps were developed and in use. In 1909, the first intrauterine device (IUD), a ring made of silkworm gut, was described.

The development and use of various means of birth control occurred despite the fact that it was illegal to provide information on contraception well into the twentieth century in the United States. Enacted in 1873, the Comstock Law specifically outlawed all contraceptive devices and information in the United States. In addition, several states had laws banning birth control. Although medical textbooks were available in the early 1900s that described contraceptive methods, it was clear that U.S. physicians were to limit the provision of contraception to "health reasons" or medical indications. As a result, women in the United States were often treated for so-called dysmenorrheal and irregular bleeding at menstrual clinics. In 1914, family planning advocate Margaret Sanger was charged with violating the Comstock Law in 1914 for providing diaphragms to poor women. Despite this, she and others continued to challenge birth control laws by opening family planning clinics during the 1920s and 1930s. These clinics were the forerunners of the Planned Parenthood Federation of America. By the 1930s, a few state health departments and public hospitals had begun to provide family planning services. However, it was not until 1965 that the U.S. Supreme Court decision in the case of *Griswold v. Connecticut* affirmed the unconstitutionality of laws prohibiting contraceptive use.

In terms of hormonal contraception, the development of the oral contraceptive was the culmination of a 10-year concerted effort to produce a physiologic hormone-based female contraceptive. Over the preceding decades, great strides had been made in the field of sex steroids through the work of such scientists as Russell Marker, Carl Djerassi, and Gregory Pincus, among others. In 1950, Margaret Sanger collaborated with social activist and wealthy heiress Katherine McCormick in an effort to fund the development of an oral contraceptive. With McCormick's financial backing, the collaboration of Drs. Gregory Pincus, John Rock, and Min-Chueh Chang produced the first oral contraceptive. By 1957, the first large clinical trials were conducted in Puerto Rico, and in 1960, the U.S. Food and Drug Administration (FDA) approved the first oral contraceptive, Enovid, made by Searle, for use as contraceptive.

However, within a few years of FDA approval, serious cardiovascular effects such as stroke, venous thromboembolism, and myocardial infarction (MI) were observed in a small proportion of users. Early epidemiologic studies of oral contraceptives containing high doses of estrogen (>50 μg) indicated increased risks of these cardiovascular events. Later studies that demonstrated the role played by certain preexisting health conditions (i.e., confounding variables), such as hypertension and smoking, in increasing the incidence of these cardiovascular events among women using oral contraceptives. As the relationship between the amount of steroid present and health risks emerged, pharmaceutical companies progressively lowered the amount of estrogen in the pill. The original pill that was approved in 1960 contained 150 μg of estrogen. By 1962, Searle had introduced a revised version of Enovid that contained 100 μg of estrogen. Subsequent formulations continued to decrease the amount of estrogen and progestin in them, such that by 1974 there were combination pills with as little as 20 μg of estrogen, and in 1973 a progestin-only pill was introduced. The early 1980s brought the development of biphasic and triphasic pills, which varied the levels of estrogen and progestin delivered over the course of a cycle. Since then, further developments have been made regarding new types of progestins, as well as new delivery systems including implants, injectables, transdermal patches, and vaginal rings. In addition, as family planning programs emerged as worldwide public health interventions, an understanding of the issues relating to convenience, compliance, and continuation also became important components of the contraceptive effectiveness equation.

Contraceptive Effectiveness

The effectiveness of contraceptive methods is usually expressed both in terms of perfect use (i.e., the lowest expected failure rate) and the typical failure rates. The former rate is based on completely compliant and correct method use on every occasion, with failure therefore being ascribed to a failure of the method itself (i.e., method failure). On the other hand, typical use or effectiveness is usually lower as a result of inconsistent or incorrect use on the part of the person using the method (i.e., user failure). Methods that are minimally influenced by the need for compliance will have typical effectiveness rates that are very close to the lowest expected (perfect use) rates of failure. Examples of such methods include the IUD or contraceptive implants. Methods that require more day to day compliance often have typical use failure rates that are substantially higher than the lowest expected failure rates (Table 7-1). Effectiveness is also often quantified by the Pearl Index, which is defined as the number of unintended pregnancies per 100 women per year. However, methods that do not require much day to day compliance on the part of the user often require involvement on the part of the provider, such as an insertion or removal procedure. Such issues can make a method "provider dependent," which can result in reduced access to the method, as opposed to a method being "user dependent," such as a condom or a diaphragm, which requires the user to do something each time she wants to use the method. User-dependent methods often have better access for users than provider-dependent methods but, because of the need for user action, are often less effective.

Requirements for Provision of Contraception

With few exceptions, the only necessary prerequisites before administering contraception are a detailed medical history and blood pressure measurement. A pelvic examination is necessary for placement of IUDs and, at present, fitting for a diaphragm or cervical cap. If pregnancy cannot be excluded by history alone, a urine pregnancy test can be performed. In addition, screening for a thrombophilic condition may be warranted if the medical history reveals a personal or strong family history of clotting disorders. Other examinations and tests, including breast exams, Papanicolaou (Pap) smears, and screening for sexually transmitted infections, while important for their intended purposes, are not necessary before the provision of contraception. This is especially important for adolescents, when the requirement for a Pap smear can impose an insurmountable barrier for some teenagers who are in need of contraception.

SYSTEMIC HORMONAL CONTRACEPTION

Systemic hormonal contraceptives can be given orally, transvaginally, or transdermally; given as an injection or implant; or released from an IUD. The systemic effect from the release of hormone from an IUD is minimal and therefore discussed separately (see Intrauterine Device section). In addition, postcoital hormonal contraception is also discussed separately (see Emergency Contraception section).

Table 7-1 Percentage of Women Experiencing an Unintended Pregnancy During the First Year of Typical Use and the First Year of Perfect Use of Contraception and the Percentage Continuing Use at the End of the First Year, in the United States

Method (1)	% of women experiencing an unintended pregnancy within the first year of use		% of women continuing use at 1 year[‡] (4)
	Typical use* (2)	Perfect use[†] (3)	
No method[§]	85	85	
Spermicides[‖]	29	18	42
Withdrawal	27	4	43
Periodic abstinence	25		51
Calendar		9	
Ovulation method		3	
Symptothermal[¶]		2	
Postovulation		1	
Cap[#]			
Parous women	32	26	46
Nulliparous women	16	9	57
Sponge			
Parous women	32	20	46
Nulliparous women	16	9	57
Diaphragm[#]	16	6	57
Condom**			
Female (Reality)	21	5	49
Male	15	2	53
Combined pill and minipill	8	0.3	68
Ortho-Evra patch	8	0.3	68
NuvaRing	8	0.3	68
Depo-Provera	3	0.3	56
Lunelle	3	0.05	56
IUD			

Method			
ParaGard (copper T)	0.8	0.6	78
Mirena (levonorgesterel containing intrauterine system)	0.1	0.1	81
Norplant and Norplant-2	0.05	0.05	84
Female sterilization	0.5	0.5	100
Male sterilization	0.15	0.10	100
Emergency contraceptive pills: Treatment initiated within 72 hours after unprotected intercourse reduces risk of pregnancy by at least 75%.[††]			
Lactational amenorrhea method: A highly effective, *temporary* method of contraception.[‡‡]			

Source: Trussell J Contraceptive efficacy. In Hatcher RA, Trussell J, Stewart F, et al (eds): Contraceptive technology, eighteenth revised edition. New York, Ardent Media, 2004.
*Among *typical* couples who initiate use of a method (not necessarily for the first time), the percentage who experience an accidental pregnancy during the first year if they do not stop use for any other reason. Estimates of the probability of pregnancy during the first year of typical use for spermicides, withdrawal, periodic abstinence, the diaphragm, the male condom, the pill, and Depo-Provera are taken from the 1995. National Surveys of Family Growth corrected for underreporting of abortion; see text for the derivation of estimates for the other methods.

[†]Among couples who initiate use of a method (not necessarily for the first time) and who use it *perfectly* (both consistently and correctly), the percentage who experience an accidental pregnancy during the first year if they do not stop use for any other reason. See text for the derivation of estimate for each method.

[‡]Among couples attempting to avoid pregnancy, the percentage who continue to use a method for 1 year.

[§]The percentages becoming pregnant in columns (2) and (3) are based on data from populations where contraception is not used and from women who cease using contraception in order to become pregnant. Among such populations, about 89% become pregnant within 1 year. This estimate was lowered slightly (to 85%) to represent the percentage who would become pregnant within 1 year among women now relying on reversible methods of contraception if they abandoned contraception altogether.

[||]Foams, creams, gels, vaginal suppositories, and vaginal film.

[¶]Cervical mucus (ovulation) method supplemented by calendar in the preovulatory and basal body temperature in the postovulatory phases.

[#]With spermicidal cream or jelly.

[**]Without spermicides.

[††]The treatment schedule is one dose within 120 hours after unprotected intercourse, and a second dose 12 hours after the first dose. Both doses of Plan B can be taken at the same time. Plan B (1 dose is 1 white pill) is the only dedicated product specifically marketed for emergency contraception. The U.S. Food and Drug Administration has in addition declared the following 18 brands of oral contraceptives to be safe and effective for emergency contraception: Ogestrel or Ovral (1 dose is 2 white pills), Alesse, Lessina, or Levlite, (1 dose is 5 pink pills), Levlen or Nordette (1 dose is 4 light-orange pills), Cryselle, Levora, Low-Ogestrel, or Lo/Ovral (1 dose is 4 white pills), Tri-Levlen or Triphasil (1 dose is 4 yellow pills), Portia, Seasonale, or Trivora (1 dose is 4 pink pills), Aviane (1 dose is 5 orange pills), and Empresse (1 dose is 4 orange pills).

[‡‡]However, to maintain effective protection against pregnancy, another method of contraception must be used as soon as menstruation resumes, the frequency or duration of breastfeeds is reduced, or the baby reaches 6 months of age.

Combined Oral Contraceptives

Oral contraceptives are the most popular method of reversible birth control in the United States. The hormonal content of combined (estrogen and progestin) oral contraceptives has decreased dramatically over the last two decades. In turn, this has led to a decrease in both side effects and cardiovascular complications, making combined oral contraceptives (COCs) a practical contraceptive option for many women from their teens until menopause. However, some caveats exist, and these are described below. COCs can be given cyclically (21 active pills followed by 7 inactive pills) or by an extended-cycle regimen (84 active followed by 7 inactive pills). When prescribed for noncontraceptive purposes such as endometriosis or just for convenience, COCs can also be given continuously.

Mechanisms of Action

Although COCs have several mechanisms of action, the primary contraceptive action is suppression of ovulation by inhibition of the midcycle surge of gonadotropin. This action is primarily mediated by the progestin component. An additional mechanism of contraceptive action is down-regulation of gonadotropin secretion during the follicular phase of the cycle, preventing follicular maturation. However, with lower-dose COCs that contain 20 to 35 μg of estrogen, a substantial number of women will continue to develop follicles while taking COCs.

Several other progestin-mediated actions contribute to contraceptive effect. These include alterations in the cervical mucus, making it thick and impervious to sperm transport. In addition, the progestin produces effects on the endometrium such that it is not receptive to ovum implantation. The progestin may also decrease normal tubal motility and peristalsis.

Contraindications

There are several situations in which a woman should not use COCs (Box 7-1). There are also situations in which the risks and benefits of COC use must be carefully weighed, or in which they should be provided with caution. These conditions include poorly controlled hypertension and migraine headaches associated with auras. Women who use anticonvulsant drug therapy (e.g., phenobarbital, phenytoin, carbamazepine) or

---

Box 7-1   Contraindications to Combined Oral Contraception Use

Previous thromboembolic event or stroke
History of an estrogen-dependent tumor
Active liver disease
Pregnancy
Undiagnosed abnormal uterine bleeding
Hypertriglyceridemia
Age older than 35 years combined with tobacco smoking*

*A consensus panel reviewing the issue of oral contraceptives and smoking suggested that COCs can be considered for women over the age of 35 years who are light smokers (fewer than 15 cigarettes/day). However, the American College of Obstetricians and Gynecologists do not support this conclusion.

other drugs that increase liver microsomal enzyme activity (e.g., rifampin) should be encouraged to use other forms of contraception because of the decreased efficacy of COCs brought about by increased drug metabolism.

Guidelines from the World Health Organization (WHO) and the American College of Obstetrics and Gynecology (ACOG) relative to COC use are summarized in Table 7-2.

Risks and Side Effects

Early side effects associated with the initiation of COC use include bloating, breast tenderness, nausea, mood changes, and breakthrough bleeding. Although bothersome, most of these side effects subside after a few months' duration. With proper counseling regarding these possible adverse effects, patients will be less likely to discontinue use because of their development. If symptoms such as breakthrough bleeding persist

Table 7-2

Guidelines for Prescribing Combined Hormonal Contraceptives*

Medical Concern	WHO Guidelines	ACOG Guidelines
Current or past DVT or PE	Unacceptable health risk[†]	Risk unacceptable unless patient is taking anticoagulant, progestin-only options or IUDs preferable
First-degree family history of DVT or PE	Advantages > risks[‡]	—
Known thrombogenic mutations	Unacceptable health risk	—
Prior stroke	Unacceptable health risk	Risk unacceptable, progestin-only options or IUDs preferred
Smoker, age < 35 years		
<15 cigarettes/day	Advantages usually outweigh risks	Risk unacceptable[#]
≥15 cigarettes/day	Risk unacceptable	Risk unacceptable
Hypertension		Appropriate in otherwise healthy, nonsmoking woman < 35 years old with careful monitoring
Blood pressure controlled	Risks > advantages[§]	
Blood pressure not controlled or with vascular disease	Unacceptable health risk[‖]	Risk unacceptable, progestin-only options or IUDs preferred
Diabetes mellitus with vascular disease	Risks > advantages/ Unacceptable health risk[¶]	Risk unacceptable, progestin-only options or IUDs preferred
Diabetes mellitus without nephropathy, retinopathy, neuropathy, other vascular disease, or more than 20 years' duration	Advantages > risks[#]	Appropriate in nonsmoking, otherwise healthy woman aged <35 years old with appropriate monitoring of blood pressure, weight, and lipids

continued

Table 7-2—Cont'd

Guidelines for
Prescribing Combined
Hormonal
Contraceptives*

Medical Concern	WHO Guidelines	ACOG Guidelines
Migraine without aura		
Age < 35 years	Advantages > risks**	Appropriate in nonsmokers
Age ≥ 35 years	Risks > advantages	Other methods preferred
Migraine with aura	Unacceptable health risk[||]	Risk unacceptable, use other methods
Headache (nonmigrainous)	No restrictions to use	—
Hyperthyroidism	No restrictions to use	—
Sickle cell disease	Advantages > risks[††]	Pregnancy carries greater risk than use of COCs; DMPA may be preferred because it reduces incidence of crises
Hypercholesterolemia	Risk acceptable if LDL cholesterol < 160 mg/dL and no other cardiovascular risks	Benefit-risk ratio depends on the presence or absence of other cardiovascular risk factors
Breast cancer		
Current disease	Unacceptable health risk	Risk unacceptable
Past disease (>5 years)	Unacceptable health risk	Risk usually outweighs benefit
Family history	No restriction	Risk acceptable

WHO, World Health Organization; ACOG, American College of Obstetrics and Gynecology; DVT, deep vein thrombosis; PE, pulmonary embolism; DMPA, depot medroxyprogesterone acetate; LDL, low-density lipoprotein.
*Combined oral contraceptives, transdermal patch and vaginal ring.
[†]Copper IUD preferred, followed by progestin only methods including LNg IUD.
[‡]Progestin-only oral contraceptives, DMPA, and IUD preferred.
[§]Progestin-only oral contraceptives and IUDs preferred.
[||]Copper IUD most preferred.
[*]Copper IUD preferred, followed by progestin-only oral contraceptives or LNg IUD.
[#]Copper IUD preferred, followed by progestin only methods or LNg-IUD.
**Copper IUD preferred.
[††]Progestin only oral contraceptives, DMPA, and IUDs preferred.

through the end of the third cycle, a switch to a different COC may be warranted. Because COCs cause the development of only a thin endometrium, amenorrhea can occur in 5% to 10% of cycles while a patient is taking COCs. Although many women believe that COCs cause weight gain, studies of currently marketed products show no causal relationship.

When COCs were first marketed, their cardiovascular effects were the subject of great scrutiny. As the specific important cardiovascular risk factors were elucidated, and as the dose of the hormones decreased over the years, these concerns have subsided. Healthy, nonsmoking women are not at increased risk for MI at any age if they use low-dose COCs. However, women older than 35 years of age who smoke (especially 15 or more cigarettes/day) or who have other risk factors for MI such as hypertension or diabetes are at increased risk of development of MI. Similarly, COCs have been linked to a small but significant increased risk for stroke in many, but not all, studies. Again, the incidence has decreased with newer formulations containing less than 50 µg of ethinyl estradiol. The absolute increase in risk for stroke with modern COCs is extremely low, especially for nonsmoking women younger than age 35 years without hypertension.

The risk for venous thromboembolism (VTE) is increased for users of both the high- and low-dose COC preparations. Overall, looking at all types of COCs, the risk of VTE is 10 to 30 events per 100,000 users, which is three to four times higher than baseline. The persons at highest risk for development of a VTE are the 1% to 2% of women with inherited risk factors for thrombophilic disorders such as deficiency in antithrombin III, protein C, or protein S and the 5% of women with activated protein C or genetic changes on the factor V chain. However, given the low absolute risk of VTE among women with thromboembolic disorders and the lack of cost-effectiveness, routine screening for thrombophilic disorders before prescription of COCs is not recommended. Rather, a detailed family and personal history can be used as a method for screening for risk factors for VTE. COCs are not recommended for any woman with a known thrombophilia or a personal history of VTE.

Initial concern regarding the possible increased risk of cancer with COCs has been replaced with reassurance regarding carcinogenesis. In fact, use of COCs has been associated with a decrease in ovarian and endometrial cancer. Women who use COCs and have persistent human papillomavirus infection may have a small increased risk of cervical cancer compared with non-users with human papillomavirus, but the absolute risk is very small and therefore routine cervical cancer screening is recommended for women who are sexually active. Large epidemiologic studies have generally not shown an association with COC use and the development of breast cancer later in life. Some studies show a small increase in breast cancer incidence among current and recent users of COCs, but these cases are more likely to be localized to the breast and are therefore more easily treatable with higher survival compared with cases of breast cancer among women who do not use COCs. COCs may also be associated with a reduction in the risk of colorectal cancer. Despite product labeling indicating a risk of hepatocellular cancer among oral contraceptive users, the most recent population-based data do not support an association. Overall, COC use is associated with a reduced risk of invasive cancer by age of 60 years.

Noncontraceptive Benefits

Besides the decrease in risk for certain cancers, including endometrial and ovarian, COCs have been associated with many other health benefits in addition to their high contraceptive efficacy. In fact, many women are prescribed COCs for their noncontraceptive benefits even if contraception is not needed. Some of these benefits are well established, whereas others are emerging with more recent research. Box 7-2 summarizes these benefits.

Box 7-2   Noncontraceptive Health Benefits of Combined Oral Contraceptives

Established benefits
Menses Related
  ↑ Menstrual cycle regularity
  ↓ Blood loss
  ↓ Iron-deficiency anemia
  ↓ Dysmenorrhea
Inhibition of Ovulation
  ↓ Ovarian cysts (true for higher-dose estrogen pills only)
  ↓ Ectopic pregnancy
Other
  ↓ Fibroadenomas/fibrocystic breast changes
  ↓ Acute pelvic inflammatory disease
  ↓ Endometrial and ovarian cancer

Emerging benefits
Positive effect on bone mass
Acne
Colorectal cancer
Uterine leiomyomata
Rheumatoid arthritis
Bleeding disorders
Hyperandrogenic anovulation
Endometriosis
Perimenopausal changes
Pelvic inflammatory disease

Adapted from Burkman R, Schlesselman JJ, Zieman M: Safety concerns and health benefits associated with oral contraception. Am J Obstet Gynecol 190:S5–S22, 2004.

Preparations

Combination pills are available in many formulations. They are generally packaged in 21- or 28-day cycles. The 28-day pack is designed to improve patient compliance by providing seven placebo pills at the end of the pack. An extended-regimen package that contains 84 days of active hormone followed by 7 days of placebo (Seasonale) is also available. More recently, a spearmint-flavored chewable oral contraceptive (Ovcon-35) has been approved by the FDA.

Monophasic pills contain the same dose of estrogen and progestin in each of the 21 hormonally active pills. "Multiphasic" preparations include biphasic pills, which contain a fixed dose of estrogen with an increasing amount of progestin, and triphasic pills, which contain varying doses of progestin or estrogen plus progestin across the pack. Multiphasic regimens are designed to slightly decrease the total steroid dose over the month; however, their clinical advantage over monophasic preparations is not proven.

Any pill containing less than 50 μg of ethinyl estradiol is considered a "low-dose" pill. The majority of COCs on the market now contain an average of 30 to 35 μg. More recently, several preparations containing only 20 or 25 μg of ethinyl estradiol are available. These very-low-dose COCs may be attractive for patients who are sensitive to the estrogenic side effects or those who may want the lowest dose possible of estrogen (e.g., perimenopausal women); however, these preparations may be less effective in obese women.

Progestins, which are testosterone derived, can bind to androgen receptors and therefore have some androgen activity. In an effort to decrease side effects and metabolic complications from these androgenic actions, more selective progestins have been developed. These newer progestins, which are contained in so-called third-generation COCs, include norgestimate and desogestrel, have structural modifications that lower their androgen activity. When compared with levonorgestrel (the most androgenic of the older progestins), these newer progestins have less affinity to bind to androgen receptors and therefore may offer potential benefits regarding androgenic side effects. However, newer COCs that contain these progestins have been shown in some studies to be associated with an increased risk of deep venous thrombosis. However, other population-based epidemiologic studies indicate that much of this effect may have been due to biases present in the smaller studies, so this finding is controversial. Nevertheless, though all COCs raise the risk of VTE to some extent, it is important to note that this risk is still three to six times lower than the increased risk of VTE associated with pregnancy. Another new progestin, drospirenone, is derived from 17 α-spirolactone and therefore has both progestogenic and antimineralocorticoid activity. Because of the potassium-sparing effects of drospirenone, caution should be used for women at risk for hypokalemia.

Vaginal Ring

The combined contraceptive vaginal ring (Nuva Ring) allows a novel method of delivering the same hormones as those used in COCs. The vaginal ring is a flexible transparent copolymer ring that is placed in the vagina continuously for 3 weeks, and then removed for a week to allow for a withdrawal bleed. The vaginal ring delivers 15 µg of ethinyl estradiol and 120 µg of etonogestrel daily. Although the ring is designed to be worn continuously for 3 weeks, it can be removed for up to 3 hours at a time without decreasing effectiveness. In addition, serum concentrations of the hormones remain at contraceptive levels through 5 weeks of continuous use if left in the vagina. The ring does not have to be fitted or placed in a specific location in the vagina, it can be worn during intercourse, and it is comfortable for both the patient and her partner. In fact, the vaginal ring can be used concomitantly with tampons, spermicide, or antimycotic comedication without adverse effects or decreased efficacy.

As a combined hormonal method of birth control, the same adverse effects and cautions that apply to traditional COCs also apply to the vaginal ring. Initial trials showed excellent cycle control with a low incidence (fewer than 5% of women) of irregular bleeding when initiating the use of a vaginal ring. Some side effects are unique to the ring, including an approximate 5% incidence in increased vaginal discharge, 5% incidence of vaginitis, and 2% incidence of vaginal discomfort. Overall, however, acceptability for the ring is quite high for both patients and their partners, with more than 90% of users recommending the method to others.

Contraceptive Patch

Another alternative method of delivering combined hormonal contraception is in the form of a transdermal patch (Ortho Evra). This thin medicated adhesive is applied to the buttocks, abdomen, upper outer arm, or upper torso (excluding the breast area), and delivers 20 μg of ethinyl estradiol and 150 μg of norelgestromin per day. The patch is changed weekly for 3 weeks, followed by a patch-free week for a withdrawal bleed.

Again, the same adverse effects and cautions that apply to traditional COCs also apply to the contraceptive patch, with the exception of a higher incidence of application site reactions (20.2%), breast symptoms during the first 2 months (18%), and dysmenorrhea (13%). Because the medication in the transdermal patch is in the adhesive itself, excellent attachment is required. Data on patch adhesion show that approximately 4.7% of patches need to be replaced because of either partial or full detachment. The efficacy of the patch is comparable to COCs, with a failure rate of less than 1%; however, clinical data indicate that contraceptive efficacy decreases in women weighing more than 90 kg (198 lb).

Progestin-Only Pill

Oral contraceptive pills that only contain progestin offer an option for women who have medical conditions contraindicating estrogen (such as thrombophilia), are intolerant to estrogenic adverse effects, or who are lactating. The progestin-only pills are associated with decreased effectiveness and increased breakthrough bleeding compared with COCs.

Injectables

Currently, the only injectable method of contraception available in the United States is depot medroxyprogesterone acetate (DMPA). This highly effective method of birth control is given as an intramuscular injection of 150 mg solution every 3 months. It works by inhibiting ovulation, as well as causing changes in the endometrium and thickening the cervical mucus because of the progestin effects.

The ideal time of administration is during the first 5 days of the menstrual cycle, and an alternative method of contraception is required for 7 days if the first dose is not given during this time period. Subsequent doses are given every 12 weeks, but ovulation is suppressed for at least 4 weeks, therefore allowing a window of time for the administration of doses. If more than 14 weeks have passed since the last dose was administered, a pregnancy test should be performed before giving the next injection because DMPA can have androgenic effects on a male fetus.

The most common adverse effects of DMPA are menstrual changes including irregular bleeding and amenorrhea. Prolonged and irregular bleeding is most common after initiation of DMPA, with amenorrhea common after 9 to 12 months of use. The other most common side effect and cause for discontinuation is weight gain, although the data on this come from studies without controls. Other side effects that have been reported include headache, breast tenderness, and psychological effects such as decreased libido, depression, nervousness, and fatigue.

DMPA is associated with increased bone resorption and, in some studies, a small but statistically significant decrease in bone density when used for more than 2 years. Although this effect appears to be transient and largely reversible, patients (especially adolescents) should be counseled regarding the recommendation for adequate calcium intake. In addition, women who may be planning to try to conceive in the future should be counseled regarding the delay in ovulation of up to 18 months after cessation of DMPA, though most women have return of fertility 6 to 9 months after the time the next injection would have been given.

A new lower-dose (104 mg) DMPA formulation that can be given subcutaneously is undergoing clinical trials. This method of administration offers the advantage of potential self-administration.

A combined hormonal injectable contraception consisting of 25 mg of medroxyprogesterone acetate and 5 mg of estradiol cypionate (Lunelle) is FDA approved. Although it requires monthly injections, the adverse effects of irregular bleeding and weight gain are less common with this combined hormonal injection. Additionally, the return to fertility is more rapid, usually within 3 to 4 months after discontinuation. Unfortunately, Lunelle was recalled by the manufacturer in October 2002, with no known plan for reintroduction to the U.S. market.

Implants Implantable, subdermal capsules that release progestins for several years provide long-acting, reversible contraception. Implants offer the advantage of no maintenance by the user and extremely high effectiveness—better than, or on par with, sterilization. Like other forms of progestin contraception, the mechanism of action occurs through a combination of suppression of ovulation, changes in the cervical mucus that make it impenetrable to sperm, and changes to the endometrium that make it thin and atrophic. Implants offer rapid onset of action, with cervical mucus changes seen within hours of placement. In general, implants can be placed during any time of the menstrual cycle, with use of backup contraception necessary for the first week of use only. After removal of implants, former patterns of ovulation and menses return rapidly. Former use of implants does not alter subsequent rates of fertility, miscarriage, stillbirth, prematurity, or congenital malformations.

Like other progestin-based methods of birth control, the most common adverse effect with implants are menstrual changes, occurring in almost three quarters of users in the first year. Bleeding patterns often become irregular, with an overall decrease in blood loss. Amenorrhea is not uncommon as well. Less common adverse effects of implants include headaches, weight gain, acne, and psychiatric or mood changes. Local skin irritation occurs in approximately 5% of implant users, but actual infection or inflammation is much less common.

Until recently in the United States, no implantable methods of birth control have been available since the six-rod implant (Norplant) was removed from the market in 2001. Containing 216 mg of levonorgestrel in six rods, Norplant was approved for use for 5 years in the United States, but two large studies have shown cumulative 7-year pregnancy rates comparable to surgical sterilization, with some decreased efficacy in women weighing more than 80 kg. Experience with Norplant has led to improvements in the contraceptive implant system, primarily by decreasing the number of implants from six to one or two. Systems with fewer implants can be inserted and removed faster and more easily. Norplant II (Jadelle) is a two-rod system containing 150 mg of levonorgestrel that is left in place for 3 to 5 years. FDA approval was obtained in 1996; however, no plans exist to market this system in the United States. However, in 2006 the FDA approved a new single-rod system implant which is now available in the United States. This system, Implanon, contains the progestin etonogestrel, which has less androgenic and more progestational activity than levonorgestrel. The single rod comes in a disposable trocar/inserter that aids subdermal placement. The duration of use is designed for 3 years. With initial studies showing only one pregnancy in over 70,000 cycles, Implanon has extremely high contraceptive efficacy.

INTRAUTERINE DEVICE

Although the IUD is the most popular method of reversible contraception worldwide, only 0.8% of American women use IUDs as their method of birth control. The use of IUDs declined during the 1980s in the United States as manufacturers discontinued marketing in response to the publicity involving the IUD and pelvic inflammatory disease (PID) and subsequent litigation. However, the increase in infectious morbidity ascribed to the IUD was largely related to the Dalkon Shield's braided multifilament tail, which allowed bacteria to ascend to the upper genital tract, bypassing the protective cervical mucus. In addition, the eligibility criteria for IUD use in the 1970s and 1980s did not adequately account for the importance of sexually transmitted disease (STD) risk factors, such as multiple sexual partners, among prospective users. As a result, women at increased risk for STDs were not adequately counseled about the risks of subsequent pelvic infection in the face of IUD use. Several well-controlled studies since the 1980s have shown that other IUDs are not associated with PID, with the exception of a slightly higher rate of infection in the time period immediately following insertion.

Types of IUDs

Three categories of IUDs exist: unmedicated (inert), copper, and hormone releasing, with only the latter two available in the United States. Specifically, the two types of IUDs currently available in the United States are the Tcu-380A (ParaGard) and the levonorgestrel IUD (Mirena). Manufacturing of another progesterone-containing IUD, Progestasert, was discontinued in 2001.

Tcu-380 (Copper) IUD
The Tcu-380A consists of a T-shaped polyethylene frame with 380 mm^2 of exposed surface consisting of fine copper wire wrapped around the

vertical stem and each of the horizontal arms. The frame contains barium sulfate for detection by x-ray.

The Tcu-380A IUD is approved for use for 10 years, although it is effective for at least 12 years. The failure rate for both perfect use (in which the user checks the strings regularly to detect expulsion) and typical use is significantly less than one per 100 women per year (see Table 7-1). The copper IUD can be used in women who cannot use hormonal methods of contraception. The main disadvantage of the copper IUD, and the most frequent reasons for its removal in the first year, are heavy menses and dysmenorrhea. Average menstrual blood loss can increase by up to 55%; however, most women do not develop iron deficiency anemia as a result.

Levonorgestrel IUD

The levonorgestrel IUD or LNg 20-IUD (Mirena) is a T-shaped polyethylene device with a collar containing 52 mg of levonorgestrel dispersed in polydimethylsiloxane attached to the vertical arm. This frame is also visible on x-ray. The device releases 15 µg of levonorgestrel daily *in vivo*.

The LNg 20-IUD is approved for up to 5 years in the United States, but is effective for up to 7 years. It is currently the most effective form of reversible contraception available (see Table 7-1). Unlike the copper IUD, the LNg 20-IUD actually reduces dysmenorrhea and decreases menstrual blood loss. Women receiving this type of IUD should be counseled regarding the altered bleeding patterns that can occur. Significant intramenstrual bleeding and spotting may occur during the first few months of use as the endometrial lining is thinning. Most women will experience lighter, shorter menses with continued use, with 20% of women becoming amenorrheic after 12 months of use. In fact, this decrease in menstrual bleeding has allowed the LNg-20 IUD to be used as an alternative to hysterectomy and endometrial ablation for the treatment of menorrhagia, as well as a means of protecting the endometrium with hormone replacement therapy and as an adjuvant therapy for tamoxifen users. The LNg 20-IUD may be a particularly useful method of contraception for women with hematologic disorders or for those who are taking chronic anticoagulants.

Mechanism of Action

Although the precise mechanism of the IUD's contraceptive action is not known, it is likely that several factors are involved. IUDs work primarily by preventing fertilization rather than by interfering with implantation. A sterile inflammatory reaction occurs when the uterus is exposed to a foreign body. This inflammatory state is toxic to the sperm and ova and prevents fertilization. It causes a production of cytotoxic peptides, enzyme activation, inhibition of sperm motility, reduced sperm capacitation and survival, and sperm phagocytosis. The free copper and copper salts released by copper-containing IUDs enhance the inflammatory reaction within the endometrium. However, this effect is local in the endometrium and cervical mucus, such that a change in serum copper levels cannot be detected. Progestin-releasing IUDs cause endometrial decidualization and glandular atrophy, in addition to thickening cervical mucus that acts as a barrier to sperm penetration. The LNg 20-IUD produces low serum concentrations of progestin, which lead to partial inhibition of follicular development and ovulation; however, at least 75% of women will have ovulatory cycles with the LNg 20-IUD.

Patient Selection and Contra-indications

Patient selection for IUD contraception is primarily aimed at decreasing the risk of infectious morbidity and other complications. Age and parity are not critical factors in selection, but rather the risk of STD acquisition is the most important consideration. There are relatively few conditions for which an IUD should not be used.

Contraindications

When anatomic abnormalities that distort the uterine cavity are present, IUDs should not be used because of the increased difficulty of insertion and the increased risk of expulsion when an IUD is placed in a uterine cavity less than 6 cm in length. Anatomic abnormalities precluding the use of an IUD can include a bicornuate uterus, cervical stenosis, and submucous leiomyomas. Special caution should be used when placing an IUD into a uterine cavity greater than 9 cm for the TCu-380A and greater than 10 cm for the LNg 20. However, nondistorting leiomyomata are not a contraindication to IUD use.

There is an increased risk of upper genital tract infection with IUD insertion in women with postpartum endometritis, postabortion infection, or active or recent STDs (within 3 months). However, there is no contraindication to use of the IUD in a woman with a distant history of PID who is no longer at risk for STDs.

IUD insertion should be avoided in anyone with a known or suspected pregnancy because IUD insertion can lead to miscarriage and increase the risk of septic abortion. However, the copper IUD can be used as a form of emergency contraception.

Because irregular bleeding can erroneously be attributed to the IUD once insertion has occurred, gynecologic problems causing irregular bleeding, including cervical and endometrial cancer, should be evaluated and diagnosed before insertion. Cervical ectropion and cervical dysplasia are not contraindications to IUD use.

Women who are immunocompromised may be at increased risk of PID with the IUD. Although some studies suggest there may be an increase in HIV transmission and acquisition with IUD use, others dispute this finding. Therefore, the IUD may be recommended for women at risk for HIV or with HIV or AIDS, especially if other methods are impractical or contraindicated.

Although no adverse events related to copper allergy or Wilson's disease have ever been reported with a copper IUD, it is recommended that copper-releasing IUDs be avoided in patients with these problems.

Conditions Requiring Caution

Caution should be exercised when considering the IUD for women with risk factors for STDs (e.g., having multiple partners or a partner with multiple partners), with a recent (within 3 months) history of treated gonorrhea or chlamydia, or with dysmenorrhea or menorrhagia (for the copper IUD only). Previous problems with an IUD including pregnancy, perforation, expulsion, pain, or heavy bleeding are not contraindications to its use.

Special Populations and Considerations

Adolescents

The IUD is one of the most effective means of birth control in women younger than 20 years of age, although pregnancies, expulsions, and removals for bleeding or pain are more frequent among women in this age group compared with older women. Rates of infection among adolescent IUD users are similar to those in adults.

Nulliparous Women

Nulliparous women in monogamous relationships are good candidates for IUDs. Compared with parous women, nulliparous women have similar rates of infection and efficacy with the IUD; however, they do experience higher rates of expulsion and discomfort that can lead to lower tolerance of the device. Fertility rapidly returns after discontinuing IUD use. Although concerns regarding infertility risks linger, a large well-designed study of nulligravid women found that the copper IUD does not appear to increase the risk of tubal infertility (see Suggested Reading).

Prior Ectopic Pregnancy

Although women who become pregnant with an IUD in place are more likely to have an ectopic pregnancy if they become pregnant, the IUD is actually protective against ectopic pregnancy because pregnancy is so rare with an IUD. The previous use of an IUD does not increase the risk of a subsequent ectopic pregnancy. Both the copper and the LNg 20-IUDs are acceptable options for women with a history of an ectopic pregnancy.

Insertion After Abortion

An IUD can be inserted safely immediately after a spontaneous or induced abortion in the first trimester without significant increased risk of perforation or expulsion. However, it is recommended to wait for uterine involution to occur before insertion of an IUD after a second-trimester abortion.

Insertion Postpartum

Immediate postpartum insertion of the copper IUD is possible after vaginal delivery or cesarean section, with a higher rate of expulsion but no increase in perforation or infection compared with interval insertion. Expulsion is less likely if the IUD is placed within 10 minutes after delivery of the placenta rather than waiting until 1 to 2 days postpartum. IUDs can also be safely inserted 4 to 8 weeks postpartum, and they are safe to use in breastfeeding women.

Chronic Medical Problems

Women with several chronic medical conditions including diabetes mellitus, cardiovascular disease, migraine headaches, breast cancer, benign breast disease, smoking, obesity, epilepsy, liver disease, gallbladder disease, or thyroid disease can use the IUD. Although valvular heart disease is not a contraindication to IUD use, prophylactic antibiotics are recommended at the time of insertion and removal to prevent endocarditis.

Several gynecologic conditions are also not contraindications to IUD use, including irregular menses (excluding menorrhagia for the copper IUD), cervical dysplasia, cervical ectropion, a history of benign ovarian cysts, past PID with a subsequent pregnancy, or history of prior cesarean delivery.

Adverse Effects and Problem Management

Copper IUDs are not associated with any systemic effects. The levonorgestrel IUD has been rarely associated with systemic effects related to the progestin; however, these are usually mild.

Abnormal Bleeding

As mentioned previously, both the copper and LNg 20 IUDs may be associated with irregular bleeding during the first few cycles after insertion. If a woman presents with excess bleeding or irregular bleeding after the first few months of insertion, certain disorders should be excluded including pregnancy, infection, partial expulsion, and gynecologic disorders of the cervix or uterus.

Pain

Cramping at the time of IUD placement is normal and may be reduced by paracervical block or administration of nonsteroidal anti-inflammatory drugs (NSAIDs) before insertion. However, severe cramping that lasts more than 15 minutes after insertion can be a sign of perforation. If a patient who already has an IUD in place develops severe cramping or abdominal tenderness, she must be evaluated for PID, ectopic pregnancy, spontaneous abortion, expulsion, or perforation. Milder menstrual cramping can be treated with NSAIDs.

Strings not Visible on Speculum Examination

If strings are not visible on speculum examination and pregnancy has been excluded, the first step is to use a cytobrush to try to draw the strings out of the endocervical canal. If this is unsuccessful, a uterine sound or the end of a sterile cotton swab can be used to explore the endocervical canal. If the IUD is present in the cervix, it should be removed at that time and replaced with a new IUD if the woman desires. If the IUD is not present at the cervix, IUD removal from the uterus can be attempted with alligator forceps or an IUD hook. Alternatively, the woman can be referred for an ultrasound or x-ray screening to determine the location of the IUD.

Expulsion

Expulsion occurs in 3% to 10% of women with the TCu-380A IUD and up to 6% with the LNg 20-IUD in the first year. Conditions that increase the risk for expulsion include nulliparity, menorrhagia, severe dysmenorrhea, prior expulsion, age younger than 20 years, or insertion immediately after second-trimester abortion or postpartum. Symptoms of expulsion include cramping, vaginal discharge, intramenstrual or postcoital bleeding, male or female dyspareunia, lengthened or absent strings, or a palpable IUD in the cervix or vagina; alternatively, expulsion may be asymptomatic.

Perforation

Uterine perforation occurs in one in 1000 IUD insertions and almost always occurs at the time of insertion. Risk factors include an inexperienced
clinician and an immobile or retroverted uterus. Clinical manifestations of
perforation include pain, a loss of resistance while inserting the IUD, or a
uterus that sounds to an unexpected depth. If perforation is suspected at
the time of insertion, the IUD should be removed, if possible, by gently
pulling on the strings. However, if there is resistance to removal, immediate laparoscopy should be performed to remove the IUD under direct visualization. Perforation may also be asymptomatic; therefore, it is important
to check the strings within a few weeks of IUD placement.

Infection

The risk of infection is greatest in the first 20 days after insertion (9.6 per
1000 women) but is otherwise rare (1.4 per 1000 women). Risk factors of
PID after insertion include the presence of bacterial vaginosis, cervicitis,
and contamination at insertion. Although antibiotics (doxycycline or azithromycin) can be given 1 hour before insertion to reduce the risk of
insertion-associated pelvic infection, there is little evidence that prophylactic antibiotics are beneficial for women at low risk of STDs.

Infections that occur more than 3 months after insertion are generally
due to a newly acquired STD. If PID is suspected, standard antibiotic treatment should be begun followed by removal of the IUD. Asymptomatic wom-
en with gonorrheal or chlamydia cervical infections and women with
trichomoniasis should receive standard treatment. Although IUD removal
is not necessary, the appropriateness of the IUD as a method of contraception
should be reassessed. Women with bacterial vaginosis and candidiasis
should receive standard treatment without IUD removal. Although there
is no increase in the incidence of bacterial vaginosis in women with IUDs,
some women do complain of increased vaginal discharge after IUD insertion.

Actinomyces, a gram-positive bacillus that is part of the normal vaginal
flora, has been associated with endometritis, PID, and pelvic abscesses. If
actinomycosis-like organisms are seen on a Pap smear of an asymptomatic
woman, there is no evidence to support antibiotic treatment or IUD removal. However, if repeat Pap smear 1 year later shows continued actinomy-
coses, the provider can either treat the woman with antibiotics (with or
without removing the IUD), remove the IUD without antibiotic treatment,
or leave the IUD in place, as long as the woman remains asymptomatic.

Pregnancy Complications

If a woman becomes pregnant with an IUD in place, the possibility of an
ectopic pregnancy must be excluded. If the pregnancy is intrauterine
and within the first trimester, the IUD should be removed if the strings
are visible on speculum examination to reduce the chance of infection
and miscarriage. If the woman desires an abortion, IUD removal can be
done at the time of the procedure. If she is having a spontaneous abortion,
the IUD should be removed and a 7-day course of antibiotics (doxycycline
or ampicillin) should be given. If pregnancy is diagnosed after the first

trimester, an ultrasound can help determine the placental and IUD locations. If the strings are visible and removal appears feasible based on the localization of the IUD, it may be removed, although removal may cause rupture of membranes or bleeding with subsequent pregnancy loss. If the IUD is left in place, the woman should be counseled regarding the increased risk of preterm labor and delivery, second-trimester fetal loss, and infection. She is not at increased risk of having a baby with birth defects.

BARRIER METHODS

Several forms of barrier methods of contraception are available, including the widely prevalent male condom, as well as female-controlled devices including the female condom, diaphragm, cervical cap, and contraceptive sponge. Barrier methods of contraception generally are less effective than hormonal contraception, and their efficacy is more dependent on the user (see Table 7-1). Nevertheless, they offer several important advantages: they generally have fewer side effects than hormonal contraception, they can be used intermittently, and they are noninvasive. Perhaps most importantly, barrier methods have been shown to decrease the risk of several STDs including chlamydia, gonorrhea, and herpes simplex virus. Male condoms have been shown to reduce the risk of transmission of HIV, and other barrier methods such as the female condom and diaphragm are being studied regarding their potential role in reducing the transmission of HIV.

Condoms

Most male condoms are made of latex, which has the disadvantage of the potential for latex sensitivity, breakage when used with oil-based lubricants, and decreased penile sensitivity. However, latex offers the advantage of protection from sexually transmitted infections including HIV. Condoms made of other materials such as polyurethane are expected to offer the same protection against STDs and HIV based on *in vitro* studies, but clinical studies have not been completed. "Natural skin" (lamb's intestine) condoms are available, but HIV and other organisms that cause STDs can penetrate condoms made from intestine.

The female condom consists of a pouch made of polyurethane that lines the vagina, with an internal ring in the closed end of the pouch that covers the cervix and an external ring that remains outside of the vagina, partially covering the perineum. These condoms are more cumbersome than male condoms, with relatively high rates of problems such as slippage. However, with experience, problems with use decrease. The female condom should be an effective barrier to STD infection; however, this issue has not been fully studied yet. This form of barrier contraception has the theoretical advantage of allowing the woman to have control in preventing STDs.

Diaphragm

The diaphragm requires fitting by a trained clinician and is only effective when used with a spermicide. It should be inserted no longer than 6 hours before sexual intercourse, and it should be left in place for approximately 6 hours (but no more than 24 hours) after coitus. Additional spermicide should be placed in the vagina before each additional act of intercourse while the diaphragm is in place. Side effects from the diaphragm are rare and minor, and they include vaginal irritation from the latex or the spermicidal jelly. In addition, urinary tract infections are twofold to threefold more common among diaphragm users compared with women using oral contraceptives.

Cervical Cap

The latex Prentif cervical cap is about as effective as the diaphragm (in nulliparous women), offers the advantage of being able to be left in place for a longer time (up to 48 hours), and does not need to be used with spermicide. However, the addition of a tablespoon of spermicide placed in the cap before insertion can improve efficacy and decrease the incidence of foul-smelling discharge common after 24 hours of use. Compared with the diaphragm, the Prentif cervical cap is somewhat harder to fit and is more difficult to insert.

Two newer cervical caps have been developed and approved by the FDA. Both are made from silicone rubber and can be left in place for up to 48 hours. Both devices are designed to be used in conjunction with a spermicide and have failure rates slightly higher than the latex diaphragm. The FemCap is shaped like a sailor's cap with a dome that covers the cervix and a brim that pushes against the vaginal fornices. It also has a strap to facilitate removal and comes in three sizes. Lea's Shield has a thick ring that extends from the dome of the cap to behind the pubic symphysis, as well as a one-way valve that allows cervical secretions to escape and creates suction to hold the cap in place. Unlike the other cervical caps and diaphragms, Lea's Shield is "one-size-fits-all."

Sponge

The Today Sponge is a soft, disposable polyurethane foam that contains the spermicide nonoxynol-9. After it is moistened with water and inserted in the vagina, it becomes effective immediately and remains effective for the next 24 hours without the need to add spermicidal cream even with repeated acts of intercourse. It does not require fitting and was available in the United States as an over-the-counter product until 1995, when it was taken off the market secondary to manufacturing problems. However, after an FDA review, the Today Sponge is currently available again in the United States.

SPERMICIDES AND MICROBICIDES

A variety of spermicidal jellies, creams, foams, gels, films, and suppositories are available without a prescription that can be used alone or in conjunction with a barrier method as contraception. All of these products on the market now contain nonoxynol-9, which was thought to decrease the risk of STDs, including HIV. However, more recent data suggest that nonoxynol-9 may in fact cause vaginal irritation and alter vaginal flora, thereby increasing the risk of HIV and STD acquisition. Several new microbicides are being developed and are in various stages of preclinical and clinical testing.

NATURAL FAMILY PLANNING

Natural family planning, or periodic abstinence, depends on avoiding intercourse during fertile days of the month. Although the highest likelihood of pregnancy occurs on the day of ovulation and the preceding 2 days, conception can occur from 6 days before ovulation until the day after ovulation. For natural family planning to work, the couple must be dedicated to remaining abstinent during this fertile period. Also, the time of ovulation must be predictable (i.e., regular menstrual cycles). In addition to tracking menstrual cycles with a calendar, women can determine the time of ovulation through other means including detection of cervical mucus changes, measuring basal body temperature, or hormone monitoring with urine luteinizing hormone kits. With good adherence to natural family planning, pregnancy rates are about the same as with the diaphragm or spermicides. To improve the efficacy and avoid a long period of abstinence, a couple can use a barrier method, spermicide, or both during the fertile period.

STERILIZATION

Sterilization is the most common method of birth control in the United States and worldwide. In the United States, 39% of women rely on female or male sterilization (28% and 11%, respectively).

Although sterilization is one of the most reliable methods of contraception, it is an option only for patients who do not wish to maintain future fertility because it is intended to be permanent and nonreversible. Accordingly, thorough counseling is needed to discuss the risks, benefits, and details about the procedure; other contraceptive options; permanence of the procedure; and the risk of failure, including the chance of ectopic pregnancy. Any discussion of female sterilization must include information regarding male sterilization as well. Regret has been reported in 3% to 25% of women; however, only 1% to 2% of all women who have undergone sterilization seek reversal. The most consistent factor associated with regret is change of marital status. A prospective study of women who underwent sterilization revealed that young age at the time of sterilization was the strongest predictor of regret, regardless of parity or marital status.

Sterilization can be performed postpartum, postabortion, as an interval procedure (unrelated to pregnancy), or in conjunction with another procedure such as cholecystectomy. Another form of contraception should be used up until the time of sterilization to reduce the possibility of a luteal-phase pregnancy. If possible, the procedure should also occur during the menstrual or proliferative phase of the cycle to reduce the chance of pregnancy at the time of the procedure. If this is not possible or practical, a sensitive urine or serum pregnancy test should be performed the day of the procedure to detect a possible luteal-phase pregnancy.

Although tubal sterilization is a very effective method of contraception, with a typical failure rate of 0.4% in the first year, a large long-term study of 10,685 women found the cumulative 10-year probability to be 18.5 per 1000 procedures. The risk of pregnancy was highest among women sterilized at a young age (younger than 28 years) with bipolar coagulation or Hulka-Clemens clip application. The failure rates with postpartum partial salpingectomy or unipolar coagulation were the lowest, though unipolar coagulation is rarely used because of safety concerns. When pregnancy does occur after tubal sterilization, the risk that it will be an ectopic pregnancy is increased (i.e., one third of all pregnancies that occur after a tubal sterilization). Nevertheless, the overall risk of an ectopic pregnancy is lowered in a woman after sterilization because of the overall greatly reduced risk of pregnancy.

Minilaparotomy

A minilaparotomy is most commonly used for postpartum sterilization, but it can be used for interval procedures as well. During the immediate postpartum period, the enlarged uterus and thinned umbilical area allow easier exposure through a minilaparotomy incision rather than laparoscopy. A 3- to 5-cm suprapubic incision can be used for an interval procedure.

Although different techniques for tubal occlusion can be used, including application of clips or rings, the more common methods of sterilization via minilaparotomy all involve removal of a portion of the fallopian tubes bilaterally. The most commonly used technique is the Pomeroy method. With this method, an isthmic "knuckle" of the tube is double ligated with plain catgut suture. Metzenbaum scissors are then used to create a defect in the mesosalpinx within the knuckle, and the ligated segment of the fallopian tube is excised. The most common complication with this method is slippage of the suture ligatures, but this risk is minimized by the placement of two sutures and exerting traction only on the distal suture. A less commonly performed technique is the Irving method, which was developed for sterilization at the time of cesarean section. With this technique, the proximal tubal stump is buried in the myometrium, whereas the distal stump is buried in the broad ligament. Because the latter part of the procedure does not increase effectiveness, it is usually omitted. Although the effectiveness of this technique is very high (with a failure rate of less than 1 per 1000 cases), the intraoperative blood loss is generally higher than with the Pomeroy method of tubal occlusion.

Another effective but complex technique of tubal sterilization is the Uchida method. With this method, the tubal serosa is dissected away from the muscularis before incision of a segment of the fallopian tube. The proximal stump of tube is subsequently buried into the mesosalpinx, and the distal stump is exteriorized or excised with the fimbria. Again, this method is associated with a higher blood loss, which along with its complexity makes this an uncommon method of sterilization.

Laparoscopic Techniques

Interval sterilization is most commonly performed by laparoscopy. The advantages of laparoscopy include rapid recovery, small incision, and the opportunity to visually explore the pelvis and abdomen. Because unexpected findings or complications can occur, the surgeon and patient must be prepared for possible conversion to laparotomy.

Although the previously described methods can be modified for use laparoscopically, the most common techniques involve application of Falope rings, clips, or electrocoagulation. Bipolar electrocoagulation is safer than unipolar electrocoagulation and is therefore preferred. Using bipolar forceps, an approximately 3-cm portion of the tube is desiccated in sequential bites along the isthmic portion of the tube. Transection of the tube is not necessary and may actually increase the chance of fistula formation. The Falope ring is a radiopaque silicon rubber ring that is applied to the fallopian tube using a ring applicator. After the ring is placed, a 1.0-cm-high knuckle of tube is seen above the ring. The ring functions to occlude the blood supply to this knuckle such that, over a period of days, the segment of tube becomes necrotic and the tubal segments separate. At times the ring will fall off of its applicator before placement, in which case it can be retrieved if easily possible or left in the abdomen without consequence. Of note, the Falope ring may not be able to be placed if the fallopian tubes are too edematous.

The other methods of occlusion are the Hulka-Clemens clip or the Filshie clip. Both are applied using a specific clip applicator. The Hulka clip consists of two toothed jaws made of plastic that are joined by a metal hinge pin. The Filshie clip, which is made of a composite of titanium and silicon rubber, is easier to apply, has a more efficient closure method, and is more effective.

Hysteroscopic Sterilization

In 2002, the FDA approved a transcervical sterilization technique (Essure) in which tiny nickel-titanium metal coils with polyethylene fibers are inserted into the fallopian tubes hysteroscopically. Over the next several months, subsequent growth of local tissue allows scar formation, which causes tubal occlusion. Initial data show that by 3 months 96% of tubes are closed, and by 6 months 100% of tubes are closed. Currently, the FDA requires that women who undergo the Essure method of sterilization continue to use an alternate form of birth control for the first 3 months after coil placement, at which time a hysterosalpingogram should be performed to confirm tubal occlusion. Although long-term data are not yet available, the initial trials show effectiveness at 99.8% among those women who are able to have coils properly placed. However, coil placement can be difficult in some women, with failure of placement in 8% of women in initial trials. Despite this shortcoming, the hysteroscopic method of tubal sterilization offers several advantages: reduced recovery time, avoidance of general anesthesia, and the ability to return to work the day after the procedure. Also, hysteroscopic sterilization is an alternative method of tubal sterilization for women in which laparoscopy or laparotomy is not preferred.

Male Sterilization

Vasectomy (i.e., ligation of the vas deferens) is a safer, easier, less expensive method of permanent sterilization that also has a lower failure rate compared with female sterilization. The procedure is usually done in a physician's office under local anesthesia. A semen analysis should be done after this procedure (typically after 30 ejaculations or 12 weeks postprocedure) to confirm azoospermia or at least the absence of motile spermatozoa. Despite earlier concerns for potential increase in prostate and testicular cancer as well as atherosclerosis, well-designed studies show no adverse consequences or harmful effects on men's health as a result of vasectomy.

181

SPECIAL CONSIDERATIONS AND SITUATIONS

Emergency Contraception

Emergency, or postcoital, *contraception* refers to any method that is used after intercourse to prevent pregnancy. The three methods available currently include high-dose progestin-only contraceptive pills, COC pills (Yuzpe method), or copper IUD insertion. Mifepristone has been studied and found to be useful as a method of postcoital contraception (as opposed to medical abortion) but is not yet approved for this use.

The Yuzpe method refers to a regimen of 100 µg of ethinyl estradiol and 0.5 mg of levonorgestrel that is taken twice, with 12 hours between doses. Until a dedicated product was made for this (Preven), various combinations of COCs were used to give the equivalent dose. This method reduces the number of anticipated pregnancies by 75% to 80%. The most common adverse effects, nausea and vomiting, can be reduced by taking meclizine 50 mg or metoclopramide 10 mg 1 hour before the first dose.

Levonorgestrel 0.075 mg given twice, with doses 12 hours apart, is a more effective method of emergency contraception, with fewer adverse effects of nausea and vomiting. The dedicated product using this regimen (Plan B) has no contraindications to its use except allergy to its components. Both of these regimens are more efficacious the earlier they are used. Although either should be used ideally within 72 hours of unprotected intercourse, the data show continued beneficial effects through 120 hours postcoital. In addition, a large WHO study demonstrated that giving a single 1.5-mg dose of levonorgestrel is as effective as two 0.75-mg doses given 12 hours apart.

With either method of emergency oral contraception used, patients should be counseled regarding the lack of protection these methods provide from STDs, as well as possible changes in menstrual bleeding. If no menstrual bleeding has occurred within 3 to 4 weeks of administration of emergency contraception, a pregnancy test should be performed. Also, women using emergency contraception should be advised that they are not protected from pregnancy if unprotected intercourse occurs after the pills have been taken. Therefore, women should be counseled to use a barrier method of contraception for the remainder of the cycle. Alternatively, oral contraceptives or another long-term form of contraception could be prescribed at that time. Women who are not using a regular method of birth control, or who are using barrier methods or natural family planning only, can be given a prescription for emergency contraception in advance.

An alternative method of emergency contraception is insertion of the copper IUD. This needs to be placed within 120 hours of unprotected intercourse. Although this method offers the advantage of providing continuing contraception after the unprotected intercourse event, it requires the provider to have an IUD available for immediate insertion. Also, candidates for emergency contraception with the copper IUD should be at low risk for acquisition of an STD.

Postpartum Period and Lactation

Of women who feed their infants exclusively via breastfeeding, 93% do not ovulate during the first 3 months postpartum because of the prolactin-induced inhibition of pulsatile gonadotropin-releasing hormone. However, women who use supplemental feedings and those who begin to menstruate are more likely to ovulate. In addition, even in women who do exclusively breastfeed, ovulation often occurs before the first menses; therefore, fertility awareness methods of contraception can be ineffective. For these reasons, many women will require contraceptive methods during the postpartum period while breastfeeding.

Because hormonal contraception may interfere with lactation and have a theoretical risk for the infant because of the transfer of hormones in the milk, nonhormonal methods of contraception (such as barrier contraception or copper IUD) are preferred. If hormonal contraception is desired, progestin-only methods are preferred because they have no significant impact on milk quality or production. The timing of initiation of progestin-only contraception in breastfeeding women is controversial because of the theoretical interference with lactogenesis with early initiation. Many authorities, such as ACOG, recommend initiating use of progestin-only pills 2 to 3 weeks postpartum and DMPA at 6 weeks' postpartum age but recognize that certain clinical situations, such as concern for patient follow-up, warrant earlier initiation of contraception. Although the clinical data are of poor quality, combined estrogen-progestin contraceptives are thought to suppress milk production. Therefore, initiation of combined hormonal contraception is generally recommended when the infant's diet is supplemented and no earlier than 6 weeks postpartum.

Perimenopause

Although fertility decreases with age, women are still at risk of becoming pregnant through menopause. In fact, the abortion ratio (the number of abortions per 1000 live births) is highest among women aged 40 years or older. Age is not a contraindication for any method of contraception, but some methods may be better suited for the needs of a perimenopausal woman. For example, the desire for permanent sterilization, the presence of underlying medical conditions, the frequency of intercourse, and the desire for noncontraceptive benefits such as control of menstrual cycle and hot flashes all influence a perimenopausal woman's choice of contraception.

In the United States, female sterilization is the most common method of contraception among perimenopausal women. IUDs offer long-term contraception that can often last through the time of menopause and have almost no contraindications related to comorbid medical conditions such as hypertension or diabetes. The LNg 20 IUD is an especially good option for perimenopausal women with irregular and heavy menses because this method has been shown to be an effective treatment for menometrorrhagia. The barrier methods may also be good options for perimenopausal women who are infrequently sexually active.

COCs are a common and useful method of contraception for perimenopausal women because of the beneficial effects on the menstrual cycle. Because COCs will mask the signs and symptoms of menopause, a common clinical dilemma is when to stop the administration of COCs. A common and viable option is to check the serum follicle-stimulating hormone (FSH) level at the end of a 7-day hormone-free (placebo) period starting at the age of 50 years. If the level is not greater than 20 IU/L, the patient should continue taking COCs and recheck the FSH level periodically in the future. Although, ideally, a 2-week hormone-free period is required for a more reliable measurement of serum FSH, this method is not as practical and puts the woman at risk for unwanted pregnancy. For women in whom estrogen is contraindicated, the progestin-only pills (POPs) are also a good option. DMPA is less ideal for perimenopausal women given the increase in irregular bleeding and increased risk of osteoporosis.

Medical Conditions

Hypertension
Women with hypertension have fewer contraceptive options than other women. Specifically, combined hormonal contraception is not recommended for women with moderate (systolic blood pressure 160 to 179 mm Hg/diastolic blood pressure 100 to 109 mm Hg) or severe hypertension because of an increased risk of cardiovascular events. However, in women with mild, controlled hypertension who are aged 35 years or younger and otherwise healthy, combination hormonal contraception may be used if blood pressure remains well controlled with monitoring several months after initiation of contraception. Progestin-only contraception can be an option, although easily reversed methods (i.e., DMPA) are preferred for women with moderate or severe hypertension. Copper and LNg 20 IUDs are good choices for women with hypertension.

Diabetes

With few exceptions, women with diabetes have the same contraceptive options as nondiabetic women. Low-dose COCs (and other combined hormonal contraception) do not have clinically significant effects on glucose metabolism or on the control of diabetes. COC use does not accelerate the progression of diabetic vascular diseases. However, in diabetic women with nephropathy, retinopathy, neuropathy, or other vascular disease, or in those who have had diabetes for more than 20 years, COCs are not recommended because of possible adverse effects on the cardiovascular system. DMPA is also not recommended because of possible negative effects on lipid metabolism that may affect the progression of neuropathy, retinopathy, or other vascular diseases. However, POPs and implants may be used safely by diabetic women with vascular disease. IUDs are also an excellent choice for diabetic women with vascular disease. Barrier methods can be used, but because of their higher rates of unintended pregnancy, caution should be used because the health risks associated with pregnancy are increased among diabetic women, especially those with vascular disease or other end-organ damage.

Sickle Cell Disease

The use of COCs by women with sickle cell disease has long been controversial. Although concern exists for the increased risk of thromboembolic events, numerous studies have shown that COC use by women with sickle cell disease is safe. The increased blood loss associated with the copper IUD could also pose a problem in women with anemia. For these reasons, the WHO recommends combined hormonal methods and the copper IUD as second choices (methods for which health benefits outweigh potential risks). All other methods of contraception are also considered acceptable for women with sickle cell disease, but a particularly good choice may be DMPA. Besides being an effective, reversible method of birth control, DMPA has been shown to reduce the incidence of painful sickling crises in women with sickle cell disease.

Epilepsy

Most anticonvulsant agents induce hepatic enzymes, which can decrease serum concentrations of the estrogen or progestin components of hormonal contraception. This effect has been observed with phenobarbital, phenytoin, carbamazepine, felbamate, and topiramate. Studies of serum levels of contraceptive steroids in women using COCs and gabapentin and tiagabine do not show a decreased level, but the anticonvulsant doses used were lower than those used in clinical practice. Valproic acid also does not alter the serum levels of contraceptive hormones. Lamotrigine does not appear to affect serum levels of oral contraceptive hormone levels, but lamotrigine levels may be reduced in women taking COCs. Because of the interaction between antiepileptic drugs and oral contraceptives, some clinicians prescribe COCs that contain 50 µg of ethinyl estradiol for women taking anticonvulsants that induce hepatic enzymes; however, no published data support this practice. Progestin-only contraceptives such as pills and implants also are affected by the increased metabolism with most anticonvulsants. However, it appears that the level of progestin with DMPA is substantially higher, such that it is still effective at preventing ovulation even in the context of coexisting antiepileptic drugs. Also, DMPA has been shown to lessen the frequency of seizures in women with partial seizures. IUDs are also a good contraceptive choice for women taking antiepileptic drugs.

KEY POINTS

1. With a few exceptions, the only requirements before administering hormonal contraception are to take a medical history and to measure blood pressure.

2. To provide the most appropriate and effective contraception for a particular woman, a thorough knowledge of all available options is essential.

3. Contraceptive effectiveness is influenced by many factors including choice, compliance, continuation, convenience, and access to a particular method.

4. Emergency contraception allows an opportunity to prevent pregnancy after unprotected intercourse.

5. Combined hormonal contraception, an extremely well-studied and safe method of birth control, is now available in multiple forms that allow patients more options to better fit their lifestyles.

6. Several highly effective progestin-only methods of birth control exist, and these are especially useful in women who cannot take estrogen.

7. Barrier methods of contraception are the only methods that offer some protection from sexually transmitted diseases in addition to preventing pregnancy.

8. The intrauterine device is a safe, cost-effective method of birth control that is often overlooked in the United States secondary to old myths about its use.

9. For women with chronic medical conditions, contraception is especially important because pregnancy may confer increased risks.

10. Many methods of birth control offer noncontraceptive health benefits.

SUGGESTED READING

Hatcher RA, Trussel J, and Stewart F, et al (eds): Contraceptive Technology. 18th rev ed. New York, Ardent Media, 2004.

Hubacher D, Lara-Ricalde R, Taylor DJ, et al: Use of copper intrauterine devices and the risk of tubal infertility among nulligravid women. N Engl J Med 345:561–567, 2001.

Peterson HB, Xia Z, Hughes JM, et al, for the U.S. Collaborative Review of Sterilization Working Group: The risk of pregnancy after tubal sterilization: findings from the U.S. Collaborative Review of Sterilization. Am J Obstet Gynecol 174:1161–1168, 1996.

Petitti DB: Clinical practice. Combination estrogen-progestin oral contraceptives. N Engl J Med 349:1443–1450, 2003.

Schiff I, Bell WR, Davis V, et al: Oral contraceptives and smoking, current considerations: Recommendations of a consensus panel. Am J Obstet Gynecol 180: S383–S384, 1999.

Speroff L, Darney PD: A Clinical Guide for Contraception, 3rd ed. Philadelphia, Lippincott Williams & Wilkins, 2001.

Stewart FH, Harper CC, Ellertson CE, et al: Clinical breast and pelvic examination requirements for hormonal contraception: Current practice vs evidence. JAMA 285:2232–2239, 2001.

World Health Organization: Medical Eligibility Criteria for Contraceptive Use, 3rd ed. Geneva, Switzerland, World Health Organization, 2004.

8

PEDIATRIC AND ADOLESCENT GYNECOLOGY

Claire Templeman and Joseph S. Sanfilippo

INTRODUCTION

The subspecialized area of pediatric and adolescent gynecology, the first experience with a gynecologic examination many girls will have, is an integral part of gynecologic care. Although some of the complaints such as vaginal discharge and bleeding are similar to those in adults, the underlying cause may be very different. Therefore, a clear understanding of normal anatomy and common gynecologic conditions affecting this age group are essential to providing appropriate care for these patients.

APPROACH TO EXAMINATION IN THE PREPUBERTAL AGE GROUP

A gynecologic examination in the pediatric age group is accomplished with the patient being "involved." In getting the child to comply, a "show and tell" approach works well; she must have control over the examination. Continued communication is essential while the process unfolds. The patient is placed in a "frog-legged position," allowing inspection of the vulva, introitus, and lower third of the vagina. Most vulvovaginitis is located in this area of the vagina. Low-power magnification as with an otoscope or colposcope is helpful. Use of a handheld mirror can be used to involve the child in the process. On completion of this segment of the examination, the patient is placed in a "knee-chest" position and asked to take a deep breath and bear down (Valsalva). Oftentimes, this provides the ability to evaluate up to the level of the cervix. Cultures and wet preparations can be obtained; it is rarely necessary to use any instrumentation. Abdominal and inguinal palpation provides further information. Any erythema, lichenification, or discharge should be noted. The configuration and intactness of the hymen should also be noted.

Tanner Classification

In the pediatric adolescent age group, quantification and characterization of pubertal milestones are important in the initial evaluation and patient follow-up. One useful method of documentation of this information is with use of the Tanner Classification (Fig. 8-1).

COMMON CONDITIONS IN PREPUBERTAL PATIENTS

Vulvovaginitis

Vulvovaginitis is the most common gynecologic condition of the prepubertal girl. The severity of the symptoms varies from child to child, but is usually distressing to both the child and the parents. It is estimated that up to 80% of gynecologic visits by premenarcheal girls result from vulvovaginitis.

Box 8-1 provides a list of factors that contribute to vulvovaginitis. A physiologic discharge is often noted around the time of puberty. It is characterized as a mucus-like, often nonodorous yellow discharge that represents ovarian hormone production. Appropriate management is reassurance. This differs from the discharge most commonly encountered in nonspecific vulvovaginitis, which typically has an odor. Nonspecific vulvovaginitis accounts for 75% of all vulvovaginitis in prepubertal girls; cultures usually reveal normal flora of the gastrointestinal tract. Nonspecific vulvovaginitis is best treated with instruction regarding vulvovaginal hygiene, wiping fecal material posteriorly away from the vaginal area, Sitz baths, and use of low-dose (1%) hydrocortisone. Additionally, Domeboro's solution can be used when acute sign and symptoms are present.

A number of bacterial organisms are responsible for "specific" vulvovaginitis in the pediatric patient. These include *Escherichia coli*, group A streptococcus, *Staphylococcus epidermidis*, *Haemophilus influenzae*, *Ureaplasma urealyticum*, and *Streptococcus pyogenes*. Appropriate antibiotics should only be administered if a particular pathogen is grown on vaginal culture. In addition, candida vulvitis may occur in prepubertal girls but is rare in the absence of diabetes or immunosuppression; routine antifungal treatment should be avoided unless this organism is seen on wet preparation or culture.

Abnormal physical examination findings are in part associated with the underlying abnormality. Table 8-1 lists the prevalence of symptoms associated with pediatric vulvovaginitis, including discharge, erythema (Fig. 8-2), and pruritus.

Pinworms

The presence of pinworms *(Enterobius vermicularis)* usually presents as intense nocturnal rectal and vulvovaginal pruritus. At night, white pin-sized worms migrate from the rectum to the vulvar skin to lay eggs. They can be diagnosed by flashlight or by dabbing clear tape on the vulvar skin and examining it under the microscope. Pinworms are treated with mebendazole as one 100-mg dose repeated 2 weeks later. Family members who are not pregnant should also be treated if there are no contraindications.

Figure 8-1

Tanner staging. (From Marshall WA, Tanner JM: Variation in the pattern of pubertal changes in girls. Arch Dis Child 44:291–303, 1969.)

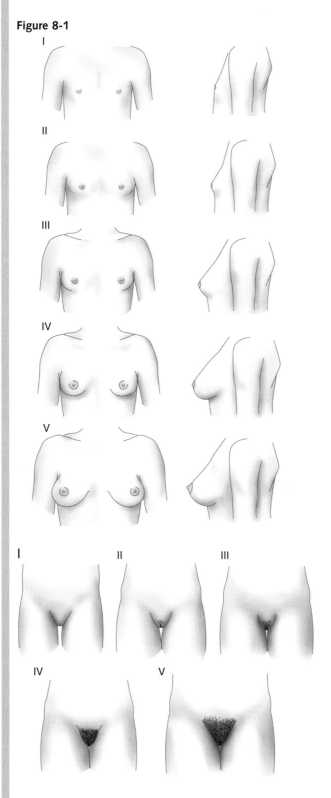

| Box 8-1 | Factors That Can Contribute to Childhood Vulvovaginitis |

Behavioral factors
Inadequate front-to-back wiping
Inattention to perineal hygiene at home or day program
Overly vigorous vulvar cleansing
Bubble baths, deodorant soaps
Sandbox play
Masturbation

Physiologic factors
Family respiratory or gastrointestinal illness
Diabetes mellitus or immunodeficiency state
Limited antibodies in vaginal secretions
Anestrogenic vaginal epithelium, neutral pH
Eczema, seborrhea, other dermatologic condition
Sexual abuse

Anatomic factors
Confining clothing
Decreased labial fat pads
Small labia minor
Thin, delicate, vulvar skin
Vulva anatomically close to anus

Adapted from Rau FJ, Muram D: Vulvovaginitis in children and adolescents. In Sanfilippo JS, Muram D, Dewhurst J, Lee PA (eds): Pediatric and Adolescent Gynecology, 2nd ed. Philadelphia, WB Saunders, 2001, pp 199–215.

Table 8-1

Symptoms Associated With Pediatric Vulvovaginitis

Problem	Prevalence (%)
Vaginal discharge	53
Erythema	33
Pruritus	32
Dysuria	12
Vaginal bleeding/spotting	5
Odor	8
Pain	4

Adapted from Rau F, Muram D: Pediatric and Adolescent Gynecology, 2nd ed. Philadelphia, WB Saunders, 2001, p 199.

Vaginal Bleeding

Vaginal bleeding in a prepubertal child usually provokes anxiety in the parents and results in a prompt visit to the physician. The common causes of the condition are listed in Box 8-2. A careful history documenting the number of episodes, the amount of bleeding, and any associated vaginal discharge or pruritus are important. Details of any witnessed fall, trauma, or suspicion of sexual abuse should be documented.

Physical examination should record vital signs along with height, weight and Tanner classification stage. On genital examination, evidence of trauma including labial tears and bruising should be noted. Hypopigmentation associated with fissuring and excoriation on the labia majora

Figure 8-2

Erythema of the vulva in a pediatric patient.

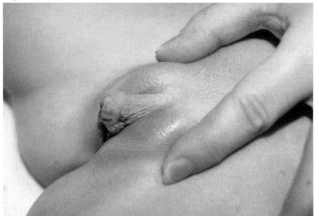

Box 8-2 Causes of Prepubertal Vaginal Bleeding
Foreign body Vaginal infections (i.e., streptococcus, shigella) Trauma Urethral prolapse Sexual abuse injuries Tumors Lichen sclerosis

and perianal area is typical of lichen sclerosis. Inspection of the urethral meatus may reveal a doughnut-shaped mass suggestive of urethral prolapse. Labial traction will help delineate the hymen and the posterior fourchette along with any present tears.

A foreign body may also be seen within the vagina through a combination of labial traction and the Valsalva maneuver. The use of a pediatric feeding tube attached to a 20-mL syringe with warmed saline is useful for performing vaginal irrigation that may reveal a foreign body, typically toilet paper. Any vaginal discharge observed should be swabbed for culture before irrigation. Suspicion for sexual abuse should prompt careful documentation of the findings and immediate discussion with child protective services in the local area. If infection is found, treatment with antibiotics to which the organism is sensitive will resolve the bleeding.

Fall-astride injuries may require repair under anesthesia. Bleeding that is persistent or recurrent will require further investigation; in particular, vaginoscopy can be performed to exclude a tumor or foreign body. Removal of the foreign body or biopsy of any suspicious mass can also be performed at this time.

Precocious puberty should be suspected in a child with a history of vaginal bleeding and signs of breast development. Investigation should include serum for follicle-stimulating hormone (FSH), luteinizing hormone

(LH), estradiol, thyroid-stimulating hormone (TSH), and prolactin. Radiologic evaluation should include a bone age obtained in a pediatric radiology facility and a pelvic ultrasound to exclude an ovarian mass such as an estrogen-secreting granulosa cell tumor.

Ovarian Cysts

Ovarian cysts in childhood are not uncommon, and therefore an understanding of the normal physiology of the ovary is essential to prevent inappropriate intervention.

Based on ultrasound data, the incidence of antenatally diagnosed ovarian cysts is estimated at 1 in 2625 female births. However, data from stillbirth and neonatal death autopsies suggest that the incidence of cysts smaller than 1 cm in diameter may be as high as 30% of all female births. Fetal ovarian cysts are typically functional because the ovary is stimulated by fetal gonadotropins, maternal estrogen, and placental human chorionic gonadotropin. The diagnosis is usually established in the third trimester of pregnancy, and improvements in ultrasound technology have resulted in this diagnosis being made more frequently. The differential diagnosis includes mesenteric and urachal cysts, mesonephric cysts, hematometra with vaginal agenesis, and gastrointestinal duplication cysts. Therefore, antenatal ultrasound examination must detail female external genitalia, a normal urinary tract (i.e., kidneys, ureter, and bladder), and a normal gastrointestinal system (i.e., stomach, large and small bowel) to confirm this diagnosis.

Because the incidence of malignancy in neonatal cysts approaches zero, postnatal management for asymptomatic, simple cysts involves observation with regular ultrasound review. Expected cyst resolution is 50% by 1 month, 75% by 2 months, and 90% by 3 months of age. Postnatal surgical intervention is reserved for cyst persistence, enlargement, symptoms, or a complex appearance on ultrasound examination. These factors are suggestive of a cyst complication such as hemorrhage or torsion.

The ovaries are active during both infancy and childhood. Cysts in patients of this age group are the result of gonadotropin stimulation producing follicular activity. The incidence decreases in early childhood and increases as puberty approaches. Ovarian cysts (mean < 7.5 mm in diameter) have been demonstrated in up to 80% of girls between 1 and 24 months of age and 68% of girls between 2 and 10 years old. In general, 90% of these are 9 mm or less in size, with an ovarian volume of 1 cm.[3]

In prepubertal patients, normal pelvic organs are usually not palpable, and "pelvic masses" are usually felt abdominally. A rectal examination may be helpful in further characterizing a mass; however, pelvic ultrasound is likely to provide the most useful information.

Ovarian cysts are occasionally functional, secreting estrogen and resulting in vaginal bleeding or breast development. This clinical presentation creates concern for precocious puberty. If ovarian cysts are associated with large café-au-lait spots and vaginal bleeding, McCune-Albright syndrome, involving gonadotropin-independent hormone secretion, should be considered. Enlarged, multicystic ovaries should prompt investigation for hypothyroidism. In both these conditions, treatment should be directed toward the underlying medical condition and not the ovarian cyst. However, ovarian torsion or a solid ovarian mass in this age group should prompt primary management of the ovarian mass.

COMMON PROBLEMS IN ADOLESCENCE

Delayed Puberty and Primary Amenorrhea

Puberty is defined as the process of developing secondary sexual characteristics indicative of endogenous hormone production. The pubertal process includes thelarche (i.e., breast development), adrenarche (i.e., axillary hair growth), and a growth spurt that precedes menarche (i.e., the onset of menses). After menarche, the hypothalamic-pituitary-ovarian (HPO) axis develops the ability to respond to both positive and negative feedback. On average, 18 months transpires between menarche and ovulatory cycles. The latter is indicative of a mature HPO axis. At the hypothalamic level, gonadotropin-releasing hormone (GnRH) is released into the portal system with the resultant release of gonadotropins. GnRH release in the anterior pituitary stimulates synthesis of FSH and LH. Although FSH and LH act synergistically, LH acts primarily on the theca cells in the ovary to produce steroidogenesis, whereas FSH acts on the granulose cells to stimulate follicular growth. Cholesterol is converted to androgens upon entrance into the theca cell. This is followed by aromatase activity and conversion of androgens to estrogens in the granulosa cell. Regulation of the HPO axis is under genetic control. Neurotransmitters including neuropeptide Y, gamma-aminobutyric acid, endorphins, interleukins, and leptins are involved in the neurohormonal axis regulation. In addition, neuregulins, epidermal growth factor, and prostaglandins (E_2 and $F_{2\alpha}$) are also involved. The prostaglandins are bioactive substances that represent a response to hormonal stimulation.

Delayed puberty is defined as the absence of secondary sex characteristics by 13.4 years of age or the absence of menarche in the presence of sex characteristics by 16 years of age. There is overlap between the differential diagnosis of delayed puberty and primary amenorrhea. Box 8-3 provides a classification of pubertal delay.

Germane to the etiology of delayed puberty is the presence of FSH receptor mutations as with ovarian resistance (i.e., Savage syndrome) or mutations of the DNA-binding domain in patients with androgen insensitivity. Other causes of delayed puberty include GnRH receptor mutations and resultant hypogonadotropic hypogonadism. When the latter is associated with anosmia, female Kallmann syndrome is the diagnosis. Mutations involving the *SRY* gene are noted in patients with Swyer syndrome.

The most common cause of delayed puberty is constitutional delay. Often there is a family history of such. Furthermore, these patients often have a relatively short upper body segment with growth delay (i.e., absence of a growth spurt). There does not appear to be an alteration in bone mineral density associated with this condition. The primary reason to

Box 8-3 Classification of Pubertal Delay and Pubertal Failure

A. Pubertal Delay
  1. Constitutional growth and pubertal delay
  2. Secondary to chronic illness
      Anorexia nervosa
      Asthma
      CNS disorders (Langerhans cell histiocytosis, congenital defects)
      Endocrine disease (hypothyroidism, hyperandrogenism, hypercortisolism, hyperprolactinemia, diabetes mellitus type I)
      Gastrointestinal disease (celiac disease, post-radiotherapy and chemotherapy, thalassemia)
      Hepatic disease
      Infections
      Intense exercise
      Malnutrition
      Renal failure
      Stress
B. Pubertal Failure
  1. Hypogonadotropic hypogonadism
      Idiopathic syndromes (Kallmann, Prader-Willi, Laurence Moon-Biedl)
      Hypopituitarism
        Isolated LH or FSH deficiency
      Panhypopituitarism
      Congenital abnormalities of CNS
      Secondary to Langerhans cell histiocytosis
  2. Hypergonadotropic hypogonadism
      Congenital
        Gonadal dysgenesis
        Biosynthesis and androgen receptor defects
        Anorchidism or cryptorchidism
        Syndromes (Klinefelter, Turner, Noonan, Alström, Steiner myotonic, Del Castillo)
  3. Hypo/hypergonadotropic hypogonadism
      Secondary to
        Surgery
        Chemotherapy/radiotherapy
        Trauma, tumors, infectious disease

CNS, Central nervous system.
Adapted from Tragiai C, Stanhope R: Delayed puberty: Best practice and research. Clin Endocrinol Metab 16(1):139–151, 2002.

treat constitutional delay is for psychological reasons. Depending on the circumstance, use of low-dose estrogens, 2 to 5 µg/day can be preceded by administration of growth hormone. This is best coordinated with either a pediatric or reproductive endocrinologist. It is important to assess thyroid function, bone age, and gonadotropin levels; karyotyping may provide additional information.

Eating Disorders

Anorexia nervosa is associated with delayed puberty. Low lean body mass has been linked to delayed puberty, and Frisch's theory of 17% total body fat being necessary for menarche and 22% for normal ovulatory cycles remains in vogue.

Endocrine Diseases

Either hypothyroidism or hyperthyroidism can result in delayed puberty. It is thought that thyroid dysfunction has a direct influence on the HPO axis. Insulin-dependent diabetes and polycystic ovarian syndrome (PCOS) can also cause delayed puberty. Treatment of the underlying disorder oftentimes results in pubertal onset.

Chronic Disease

Medical problems such as asthma, inflammatory bowel disease, or renal failure may delay the onset of puberty. The mechanism of action appears to be primarily at the hypothalamic level, adversely affecting GnRH release. This results in amenorrhea. Other problems include the intense exercise, oncologic disease, and congenital or acquired defects of the central nervous system.

Hypo-gonadotropic Hypogonadism

Idiopathic hypogonadotropic hypogonadism is associated with low levels of gonadotropins with resultant low levels of sex steroids. Current thinking ascribes the etiology of hypogonadotropic hypogonadism to mutations in a number of genes. Specifically, these genes include *KAL* gene (X-linked Kallmann syndrome), *DAXI* gene (X-linked adrenal hypoplasia) and related orphan nuclear receptor, steroidogenic factor-I, leptin, and prohormone convertase-I. The last of these affects GnRH release. Other problems in this category include GnRH receptor defects and transcription at the pituitary level with regard to *HESX-I, LHX3,* and *PORP-I.* LH and FSH receptor defects are also implicated.

Hyper-gonadotropic Hypogonadism

The category of hypergonadotropic hypogonadism is primarily indicative of gonadal dysgenesis, with Turner's syndrome the most common type. With the latter, 45X karyotype or a mosaic is responsible. Perrault syndrome is characterized by 46XX and pure gonadal dysgenesis. This syndrome is associated with gonadal failure and sensorineural deafness. XY gonadal dysgenesis and multiple X chromosomes are other related forms of hypergonadotropic hypogonadism.

The other major type is Klinefelter's syndrome, which is characterized by seminiferous tubule dysgenesis and either 47XXY or other varieties with additional chromosomes. The characteristic phenotype is small external genitalia, radial-ulnar synostosis, mental retardation, and dysmorphic features that include hypertelorism, prognathia, and strabismus. In general, these patients are tall and have gynecomastia.

Chemotherapy

Delayed puberty can also result from chemotherapy. Of interest, pre- and postpubertal ovaries are generally more resistant to cyclophosphamide than are adult ovaries. However, there appears to be a dose-related response that may be reversible. The addition of busulfan almost always results in ovarian failure. Radiotherapy can cause injury to the gonads and result in a hypergonadotropic state when the ovaries are involved. On the other hand, hypogonadotropic states can result with central nervous system irradiation as well as with acute leukemia. In general, central nervous system radiation doses of more than 40 Gy result in delayed or failed onset of puberty.

Androgen Insensitivity Syndrome

This problem resulting in primary amenorrhea is a reflection of defects in the androgen receptor. The key characteristic is that of a phenotypic female with a karyotype containing a Y-bearing line. The circulating androgens (i.e., total testosterone) are in the male range. These patients ideally undergo gonadectomy to minimize the risk of malignancy.

Evaluation and Management of Delayed Puberty and Primary Amenorrhea

The algorithm in Figure 8-3 provides an orderly method of assessment for delayed puberty and primary amenorrhea. Treatment will vary depending on the underlying etiology of the delayed onset. It is important that the patient be kept in step with peers. Low-dose estrogens may be used to initiate pubertal development, as noted in the constitutional delayed section.

Secondary Amenorrhea

An adolescent presenting with secondary amenorrhea must always have pregnancy ruled out; a pregnancy test should routinely be obtained. At

Figure 8-3

An algorithm for the evaluation of delayed puberty and primary amenorrhea. GHD, Growth hormone deficiency; Gn def., gonadotropin deficiency; GnRH, gonadotropin-releasing hormone; hCG, human chorionic gonadotropin; AIS, androgen insensitivity syndrome.

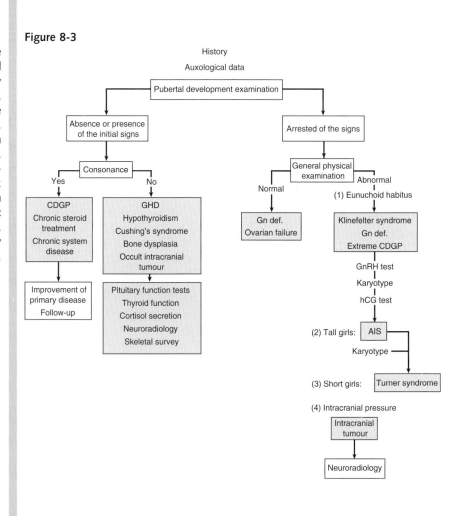

times, the adolescent may deny being sexually active, especially if asked in the presence of a parent. Evaluation and management of non–pregnancy-related secondary amenorrhea are best undertaken as they are in an adult patient.

Polycystic ovary syndrome (PCOS) in an adolescent is worthy of discussion. Although PCOS is often not diagnosed until adulthood, careful questioning may uncover symptoms beginning in adolescence. A detailed history reveals onset of menstrual irregularity, primarily in the form of oligomenorrhea, and hirsutism beginning in adolescence. Stemming from the original description by Stein and Leventhal in 1935 as a syndrome consisting of amenorrhea, hirsutism, and obesity associated with polycystic ovaries, our knowledge today includes a better understanding of the disease process in the adolescent.

Although an increased ratio of LH to FSH is of interest, the diagnosis is a clinical one and not predicated on the presence or absence of a 2:1 or greater ratio. The condition affects 6% to 8% of the population and is characterized by hyperandrogenism and insulin resistance. Current thinking reflects that the hyperinsulinemia effect at the ovarian level is responsible for the metabolic aberration and an increase in ovarian androstenedione and testosterone production. This leads to peripheral conversion of androgens to estrone and a resultant "positive feedback" at the hypothalamic-pituitary level. The effect of the latter is increased LH release and ovarian inhibin production (Fig. 8-4).

Metformin has become a mainstay of therapy in adolescent patients. This insulin sensitizer is frequently responsible for the onset of regular menses, in part a reflection of the metabolic correction at the ovarian level. The long-term consequences of PCOS must be emphasized and should include adult-onset (type II) diabetes mellitus and cardiovascular profiles resembling that of men with early-onset cardiovascular disease. Although the data are not clear-cut, the earlier use of insulin sensitizers theoretically may avert these adult-related problems. Currently, the U.S. Food and Drug

197

Figure 8-4

Pathophysiology of polycystic ovarian syndrome according to the "estrone hypothesis." PCO, Polycystic ovary; LH, luteinizing hormone; FSH, follicle-stimulating hormone.

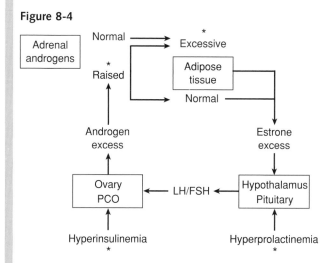

Administration approves metformin for the treatment of type II diabetes, and the patient and parent should be informed accordingly. Although gastrointestinal adverse effects are not uncommon, the more profound but rarer problem is that of lactic acidosis in association with metformin use.

Alternative treatments in adolescent patients include use of oral contraceptives to increase sex hormone–binding globulin and thus decreased effects of free androgen. Other preparations, such as 5α-reductase inhibitors and spironolactone, are used to treat the hirsutism aspect of the disease but are not well studied in adolescents.

Ovarian Cysts in Adolescence

The early postmenarcheal period is often associated with anovulation. Ovarian cysts in this age group may be the result of anovulation or failure of involution. These cysts are often detected on a pelvic ultrasound scan performed to diagnose the cause of pain and typically will resolve spontaneously. However, if there is concern over the etiology, a follow-up ultrasound scan 4 to 6 weeks later can be helpful. Persistent ovarian cysts raise the possibility of paratubal masses, benign tumors, endometriomas, complications of pelvic inflammatory disease including tubo-ovarian abscess or hydrosalpinx, and rarely, germ cell malignancies. The possibility of pregnancy must always be considered in the case of a teenager with an adnexal mass. Each of these conditions may have similar symptoms, making history and physical examination important in determining the likely etiology.

Management will depend on the diagnosis; however, preservation of ovarian tissue should be the primary concern. This approach is reasonable given a reported ovarian malignancy rate of 4.4% in girls between the ages of 15 and 21 years.

The presence of abdominal pain in a patient with an ovarian mass should increase concern for ovarian torsion. This diagnosis should still be considered even in the presence of flow on Doppler examination. Once confirmed at surgery, detorsion and preservation of the ovary should be pursued unless the ovary is obviously necrotic.

Pelvic Pain

Pelvic pain is a common clinical challenge for all physicians due to the large number of potential causes. Pelvic pain is defined as acute if it has been present less than 1 week and chronic if it has been present 3 to 6 months. This distinction is important because it will provide insight into the likely etiology. Possible gynecologic etiologies for acute and chronic pain are listed in Box 8-4.

A detailed history of the pain characteristics and associated symptoms is an important first step. This should be completed in addition to a gynecologic, sexual, and general medical history. Age at menarche and any relationship of the pain to menstruation should be documented. Physical examination should initially concentrate on Tanner stage development, since this will allow the physician to illuminate possible diagnoses. For example, if the patient is at Tanner developmental stage I for breast and

---

> **Box 8-4** Gynecologic Causes of Acute and Chronic Pelvic Pain in Adolescence
>
> **Causes of acute pain**
> Infectious disease (i.e., acute pelvic inflammatory disease)
> Pregnancy complication (i.e., spontaneous abortion, ectopic pregnancy)
> Ovarian cyst accident (i.e., torsion, rupture, hemorrhage)
> Musculoskeletal injury
> Obstructive uterovaginal anomaly
>
> **Causes of chronic pain**
> Endometriosis

pubic and axillary hair, then a hematometra from an obstructed uterine anomaly is unlikely because menarche is the final event on the pubertal timeline. The decision to perform a pelvic examination will often depend on the age of the patient.

In early adolescence, the patient should be given the option of pelvic examination in the absence of the parents; this will allow the physician additional time to gain information about sexual activity including previous sexually transmitted disease, contraceptive habits, and pregnancy history. An explanation of the procedure and instruments used for a pelvic examination is essential, especially if this is the first pelvic examination the patient has undergone. An assurance that the examination will stop at the patient's request is important in making her feel in control and is likely to enhance adequate pelvic examination.

Careful inspection of the external genitalia may reveal a hymeneal bulge at the fourchette or evidence of discharge. Speculum examination will allow for the collection of specimens for the detection of chlamydia and gonorrhea. Alternatively, if there is strong suspicion in a patient who will not consent to a pelvic examination, urine sampling can be performed to test for these organisms. Pelvic examination may reveal tenderness indicative of inflammation and infection.

An often overlooked cause of pelvic of abdominal pain is injury to the musculoskeletal system. It is important to actively explore this possibility, since it may prevent unnecessary surgical intervention. These injuries may be the cause of either acute or chronic pain. Typically, examination reveals "trigger points" of focal tenderness. These areas may cause referred pain through taut bands of muscle; this condition is known as *myofascial syndrome*. Potential treatments include local anesthetic injection of these areas and physical therapy performed by a therapist who is experienced in treating pelvic pain conditions.

Endometriosis

Traditionally, endometriosis had been thought to occur only rarely in adolescence. However, recent studies suggest that, among teenagers with pelvic pain unresponsive to medical therapy, 67.4% to 73% have endometriosis diagnosed at laparoscopy. Using the revised American Fertility Society (now termed *American Society for Reproductive Medicine*) classification, adolescent endometriosis has typically been reported as being stage 1 (mild) or 2 (moderate) unless there is an associated outflow tract obstruction. Overall, 6.9% of patients may have a family history of the disease.

Current assessment of an adolescent presenting with chronic pelvic pain includes a detailed history including pain characteristics along with previous and current treatments. Physical examination may illicit evidence of musculoskeletal and cul-de-sac tenderness along with levator muscle spasm. A pelvic ultrasound scan should be obtained to exclude an ovarian mass or uterovaginal anomaly.

In adolescents, the current standard of care in the management of dysmenorrhea or pelvic pain unresponsive to conservative therapy (i.e., nonsteroidal anti-inflammatory drugs and a trial of oral contraceptives) is laparoscopy. This provides for the diagnosis and treatment of any endometriotic lesions; biopsy of any evident disease is important to establish the diagnosis. Changes in the appearance of endometriosis with age have been described. These changes include an evolution of subtle forms of the disease (e.g., red lesions, clear or white vesicles) in adolescence evolving into more typical blue or black lesions a decade later. Therefore, a surgeon investigating pelvic pain in adolescents must be familiar with atypical forms of endometriosis.

There is currently no marker predictive of endometriosis progression. Therefore, in the absence of obvious residual disease, it is difficult to determine which patients may benefit from postoperative treatment. In adolescents, whose primary concern is usually pain instead of infertility, postoperative medical treatment may be used as a means for delaying the time to symptom recurrence by producing amenorrhea.

In patients with intractable pelvic pain, the benefits of a multidisciplinary pain team approach can be invaluable. The use of physical therapy alone or in association with transcutaneous nerve stimulators may be helpful. Alternative therapies such as acupuncture have also proved successful in some patients.

Uterovaginal Anomalies

An understanding of müllerian anomalies and their presentation requires a thorough understanding of reproductive embryology and the classification of uterovaginal anomalies. A classification that categorized uterine anomalies into six groups was developed in the past. This classification was revised by the American Fertility Society in 1988 to include associated variations in the vagina, cervix, and fallopian tubes.

An extensive discussion regarding uterovaginal anomalies is beyond the scope of this chapter; however, knowledge of the presentation and management in adolescence is important. Obstructive müllerian anomalies may coexist with endometriosis, increasing the severity of the pain symptoms. Typical presenting complaints in adolescence include the following:

1. Primary amenorrhea with cyclic abdominal pain: Adolescents with these symptoms will usually have normal secondary sexual

characteristics, and genital examination may reveal vaginal agenesis, a transverse septum, or rarely, cervical agenesis. If a bluish bulging mass is seen at the introitus, an imperforate hymen should be suspected. Rectal examination may confirm the presence of a pelvic mass that may be bulging above the level of obstruction, suggestive of hematometra (i.e., collection of blood in the uterine cavity) or hematometrocolpos (i.e., collection of blood in the uterine cavity and vagina). Patients with primary amenorrhea, vaginal agenesis, and no bulging mass may have müllerian agenesis with a functional endometrial cavity in one of the smaller residual horns.

2. Normal cyclic menstruation with increasing abdominal and pelvic pain: Patients with these symptoms will also have normal secondary sexual characteristics; pelvic examination results may be normal or may reveal an adnexal mass indicating the possibility of an obstructed, noncommunicating uterine horn. Careful palpation for tense, lateral masses in the vagina is important in this clinical setting, since this indicates the possibility of an obstructed hemi-vagina.

3. Normal cyclic menstruation in the absence of abdominal pain, but discomfort with tampon insertion or intercourse: Adolescents with these symptoms may have hymeneal septum or perforated transverse vaginal septum through which menstruation can occur.

A differential diagnosis for uterovaginal anomalies can usually be established after clinical examination; imaging is essential before any proposed surgery. Pelvic ultrasound is widely available and will detect hematometra, hematocolpos, and adnexal masses. It should be accompanied by renal ultrasound due the high incidence (25%) of coexistent anomalies. Magnetic resonance imaging is useful for delineating the presence of a cervix or transverse septum and in patients with complex anomalies. The timing of surgery will depend upon the urgency of the clinical situation.

An imperforate hymen or pregnancy in a noncommunicating horn will require immediate attention. In nonemergent situations, the age at presentation and maturity of the patient are important considerations. If postoperative use of vaginal dilators is required, it is essential that the patient feel comfortable with their use and understand the commitment required. Noncompliance will yield vaginal stenosis and an unsatisfactory outcome. If the patient is not comfortable with vaginal dilators at the time of diagnosis and has an obstructive anomaly, menstrual suppression with a GnRH agonist, depot medroxyprogesterone acetate, or oral contraceptive pills may allow time for counseling and practice in vaginal dilator use.

Menorrhagia and Abnormal Uterine Bleeding in Adolescence

Excessive, prolonged, or irregular bleeding from the uterine cavity is termed *abnormal uterine bleeding*; in the absence of anatomic causes, it is called *dysfunctional uterine bleeding*. In adolescents, immaturity of the HPO axis produces anovulation, which often results in excessive bleeding. This pattern decreases with time and occurs in fewer than 20% of girls 5 years from menarche. The potential causes of abnormal bleeding are listed in Box 8-5.

> **Box 8-5** Causes of Abnormal Uterine Bleeding in Adolescence
>
> Pregnancy complications
> Benign and malignant neoplasms of the genital tract
> Ovarian tumors such as granulosa cell tumors
> Cervical polyps or malignancy
> Leiomyomas
> Genital tract infection
> Endocrinopathy
> Polycystic ovarian disease
> Hyperprolactinemia
> Thyroid disease
> Trauma
> Exogenous drugs and hormones
> Chronic systemic disease

Coagulopathy is the second most common cause of abnormal uterine bleeding in adolescents. This may be the initial presentation of a hematologic disease in up to 3% of patients—most commonly, von Willebrand's disease. Other possible diagnoses include immune-mediated thrombocytopenia, Glanzmann's disease, Fanconi anemia, and thalassemia major. Menorrhagia in patients with known hematologic disease is more common, occurring in up to 30% of these adolescents, particularly when platelet nadir is present.

Evaluation of abnormal uterine bleeding in adolescents involves taking a careful history and performing a physical examination, including the collection of genital cultures. Investigation may include a complete blood count and smear, a coagulation profile including a prothrombin and partial thromboplastin times, and ristocetin cofactor as a functional marker of von Willebrand's disease. Endocrine evaluation to assess for thyroid disease (TSH and thyroxine) is also important.

Management should be directed toward treatment of any acutely reversible cause, such as genital trauma. Otherwise, the management should proceed according to the severity of the bleeding, as outlined in Table 8-2.

CONCLUSIONS

An understanding of normal genital anatomy and physiology is important for practitioners who manage gynecologic problems in children and adolescents.

Vaginal discharge in prepubertal girls is most commonly due to nonspecific vulvovaginal vaginitis resulting from poor hygiene. Antifungal treatments, commonly used in adult women, are rarely indicated in children. In adolescents, progressive dysmenorrhea should prompt investigation for endometriosis or a uterovaginal anomaly. Menorrhagia in young women may be indicative of an underlying coagulation disorder, and laboratory investigation should commence before hormonal treatment.

Table 8-2

Management of
Abnormal Uterine
Bleeding in the
Adolescent

Hemoglobin Value (g/100 mL)	Management
>12	Reassurance
	Menstrual calendar
	Iron supplements
	Periodic reevaluation
10–12	Reassurance and explanation
	Menstrual calendar
	Iron supplements
	Cyclic progestins or oral contraceptives
	Reevaluate in 6 months
<10, with no active bleeding	Evaluate for coagulation defect
	Transfuse, give iron supplements
	Oral contraceptives
	Reevaluate in 3 months
Acute hemorrhage	Evaluate for a coagulation defect
	Transfuse
	Consider intravenous estrogens with progestin therapy
	Consider dilatation and curettage
	Oral contraceptive for 6–12 months

Adapted from Templeman C, Hertweck SP, Muram D, Sanfilippo J: Vaginal bleeding in childhood and menstrual disorders in adolescence. In Sanfilippo JS, Muram D, Dewhurst J, Lee PA (eds): Pediatric and Adolescent Gynecology, 2nd ed. Philadelphia, WB Saunders, 2001, pp 237–247.

203

SUGGESTED READING

Bertelloni S, Baroncelli G, Ferdeghini M, et al: Normal volumetric bone mineral density and bone turnover in young men with histories of constitutional delay of puberty. J Clin Endocrinol Metab 83:4280–4283, 1998.

Burstein GR, Hunt KV: What's new in the new CDC HIV and STD guidelines? J Pediatr Adolesc Gynecol 16:57–60, 2003.

Frisch R, McArthur J: Menstrual cycles: Fatness as a determinant of minimum weight for height necessary for their maintenance or onset. Science 185: 949–951, 1974.

Kumar R, Biggart J, McEnvoy J, McGeown MT: Cyclophosphamide and reproductive function. Lancet 1:1212–1214, 1972.

Rappaport R, Brauner R, Czernichow P, et al: Effect of hypothalamic and pituitary radiation on pubertal development in children with cranial tumors. J Clin Endocrinol Metab 54:1164–1168, 1982.

REVISED ENDOMETRIOSIS CLASSIFICATION

Revised American Society for Reproductive Medicine: Classification of endometriosis: 1996. Fertil Steril 67:817–821, 1997.

Sanders J: The Seattle Marrow Transplant Team: The impact of marrow transplant preparative regimens on subsequent growth and development. Semin Hematol 28:244–249, 1991.

Timmreck L, Reindollar R: Contemporary issues in primary amenorrhea. Obstet Gynecol Clin North Am 30:287–302, 2003.

Traggiai C, Stanhope R: Delayed puberty: Best practice and research. Clin Endocrinol Metab 16(1):139–151, 2002.

UTEROVAGINAL AMERICAN SOCIETY OF REPRODUCTIVE MEDICINE CLASSIFICATION

Buttram VC Jr, Gibbons WE: Mullerian anomalies: A proposed classification (an analysis of 144 cases). Fertil Steril 32:40–46, 1979.

9

CONGENITAL AND DEVELOPMENTAL ANOMALIES

Marjan Attaran and Gita P. Gidwani

AMBIGUOUS GENITALIA IN NEWBORNS

Although most obstetricians will rarely see an infant with ambiguous genitalia at the time of delivery, the need to assess the situation quickly is important if this unfortunate developmental anomaly occurs. Any deviation from the normal male or female genitalia should prompt an investigation because ambiguous genitalia may reflect a discrepancy between genetic sex, gonadal sex, and phenotypic sex. The recognition of ambiguous genitalia poses a medical and psychological emergency.

The clinical examination alone seldom determines the precise diagnosis of the underlying intersex condition but should be performed in a systematic fashion. The clitoris or phallus is usually enlarged; the length and the transverse diameter must be measured and compared with norms. The normal length and transverse diameter of the clitoris in a newborn is 3 mm. The location of the urethra should be determined. It is usually seen on the ventral surface of the base of the clitoris or on the perineum. Rarely, a second opening of the vagina may be identified. Labia should be identified; these may show a variable degree of masculinization from mild thickening to formation of a scrotal sac (i.e., scrotalization) (Fig. 9-1). A palpable gonad is most commonly a testis, though an ovary in a hernial sac may rarely be present. A rectal examination should be performed to palpate for the presence or absence of the cervix and uterus.

Immediate issues in a newborn with ambiguous genitalia include the following:

1. Identify possible life-threatening disease such as congenital adrenal hyperplasia (CAH) resulting from 21-hydroxylase deficiency.
2. Assign appropriate gender. It is critical not to make a gender assignment in the delivery room and to postpone the determination until test results become available. Most parents will be upset and dismayed; it is important to reassure the parents that they have a healthy baby but that the development of external genitalia is incomplete and that further tests are necessary. The baby should be

Figure 9-1

Ambiguous genitalia.

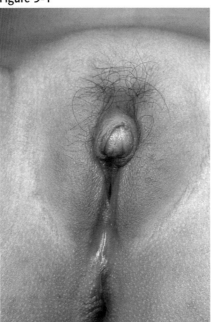

examined in the presence of the parents and normal genital development explained.

3. Initiate necessary surgical, medical, and psychological interventions.

The evaluation and differential diagnosis of the ambiguous genitalia are shown in Boxes 9-1 and 9-2.

Box 9-1 Evaluation of Ambiguous Genitalia

History
Pregnancy medications
Pregnancy illnesses
Family history

Physical examination
Location of urethral meatus
Degree of fusion of the labioscrotal folds
Length of phallus
Palpable gonads
Presence of vagina/urogenital sinus
Evidence of hyperpigmentation

Laboratory
17-hydroxyprogesterone
Karyotype
Serum electrolytes
Serum androgens

Imaging studies
Pelvic ultrasound
Genitogram
Magnetic resonance imaging of pelvis

Box 9-2   Differential Diagnosis of Ambiguous Genitalia

Female pseudohermaphroditism
Congenital adrenal hyperplasia
Maternal disease
Drug intake

Male pseudohermaphroditism
Abnormalities in androgen synthesis
Abnormalities in androgen action

True hermaphrodite
Gonadal dysgenesis

CAH is the most frequent cause of ambiguous genitalia. The most common form of CAH is the autosomal-recessively transmitted 21-hydroxylase deficiency. Mutations in the *CYP21* gene generate defective protein products that cannot adequately convert 17-hydroxyprogesterone to 11-deoxycortisol. Buildup of the precursors results in accumulation of adrenal androgens, dehydroepiandrosterone, and androstenedione, which are peripherally converted to testosterone. This, in turn, causes virilization of the female external genitalia. The karyotype is 46XX and the physical examination and ultrasound show a normal uterus and ovaries. Female infants may have varying amounts of genital ambiguity. The timing, duration, and amount of androgen exposure determine the degree of labioscrotal fusion, clitoral enlargement, and malposition of the urethra. Within the first few days of life, patients with the salt-losing type of CAH present with symptoms of poor feeding, vomiting, weight loss, and dehydration. These babies have hyponatremia and hyperkalemia and may develop hypotension due to volume depletion.

The surgical and medical treatment of these babies requires the expertise of subspecialists in endocrinology, urology, surgery, neonatology, and genetics. If left untreated, patients with simple virilizing CAH will show progressive signs of virilization. Pubic, axillary, and body hair will develop very early. Adult height is shortened due to early epiphyseal closure and, if left unchecked, the female eventually develops a male body habitus and will present with primary amenorrhea.

Management of Ambiguous Genitalia

The results of the blood tests and karyotype are usually available within 3 days (see Box 9-1). Radiographic studies such as pelvic ultrasound, genitogram, and pelvic magnetic resonance imaging (MRI) will also help decide the sex of the baby. Although diagnosis of the baby's condition requires knowledge of these studies, sex assignment is best based on other criteria as well. The parents need to be included in the discussion and decision making. The timing of surgery also needs to be discussed. Recent reports show that sexual reversal is not a trivial issue—gender appearance, sexual functioning, and potential fertility all need to be evaluated before final gender assignment is made. The multidisciplinary academic centers are best suited for these decisions.

Once the gender assignment has been determined, the physicians should help the family put aside issues of sexual ambiguity. The parents should be encouraged to use gender-specific names for the boy or girl. As long as the parental attitudes toward the chosen sex remain unequivocal, the child usually assumes his or her gender without difficulty.

Thus, the obstetrician must have an understanding of the problems faced when ambiguous genitalia are encountered. In addition to gender assignment, the emergent nature of managing the metabolic issues becomes crucial in the first few days after such a birth.

UTERINE AND VAGINAL ANOMALIES

208

Incidence

Developmental anomalies of the female reproductive system may come to attention at the time of birth, during puberty, or when the patient presents with reproductive difficulties. The reported incidence of müllerian anomalies varies widely, depending on the population under study. In one study, the rate of müllerian anomalies in women undergoing tubal ligation was 3.2%. However, the rate of anomalies in women with recurrent miscarriages may be as high as 12%. In all likelihood, the true incidence of müllerian anomalies has been underestimated, since many women with these anomalies remain undetected.

Classification

To describe the anomaly concisely and compare modes of therapy, a classification system for müllerian anomalies is necessary. Due to the seemingly endless variety of anomalies encountered, classification has proved to be difficult. A review of the literature reveals many different classification systems, but the most widely accepted and used classification system was described by the American Society of Reproductive Medicine (Box 9-3). Rock's classification is more descriptive and probably more helpful than other classification systems in understanding the possible pathogenesis of the abnormality. Since the vagina evolves from both the müllerian ducts and the urogenital sinus, müllerian anomalies may present with vaginal abnormalities in addition to anomalies of the uterus. Hence, classification of vaginal abnormalities should also be considered. One example of such a classification is presented in Box 9-4.

Müllerian Agenesis

Müllerian agenesis (Mayer-Rokitansky-Küster-Hauser syndrome) involves agenesis of the uterus and upper two thirds of the vagina; it has been observed in 1 in 5000 females. This diagnosis is typically considered when the patient presents during her mid to late teens with a complaint of primary amenorrhea. After gonadal dysgenesis, it is the second most common cause of primary amenorrhea. Since their ovaries function normally, these patients progress through all normal pubertal phases except menarche. Pain is an infrequent complaint. Since the hypothalamic-

Box 9-3 American Society of Reproductive Medicine Classification of Müllerian Anomalies

Agenesis/hypoplasia
Vaginal
Cervical
Fundal
Tubal
Combined anomalies

Unicornuate
Communicating
Noncommunicating
No cavity
No horn

Didelphys

Bicornuate
Complete
Partial

Septate
Complete
Partial

Arcuate

DES related

DES, Diethylstilbestrol.
Adapted from The American Fertility Society classifications of adnexal adhesions, distal tubal occlusion, tubal occlusion secondary to tubal ligation, tubal pregnancies, müllerian anomalies and intrauterine adhesions. Fertil Steril 49(6):944–955, 1988.

Box 9-4 Vaginal Septa Classification

Transverse
Obstructing
Nonobstructing

Longitudinal
Obstructing
Nonobstructing

Other
Stenosis
Iatrogenic
Complex

Adapted from Attaran M, Falcone T, Gidwani G: Obstructive mullerian anomalies. In Gidwani G, Falcone T (eds): Congenital Malformations of the Female Genital Tract. Philadelphia, Lippincott, Williams and Wilkins, 1999, pp 145–168.

pituitary-ovarian axis remains unaffected, their cycles are ovulatory and thus they may experience mittelschmerz pain. If functioning endometrial tissue is present in the müllerian remnants, the patient may rarely complain of severe cyclic pain. Associated renal anomalies are noted in 40% of patients. Abnormalities may include the absence or malposition of the kidney. Spine, limb, and rib anomalies are noted in 12% of the patients, and congenital deafness has also been reported.

On physical examination, patients with vaginal agenesis have fully developed secondary sexual characteristics. The external genitalia appear normal, but only a vaginal dimple or blind ending vaginal pouch is noted. A hymenal fringe is frequently seen. Rectal examination usually fails to demonstrate any obstructive pathology or müllerian structures.

The pathogenesis of müllerian agenesis is unknown. Although some investigators consider this entity to be inherited in a multifactorial mode, most believe that it is sporadic in origin. No müllerian anomalies have been noted in female infants born to mothers with müllerian agenesis via surrogacy and *in vitro* fertilization.

Once the history and physical examination raise suspicion of müllerian agenesis, imaging of the pelvis must be performed. In most cases, ultrasound provides enough information, but communication with the radiologist must occur. Many times, a small remnant of müllerian tissue will incorrectly be read a uterus, unless the radiologist is made aware of patient's postpubertal status. Ovaries appear normal, although they may be located somewhat higher in the pelvis. MRI is the best modality for detecting functioning endometrium within the müllerian remnants. Laparoscopy is usually not necessary to make the diagnosis of müllerian agenesis. However, if the patient is experiencing pain and the radiologic findings are inconsistent, laparoscopy may be considered.

The presentation of müllerian agenesis is very similar to complete androgen insensitivity syndrome (AIS) and must be differentiated from it. Table 9-1 summarizes the similarities and differences between these entities. After gonadal dysgenesis and müllerian agenesis, AIS is the third most common cause of primary amenorrhea. Patients with AIS have a 46XY karyotype and produce normal male quantities of androgens. However, a defect in the androgen receptor leads to a physiologic inability to detect androgens and a lack of male development of the external genitalia. Although close inspection of the external genitalia in patients with AIS may reveal underdeveloped labia minora and sparse or lack of pubic hair, the general phenotypic appearance is of a normal female. These patients commonly have a blind-ending vaginal pouch and breast development, which on close inspection may reveal a subtle abnormality of the areola. Their sexual identity

Table 9-1

Differentiating Müllerian Agenesis From Androgen Insensitivity Syndrome

Characteristics	Müllerian Agenesis	Androgen Insensitivity Syndrome
Primary amenorrhea	Yes	Yes
Female external genitalia	Yes	Yes
Breasts	Yes	Yes
Blind-ending vaginal pouch/dimple	Yes	Yes
Normal axillary and pubic hair	Yes	Variable
Gonads	Ovaries	Testicles
Karyotype	46XX	46XY

is female, and thus great care must be taken to use an appropriate choice of words when describing the disorder. Because of their Y chromosome and risk for development of gonadal tumors, a gonadectomy must be performed, followed by subsequent hormone replacement therapy.

Dilation, a nonsurgical mode of vaginoplasty, has a chance of success greater than 80%. Since the complication rate is almost nonexistent, this is the preferred method of vaginoplasty in patients with müllerian agenesis or complete AIS. RT Frank originally presented the concept of active dilation of the vagina in 1938. Several decades later, JM Ingram proposed passive dilation of the vagina. Graduated Lucite dilators are placed against the vaginal dimple for 30 min/day. Once one dilator fits completely, the patient moves on to the next size dilator. In this fashion, a vagina may be created over a 3-month time span. Encouragement and emotional support provided through frequent follow-up visits leads to high success rates.

If vaginal dilation fails or is not attempted, surgical construction of the vagina can be performed. Vaginal construction is usually performed on patients between the ages of 16 and 22 years to ensure the presence of endogenous estrogen and the mental maturity of maintaining the vagina after its creation. Many surgical techniques have been devised for the formation of the vagina. In most cases, an opening is created in the area of the vaginal vestibule between the urethra and rectum, followed by placement of a tissue such as skin graft, amnion, bowel, or peritoneum in the neovagina. The most commonly used surgical mode of vaginoplasty is the McIndoe procedure, first described in 1938. After a transverse incision is made in the space between the urethra and rectum, the areolar tissue is dissected up to the peritoneal cavity. The created cavity is then lined with a skin graft that has been wrapped around a mold. The stent is kept in the neovagina for a duration of 1 week, during which the patient is hospitalized and administered antibiotics, an indwelling urinary catheter, strict bed rest, and a low-residue diet. Upon return to the operating room, the mold is removed and the tissue lining the cavity is evaluated for adherence and viability. Excess tissue is trimmed, and another vaginal dilator is placed inside the newly created vagina. The patient must be prepared to wear this dilator continually for 3 months. In the subsequent 6 months, she may switch to wearing the dilator just at night, unless she is sexually active. Failure to comply with postoperative dilator use will lead to vaginal stenosis. Very high success rates are reported in compliant patients.

The diagnosis of müllerian agenesis or AIS must be presented with extreme sensitivity and tact to the patient and her parents. Many times, the young patient cannot voice her fears regarding the long-term implications of this diagnosis. The normal appearance of the external genitalia and ability to have normal intercourse with creation of the neovagina must be stressed. Indeed, long-term studies indicate a high sense of satisfaction with sexual function. Most couples' sense of disappointment stems from their inability to bear children. *In vitro* fertilization and surrogacy can provide a means of overcoming the lack of a uterus in patients with müllerian agenesis. These options should be articulated to the adolescent and her parents.

Other Müllerian Anomalies

Abnormal fusion of the müllerian ducts leads to an infinite variety of uterine anomalies (Fig. 9-2). As already stated, many of these defects will escape detection. However, patients with recurrent pregnancy wastage, pelvic pain, or abnormal bleeding will eventually seek medical care. The presentation, diagnosis, and management of some of these anomalies are discussed, as follows.

Communicating and Non-communicating Uterine Horns

A unicornuate uterus may have an associated rudimentary horn. If the rudimentary horn does not have an endometrial lining and the patient is asymptomatic, no further therapy is recommended. The patient will be symptomatic if the uterine horn has functioning endometrial tissue and is not communicating with the uterus (Figs. 9-3 and 9-4). Her complaints may include severe dysmenorrhea, which may result from hematometra (blood accumulation in the noncommunicating horn), or endometriosis, which has occurred as a result of retrograde menstruation. Pelvic examination may reveal a pelvic mass, which imaging studies will confirm. As already mentioned, the renal system must be evaluated for associated anomalies.

Excision of the functioning noncommunicating uterine horn is indicated. Although endometriosis is commonly noted, its full excision and

Figure 9-2

Müllerian anomalies of the uterus.

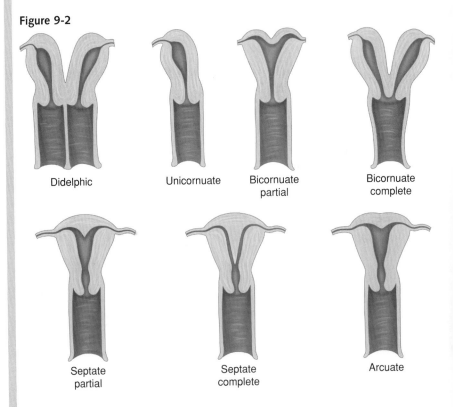

| Didelphic | Unicornuate | Bicornuate partial | Bicornuate complete |

| Septate partial | Septate complete | Arcuate |

Figure 9-3

Noncommunicating horn.

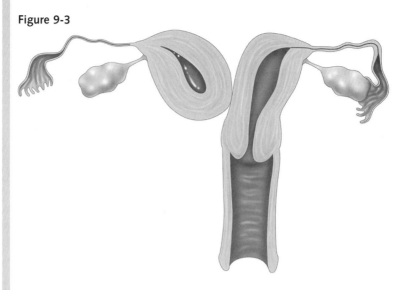

Figure 9-4

Laparoscopic image of noncommunicating horn.

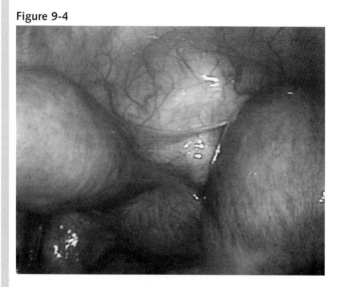

coagulation is not mandated since resection of the obstructed horn usually leads to resolution of the endometriosis. At the time of surgery, the non-communicating horn may be linked to the unicornuate uterus via fibrous or myometrial tissue. It is controversial whether a communicating horn with functional endometrium should be removed. However, pregnancy in a uterine horn can be a life-threatening condition, typically due to its late detection and risk for rupture.

Bicornuate and Septate Uteri

The incidence of bicornuate uterus in the fertile population ranges from 0.1 to 0.6%. It is believed to account for 20% of all uterine anomalies. Both bicornuate and septate uteri are associated with higher rates of early spontaneous abortion and preterm delivery. Uteroplacental insufficiency and cervical incompetency account for the higher fetal wastage rate in such patients. The diagnosis of a bicornuate uterus is typically entertained when a hysterosalpingogram is performed during an infertility or recurrent pregnancy loss investigation. It is difficult to differentiate a septate uterus from a bicornuate uterus via hysterosalpingogram (Fig. 9-5). Hence laparoscopy may be necessary to assess the uterine contour. Occasionally, uterine contour can be assessed adequately with ultrasound. However, a pelvic MRI is a more accurate means of assessing müllerian anomalies than pelvic US. It provides information about both the uterine contour and characteristics of the septal/myometrial tissue between the two uterine cavities.

The differentiation between bicornuate and septate uterus is important because the surgical management differs. In the past, both were managed via abdominal metroplasty. Uterine septa are currently removed via operative hysteroscopy; abdominal metroplasty is not recommended for bicornuate uterus unless the patient has experienced repetitive second-trimester losses.

Didelphic and Unicornuate Uterus

A review of the literature reveals a low incidence of didelphic and unicornuate uterus. Occasionally, detection of a longitudinal vaginal septum during routine gynecologic examination will lead to identification of a didelphic uterus; usually these anomalies are recognized when the patient presents with a poor reproductive outcome. Many times they are found incidentally at the time of laparoscopy or cesarean section. Because many go undiagnosed, the true incidence of these anomalies is likely underestimated. An increase in the rate of spontaneous abortion and preterm labor has been reported with didelphic and unicornuate uteri. In addition, there is a higher rate of malpresentation and subsequent cesarean section.

214

Figure 9-5

Hysterosalpingogram of bicornuate or septate uterus.

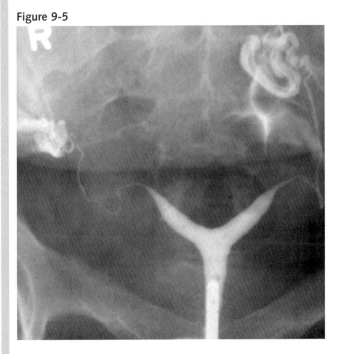

Of all the uterine anomalies, uterine didelphys is associated with the fewest obstetric problems. Thus, surgical unification of the didelphic uterus is not indicated. The placement of prophylactic cervical cerclage in such patients is controversial, and the indications for cerclage are similar to the indications in other pregnancies.

Uterine Didelphys with Obstructing Longitudinal Vaginal Septum

Patients with complete obstructing longitudinal vaginal septa present with cyclic periods associated with increasingly severe dysmenorrhea (Fig. 9-6). Vaginal examination usually reveals a paravaginal mass, and pelvic ultrasound shows hematometra and hematocolpos on the obstructed side (Fig. 9-7). Patients with incomplete longitudinal vaginal septa may

Figure 9-6

Obstructing longitudinal vaginal septum.

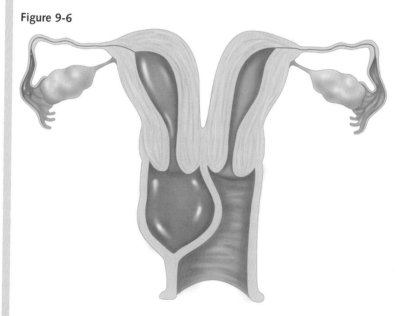

215

Figure 9-7

Ultrasound of hematometra resulting from obstructing longitudinal vaginal septum.

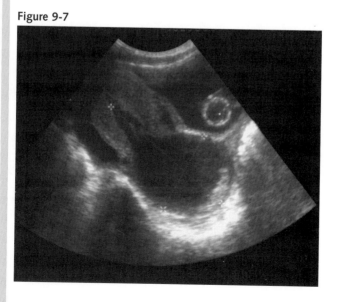

present with irregular bleeding and varying amounts of vaginal discharge (Fig. 9-8). Depending on the degree of communication between the two vaginas, a bulge may not be easily palpable. A pelvic ultrasound scan revealing a didelphic uterus should raise the index of suspicion regarding this entity. Associated anomalies include renal agenesis, usually on the same side as the obstruction.

The septum is excised in its entirety, and the upper and lower vaginal epithelium are reapproximated. The cervix in the obstructed vaginal canal usually has an erythematous glandular appearance. The goal of surgery is to relieve the obstruction and visualize both cervices so that Papanicolaou smears can be easily performed. Pregnancy rates of 87% and live birth rates of 77% have been reported, which are equivalent to the rates in women with didelphic uteri and nonobstructing longitudinal septa.

Longitudinal Vaginal Septum

Nonobstructing vaginal septa are typically asymptomatic. Occasionally, patients may note continued spotting and bleeding despite the use of a tampon. Others may present with complaints of difficulty with intercourse or problems with removal of a tampon if the septum is incomplete. The diagnosis can easily be missed, since in many cases the two vaginal cavities are unequal in size. The septum may be complete or partial. Once the diagnosis is made, the müllerian and renal system must be evaluated for any associated anomalies. Resection of the septum is indicated if the patient has pain with intercourse or wants to use a tampon more effectively. There is limited scientific evidence to mandate removal of every longitudinal vaginal septum before pregnancy occurs. However, in cases where the septum is thick and the vaginal cavities are equal in size, some advocate removal of the septum to avoid dystocia during delivery and tearing of the septum. Patients presenting with infertility may benefit from removal

Figure 9-8

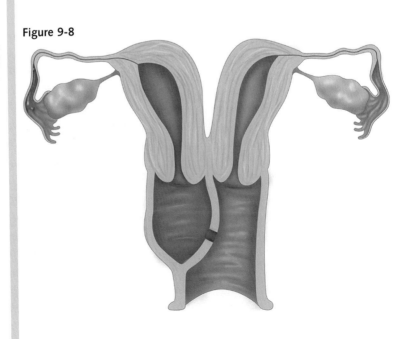

Incomplete longitudinal vaginal septum.

is of legal age and can make her own decisions regarding surgical treatment. Most advocate hysterectomy in cases where both the vagina and cervix have failed to develop. Multiple authors have reported cervical canalization and vaginoplasty, but patency rates are less than 50% and many patients require multiple surgeries. In addition, severe complications including sepsis and death have been reported after this procedure. However, both spontaneous and *in vitro* fertilization pregnancies have been reported in a few patients who have undergone uterine-sparing procedures.

Transverse Vaginal Septum

The failure of fusion of the urogenital sinus with the müllerian ducts may be the cause of transverse vaginal septa. It is reported to occur from 1 in 2100 to 1 in 72,000 women, with the majority of transverse septa being located in the upper third of the vagina. The septum may be complete or incomplete, and the diagnosis is typically made during or after puberty. Occasionally, however, an infant may have a mucocolpos or mucometrium that presents as an abdominal mass.

Patients with a complete transverse septum usually present with primary amenorrhea and cyclic pelvic pain, depending on the location of the obstruction; the higher the location of the septum, the earlier the patient presents with symptoms. Endometriosis has been noted in such patients. Physical examination reveals normal secondary sexual characteristics. Unlike imperforate hymen, bulging of the introitus is usually not noted. The external genitalia may appear normal, but a rectal examination will frequently identify a pelvic mass, which is consistent with a hematocolpos. Patients with incomplete transverse septa frequently complain of abnormal bleeding or foul-smelling vaginal discharge. The goal of imaging is to clarify the diagnosis and to determine the location and thickness of the septum. A transperineal ultrasound or pelvic MRI scan can be helpful in determining the thickness of the vaginal septum. A transabdominal ultrasound should be able to show the hematocolpos/hematometra. Most important, the cervix must be identified via imaging to help prepare the patient for the correct surgery.

If the septum is thin, it is removed in its entirety and the upper and lower vaginal epithelia are reapproximated. If the septum is thick and high, the patient must be prepared for the possible need of a split-thickness graft to line the area of defect once the septum is removed. In such cases, the patient must use a dilator for an extended period of time after the surgery to avoid stenosis at the site of the excised septum. Despite extensive counseling, young patients may have difficulty placing the dilator in the vagina, thus jeopardizing the successful outcome of this surgery. In such situations, it may benefit the patient to suppress her menstrual cycle for several years until she matures and is able to assume responsibility for her body. Vaginal dilation before surgery has been advocated by some to avoid the need to use a graft for patients with thick, high vaginal septa. The dilation process helps lengthen the proximal vaginal epithelium, whereas the hematocolpos lengthens the upper vaginal epithelium; the extended vaginal epithelial tissue may now be long enough to reapproximate.

of the septum, since sperm deposition may occur in the hemivagina contralateral to the ovulating ovary, leading to a low probability of conception.

Cervical Agenesis

Obstructive symptoms present relatively early (close to the time of presumed menarche) in patients who have cervical agenesis (Fig. 9-9). Girls present in their early teens, primarily with pelvic/abdominal pain and associated primary amenorrhea. Pediatricians and gastroenterologists have usually performed a complete abdominal pain investigation on such premenarchal patients before their presentation to the gynecologist. They may or may not have associated vaginal atresia; thus, examination of the external genitalia may not be helpful. An ultrasound scan of the pelvis is likely to be the first imaging study to reveal a hematometra as the cause of the patient's pain. Since patients with high, thick transverse septa are likely to have a similar presentation, it is important to clarify the existence of a cervix via MRI. Such patients may present with endometriosis, endometriomas, and hematosalpinges as a result of the obstruction.

Significant controversy exists regarding management of such patients. In situations in which a vagina is present and MRI reveals a portion of a cervix, canalization of the cervix can be attempted. Although some authors attempt to differentiate among four types of cervical anomalies (ranging from complete agenesis to cervical dysgenesis, wherein a portion of the cervix is present), it is clinically very difficult to determine the amount and quality of cervix present, especially when the anatomy is distorted because of hematometra.

When cervical agenesis is diagnosed, the first line of therapy is to suppress endometrial shedding and control pain with continuous oral contraceptive pills, medroxyprogesterone acetate (Depo-Provera) or gonadotropin-releasing hormone agonist (Depo-Lupron). Since these patients are very young, they are not psychologically ready to understand or accept the responsibility of a surgical procedure. Medical therapy is continued until the patient

217

Figure 9-9

Cervical agenesis.

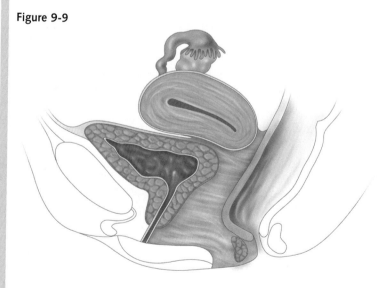

In addition, presurgical dilation prepares and teaches the young patient how to comfortably use a dilator.

Few studies have been performed on the long-term outcomes of such patients. Compared with patients with imperforate hymen, the pregnancy rate of patients with transverse septa was significantly lower and the miscarriage rate was higher. This discrepancy may be due to a higher rate of endometriosis in the latter group.

ANOMALIES OF THE EXTERNAL GENITALIA

Clitoris

Clitoromegaly

The average length of a normal clitoral shaft and glans is 1.5 to 2.0 cm. Because it is difficult to measure the length of the glans accurately, the diameter is commonly used to determine normalcy. The mean transverse diameter of the clitoral glans ranges from 3.5 to 4 mm; a diameter greater than 1 cm is considered abnormal. Rarely, hypertrophy may be seen as an isolated anomaly with no underlying pathology. More commonly, an enlarged clitoris is associated with androgen overproduction. Depending on the timing of exposure to excess androgens, labial scrotalization (as seen with ambiguous genitalia developed while *in utero*) and associated abnormalities in the location of the urethra may be present. Exposure to excess androgens after the complete development of the external genitalia leads to isolated clitoromegaly (Fig. 9-10). The treatment of clitoromegaly may include

Figure 9-10

Clitoromegaly.

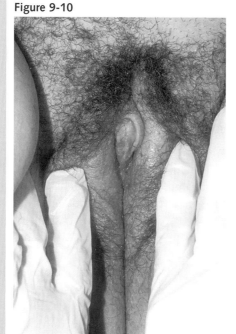

cosmetic reduction clitoroplasty with conservation of the neurovascular bundle.

Splitting or Cleavage of the Clitoris

Splitting or cleavage of the clitoris are very rare anomalies and are typically seen in conjunction with other major congenital anomalies such as extrophy of bladder, hypospadias, splitting of the urethra, or absence or cleavage of symphysis pubis.

Labia Minora

Labial Hypertrophy

Labial hypertrophy involves enlargement of the labia minora and is often asymptomatic. Generally, the labia are considered hypertrophic when they are elongated beyond the labia majora or when their width from the base is greater than 5 cm. The etiology of this condition is usually unknown, but it may occasionally be associated with mechanical pulling of the labia. Reassurance of the patient is all that is necessary in most instances. In cases in which patients experience persistent local irritation or excoriation, surgical reduction may be necessary. In the past, the excess tissue was trimmed such that the line of incision comprised the new labial edge. More recently, authors have described removal of the posterior quadrant of the labia minora, leaving an anterior flap, which is then secured to the base. This technique ensures that the surgical scar is at the base of the labia.

Fused Labia

The most common cause of labial fusion is CAH. When it occurs *in utero*, it is secondary to excess androgen exposure or associated with abdominal wall defects. This term has erroneously been used to describe labial adhesions in young children.

Hymen

Imperforate Hymen

Examination of a newborn's external genitalia should provide information on the patency of the vaginal canal. Thus, an imperforate hymen should be detected at the time of birth. Although the newborn is usually asymptomatic, a mucocolpos may occasionally be diagnosed. In these cases, exposure of the infant to maternal levels of estrogen leads to cervical secretions, which accumulate behind the imperforate hymen. This anomaly may be diagnosed *in utero* and may be associated with other anomalies. Occasionally, the mucocolpos is large enough to cause obstruction of the bladder and urethra, causing urinary retention. In the case of urinary symptoms, surgical management is necessary. The infant is placed in the dorsal lithotomy position, local anesthetic is applied, and a cruciform incision made over the bulging membrane. The margins are then excised; hemostasis is rarely a problem.

Imperforate hymen discovered incidentally in a prepuberal child can be managed expectantly because it is important that thelarche has started before surgery is attempted. Adequate amounts of estrogen in a young girl help with healing and may counter the need for reoperation.

In most instances, the imperforate hymen is detected in the perimenarchal years. The patient presents with cyclic abdominal pain and primary amenorrhea. Physical examination of the external genitalia shows the imperforate hymen bulging with a bluish hue. Occasionally there will be an abdominal mass, which is the uterus being pushed forward by the distended vagina. Some patients will present with urinary retention, abdominal pain, or urinary tract infection in the doctor's office or emergency department. Diagnosis is made by physical examination and an ultrasound scan to visualize the hematocolpos in the vagina with a normal-appearing uterus. In unusual cases, MRI may be needed.

The treatment is surgical and must be done in the operating room with the patient under anesthesia. The hymen is excised and the accumulated blood drained. There is no need to visualize the cervix because the distended vagina often makes it a difficult task. Transvaginal needle drainage of the blood should not be attempted in the emergency department because of the high risk of infection.

Septate, Cribriform, and Microperforate Hymen

Many variations in the appearance of the hymen have been described. As long as a small opening is present for efflux of blood and vaginal secretions, the patient is asymptomatic. Septate and cribriform hymen are diagnosed on routine examination or when the patient complains of difficulty with the introduction of tampons (Fig. 9-11).

Microperforate hymen can be easily confused with imperforate hymen in prepuberal girls (Fig. 9-12). However, as the girl enters thelarche, secretions from the vagina make the diagnosis clear. Excision is indicated to prevent difficulty with intercourse and if she desires the use of tampons.

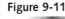
Figure 9-11

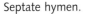
Septate hymen.

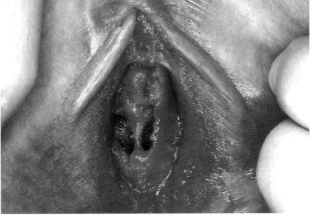

Figure 9-12

Microperforate hymen.

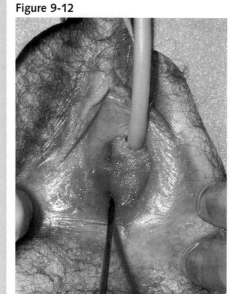

KEY POINTS

1. The most frequent cause of ambiguous genitalia in newborns is congenital adrenal hyperplasia.
2. After gonadal dysgenesis, müllerian agenesis is the second most common cause of primary amenorrhea.
3. Müllerian anomalies are often associated with renal anomalies.
4. Vaginal dilation is the primary mode of creating a vagina in patients with müllerian agenesis.
5. Patients with complete androgen insensitivity syndrome must undergo gonadectomy.
6. Bicornuate and septate uteri must be differentiated from each other since their management differs.
7. Of all uterine anomalies, uterine didelphys is associated with the fewest obstetric problems.
8. The first line of therapy in patients with obstructive müllerian anomalies is to shut down endometrial shedding and to control pain.
9. When removing a transverse vaginal septum, the septum must be excised in its entirety and the upper and lower vaginal epithelium reapproximated.
10. Detection of clitoromegaly should trigger an evaluation for hyperandrogenism.
11. An imperforate hymen in a perimenarchal girl is excised in the operating room.

SUGGESTED READING

American College of Obstetrics and Gynecology: ACOG committee opinion. Nonsurgical diagnosis and management of vaginal agenesis. Number 274, July 2002. Committee on adolescent health care. American College of Obstetrics and Gynecology. Int J Gynaecol Obstet 79(2):167–170, 2002.

American Fertility Society classifications of adnexal adhesions, distal tubal occlusion, tubal occlusion secondary to tubal ligation, tubal pregnancies, müllerian anomalies and intrauterine adhesions. Fertil Steril 49(6):944–955, 1988.

Bugmann P, Amaudruz M, Hanquint M, et al: Utericervicoplasty with bladder mucosa layer for the treatment of complete cervical agenesis. Fertil Steril 77(4):831–835, 2002.

Candiani S, Fedel GB, Candiani L: Double uterus, blind hemivagina, and ipsilateral renal agenesis: 36 cases and long term follow up. Obstet Gynecol 90:26–32, 1997.

Edmonds DK: Congenital malformations of the genital tract. Obstet Gynecol Clin North Am 27(1):49–62, 2000.

Edmonds DK, Muram D: Sexual development anomalies and their reconstruction: Upper and lower tracts. In Sanfilippo JS, Muram D, Dewhurst J, Lee PA (eds): Pediatric and Adolescent Gynecology, 2nd ed. Philadelphia, WB Saunders, 2001,pp 553–583.

Emans SJ, Laufer MR, Goldstein DP: Pediatric and Adolescent Gynecology. Philadelphia, Lippincott-Raven, 1998, pp 303–362.

Gidwani DP, Falcone G: Congenital malformations of the female genital tract. Philadelphia, Lippincott Williams and Wilkins, 1999.

Haddad B, Louis-Sylvestre C, Poitout C, et al: Longitudinal vaginal septum: A retrospective study of 202 cases. Eur J Obstet Gynecol Reprod Biol 74(2): 197–199, 1997.

Heinonen PK: Clinical implications of didelphic uterus: Long term followup of 49 cases. Eur J Obstet Gynecol Reprod Biol 91(2):183–190, 2000.

Hurst BS, Rock JA: Preoperative dilation to facilitate repair of the high transverse vaginal septum. Fertil Steril 57(6):1351–1353, 1992.

Klingele JA, Gebhart CJ, Croak JB, et al: McIndoe procedure for vaginal agenesis: Long-term outcome and effect on quality of life. Am J Obstet Gynecol 189:1569–1573, 2003.

Nelson AJ, Gearhart CP: Current views on evaluation, management, and gender assignment of the intersex infant. Nat Clin Pract Urol 1:138–143, 2004.

Petrozza JC, Gray MR, Davis MR, et al: Congenital absence of the uterus and vagina is not commonly transmitted as a dominant genetic trait: Outcomes of surrogate pregnancies. Fertil Steril 67(2):387–389, 1997.

Rock JA, Breech L: Surgery for anomalies of the müllerian ducts. In Rock JA, Jones HW (eds): TeLinde's Operative Gynecology. 9th ed. Philadelphia, Lippincott-Raven Publishers, 2003,pp 705–752.

223

10

PREGNANCY LOSS AND TERMINATION

Allison A. Cowett and E. Steve Lichtenberg

Early Pregnancy Loss

Epidemiology

As many as 10% to 15% of pregnancies diagnosed by ultrasound or chemical testing fail spontaneously by 20 weeks' gestation, and it is likely that the rate of undiagnosed early pregnancy loss is 50% or greater. Diagnosed early pregnancy loss is generally recognized 1 or more weeks after the pregnancy demise. One in four women will experience such a loss in her lifetime. An individual woman's risk increases with increasing age, number of previous losses, and certain medical conditions, including thrombophilia and immunologic and infectious etiologies. The majority of early pregnancy loss is the result of aneuploidy and is therefore recognizable by chromosome analysis.

Diagnosis

Before the widespread use of ultrasound to evaluate early pregnancy failure, diagnosis was based on symptoms, urine pregnancy testing, and physical examination. Using these diagnostic tools, spontaneous abortions were categorized as threatened, inevitable, incomplete, or complete. A *threatened abortion* referred to the clinical presentation of bleeding in the presence of a closed cervical os. The term *inevitable abortion* was invoked in the setting of bleeding and an open cervical os before the passage of pregnancy tissue. *Incomplete abortion* referred to bleeding, an open cervical os, and the passage of a portion of the pregnancy, whereas *complete abortion* was defined as a closed cervical os following bleeding and passage of all products of conception.

With the advent of ultrasound and its widespread use in early pregnancy, it was recognized that these categories described a heterogeneous group of sonographic findings. Using ultrasound, it is possible to more precisely categorize early pregnancy failure or any abnormal intrauterine first-trimester pregnancy into *incomplete abortion* (i.e., passage of some pregnancy elements), *anembryonic pregnancy* (i.e., gestational sac devoid of embryo and yolk sac), or *embryonic demise* (i.e., presence of nonviable embryo). Technically, the term *missed abortion* denotes any nonviable pregnancy that is retained within the uterus for 4 weeks after the pregnancy's demise, although in common parlance it denotes a failed pregnancy of any duration with products retained. The term *blighted ovum* is a misnomer since nonmolar fertilization requires the union of elements from both ovum and sperm.

The presentation of early pregnancy failure is variable. Symptomatic patients may present with any combination of the following symptoms: vaginal bleeding, lower abdominal or pelvic cramping, passage of pregnancy tissue and, occasionally, fever in the absence of instrumentation. Asymptomatic patients may be found to have a discrepancy between reported last menstrual period (LMP) and uterine size on bimanual pelvic examination. A quantitative beta human chorionic gonadotropin (βhCG) level that does not rise appropriately over time or a low progesterone level may be an indication of a nonviable gestation. Levels of βhCG vary widely at the same gestational age and should not be used singly. For gestations at even the earliest stage, the minimal rise in βhCG levels required to sustain a diagnosis of viability is 24% at 1 day and 53% at 2 days. Definitive diagnosis of viability is made by ultrasound scan (i.e., visible cardiac motion or appropriate serial growth) and is often used in conjunction with gestational age dating by reported LMP and βhCG levels.

In a viable pregnancy, use of transvaginal ultrasound generally reveals a gestational sac between 32 and 37 days post-LMP. When the gestational sac measures 8 to 10 mm, a yolk sac will be present. Absence of a yolk sac, embryonic pole, or both when the gestational sac measures greater than 1.5 to 2.0 cm is indicative of anembryonic pregnancy. Similarly, absence of cardiac activity in the presence of an embryo measuring 5 mm, or approximately 7 weeks post-LMP, is highly suspicious for embryonic demise. Other ultrasonographic findings that raise suspicion of early pregnancy loss include debris within the gestational sac, an irregularly shaped sac, a retroplacental clot, or cardiac activity of less than 100 beats/min. Because ultrasound findings are highly dependent on operator skill, quality of equipment, and anatomic variation, reevaluation before definitive treatment of early pregnancy failure may be appropriate in the setting of a desired pregnancy. Therefore, the decision to act on the basis of a single ultrasound evaluation is contingent upon certainty of the clinical presentation, clinician experience, and the level of patient acceptance.

Management

Nonviable pregnancy diagnosed early in gestation can be managed surgically, medically, or expectantly. Management should be guided by the patient's clinical presentation and preference. Clinically stable patients should be counseled regarding each option and may play an active role in the management decision.

Surgical management has long been considered the standard of care for early pregnancy failure and represents two thirds of all outpatient gynecologic procedures performed in the United States. Surgical evacuation of the uterus is accomplished using either electric suction evacuation or manual vacuum aspiration. It is the treatment of choice in the setting of hemodynamic instability, uncontrolled vaginal bleeding, infection, discomfort unresponsive to analgesia, or patient preference. Complications from curettage include incomplete evacuation, uterine perforation, pelvic infection, and hemorrhage requiring transfusion, but complications are the exception.

Although surgical intervention is common, medical management is often an option. Interest in medical management has grown with the development of medical abortion regimens. Both mifepristone (an antiprogesterone) and methotrexate (an antimetabolite of folic acid synthesis) have been used in combination with prostaglandin analogues such as misoprostol to effect medical evacuation of the uterus for early failed gestation. The use of misoprostol (a prostaglandin E_1 analogue) alone for medical evacuation of the uterus in the setting of early pregnancy failure has been studied more extensively than either of the combined regimens. It has been used in varying doses and routes, and widely disparate success rates have been reported based on dose, route of administration, ultrasonographic diagnosis, and period of time to pregnancy expulsion. Success rates are higher with vaginal versus oral administration. Misoprostol 800 μg in a single dose and in repeat doses 24 hours apart have been shown to effect uterine evacuation in 80% to 90% of cases. Success rates are likely higher with incomplete abortion vs. embryonic demise or anembryonic gestation. The rate of complications (i.e., need for emergent surgical evacuation or transfusion) is low. Patients may be followed up with serial ultrasound scans, βhCG measurements, or both, to ensure complete uterine evacuation, but a reassuring patient history coupled with a normal bimanual examination may be sufficient.

Expectant management of early nonviable pregnancy is appropriate in selected settings. The use of ultrasonography to distinguish incomplete abortion, embryonic demise, and anembryonic gestation can be used to predict the likelihood of success without surgical or medical intervention. Rates of completed spontaneous abortion have been reported as 84% for incomplete abortion, 59% for embryonic demise, and 52% for anembryonic gestation after 2 weeks of expectant management. Rates of spontaneous resolution as high as 89% for embryonic demise and 79% for anembryonic gestation are reported when expectant management is extended to 4 weeks after diagnosis. Counseling about the relative success of expectant management may decrease the number of women undergoing surgical and medical intervention for early pregnancy failure. As with medical management, expectant management is appropriate only when emergent surgical management is readily available.

Finally, regardless of the management approach, the psychological impact of early pregnancy failure should not be overlooked. Tending to patients' emotional state in the setting of pregnancy loss is essential given its prevalence in the population. It is appropriate to counsel the majority of patients that early pregnancy failure is a sporadic event that is unlikely to recur and will not adversely affect future childbearing potential.

Recurrent Pregnancy Loss

Approximately 1% of women of reproductive age will experience recurrent pregnancy loss, strictly defined as three or more clinically recognized pregnancy losses before 20 weeks' gestation or of fetal weight less than 500 g. Most commonly, these losses occur in preimplantation and post-implantation embryos, with recurrent pregnancy loss after 14 weeks being uncommon. Although three losses has traditionally defined recurrent pregnancy loss, it is reasonable to initiate a diagnostic workup in patients having experienced only two losses, especially in the setting of advanced maternal age, infertility, and losses occurring after the confirmation of fetal cardiac activity.

Etiologies

Genetic

Between 2% and 8% of recurrent pregnancy losses are caused by an abnormality in the parental chromosomal complement. In the case of an abnormal karyotype, balanced reciprocal or robertsonian translocation is the most common finding, although mosaicism, single-gene mutations, and inversions are also prevalent. Chromosomal abnormalities are seen in a 2:1 female-to-male ratio in the setting of recurrent pregnancy failure.

Anatomic

Anatomic abnormalities distorting the uterine cavity may be either congenital or acquired. Congenital etiologies include müllerian duct anomalies, such as uterine septae, bicornuate or unicornuate uterus, and the sequelae of diethylstilbestrol exposure. These anatomic variations are traditionally associated with second-trimester pregnancy loss, although they may also play a role in recurrent early pregnancy failure. Acquired anatomic causes include intrauterine adhesions following metallic curettage, hysteroscopic surgery or tubercular infection, and deformations of the cavity and lining due to submucosal leiomyomata. The mechanism by which anatomic aberrations in the uterine cavity lead to pregnancy wastage is not entirely clear, although they are hypothesized to lead to impaired implantation or insufficient vascularization of the developing pregnancy. Endometriosis has also been adduced as an acquired anatomic etiology of recurrent pregnancy loss, but this has not been well described or substantiated. Anatomic causes are thought to comprise 10% to 15% of all recurrent pregnancy losses.

Endocrinologic

Endocrinologic factors include deficiency in the luteal phase, poorly controlled diabetes mellitus, hypothyrodism and hyperthyroidism, and hyperprolactinemia. These conditions affect the delicate sequence of hormonal interactions needed to establish and maintain a pregnancy. However, evaluation for endocrinologic dysfunction should be limited to symptomatic patients given that subclinical disease is unlikely to be the underlying etiology of recurrent loss.

Infectious

Numerous infectious agents including species of mycoplasma, ureaplasma, β-hemolytic streptococcus, chlamydia, *Toxoplasma gondii*, *Listeria monocytogenes*, rubella, coxsackievirus, measles, herpesvirus, and cytomegalovirus have been associated with recurrent pregnancy loss. However, with the exception of *Mycoplasma* species, none have been well substantiated. The mechanism by which microbes affect pregnancy failure is likely immunologic in nature.

Thrombophilic

The growing number of abnormalities associated with congenital and acquired hypercoagulable states such as factor V Leiden mutation, prothrombin gene mutation, antithrombin III deficiency, protein S and C deficiencies, and homozygosity for methylene tetrahydrofolate reductase deficiency may be associated with adverse pregnancy outcomes including second- and third-trimester loss. However, current evidence does not support an association between the thrombophilias and recurrent early pregnancy failure.

Immunologic

Immunologic causes of recurrent pregnancy loss are the result of both alloimmune and autoimmune factors. When alloimmune factors are at play, the abnormal cellular response is thought to be mediated by the cytokines such as interferon-γ and tumor necrosis factor. These cytokines are released by inflammatory cells within the trophoblastic tissue and inhibit normal development of the growing conceptus, leading to recurrent loss. These mechanisms are poorly understood. Consequently, diagnosis and treatment of cell-mediated immunologic factors in the setting of recurrent pregnancy failure have been largely unsuccessful to date.

Antiphospholipid antibodies, acting against cardiolipin or phosphatidylserine, have been implicated in a myriad of obstetric complications such as early spontaneous pregnancy loss, intrauterine growth restriction, preeclampsia, and intrauterine fetal demise. The mechanism is thought to involve increases in thromboxane, decreases in prostacyclin, and overactive platelet aggregation resulting in microinfarction of the placental vasculature. A number of other autoantibodies such as antithyroid, antisperm, and antitrophoblast are being studied as a possible cause of recurrent pregnancy loss.

Environmental, Social, and Behavioral

Organic solvents, heavy metal toxicity by lead and mercury, and medications such as inhalational anesthetics and chemotherapeutic agents have been associated with recurrent pregnancy loss. Tobacco, cocaine, and ethanol exposure are positively associated with recurrent pregnancy loss and are likely to have a dose response relationship with pregnancy failure. An association between caffeine ingestion and pregnancy loss has been studied but not substantiated.

Diagnosis and Treatment

A thorough evaluation examining each of the above noted etiologies should be undertaken when the decision is made to initiate a workup for recurrent pregnancy failure. The evaluation includes a complete history, physical examination, and laboratory studies. Therapy is tailored to each patient according to the results of the diagnostic evaluation (Table 10-1). Before the initiation of the evaluation, the patient and her partner should be counseled that the rate of *unexplained* recurrent pregnancy loss, even after a complete evaluation, may be as high as 50% to 60%. Couples are more likely to have unexplained recurrent losses in the setting of maternal age over 35 years, no recent history of a live birth, and normal chromosomal findings in the abortuses.

Table 10-1

Etiology	Diagnostic Tests	Abnormal Results	Treatment
Genetic	Parental karyotype	3% to 5%	Genetic counseling, donor gametes
Anatomic	Hysterosalpingogram Hysteroscopy Sonohysterography	15% to 20%	Surgical repair Cervical cerclage
Endocrine	Endometrialbiopsy Serum thyroid-stimulating hormone	5% to 8%	Clomiphene citrate Thyroid hormone replacement
	Serum prolactin		Bromocriptine
Infectious	Cervical cultures	5% to 10%	Antibiotics
Immunologic	Lupus anticoagulant, antiphospholipid antibodies	15% to 25%	Heparin and aspirin in pregnancy
Environmental/ Behavioral/ Social	Interview, questionnaire	Unknown	Counseling to alter exposure or behavior, treatment of depression as indicated

Adapted from Kutteh WH: Recurrent pregnancy loss: An update. Curr Opin Obstet Gynecol 11(5):435–439, 1999.

Despite the high rate of unexplained recurrent pregnancy loss and the remaining unanswered questions about the benefits of many established therapies, the majority of couples with a history of recurrent pregnancy loss will ultimately experience a live birth. Rates of live birth by number of previous losses and etiology of recurrent loss are listed in Table 10-2.

PREGNANCY TERMINATION

Epidemiology of Unintended Pregnancy and Abortion

Forty-nine percent of all pregnancies conceived in the United States are *unintended*, defined as a pregnancy that is mistimed or unplanned. Women with unintended pregnancies are more likely to be young, unmarried, of non-white race, and living in poverty. Just under half of these women report using contraception in the month before conception. Excluding spontaneous miscarriages, 54% of unintended pregnancies end in abortion, and the remaining 46% result in live births. Women choosing to terminate an unintended pregnancy are more likely to be unmarried and older and to have used contraception in the month before conception than women who opt to continue the pregnancy. Almost half of all women will have an unintended pregnancy between the ages of 15 and 44 years, and 43% of women in the United States will have undergone an abortion by the age of 45 years.

Table 10-2

Number of Spontaneous Losses	Live Birth Rate (%)
1	76
2	70
3	65
4	60
Etiology of Recurrent Loss	
Genetic	20–80
Anatomic	60–90
Endocrine	>90
Infectious	70–90
Immune	70–90
Idiopathic	40–90

From Hill JA: Recurrent spontaneous early pregnancy loss. In Berek JS, Adashi EY, Hillard PA (eds): Novak's Gynecology, 12th ed. Baltimore, MD, Williams & Wilkins, 1996, pp 963–979.

As a result of these statistics, induced abortion is one of the most common surgical procedures performed in the United States. After legalization of abortion, the number of abortions per 1000 women aged 15 to 44 years rose steadily from 16.3 in 1973 to 29.3 in 1980. Since that time, the United States has seen a gradual decline in the rate of induced abortion to 21.3 in the year 2000, the lowest rate since 1974. This corresponds to approximately 1.3 million abortions performed per year, or 21% of all pregnancies.

Along with the falling number of abortions, the availability of abortion providers is also decreasing. Providers are concentrated in metropolitan areas, and abortion services are not available in 87% of all U.S. counties. In contrast, other reproductive health services such as general obstetrics and gynecology are available in half of all counties. The distance women must travel to receive abortion services is one of the most significant barriers to procedure accessibility. One in every four women travels over 50 miles to obtain an abortion. Other barriers to accessibility include denial of public funding, mandatory waiting periods, physical plant requirements, and parental involvement laws.

Fifty-four percent of all abortions performed in the United States occur prior to 9 weeks' gestation, and 88% take place before 13 weeks. Only 1.4% are performed after 20 weeks. The vast majority of first-trimester abortions are performed by suction curettage, although the number of medical abortions is steadily increasing since the U.S. Food and Drug Administration's approval of mifepristone for early medical abortion in the year 2000. Abortions in the second trimester are primarily performed by dilation and evacuation or induction. More than 90% of U.S. abortions are currently performed in outpatient clinics, the majority of which primarily provide abortion services. A smaller percentage occur in hospitals and physicians' offices. Morbidity and mortality from induced abortion in all three settings are low.

Counseling for Pregnancy Termination

The decision to voluntarily terminate a pregnancy is a profoundly personal one. The benefits of comprehensive counseling before abortion are multifold. Counseling provides the patient the opportunity to explore all pregnancy options, to identify and manage difficult and intense emotions, to gather information about the medical aspects of the abortion, and to develop a rapport with the health care providers. Counseling should be conducted in a nonjudgmental, accepting, and empathetic manner because it frames the entire abortion process and has a profound impact on patient experience and emotional resolution. Successful counseling empowers the patient to make an informed decision about her current pregnancy and to understand options for contraception and the prevention of future unintended pregnancy.

As with any medical procedure, informed consent is an essential part of the counseling process. The patient must have a full understanding and knowledge of the risks of the procedure as well as its alternatives. She must be voluntarily ending her pregnancy without evidence of coercion by a parent, partner, or other external force. Counseling also identifies common feelings in women seeking abortion, including fear of the medical procedure, fear of pain, concerns about future fertility, guilt, sadness, and loss. For the majority of women, these negative reactions are short-lived and successfully overcome. Studies have shown that the majority of women voluntarily seeking abortion services experience positive feelings of confidence in their decision as well as relief when the process is over. The potential for long-term psychological sequelae after induced abortion is small and has been frequently overstated. Risk factors for negative reactions to abortion include low self-efficacy, poor self-esteem, preexisting mental illness, ambivalence regarding the decision to end the pregnancy, lack of social support, perceived coercion, an experience of social stigma connected to abortion, and medically indicated termination of pregnancy for maternal or fetal indications.

Counseling for *medical* abortion requires detailed information about the timing and range of symptoms encountered during the medication-induced miscarriage event as well as precise triggers for contacting medical personnel for bleeding, cramping, and fever. *Second-trimester abortion* counseling calls for added instruction about inherently increased medical risks, cervical preparation, and postoperative care.

First-Trimester Surgical Abortion

Diagnosis of Pregnancy and Gestational Age Determination

Accurate diagnosis of pregnancy, pregnancy location, and gestational age are critical to avoiding unnecessary intervention, choosing the best management, and minimizing complications. The diagnosis of pregnancy is made based on a history of amenorrhea and confirmed by laboratory evaluation. Common symptoms of early pregnancy include breast tenderness, nausea, emesis, and fatigue; however, symptoms are highly variable and should not be used to diagnose pregnancy without laboratory confirmation. hCG is present in maternal serum approximately 1 week after fertilization at the time of blastocyst implantation. hCG is produced only by fetal and trophoblastic tissue and is present in almost equal concentrations in maternal serum and urine. It therefore provides an excellent laboratory marker for pregnancy evaluation. In the setting of normal pregnancy development, levels of hCG should double every 1.4 to 2 days. Levels of hCG peak between 7 and 10 weeks of pregnancy at 20,000 to 200,000 mIU/mL and gradually decline thereafter. Modern sensitive urine pregnancy tests use an enzyme-linked immunosorbent assay technique that contains antibodies to the βhCG subunit and achieves 98% sensitivity at 7 days postimplantation (25 to 50 mIU/mL). Evaluation of quantitative serum βhCG, accomplished by radioimmunoassay, is sensitive to 2 to 10 mIU/mL and is used in the evaluation of suspected abnormal pregnancy and surveillance after diagnosis of hydatidiform mole.

Gestational age determination is based on history of the LMP, pelvic examination, and ultrasound evaluation. Bimanual examination is relatively imprecise at measuring gestational age in the first trimester and is more reliable after 12 weeks of gestation when the uterus grows beyond the pelvis into the abdomen. This imprecision is lessened in the setting of regular menses, patient confidence in LMP dating, and physical examination findings consistent with dating by history. Ultrasound measurement is particularly useful when menstrual dating is unreliable, conception occurred while using hormonal contraceptive methods, a discrepancy exists between menstrual dating and physical examination findings, or gestational age is beyond the first trimester.

The gestational sac is the earliest ultrasonographic evidence of intrauterine pregnancy, appearing in the fourth or early in the fifth week of pregnancy when using a vaginal transducer. The gestational sac consists of a sonolucent center with a "double" echogenic ring representing (1) early placental formation and (2) thickening of the endometrium in response to invasion by trophoblastic tissue. Transvaginal findings in normal pregnancy are listed in Table 10-3. The absence of a gestational sac in a patient with a quantitative βhCG exceeding the discriminatory zone should prompt evaluation for ectopic gestation. Absence of other developmental milestones raises suspicion for early pregnancy failure, and management of the patient should proceed according to the diagnosis. Ultrasound measurements used for gestational age determination are listed in Table 10-4.

Table 10-3

Transvaginal Ultrasound Findings in Normal Pregnancy

Gestational sac	Visualized at hCG level of 1500–2000 mIU/mL (discriminatory zone) or ∼5 weeks from LMP
Yolk sac	Visualized when gestational sac diameter 8–10 mm or ∼6 weeks from LMP
Cardiac activity	Visualized when embryo measures ≥5 mm or ∼7 weeks from last menses

hCG, Human chorionic gonadotropin; mIU, milli-international units; LMP, last menstrual period.

Table 10-4

Ultrasound
Gestational Age
Determination

Ultrasound Appearance	Measurement
Prior to visualization of embryo	Mean sac diameter (mm) + 30
Embryo measuring <25 mm	Embryonic length (mm) + 42
Embryo measuring 25–55 mm	Crown-rump length
Beyond 12 weeks' gestation	Biparietal diameter and femur length

Preoperative Evaluation

Preoperative evaluation of the patient before abortion includes a complete medical history to identify any pertinent chronic conditions. There are almost no medical conditions in which abortion in the first trimester is contraindicated and relatively few conditions in which abortion should not be performed in an outpatient setting. However, chronic medical conditions may require particular management at the time of abortion, and this information should be elicited (Table 10-5). Physical examination is targeted to a patient's current or recent symptoms and chronic conditions and includes a pelvic examination for estimation of gestational age, uterine size and contour, and evidence of cervical inflammation or discharge. Mandatory laboratory evaluation includes a urine pregnancy test or ultrasound to validate pregnancy and determination of Rh status. Unsensitized Rh-negative women should receive immunoglobulin D (RhoGAM) to prevent isoimmunization at the time of the abortion. Although a pregnancy at 7 weeks' gestation or earlier may be at little or no risk of causing sensitization, definitive clinical evidence to support the withholding of immunization is lacking. Many providers will also evaluate baseline hemoglobin or hematocrit levels before abortion.

Mandatory screening for sexually transmitted diseases is beneficial in settings where universal periabortal antibiotic prophylaxis is not practiced. Treatment should be initiated for known or suspected chlamydial or gonorrheal cervicitis and bacterial vaginosis, given the increased rate of postoperative infections when any of these pathogens is present. Universal short-course oral prophylaxis with tetracyclines, penicillins, macrolides, and other commonly used antibiotic classes markedly reduces postabortal infectious morbidity.

Surgical Technique

Before 1960, metallic dilation and sharp curettage was the predominant method of uterine evacuation for induced and spontaneous abortion. The introduction of vacuum aspiration techniques in the early 1960s, the adoption of modest serial metallic dilation, and the enormous experience gained after the legalization of abortion in 1973 have lead to a 50% reduction in abortion mortality in the United States. In addition, preoperative ripening of the cervix with osmotic dilators or medications is employed by some abortion providers and may decrease the already low incidence of uterine injury and increase the ease of dilation at the time of surgery. Two percent of North American abortion providers routinely

Table 10-5

Condition	Management
Asthma	Inhaled bronchodilators available; prophylactic dose before procedure
Coagulopathy	
Inherited or acquired factor deficiency	Laboratory evaluation to determine deficit factors; factor replacement before procedure if indicated
von Willebrand disease	Desmopressin acetate before procedure for selected cases
Medication induced	Continue normal anticoagulation regimen; proceed with procedure when coagulation studies are in the therapeutic range
Diabetes mellitus, insulin dependent	Administer one half of usual morning insulin regimen; perform procedure in morning; allow patient to eat/resume regular insulin regimen postoperatively
Heart disease	
Severe, with compromised function	Perform procedure in setting where invasive cardiac monitoring is available for intra- and postoperative use
At high risk for bacterial endocarditis	Prophylactic antibiotics not indicated for abortion in the absence of infection or prosthetic valve, although treatment is routine care in many settings
HIV, hepatitis B or C infection	Continue any regular medication regimen; consider screening for sexually transmitted infections; universal precautions for tissue handling and instrument sterilization
Hypertension	Continue regular medication regimen; avoid vasoconstricting uterotonic agents; rule out preeclampsia in patients at later gestation
Seizure disorder	Continue regular medication regimen; consider administration of benzodiazepine or antiepileptic agent at time of procedure to increase seizure threshold
Sickle cell disease	Consider transfusion if red blood cell percentage is below usual baseline
Substance abuse	Anticipate altered pain tolerance; postpone procedure if patient is intoxicated or requires dangerously increased analgesic requirements

Adapted from Poehlmann DS, Ferguson B: Medical evaluation and management. In Paul M, Lichtenberg ES, Borgatta L, et al (eds): A Clinician's Guide to Medical and Surgical Abortion. Philadelphia, Churchill Livingstone, 1999, pp 52–61.

use osmotic dilators, predominantly laminaria tents, for first-trimester termination. The prostaglandin analogue misoprostol is also effective for cervical ripening when administered as a 400-μg dose either vaginally, sublingually, or orally 2 to 4 hours before the procedure.

Care should be taken to position the patient properly before the procedure. The "no touch" technique, avoiding direct contact with any portion of an instrument that will enter the uterine cavity, should be practiced. Although widely employed, use of an antiseptic solution to clean the cervix has not been shown to decrease the incidence of postoperative febrile morbidity or endometritis, since these agents are not bacteriostatic unless complete drying has occurred. Cervical dilation is accomplished by gentle insertion of graduated dilators through the cervical os. Historically, the cervix has often been dilated to the number of millimeters corresponding to the patient's estimated gestational age (e.g., 12 mm for 12 weeks' gestation). However, evacuation of the products of conception is often easily accomplished using less dilation. The cervix should never be forcibly dilated because this magnifies the risk of cervical laceration and uterine perforation. After adequate dilation, a suction cannula of appropriate size is inserted into the intrauterine cavity and connected to the vacuum source. The procedure is complete when a gritty surface is appreciated throughout the cavity and increased tension on the cannula indicates that uterine involution has begun. Routine use of the uterine sound adds little benefit in most cases and can usually be omitted; however, it can be a helpful guide into the uterine cavity when the cervix is narrow, stenotic, or tortuous. Gentle, sharp "check" curettage to reassure the physician that evacuation is complete carries little risk of perforation in experienced hands. The use of uterotonic agents at the time of surgery is not universal; however, intravenous, intramuscular, or intracervical administration of such agents has been shown to decrease operative blood loss and postoperative complications, an effect that is more pronounced in the late first trimester and beyond. Use of intraoperative ultrasound may be used for more challenging cases, such as in a patient with cervical stenosis, uterine anomaly, or obesity, and in teaching settings, but its routine use has not been evaluated for safety in a comparative or randomized way.

Manual vacuum aspiration, use of a self-contained vacuum syringe attached to a cannula, has typically been used in earlier gestational ages and in the developing world where electricity is either not available or not reliable. Manual vacuum aspiration has improved the provision of early abortion because it allows for removal of an intact gestational sac, easing tissue examination compared with conventional suction abortion. It is less noisy than electric vacuum aspiration and may also improve satisfaction for the patient undergoing abortion without sedation. In small randomized trials at teaching institutions, it has been shown to be as safe and effective as electric vacuum aspiration in the hands of both experienced and novice providers.

Pain Management
The importance of adequate pain management at the time of induced abortion cannot be overstated. Patients experience both physical and psychological aspects of pain differently. Effective management of pain improves patient experience and satisfaction. Nulliparous patients have been found to have an increased amount of pain at the time of first-trimester abortion compared with patients with a history of prior delivery. Factors not found to be associated with patients' subjective perception of pain include a history of prior abortion, prior pelvic examination, amount of cervical dilation, and size of the cannula used to perform the procedure.

The majority of first-trimester abortions in the United States are performed with the patient under local anesthesia or with intravenous sedation in the outpatient setting. In a 1997 survey of U.S. abortion clinics, 17% offered general anesthesia, 13% offered nitrous oxide and local anesthesia, 65% intravenous sedation and local anesthesia, and 40% local anesthesia with or without the addition of oral medications. The choice of anesthetic options is based on patient and provider preference, clinic resources, and clinical contraindications.

The local anesthetics most commonly used for paracervical blockade are amino amides such as lidocaine (Xylocaine) and mepivacaine (Carbocaine). They are stable, inexpensive, and rarely cause allergic reaction or overdose. Inadvertent intravascular injection can result in lightheadedness, perioral numbness, and metallic taste. Significant overdose can lead to seizures, coma, respiratory arrest, and cardiovascular collapse. The amino esters such as procaine (Novocain) and 2-chloroprocaine (Nesacaine) are used less frequently and are contraindicated in patients with a history of pseudocholinesterase deficiency, but they provide valuable alternatives for patients with allergies to the amino amides.

Techniques used for paracervical blockade differ widely. Local anesthetics are rapidly absorbed due to the highly vascular nature of the parametrium during pregnancy, and unilateral cervical block rapidly suffuses the contralateral nerve plexus. Therefore, the maximum dose of procaine-analogue drugs recommended for paracervical block is 200 mg or 20 mL of a 1% solution. Administering a larger volume of a more dilute solution may increase the safety and efficacy of a paracervical block, although the increased efficacy of this technique may be related to distension of tissue rather than the anesthetic property of the medication. The use of vasopressin in addition to a local anesthetic in the paracervical block is a widespread technique that may decrease procedural blood loss. A buffer solution may be added to the local anesthetic to decrease the pain at the injection site, but this has not been shown to add an advantage in terms of safety or efficacy. Oral analgesics used in combination with paracervical block include nonsteroidal anti-inflammatory agents (NSAIDs), orally active narcotics, and benzodiazepines.

Intravenous sedation for abortion typically includes a combination of a benzodiazepine and a narcotic. Using one or both types of agents, patients receive significant relief of pain but remain easily arousable and able to communicate and follow simple commands. Commonly used medications are midazolam, a short-acting benzodiazepine, and fentanyl, a narcotic with rapid onset and short duration of action. Administration of these medications in consciousness-altering doses should be provided only in the presence of pulse oximetry monitoring during surgery and in the immediate postoperative period because of the potential for respiratory depression.

In contrast to intravenous sedation, general or deep-sedation anesthesia involves the administration of medications leading to partial or complete ablation of breathing reflexes and consciousness. This kind of anesthesia often involves the administration of an induction agent, an anxiolytic drug and a narcotic medication. Induction agents cause dose-dependent central nervous system depression. Commonly used induction agents are the ultra-short-acting barbiturates methohexital and (less often) thiopental as well as the most popular sedative hypnotic medication, propofol. Other classes of medications that may be added include neuromuscular-blocking agents such as succinylcholine (commonly used for tracheal intubation) and inhalation anesthetics such as nitrous oxide. However, the halogenated ethers should be avoided given their tocolytic effect on myometrium and strong propensity to induce increased intraoperative and postoperative bleeding.

When intravenous sedation or general anesthesia is planned, precautions should be taken to decrease the risk of pulmonary aspiration. As a general practice, but subject to individualized exceptions, patients should abstain from intake of clear liquids for 2 hours and from full liquids or solid food for at least 6 hours before the procedure because gastric emptying is delayed in pregnancy. Postoperatively, patients should not be permitted to operate a motor vehicle until the effects of all medications have abated.

Studies including data primarily collected in the first decade of legal abortion in the United States indicated that general anesthesia resulted in increased mortality and complication rates compared with local anesthesia. However, more recently published studies have been reassuring and indicate that local anesthesia, intravenous sedation, and general anesthesia are all safe and appropriate options for pain management at the time of induced abortion. This paradigm shift is likely a result of improvements in the safety of general anesthesia, including advanced monitoring and improved training of personnel. The safety of each anesthetic option hinges most crucially on the training and skill of personnel as well as monitoring, medication, and equipment availability. Institutional decisions to offer deeper levels of anesthesia should therefore prompt a concerted effort to educate, train, and equip all clinical personnel appropriately.

Examination of the Products of Conception

Examination of the products of conception after suction abortion is essential to decrease the risk of retained pregnancy tissue as well as to identify cases of failed abortion and possible ectopic or molar pregnancy. Before 9 weeks' gestation, the gestational sac is identified as a thin, transparent membrane fringed with lacy projections representing chorionic tissue. After 8 to 9 weeks' gestation, fetal parts become visible. Ultrasound investigation for retained tissue should be performed if careful tissue examination fails to identify expected findings. If the uterus appears empty and the gestational sac is not located in the tissue obtained on aspiration, a workup for ectopic pregnancy should be initiated.

Incidence and Management of Complications

In developed countries, the mortality rate from legal, induced abortion in the first trimester is less than 1 in 100,000 procedures, making the procedure safer than pregnancy and childbirth. Large studies have shown extremely low rates of both minor complications (< 9 in 1000) as well as complications requiring hospitalization (< 1 in 1000). Recognized complications and their respective complication rates are listed in Table 10-6. Symptoms, risk factors, prophylactic measures, and management options are listed in Table 10-7.

Second-Trimester Surgical Abortion

Twelve percent of abortions in the United States are performed after 12th week of pregnancy, and 95% of these are surgical, rather than induction procedures. Only 1% of abortions occur after 20 weeks' gestation, 80% of which are accomplished surgically. Common reasons for delay of elective termination of pregnancy into the second trimester include undiagnosed pregnancy resulting from irregular menses, patient ambivalence, financial and accessibility constraints, and sudden changes in family and partner support. A smaller percentage of second-trimester procedures are necessitated by maternal illness, fetal anomalies, and obstetric indications that are often diagnosed after the first trimester.

Before the early 1970s, second-trimester abortion was accomplished primarily by hysterotomy and intra-amniotic instillation of saline, two procedures with relatively high complication rates. At the time that abortion was legalized in the United States, dilation and evacuation (D&E) as a technique for second-trimester abortion was developed and perfected in Europe and was found to be far safer than previously used procedures. By the 1980s, D&E was the predominant method of second-trimester abortion in the United States, providing a significant improvement in the safety profile of abortion in the second trimester.

Many of the same principles safeguarding first-trimester surgical abortion apply to D&E as well. Patients must be adequately counseled regarding pregnancy options, the abortion process, and procedural risks, and informed consent must be obtained. An ultrasound scan is essential for gestational age determination because the results guide the practitioner about the extent of preoperative cervical preparation. Preoperative medical evaluation and laboratory tests are identical to those required for first-trimester procedures. Options for pain management are also similar to those available in the first trimester, with the understanding that surgical abortion in the second trimester is generally a longer, more extensive operation than suction dilation and curettage. Therefore, practitioners of

Table 10-6

First-Trimester Surgical Abortion Complication Rates

Complication	Rate*
Failed abortion	0.5–2.3
Retained products of conception	2.9–19.6
Postabortal hematometra	1.5–2.0
Hemorrhage (>250 mL blood loss)	0–1.5
Disseminated intravascular coagulopathy	0–0.8
Endometritis	1.0–4.6
Perforation/high cervical tears	0.1–1.7
Asherman syndrome	0.16–0.5

*Per 1000 procedures.

Table 10-7 Surgical Abortion Complications: Symptoms, Risk Factors, and Management

Complication	Symptoms	Risk Factors	Prophylaxis	Management
Failed abortion	Ongoing pregnancy symptoms	Uterine anomalies, multiple gestation, early gestation, operator inexperience	Meticulous tissue exam; intraoperative or postoperative ultrasound	Respiration
Retained products	Bleeding, cramping, infection	Uterine anomalies, large cavity	Same as for failed abortion	Respiration
Postabortal hematometra	Pelvic pressure, cramping 15–60 minutes postoperatively		Uterotonics	Respiration
Hemorrhage (>250 mL blood loss)	Excessive bleeding			
Atony		Gestational age >10 weeks, advanced maternal age, increasing parity, prior cesarean section, history of postabortal or postpartum hemorrhage	Uterotonics	Bimanual uterine massage, oxytocin, ergotamines, vasopressin, 15 methyl $PGF_{2\alpha}$, misoprostol
Disseminated intravascular coagulopathy		Increased gestational age, prolonged demise, amniotic fluid embolism, sepsis		Clotting factor and volume replacement

	Symptoms/Signs	Risk factors	Prevention	Treatment
Endometritis	Pelvic pain, fever	Age <20 years, nulliparity, previous pelvic inflammatory disease, cervicitis	Aseptic technique, treatment of cervicitis, routine use of periabortal antibiotics	Broad spectrum antibiotics (gentamicin and clindamycin)
Uterine injury				
Cervical tear, external os	Bleeding	Operator inexperience, increased parity, increased gestational age, cervical resistance to dilation or ripening	Gentle surgical technique	Silver nitrate, Monsel's solution, surgical repair.
Perforation/ high cervical tears	Bleeding, loss of resistance, aspiration of bowel or omentum			In the first trimester, conservative management—in the absence of bleeding or suspected visceral injury—and laparoscopy or laparotomy—in the setting of active bleeding, instability, or suspected visceral injury. In the second trimester, prolonged tamponade, vaginal repair, abdominal repair and, in selected cases, angiographic embolization.
Asherman's syndrome	Persistent amenorrhea	Sharp curettage	Avoidance of excessive metallic curettage	Cervical dilation, hysteroscopic lysis of adhesions, estrogen therapy

*Per 1000 procedures.

PGF, prostaglandin F.

Adapted from Lichtenberg ES, Grimes DA, Paul M: Abortion complications: Prevention and management. In Paul M, Lichtenberg ES, Borgatta L, et al (eds): A Clinician's Guide to Medical and Surgical Abortion. Philadelphia, Churchill Livingstone, 1999, pp 197–216.

second-trimester surgical abortion frequently opt for intravenous sedation or regional or general anesthesia over local anesthesia alone. Major differences between first- and second-trimester procedures are the importance of preoperative cervical preparation, operative technique, and the rate and extent of operative complications.

Preoperative Cervical Preparation

D&E involves the removal of the fetus and placenta from the intrauterine cavity using a combination of instrumental extraction and suction evacuation. The cervical dilation required to accommodate the necessary instruments and the products of conception corresponds to the gestational age of the pregnancy. Studies have shown that the use of osmotic dilators decreases the risk of intraoperative cervical laceration and uterine perforation compared with historical complication rates using only metallic dilation for cervical expansion. The major types of osmotic dilators and their properties are listed in Table 10-8. Practitioners of second-trimester abortion use a wide variety of protocols to achieve cervical dilation. These typically involve a single insertion of multiple dilators or serial insertions 24 to 48 hours before the procedure. The number and size of dilators used is based both on gestational age and cervical compliance. Depending on the level of patient discomfort, mild oral analgesics, partial or full-dose paracervical block anesthesia, or both may be used for dilator insertion. Occasionally, a narcotic injection is necessary and, rarely, deep sedation or general anesthesia is required. Patients frequently experience mild to moderate pain and cramping after osmotic dilator placement. NSAIDs or acetaminophen are generally sufficient for postinsertion pain management, but sometimes a short course of oral narcotics is necessary. Light vaginal bleeding or spotting is also common, whereas heavy bleeding after osmotic dilator insertion is rare and usually the result of cervical expansion (equivalent to bloody show in labor). Placental incursion to the cervical os (placenta previa) may also be a cause of bleeding during dilator placement but can be tamponaded with additional dilators. Studies have shown placenta previa poses no increased risk of hemorrhage during second-trimester D&E abortion.

The relative discomfort, expense, and inconvenience of osmotic dilator insertion have led providers of D&E to search for alternative means of safe and effective cervical preparation. A number of prostaglandin derivatives have been used to effect cervical ripening prior to D&E. Misoprostol has

Table 10-8

Osmotic Dilators

Name of Dilator	Composition	Size Range	Expansion
Laminaria japonica	Dried, compressed seaweed	2–10 mm	3–4 times
Lamicel	Polyvinyl alcohol sponge impregnated with magnesium sulfate (active ingredient)	3 or 5 mm	None
Dilapan-S	Polyacrylonitrile rod (Hypan)	4 mm	Up to 15 mm

242

been used in a variety of dosages orally, sublingually, vaginally, and buccally in an effort to circumvent osmotic dilator use up to 18 weeks' gestation. Prostaglandins may also be used in combination with osmotic dilators for enhanced cervical preparation with the proviso that overnight use of misoprostol may result in unscheduled delivery and therefore is used very selectively by most providers.

Surgical Technique

As with first-trimester surgical abortion, proper patient positioning is essential for ease of performing D&E. Modified specula allowing for more expansive visualization of the cervix can be used. Because the cervix is highly vascular with increasing gestational age, many practitioners opt to grasp the cervix with a ring forceps or atraumatic tenaculum. Osmotic dilators are removed before evacuation of the uterine contents.

Surgical evacuation may be accomplished in the early second trimester with large-bore suction tubing connected to a vacuum source. Beyond 16 weeks' gestation, use of extraction forceps in addition to suction evacuation is generally required. Extraction forceps such as the Van Lith, Sopher, and Bierer models have been developed for D&E; they possess varying surface areas, heft, length, and pelvic curvature. The minimum cervical dilation required to accommodate these instruments varies from 12 to 17 mm. After evacuation of fetal parts and the placenta with extraction forceps, suction is used to ensure complete emptying of the intrauterine cavity. Surgical completion is indicated by a tactile sense of uterine involution and a gritty sensation throughout the cavity, which may be diminished or absent in patients with uterine leiomyomata or a history of uterine surgery. At the completion of the procedure, a digital examination of the cervical os is performed to ensure the integrity of the cervical mucosa (absence of a high cervical tear). Finally, the operator should inventory the fetal parts and placenta to ensure that the evacuation is complete.

When adequate cervical dilation is achieved preoperatively, D&E may be accomplished with the fetus intact. Intact procedures reduce the need for uterine instrumentation and therefore theoretically decrease the risk of cervical laceration and uterine perforation. Intact procedures also allow for more comprehensive autopsy evaluation in the setting of pregnancy termination for congenital anomalies and may more readily permit bonding postevacuation to help parents achieve emotional resolution. Studies comparing intact and nonintact procedures are limited; however, a large case series of intact procedures has recorded similar complication rates to nonintact procedures.

Special Considerations

Intrauterine fetal demise results in softening of cortical bone and may enhance cervical ripening. This knowledge has led some providers of second-trimester abortion to advocate fetocidal techniques before surgery. Transabdominal intra-amniotic or intrafetal injection of either potassium chloride or digoxin can be used for this purpose and has been shown to be safe in a case series. However, improved safety and efficacy over the standard technique of surgical abortion after fetocidal injection has not been proved.

As in the case of first-trimester surgical abortion, the use of intraoperative and postoperative uterotonic agents to decrease blood loss varies widely among abortion providers. Most providers use some form of uterotonic therapy. The addition of vasopressin to the paracervical block has been shown to decrease intraoperative blood loss after 15 weeks' gestation. Dilute intravenous oxytocin and vasopressin may also be used prophylactically to reduce the risk of uterine atony and intraoperative hemorrhage.

Some providers of second-trimester abortion routinely use intraoperative ultrasound. One small study has shown a decreased rate of uterine perforation when intraoperative ultrasound was used in a residency training setting. It is unclear whether the routine use of intraoperative ultrasound decreases the rate of potential complications when the operator is experienced in performing D&E. Certainly, judicious use of ultrasound is valuable to confirm complete uterine evacuation when the operator believes the uterus to be empty by tactile sensation, but not all products of conception have been identified.

Incidence and Management of Complications

Complication rates for surgical abortion increase with advancing gestational age. The mortality rate associated with D&E is approximately four per 100,000 cases. Hysterectomy is required in 1.3 to 4 per 10,000 cases. Rates of other recognized complications of second-trimester surgical abortion are listed in Table 10-9. Management of complications is similar to management in the first trimester (*see* Table 10-7), but suspicion of tissue injury must be evaluated in a timely and rigorous manner given the added risk of hemorrhage and sepsis during the second trimester.

Care After Surgical Abortion

The level of care provided in the immediate postoperative period after pregnancy termination should be tailored to the complexity and duration of the procedure as well as the type of anesthesia used. Postoperative surveillance should include monitoring of vital signs, vaginal bleeding, and uterine tone. Pain management may include nonpharmacologic measures

Table 10-9

Dilation and Evacuation Complication Rates

Complication	Rate*
Retained products of conception	4–20
Hemorrhage (>450 mL blood loss)	7
Disseminated intravascular coagulopathy	1.9–5.0
Endometritis	6–20
Uterine injury	
Cervical tear, confined to external os	22–40
Perforation/high cervical tears (involving internal os, lower segment, corpus or fundus)	2

*Per 1000 procedures.

such as application of heat to the abdomen for relief of uterine cramping and reassurance. NSAIDs, acetaminophen, and a short course of oral narcotics are frequently used for postoperative pain management. Patients differ widely in their postoperative medication requirements. Antiemetics may also be used for symptomatic relief in the immediate postoperative period, although most postoperative emesis is transient and nonrepetitive.

Postoperative care after second-trimester surgical abortion is similar to that after a first-trimester procedure in that it should be suited to the length and complexity of the surgery as well as the type of anesthesia used. Postoperative surveillance usually involves evaluation of vital signs and postoperative bleeding for at least 1 hour in the mid second trimester and for 2 hours in later gestations.

A meta-analysis of the use of prophylactic antibiotics after induced abortion up to 15 weeks' gestation revealed a significant reduction in postoperative infection in both low- and high-risk patients who received a course of perioperative antibiotics. This has led to the widespread use of prophylactic antibiotics after abortion. Doxycycline is active against chlamydial, gonorrheal, and mycoplasma species and has traditionally been used for a 7-day course. However, a randomized trial of prophylactic doxycycline given for 3 vs. 7 days after first-trimester surgical abortion found no difference in postoperative infection rates, indicating that 3 days of prophylaxis may be sufficient. Some providers also prescribe a short course of prophylactic uterotonic medication such as methylergonovine (Methergine) to decrease postoperative bleeding. Rh immune globulin (RhoGAM) is administered to Rh-negative patients to prevent isoimmunization. Although the evidence for isoimmunization after first-trimester abortion is theoretical, the benefits of preventing isoimmunization likely outweigh the minimal risks associated with its administration.

Counseling regarding the normal postoperative course is essential in caring for a patient undergoing abortion. Patients should be provided with a list of warning signs (Box 10-1) and a 24-hour emergency contact number. Patients may return to normal physical activity 1 to 2 days after the normalization of bleeding with the exception of vaginal intercourse, which should be avoided for 1 to 2 weeks. After second-trimester abortion, patients should be counseled that breast engorgement and milk letdown may occur. They should be encouraged to suppress lactation by wearing a tight bra, using NSAIDs for symptomatic relief, adding cold packs if needed, and

---

Box 10-1   **Warning Signs Following Induced Abortion**

Vaginal bleeding that saturates 2 sanitary pads in 2 hours
Temperature >100.4°F
Severe abdominal pain or cramping
Ongoing pregnancy symptoms unresolved after 1 week
Vaginal bleeding lasting >2 weeks
Failure to resume regular menses (in the absence of progesterone-only
   contraception) within 6 weeks

avoiding breast stimulation. Finally, postabortion care should include a review of the patient's contraceptive choice and a complete understanding of how she plans to implement this choice. Many abortion providers offer and recommend a postoperative visit 1 to 2 weeks after the procedure. However, in uncomplicated cases, detailed patient counseling about normal recovery and warning signs of possible complications with follow-up telephone communication are likely to be just as effective and more efficient alternatives. Women at high risk for complications should be encouraged to seek follow-up care in a time course that matches the development of the complication.

Second-Trimester Abortion by Induction of Labor

Second-trimester abortion by labor induction involves the use of medications or mechanical devices to induce labor, dilate the cervix, and cause expulsion of the fetus and placenta. Although complete epidemiologic data are lacking, an estimated 1% of abortions in the United States are performed by labor induction. However, in countries with subsidized health care services or low resources, induction abortion is more widely practiced. A myriad of different medications and procedures have been used to induce labor in the second trimester, including a number of instillation agents, oxytocin, mechanical devices, and prostaglandins. Although there are numerous published studies describing and comparing the safety and efficacy of several of these agents, the majority of trials are small and involve the use of multiple induction medications, making the studies difficult to compare.

Instillation Agents

The U.S. Centers for Disease Control and Prevention estimated that 57% of second-trimester abortions performed in 1974 involved instillation procedures. These numbers have declined dramatically (to an estimated 4% in 1994) due to the advent of newer, safer methods of induction as well as improved techniques for D&E. Instillation of hypertonic saline involves the withdrawal of 35 to 200 mL of amniotic fluid by amniocentesis and instillation of 200 mL of 20% saline into the intrauterine cavity at more than 16 weeks' gestation. This process causes damage to decidual cells, the release of prostaglandins, and resultant cervical softening and is used in combination with oxytocin to induce labor. Adverse effects include fever, nausea, vomiting, hemorrhage, and infection and occur in 5% to 12% of patients. The rate of serious complications (e.g., hemorrhage requiring transfusion, fever for more than 2 days, or unintended surgery) is 2%. Disseminated intravascular coagulopathy has been reported to occur as frequently as 6.6 per 1000 cases. Rare complications including seizures, uterine necrosis secondary to intramyometrial injection of saline, hypernatremia, coma, and death have also been reported.

Hyperosmolar urea has also been used for labor induction in the second trimester. Similar to saline instillation, 200 mL of amniotic fluid is removed by amniocentesis and 135 mL, or 80 g, of urea is instilled by gravity into the uterine cavity. Labor induction is accomplished in combination with prostaglandins or oxytocin. A third instillation agent, prostaglandin $F_{2\alpha}$, is associated with a decreased risk of disseminated intravascular coagulopathy and a shorter instillation-to-abortion time compared with the use of saline. However, 30% of patients experience adverse effects including nausea, vomiting, diarrhea, and fever. Rare complications such as cardiac arrhythmias, myocardial infarction, and hemorrhagic stroke have also been recorded. The use of instillation agents has essentially been abandoned in the United States because of unacceptable major complication rates and the advent of newer, safer techniques.

Oxytocin

Oxytocin is administered either intravenously or intramuscularly, causing stimulation of myometrial receptors and resultant uterine contractions. However, because the uterus in the second trimester contains fewer oxytocin receptors than myometrial tissue in the third trimester, oxytocin is considered less effective in the mid trimester, and higher doses of medication are required. Oxytocin can be used as a single agent or in combination with prostaglandins or mechanical dilators for second-trimester induction abortion. Stepwise escalations of 50 units infused over 3 hours with 1-hour breaks to prevent water intoxication is a time-tested, safe, and popular regimen.

Prostaglandins

A number of prostaglandins have been used for second-trimester labor induction. Fifteen-methyl prostaglandin $F_{2\alpha}$ ($PGF_{2\alpha}$) (carboprost tromethamine) may be administered intramuscularly or intravaginally to induce labor, but its use is limited by unacceptably high rates of gastrointestinal side effects. The PGE_2 analogue sulprostone also exhibits significant gastrointestinal side effects and has been associated with cardiovascular-related deaths; it is not available in the United States. The natural prostaglandin dinoprostone (Prepidil, Cervidil) is a vaginal suppository administered every 3 hours for labor induction. Its use is limited by its relative expense and the necessity of refrigeration.

Misoprostol

Misoprostol is a PGE_1 analogue initially developed for the prevention of gastric ulcers that is widely available, inexpensive, and stable at room temperature. Misoprostol has lower rates of gastrointestinal and other adverse effects compared with other prostaglandin analogues and has become the most commonly used agent for labor induction. A second PGE_1 analogue, gemeprost, is widely used outside the United States and has been associated on rare occasions with nonfatal cardiac arrhythmias. Multiple studies have examined the use of misoprostol for second-trimester labor induction, comparing various dosing regimens, routes of administration, and outcomes such as time to abortion, side effects, and complications. Vaginal administration has been shown to be more efficacious than oral administration, leading to shorter induction-to-abortion intervals in a number of studies.

Shorter induction-to-abortion intervals are also commonly seen with spontaneous *in utero* fetal demise compared with live gestations, regardless of induction regimen. In a study of patients undergoing labor induction between 12 and 22 weeks' gestational age using misoprostol 200 μg administered vaginally every 12 hours, the mean induction to abortion time was 10.4 hours for patients with fetal demise and 15.4 hours for patients with live fetuses.

A range of misoprostol doses has been studied, including 200, 400, and 600 μg administered between every 4 and 12 hours. Given the varying gestational ages and the differing percentages of patients with fetal demise vs. live gestations in these studies, direct comparison to determine the optimal dosing regimen has proven challenging. For comparison, Table 10-10 lists common adverse effects, induction-to-abortion intervals, and rates of complete abortion (passage of both fetus and placenta) of several commonly used regimens.

The most common complication associated with misoprostol induction of labor in the second trimester is curettage for retained products of conception, reported in 8% to 67% of cases. The percentage of failed induction or the need to abandon labor induction in favor of a surgical procedure is approximately 7%. Other major complications including hemorrhage requiring transfusion, endometritis, cervical laceration, and uterine rupture are uncommon occurrences and are rarely reported given the small sample size of the majority of studies.

Although the American College of Obstetricians and Gynecologists proscribes use of misoprostol in the third trimester for women with prior cesarean delivery because of the risk of uterine rupture, misoprostol may be used with caution for second-trimester labor induction in patients with a history of uterine surgery. Given the rarity of case reports of rupture, the greater thickness of the fundus in the second trimester, and the lower intrauterine pressures generated by a standard labor pattern, it is unlikely that the risk of uterine rupture is equal to the third-trimester risk. However, some misoprostol studies in the second trimester exclude patients with a scarred uterus, and the actual rate of rupture is unknown. Therefore, judicious use of small doses at longer intervals with close surveillance is imperative.

Special Considerations

Cervical preparation before labor induction decreases the induction-to-abortion interval and likely reduces the overall rate of complications. Some providers of second-trimester labor induction routinely use osmotic dilators for cervical preparation before prostaglandin induction. The use of mifepristone, an antiprogesterone agent used for early medical abortion, softens the cervix and sensitizes the myometrial receptors to prostaglandins. In European studies, its use 48 hours before induction abortion has been shown to significantly decrease induction-to-abortion time as well as the dose of prostaglandin required to effect complete abortion.

Studies have also shown that induction-to-abortion time is significantly decreased in the setting of fetal demise. This has prompted some abortion providers to advocate fetocidal procedures before labor induction. In

Table 10-10

Common Dosing
Regimens for
Misoprostol Induction
of Labor in the
Second Trimester,
Associated Side
Effects, Induction-to-
Abortion Interval,
and Complete
Abortion Rates

Dosing Regimen	Side Effects (%)			Mean Induction-to-Abortion Interval (Hours)	Complete Abortion Rate (%)
	Nausea ± Vomiting	Diarrhea	Fever ≥ 38°C		
200 µg every 6 hours*,†	9–47.2	0–2	23.4–26	13.8–16.9	43.9–62.2
200 µg every 12 hours*,‡,§,‖	3.9–11	0–8	0–11	12–45	33.3–64.7
400 µg every 4 hours¶	0	0	25	19.6	92
400 µg every 6 hours#	3.75	0	0	14.5	57.1
400 µg every 12 hours‡,**	12–16.2	6–20.6	2–67.6	33.4–35.8	72–89.7
600 µg every 12 hours‡	20	22	28	22.3	78

249

*Jain JK, Kuo J, Mishell DR: A comparison of two dosing regimens of intravaginal misoprostol for second-trimester pregnancy termination. Obstet Gynecol 93:571–575, 1999.
†Dickinson JE, Godfrey M, Evans SF: Efficacy of intravaginal misoprostol in second-trimester pregnancy termination: A randomized controlled trial. J Matern Fetal Med 7:115–119, 1998.
‡Herabutya Y, O-Prasertsawat P: Second trimester abortion using intravaginal misoprostol. Int J Gynecol Obstet 60:161–165, 1998.
§Nuutila M, Toivonen J, Ylikorkala O, Halmesamki E: A comparison between two doses of intravaginal misoprostol and gemeprost for induction of second-trimester abortion. Obstet Gynecol 90:896–900, 1997.
‖Jain JK, Mishell DR: A comparison of intravaginal misoprostol with prostaglandin E2 for termination of second-trimester pregnancy. N Engl J Med 331:290–293, 1994.
¶Bebbington MW, Kent N, Lim K, et al: A randomized controlled trial comparing two protocols for the use of misoprostol in midtrimester pregnancy termination. Am J Obstet Gynecol 187:853–857, 2002.
#Dickinson JE, Evans SF: A comparison of oral misoprostol with vaginal misoprostol administration in second-trimester pregnancy termination for fetal abnormality. Obstet Gynecol 101:1294–1299, 2003.
**Pongsatha S, Tongsong T, Suwannawut O: Therapeutic termination of second trimester pregnancy with vaginal misoprostol. J Med Assoc Thai 84:515–518, 2001.

addition to this advantage, fetocidal injection before induction prevents the live birth of a nonviable infant that may be distressing to patients and health care providers and may prompt heroic efforts for fetal salvage.

The choice to perform surgical vs. induction abortion in the second trimester is based on several factors. Although large, randomized studies comparing the safety and efficacy of D&E to induction abortion have not been performed, the available body of evidence suggests that D&E has a lower rate of overall complications in the hands of experienced operators. Therefore, the choice of procedure may be made solely on the availability of adequately trained providers. On occasion, safety considerations clearly favor the more rapid process of D&E; that is, in the setting of obstetric emergencies such as severe preeclampsia; eclampsia; hemolysis, elevated liver enzymes, and low platelet count (HELLP syndrome); or suspected placenta accreta, and severe preexisting maternal medical conditions.

However, when both procedures are medically acceptable and available, patient preference is extremely important and should be considered.

Patients terminating desired pregnancies because of pregnancy-related complications, fetal anomalies, or maternal illness may prefer induction of labor because it provides an opportunity to bond after delivery with the fetus or newborn. Finally, when performed in a hospital setting, induction of labor is significantly more costly than D&E as a result of lengthy induction-to-abortion intervals.

Early Medical Abortion

The desire of many women seeking abortion to avoid surgical intervention and the attempt to increase its accessibility has led to the development of medical abortion regimens. Natural prostaglandins (e.g., PGE_2 and $PGF_{2\alpha}$) as well as synthetic prostaglandin analogues (e.g., misoprostol, gemeprost, sulprostone) have been used to effect medical abortion. However, use of prostaglandins alone requires high doses of medication and may be limited by unacceptable rates of gastrointestinal adverse effects. Mifepristone (also known as RU-486), a norethindrone derivative with affinity for the progesterone receptor that acts as an antiprogesterone, was developed in 1982. Its use in combination with prostaglandin analogues for medical abortion allows for decreased doses of prostaglandins and therefore fewer adverse effects. In 1988, both China and France approved mifepristone for use in medical abortion up to 49 days post-LMP. This was followed by approval up to 63 days in the United Kingdom and Sweden. Mifepristone first became available for use in medical abortion in the United States in September 2000. It is now also available in a number of countries in Europe and Asia.

Mifepristone
Mifepristone acts on decidual capillary endothelial cells causing separation from trophoblasts as well as prostaglandin release. Its administration also results in softening of the cervix in preparation for pregnancy expulsion. Early studies of mifepristone alone in single or divided doses of 50 to 400 mg/day for 4 days led to successful medical abortion in 60% to 80% of women at ≤49 days post-LMP. Use of mifepristone in combination with prostaglandins notably improves the rate of complete abortion. A number of different prostaglandin analogues have been used. Misoprostol has become the predominant medication used in combination with mifepristone for medical abortion in the United States and widely around the world.

Initial medical abortion studies performed in the United States were large, multicenter trials using the French protocol of mifepristone 600 mg given orally followed by misoprostol 400 μg by mouth 48 hours later. Patients remained in the clinic or hospital setting for 4 hours after misoprostol administration. This regimen resulted in a successful abortion rate that was gestational-age dependent: 96% to 98%, 91% to 95%, and less than 90% for patients less than or equal to 42, 43 to 49, and more than 49 days post-LMP, respectively. The remaining patients required surgical intervention for completion of the abortion. Close to half of all patients studied aborted within 4 hours of misoprostol administration, and 75% completed the abortion within 24 hours. Complication rates were low.

The French protocol was the basis for the protocol approved by the U.S. Food and Drug Administration in 2000.

Subsequent studies have led to significant changes in the medical abortion regimen currently used in the United States. Studies have shown mifepristone in a 100- or 200-mg oral dose to be equivalent to the 600-mg dose in efficacy. Vaginal (in preference to oral) administration of misoprostol results in fewer gastrointestinal side effects, decreased time to complete abortion, and improved rates of complete abortion. These findings are consistent with pharmacokinetic studies of misoprostol that show a slower peak onset and longer duration of action for the vaginal vs. oral route. U.S. studies examining patient home self-administration of vaginal misoprostol found this change in the regimen to be safe, efficacious, and acceptable to patients. Finally, studies examining time between mifepristone and misoprostol administration showed similar safety and efficacy for a window of 24 to 72 hours between medications. A large randomized trial has shown that giving misoprostol 8 hours after mifepristone achieves nearly equal success and possibly lower side effects compared with 24-hour administration. A large trial is now in progress testing efficacy, side effects, and acceptability of simultaneously administered 200 mg of mifepristone and 800 µg of vaginal misoprostol. These studies have led to the expansion of medical abortion provision that has decreased costs and side effects while improving efficacy, patient acceptability, and convenience.

Mifepristone/Misoprostol Abortion Provision

Medical abortion provision requires preoperative options counseling similar to that provided with surgical abortion. Patients should be sure of their decision to terminate the pregnancy before proceeding with mifepristone administration. Most importantly, patients choosing medical abortion over the surgical method should be thoroughly counseled that vaginal bleeding and abdominal cramping similar to spontaneous miscarriage will occur after administration of misoprostol. Patients who lack sufficient pain tolerance, maturity, social support, or privacy to successfully pass the pregnancy outside the medical setting should be counseled in favor of surgical abortion (Box 10-2). A complete medical history and targeted physical examination should be completed. Contraindications to medical abortion (Box 10-3) do not preclude surgical abortion provision in the outpatient setting.

Documentation of pregnancy and gestational age determination are accomplished by physical examination, urine pregnancy test, and transvaginal ultrasound evaluation. Although the use of ultrasound is not universal in

---

Box 10-2   Psychosocial Contraindications to Medical Abortion

Unwillingness to pass pregnancy at home
Desire for immediate abortion
Inability to return for follow-up
Unwillingness to undergo surgical intervention for complications or failure
Lack of access to telephone or transportation to emergency facility

Box 10-3   Medical Contraindications to Mifepristone/Misoprostol Abortion
Coagulopathy
Severe anemia
Current anticoagulation therapy
Chronic renal failure
Current, long-term systemic corticosteroid therapy
Confirmed or suspected ectopic pregnancy
Undiagnosed adnexal mass
Inherited porphyrias
Intrauterine device *in situ*
History of allergy to mifepristone, misoprostol, or other prostaglandin

Adapted from Creinin MD: Early Medical Abortion with Mifepristone or Methotrexate: Overview and Protocol Recommendations. Washington, DC, National Abortion Federation, 2001.

gestational age determination before medical abortion, all major U.S. trials have used ultrasound for dating, and its use in clinical practice is widespread. Medicolegal concerns in the United States about missing an ectopic pregnancy play an important role in the decision to use ultrasound for pre-enrollment dating. Laboratory evaluation of Rh status and baseline hemoglobin or hematocrit should be performed. As in the case of surgical abortion, Rh-negative patients should receive Rh immune globulin (MICRhoGAM or RhoGAM) to prevent isoimmunization. Finally, all patients should be counseled regarding postabortal contraception.

Patients undergoing medical abortion in the United States are commonly treated with an evidence-based regimen of 200 mg of mifepristone orally administered in the clinic or office setting followed by 800 µg of misoprostol self-administered vaginally in 24 to 72 hours. Pain management regimens may include NSAIDs and a short course of orally active narcotics. Patients are counseled to seek medical attention for excessive bleeding, sustained fever, or lack of vaginal bleeding 24 hours after vaginal misoprostol administration. Follow-up evaluation is scheduled for 1 or 2 weeks, with the option of more rapid follow-up if the patient believes the pregnancy has passed. Transvaginal ultrasound revealing an absent gestational sac is consistent with complete medical abortion. A thickened endometrial stripe or the appearance of accumulated blood clots in the endometrial cavity in the absence of significant vaginal bleeding is not associated with the need for surgical intervention. A patient with incomplete medical abortion, as evidenced by a persistent gestational sac on ultrasound, may be treated with additional misoprostol or surgical intervention, depending on the patient's clinical presentation and patient and provider preference.

Complications of Mifepristone/Misoprostol Medical Abortion
Vaginal bleeding and cramping are fully anticipated after medical abortion and should not be considered procedural complications. The rates of minor, self-limited gastrointestinal and other adverse effects vary with medication protocols and are listed in Table 10-11. The rate of surgical

Table 10-11

Side Effect	Rate (%)
Nausea	36–67
Headache	13–37
Vomiting	13–34
Diarrhea	8–27
Dizziness	12–37
Fever or chills	4–37

Adapted from Stewart FH, Wells ES, Flinn SK, Weitz TA: Early Medical Abortion: Issues for Practice. San Francisco, UCSF Center for Reproductive Health Research and Policy, 2001.

intervention for failed or incomplete medical abortion or significant bleeding is between 2% and 5%—increasing with gestational age and decreasing with provider experience. Blood transfusion is required in one to three per 1000 cases. Infection is a rare complication of medical abortion, reported as 0.09% to 0.5%. A few studies have reported empiric antibiotic use for presumed endometritis in as many as 5% to 11% of patients. There is no evidence to support use of routine periabortal antibiotic prophylaxis in first-trimester medical abortion.

Methotrexate/Misoprostol Medical Abortion

By blocking dihydrofolate reductase and inhibiting DNA synthesis, methotrexate acts against rapidly dividing cell lines and has been used to successfully treat neoplasms (including gestational trophoblastic tumor), autoimmune disease, and unruptured ectopic pregnancy. Although methotrexate has significant toxicity at high doses, low doses similar to those used to treat ectopic pregnancy are well tolerated with few adverse effects. Studies have shown 50 mg/m^2 of intramuscular methotrexate followed by 800 µg of misoprostol administered vaginally 3 to 4 days later to be effective for early medical abortion. Success rates are improved by administering a second dose of misoprostol 24 hours after the initial dose and *increasing* the time interval between methotrexate and misoprostol administration to as long as 1 week. As with mifepristone/misoprostol abortion, rates of complete abortion decrease with advancing gestational age and are in the range of 92%, 89%, and 82% for 49 or fewer, 50 to 56, and 57 to 63 days post-LMP, respectively. Oral administration of methotrexate has been associated with increased adverse effects over intramuscular administration. Although notably less costly, methotrexate is much less widely used as an abortifacient since the approval of mifepristone due to its lower efficacy and due to the rare occurrence of serious adverse effects. Medical contraindications to methotrexate are listed in Box 10-4.

Misoprostol Alone for Medical Abortion

Misoprostol alone has been used for medical abortion in areas where additional medications are not available or inaccessible due to cost. As with the combined regimens, success rates decrease with increasing gestational age. For pregnancies up to 63 days post-LMP, success rates range from

Box 10-4 Medical Contraindications to Methotrexate/Misoprostol Abortion
Acute or chronic renal disease
Acute or chronic hepatic disease
Coagulopathy
Severe anemia
Acute inflammatory bowel disease
Uncontrolled seizure disorder
History of allergy to methotrexate, misoprostol, or other prostaglandins

Adapted from Creinin MD: Early Medical Abortion with Mifepristone or Methotrexate: Overview and Protocol Recommendations. Washington, DC, National Abortion Federation, 2001.

80% to 90% when up to three 800-μg doses of misoprostol are administered vaginally at 24-hour intervals. Similar regimens have shown encouraging results at up to 13 to 14 weeks of gestation. When used alone without pretreatment with mifepristone or methotrexate, higher doses of misoprostol are required to achieve equal rates of complete abortion. Higher doses of misoprostol are associated with increased adverse effects, which may limit the use of misoprostol alone in settings where other regimens are available.

Long-Term Effects of Pregnancy Termination

Given the incidence of induced abortion, concerns have been raised regarding the long-term sequelae of the procedure. The evidence suggests that first-trimester induced abortion does not adversely affect future reproductive potential. In particular, studies have shown no increase in the rate of infertility, early pregnancy failure, ectopic pregnancy, low birth weight, or preterm delivery. Similarly, multiple vacuum abortions in the first trimester using judicious dilation are not more likely to cause future reproductive complications than a single procedure. Studies examining reproductive outcomes after second-trimester terminations are few and contain smaller numbers of patients, but are reassuring. Likewise, a large study examining pregnancy after mifepristone/misoprostol abortion found no adverse effects of early medical termination on subsequent pregnancy.

There has been significant debate regarding the association between induced abortion and the risk of subsequent malignancy. No definitive relationship between pregnancy termination and nongynecologic malignancy has been established. Many of the studies evaluating the risk of gynecologic malignancies after induced abortion have methodologic issues limiting the utility of their findings. Studies show conflicting results, some finding an increased association and others a protective effect. There is currently no definite evidence that induced abortion increases the risk of developing cancer of the cervix, ovary, or uterus. Perhaps the most widely debated association has been the risk of breast cancer after induced abortion. As with the gynecologic malignancies, conflicting studies have been published. However, very large studies done prospectively in Sweden and Denmark have failed to show an association between induced abortion and subsequent increased risk of breast cancer. Induced abortions in these countries are legal, accessible, federally funded, and recorded in a national registry as are obstetric deliveries, bypassing the potential methodologic problems associated with recall bias by women diagnosed with breast cancer. A recent British report of 83,000 women with breast cancer that collated data in 53 epidemiologic studies from 16 counties found that women who were not vulnerable to recall bias (information on past abortions was recorded before the diagnosis of breast cancer) had no increase in breast cancer incidence after either spontaneous or induced abortion.

Finally, with respect to the long-term psychological sequelae of elective abortion, there is no substantive evidence for the existence of a post-traumatic syndrome related to this event. Grief and remorse are apt to be more severe and lasting in those with low self-efficacy, poor self-esteem, preexisting mental illness, ambivalence about their decision, lack of social support, perceived coercion, experience of social stigma connected to abortion, or medically indicated termination of pregnancy for maternal or fetal reasons. Patients manifesting profound depression or self-blame should receive the option of referral to a licensed counselor who respects personal autonomy.

KEY POINTS

1. Early pregnancy failure occurs in 10% to 15% of clinically recognized pregnancies and 50% of all conceptions. Management may be surgical, medical, or expectant based on clinical presentation, physician expertise, and patient preference.

2. The majority of cases of recurrent pregnancy loss are idiopathic, and 40% to 90% of patients with this diagnosis will achieve viable birth without treatment.

3. Approximately one half of all pregnancies conceived in the United States are unplanned, and just over 50% of these pregnancies will end in abortion. The vast majority (88%) of induced abortions occur before 13 weeks' gestation.

4. First-trimester dilation and suction curettage is the one of most common surgical procedures performed in the United States. The incidence of both major complications requiring hospitalization and minor complications are low, less than 0.1% and 1%, respectively.

5. Accurate assessment of gestational age is essential to minimize the risk of abortion-related complications. Reported last menstrual period, physical examination, and ultrasound evaluation are used to determine gestational age.

6. The majority of chronic medical conditions do not preclude performance of induced abortion in the outpatient setting.

7. A short course of prophylactic tetracyclines, penicillins, or macrolide antibiotics decreases the risk of postabortal infectious morbidity in both high- and low-risk patients.

8. Manual vacuum aspiration involves the use of a self-contained vacuum syringe that can be used in place of electric vacuum aspiration for suction curettage in the first trimester.

Continued

KEY POINTS—CONT'D

9. Local anesthesia, intravenous sedation, and general anesthesia (i.e., deep sedation) are safe and appropriate options for pain management for patients undergoing induced abortion, provided adequately trained personnel and monitoring equipment are available.

10. The majority of abortions after 13 weeks' gestation are dilation and evacuation (D&E) procedures. The D&E associated mortality rate is four per 100,000 cases.

11. An estimated 1% of abortions in the United States are performed by labor induction. Several medications and procedures have been used to induce labor in the second trimester, including instillation agents, oxytocin, and prostaglandins.

12. Evidence suggests that D&E has a lower rate of overall complications than induction abortion in the hands of adequately trained, experienced operators.

13. The combination of oral mifepristone and vaginal misoprostol for medical abortion is highly efficacious at up to 63 days post-LMP. Rates of successful medical abortion are gestational-age dependent, and the incidence of complications is low.

14. There is no evidence to support an association between induced abortion and an increased risk of future adverse pregnancy events, gynecologic or nongynecologic malignancy (including breast cancer), or psychological sequelae.

SUGGESTED READING

Autry AM, Hayes EC, Jacobson GF, Kirby RS: A comparison of medical induction and dilation and evacuation for second-trimester abortion. Am J Obstet Gynecol 187:393–397, 2002.

Barnhart KT, Samuel MD, Rinaudo PF, et al: Symptomatic patients with an early viable intrauterine pregnancy: hCG curves refined. Obstet Gynecol 104:50–55, 2004.

Chasen ST, Kalish RB, Gupta M, et al: Dilation and evacuation at >20 weeks: Comparison of operative techniques. Am J Obstet Gynecol 190:1180–1183, 2004.

Collaborative Group on Hormonal Factors in Breast Cancer: Breast cancer and abortion: Collaborative reanalysis of data from 53 epidemiologic studies, including 83,000 women with breast cancer from 16 countries. Lancet 363:1007–1016, 2004.

Finer LB, Henshaw SK: Abortion incidence and services in the United States in 2000. Perspectives on Sexual and Reproductive Health 35(1):6–15, 2003.

Grossman D, Ellertson C, Grimes DA, Walker D: Routine follow-up visits after first-trimester induced abortion. Obstet Gynecol 103:738–745, 2004.

Hakim-Elahi E, Tovell HM, Burnhill MS: Complications of first trimester abortion: A report of 170,000 cases. Obstet Gynecol 76:129–135, 1990.

Henshaw SK: Unintended pregnancy in the United States. Family Planning Perspectives 30(1):24–46, 1998.

Kutteh WH: Recurrent pregnancy loss: An update. Curr Opin Obstet Gynecol 11(5):435–439, 1999.

MacIsaac L, Darney P: Early surgical abortion: An alternative to and backup for medical abortion. Am J Obstet Gynecol 183:S76–S83, 2002.

Newhall EP, Winikoff B: Abortion with mifepristone and misoprostol: Regimens, efficacy, acceptability and future directions. Am J Obstet Gynecol 183:S44–S53, 2000.

Paul M, Lichtenberg ES, and Borgatta L, et al (eds): A Clinician's Guide to Medical and Surgical Abortion Philadelphia, Churchill Livingstone, 1999.

Sawaya GF, Grady D, Kerlikowske K, Grimes DA: Antibiotics at the time of induced abortion: The case for universal prophylaxis based on a meta-analysis. Obstet Gynecol 87:884–890, 1996.

11

ECTOPIC PREGNANCY
Eric M. Heinberg

INTRODUCTION

Ectopic pregnancy (EP) is defined as the implantation and development of a fertilized ovum anywhere outside of the uterine cavity. The insidious and potentially catastrophic nature of EP has historically made it one of the most feared conditions to occur in women of reproductive age. Because an undiagnosed EP can quickly result in the untimely death of an otherwise healthy patient, the diagnosis and treatment of this condition have been extensively studied. Mastery of the most current clinical and scientific knowledge surrounding this topic is important for all health practitioners who treat women and essential for those practitioners who focus exclusively on women's reproductive health.

EPIDEMIOLOGY

Incidence

Due to the significant number of unreported spontaneous and elective abortions and the unknown number of asymptomatic EPs that resolve without therapy, the true incidence of EP can only be roughly estimated. The reported incidence of EP worldwide appears to vary significantly between industrialized and developing countries. Although differing denominators used by individual investigators make direct comparisons difficult, the highest EP incidence rates seem to occur on the African continent. Surveillance by the U.S. Centers for Disease Control and Prevention indicate that in the United States the incidence of EP has increased almost five-fold since 1970, from 4.5 per 1000 pregnancies to 20 per 1000, or 2% of all pregnancies, in 1992 (Fig. 11-1). Because these data do not include patients who were medically treated for EP in physicians' offices, the true incidence of this condition is likely even greater. The increase in incidence of EP in the United States parallels four evolving circumstances: an increased incidence of acute sexually transmitted salpingitis, the increased use of assisted reproductive techniques, more frequent tubal sterilization, and the development of more sensitive means of early diagnosis of EP. When calculated as an incidence per 1000 reported conceptions, the rate of EP in the United States increases with maternal age. More than 85% of EPs occur in multigravid women.

Figure 11-1

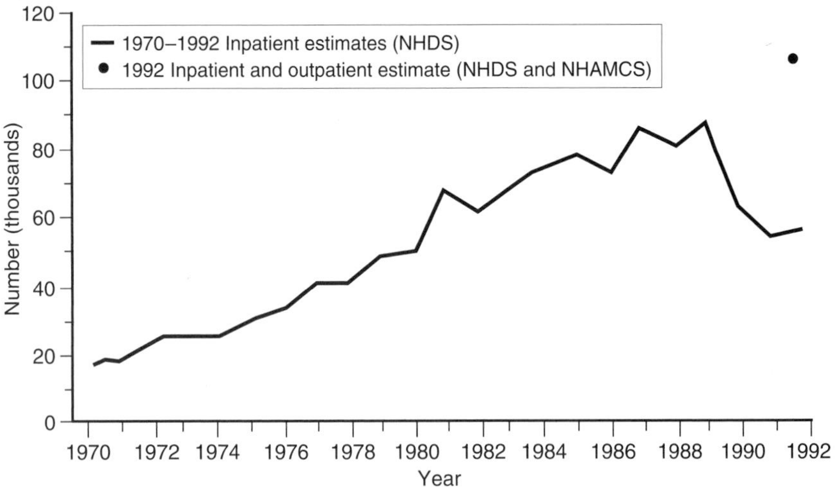

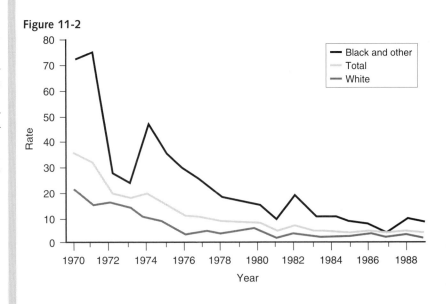

Number of ectopic pregnancies, United States, 1970–1992. (From Centers for Disease Control and Prevention: Ectopic Pregnancy—United States, 1990–1992. MMWR 44 [Suppl 3]:46–48, 1995.)

Mortality

Although the death-to-case rate for EP in the United States continued to decrease from 35 per 10,000 in 1970 to 3.8 per 10,000 in 1989, by 1992 EPs still accounted for 9% of all pregnancy-related deaths. The relative risk of death from EP in the United States is 10 times the risk of death from childbirth and 50 times the risk of death from legally performed surgical abortion, making EP the most common cause of death in the first half of pregnancy. Non-white and black women are disproportionately affected by EP. From 1970 to 1989, non-white and black women in the United States were 1.4 times more likely to have an EP than white women, and five times more likely to die from the condition (Fig. 11-2). Thus, EP is the single most important cause of all maternal deaths among non-white and black women in the United States. Such discrepancies among

Figure 11-2

Ectopic pregnancy death rates, by race, United States, 1970–1989. (From Centers for Disease Control: Ectopic Pregnancy—United States, 1988–1989. MMWR 41 [Suppl 32]:591–594, 1992.)

racial groups are only partially explained by the higher incidence of EP within the non-white population, with various other social and economic factors thought to contribute as well.

In their examination of clinical factors associated with death from EP, Atrash et al. found that hemorrhage was the primary cause of death in 88% of fatal cases; three fourths of these patients perished in the first trimester of their gestation. Dorfman et al. also studied EP-related deaths during the same period and noted that 80% of ectopic gestations were located within the fallopian tube, with the other 20% being either interstitial or abdominal EPs. Because interstitial and abdominal pregnancies are relatively rare and tend to produce symptoms later in gestation, they are more commonly associated with substantial pelvic hemorrhage and have a rate of fatality that is five times higher than the mortality rate associated with tubal EPs.

PATHOGENESIS AND RISK FACTORS

Tubal Injury and Salpingitis

Normal passage of the newly formed zygote into the uterine cavity is dependent on proper functioning of the fallopian transport mechanisms. Any factor that structurally or functionally alters these mechanisms may contribute to the occurrence of an ectopic implantation. Table 11-1 lists risk factors for EP and their associated odds ratios as derived from meta-analyses.

Inflammatory changes in fallopian tube architecture consist primarily of agglutination of the delicate longitudinal folds (plicae) of the endosalpinx

Table 11-1

Risk Factors for Ectopic Pregnancy

Risk Factor	Odds Ratio*
High Risk	
Tubal surgery	21.0
Tubal sterilization	9.3
Previous ectopic pregnancy	8.3
In utero diethylstilbestrol (DES) exposure	5.6
Intrauterine device	4.2–45.0
Documented tubal pathology	3.8–21.0
Moderate Risk	
Infertility	2.5–21.0
Previous genital infection	2.5–3.7
Multiple sex partners	2.1
Low Risk	
Previous pelvic/abdominal surgery	0.9–3.8
Smoking	2.3–2.5
Vaginal douching	1.1–3.1
Age < 18 years at first sexual intercourse	1.6

*Single values are common odds ratios from homogeneous studies; double values are ranges of values from heterogenous studies.

(Fig. 11-3). Such adhesions create pockets of tissue that may trap the developing morula within the tube. The ciliary action of the tubal epithelium may also be diminished by inflammation. A 20-year longitudinal study of 900 women by Weström et al. showed that the morphologic alterations resulting from prior episodes of acute tubal inflammation contributed to roughly half of the initial cases of EP in their study population, a finding that has been supported in subsequent studies. These same investigators demonstrated that the risk of subsequent EP increased six-fold after an episode of acute salpingitis, compared with a control group of women who had no clinical history of salpingitis. Recurrent upper genital tract infections increased the chance of tubal damage: 12.8% of women suffered tubal damage after a single episode of upper genital tract infection, 35.5% of women suffered tubal damage after two episodes of upper genital tract infection, and 75% of women suffered tubal damage after three or more episodes of upper genital infection. The American College of Obstetricians and Gynecologists considers *Chlamydia trachomatis* to play an important causative role in the development of EP because the same degree of tubal damage occurs after asymptomatic chlamydial upper genital tract infections as occurs after acute chlamydial pelvic inflammatory disease.

Functional Factors

In patients with EP in whom no inflammatory sequelae are identified, the cause may be attributed to a physiologic disruption of tubal functioning. Such a disruption may result from elevated serum levels of either estrogen or progesterone, both of which can exert direct effects on tubal smooth muscle, thereby altering tubal contractility. This phenomenon may

Figure 11-3

This cross-section of the ampulla demonstrates plical agglutination with fluid accumulation, resulting in a pattern known as follicular salpingitis (named for tis resemblance to ovarian follicles). (From Stock RJ: The fallopian tubes. In Hernandez E, Atkinson BF [eds]: Clinical Gynecologic Pathology. Philadelphia, WB Saunders, 1996, p 385.)

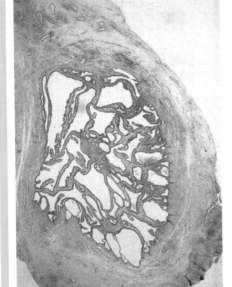

account for the increased incidence of EP associated with progestin-only oral contraceptives and progestin-secreting intrauterine devices (IUDs), following use of postovulatory high-dose estrogens to prevent conception, and after pharmacologic ovulation induction using either clomiphene citrate or human menopausal gonadotropin.

Tubal Surgery and Sterilization

Any surgical procedure performed on the oviduct, including reconstructive procedures on previously damaged or malformed fallopian tubes and routine tubal sterilization, can alter tubal architecture and increase the risk of a future EP. As summarized in an excellent review by Pisarska and Carson, meta-analyses have shown that corrective tubal surgery conveys a 21-fold increase in the risk of subsequent EP, whereas tubal sterilization increases the risk nine-fold in those women who subsequently become pregnant. The incidence of EP after tubal reanastomosis after sterilization procedures is around 4%, though it may be as high as 15% to 25% after corrective procedures for distal tubal disease. Data from the U.S. Collaborative Review of Sterilization suggest that one third of pregnancies that occur after tubal sterilization are ectopic. This risk is particularly high among women who are sterilized before the age of 30 years, since risk of EP in this population is almost twice that of older women. The technique of bipolar tubal coagulation has been associated with a risk of EP that is significantly higher than that associated with other methods of surgical sterilization.

Failed Contraception

Because the overall number of pregnancies is decreased, the proper use of virtually any method of contraception reduces a woman's risk of EP by 90%. However, the failure of certain methods of contraception imparts an increased risk of EP compared with pregnant control subjects. Copper and, more importantly, progesterone-secreting IUDs have been shown in various large studies to be associated with significantly increased risks of EP. Although combined oral contraceptive failure does not appear to be associated with an increased risk of EP, pregnancy that occurs while progestin-only oral contraceptives are being used carries a 5% chance of being ectopic.

Infertility and Assisted Reproduction

Infertility is associated with a moderately increased risk of EP, particularly when pregnancy results from methods of assisted reproduction techniques (ART). Almost 100,000 cycles of ART treatment were performed in the United States in 2000. The rate of EP resulting from *in vitro* fertilization and tubal transfer procedures was 2.1% in the year 2000, down from 2.8% in 1995 and about 5% in 1992. There is a strong relationship between the risk of EP in infertile women and tubal causes of infertility. Tubal infertility, and hydrosalpinx in particular, conveys a four-fold increased risk of EP compared with incidence in women with normal fallopian tubes. Tubal surgery in these patients increases this risk another 10%. Ovulation agents are themselves independently associated with EP via the marked hormonal influences they impart. Operator technique in embryo transfer has also been shown to be a factor in the development of EP.

Other Factors

Prior EP conveys a six- to eight-fold risk of subsequent ectopic gestation. This risk increases in direct proportion with the number of prior EPs and decreases similarly with intrauterine pregnancies that follow the initial EP.

Lifestyle factors such as multiple sexual partners and early initiation of sexual intercourse understandably carry an increased risk of EP. Handler et al. demonstrated that cigarette smoking imparted a two-fold increased risk of developing an EP after controlling for other factors. This risk was dose dependent and correlated directly with the number of cigarettes smoked per day. The risk increased four-fold in women smoking more than 30 cigarettes per day. Possible mechanisms for this increased risk include direct alteration of tubal motility, increased susceptibility to tubal infection due to overall immune suppression, or other factors related to lifestyle.

The histopathologic condition salpingitis isthmica nodosa has been identified by several investigators in up to one half of specimens after salpingectomy for EP. The term *salpingitis isthmica nodosa* is somewhat confusing both because the condition is not an inflammatory one and because it is not confined to the tubal isthmus. Classically, the condition consists of diverticula extending from the tubal lumen into the muscularis. These diverticula are surrounded by pronounced muscular hypertrophy. Salpingitis isthmica nodosa appears to disrupt the functioning of tubal transport without mechanical obstruction. The condition is believed by some experts to result from chronic salpingitis, whereas others believe it is congenital in nature.

In utero exposure to diethylstilbestrol (DES) is associated with various congenital malformations of the fallopian tubes including hypoplasia, diverticula, and accessory ostia. These malformations may account for the four- to five-fold increase in the incidence of EP seen in women who have experienced this exposure.

NATURAL HISTORY AND CLINICAL PRESENTATION

Location

Ninety-eight percent of EPs occur in the oviducts (Fig. 11-4). Of these tubal pregnancies, 80% are ampullary, 12% are isthmic, 6% occur within the fimbriae, and 2% are interstitial. EPs not involving the fallopian tubes are comparably rare, with 1.4% being abdominal, 0.15% cervical, and 0.15% ovarian. Although still the most common site, the percentage of EPs occurring in the fallopian tubes of patients receiving infertility treatment following ART is only 82%; interstitial EPs constitute 7%, ovarian EPs 5%, and cervical EPs 1.5% of the remainder of these ectopic gestations. Due to the more widespread use of multiple embryo transfers, once rare heterotopic pregnancies now compose almost 12% of EPs that result from ART.

Tubal Abortion

Tubal abortion is one of the two most common outcomes of tubal EP and is more likely to be associated with an ampullary EP. Tubal abortion results from tubal hemorrhage that causes the implanted conceptus to be dislodged from its site within the tube and expelled from the fimbriated

Implantation sites for ectopic pregnancies after natural cycles (left) and assisted reproduction techniques (ART) (right).

Figure 11-4

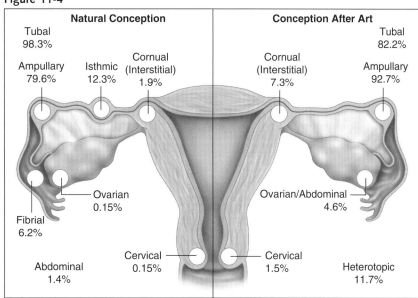

extremity. Tubal abortion is complete when the trophoblastic tissue separates cleanly from the tubal wall and the products of conception fall freely into the peritoneal cavity. This may ultimately result in complete resolution or, rarely, reimplantation of the EP anywhere within the peritoneal cavity. When clean separation does not occur and part or all of the placenta remains in the tube, bleeding will continue.

Tubal Rupture

It was long believed that, in tubal EP, growth of the developing morula occurred within the tubal lumen after implantation in the oviduct. Histopathologic studies have demonstrated that this is not the case, however. Trophoblastic tissue implanted on the mucosal surface within the tube invades both the lamina propria and tubal muscularis to enter and grow between the tube and its peritoneal surface (Fig. 11-5). Growth within this potential space proceeds as the trophoblast invades the rich tubal vasculature, ultimately causing either retroperitoneal or intra-peritoneal hemorrhage, or both. Distension of the tubal peritoneum is the source of paroxysmal abdominal pain that precedes necrosis and subsequent rupture of the tissue, often resulting in significant hemorrhage. EPs situated in the isthmic portion of the oviduct will often rupture in the first few weeks after implantation, as opposed to EPs localized to the tubal interstitium, which typically rupture later. Tubal rupture most often occurs spontaneously; however, it may be precipitated by trauma such as that which occurs during coitus or bimanual examination. Rupture can result in partial, complete, or no extrusion of the EP from the damaged tube, and significant hemorrhage may occur in any of these scenarios. A population-based study by Job-Spira and colleagues determined a three-fold risk of tubal rupture when the initial human chorionic gonadotropin (hCG) level was greater than 10,000 mIU/mL. A recent retrospective study of 221 cases of tubal

Figure 11-5

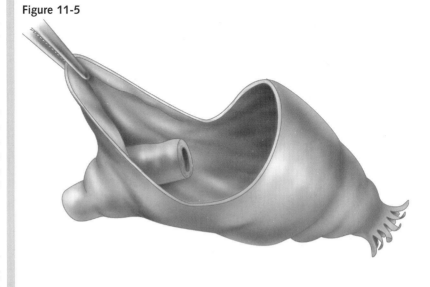

Dissected ampullary ectopic pregnancy showing space between the tube and peritoneum, revealed when blood clots and placenta were removed. Toward the fimbriated end, no dissection was performed and the external appearance is that of a dilated tube. (From Budowick M, Johnson TRB, Genadry R, et al: This histopathology of the developing tubal ectopic pregnancy. Fertil Steril 34:169–171, 1980. Reproduced with permission of the publisher, The American Fertility Society.)

EP by Bickell et al. noted that the greatest risk of tubal rupture, 5% to 7%, occurred within the first 48 hours after the onset of symptoms (relative risk, 2.1; 95% confidence interval [CI], 1.0–4.2). Beyond 48 hours, the risk leveled off at 2.5% per additional 24 hours.

Symptoms and Signs

Tables 11-2 and 11-3 list symptoms and physical signs that suggest EP. In the classical clinical picture of EP, a normal menstrual period is followed

Table 11-2

Symptoms of Ectopic Pregnancy

Symptom	% Patients with Symptom
Abdominal pain	90–100
Amenorrhea	75–95
Vaginal bleeding	50–80
Dizziness/fainting	20–35
Urge to defecate	5–15
Symptoms of pregnancy	10–25
Passage of tissue	5–10

Table 11-3

Physical Signs of Ectopic Pregnancy

Sign	% Patients with Sign
Adnexal tenderness	75–90
Abdominal tenderness	80–95
Adnexal mass*	50
Uterine enlargement	20–30
Orthostatic changes	10–15
Fever	5–10

*Twenty percent present on the side contralateral to EP.

by delayed vaginal "spotting." This precedes the sudden onset of severe, stabbing low-abdominal pain, followed by hemodynamic instability caused by significant blood loss. Marked abdominal tenderness and pain with vaginal or cervical manipulation are present. The posterior vaginal fornix may be palpably full due to blood in the cul-de-sac, the uterus is slightly enlarged, and a boggy mass may be felt within either adnexum. Blood irritating the diaphragm may cause pleuritic pain or pain in the shoulder or neck. Thankfully, in the contemporary setting of sensitive pregnancy tests, transvaginal ultrasonography, and better understanding of risk factors for EP, the diagnosis is frequently made before the onset of significant symptoms. It has become uncommon for the condition to first be recognized when a woman presents to an emergency department in hypovolemic shock after tubal rupture.

Symptoms typical of early pregnancy such as amenorrhea, nausea and vomiting, breast tenderness, and fatigue are often associated with EP. The most common symptoms of EP, abdominal pain and irregular vaginal bleeding, tend to develop 6 weeks after normal menses. Pain may initially be a vague, colicky soreness, only to become acutely severe at the time of rupture of the oviduct. The location of the patient's abdominal pain can be highly variable. It is noteworthy that more than 50% of women with EP are asymptomatic before tubal rupture. Syncope occurs in one third of women who experience this complication.

About one quarter of women with EP do not report amenorrhea. Instead, they mistake for true menses the sloughing of the intrauterine tissue that occurs when hormonal support of the endometrium wanes. This results in scant, dark-colored vaginal bleeding that may be intermittent or continuous. Heavy vaginal bleeding is more suggestive of a spontaneous abortion. Between 5% and 10% of women with EP will report the passage of a decidual cast.

Abdominal tenderness to palpation, together with adnexal tenderness elicited through a bimanual pelvic examination, is present in virtually all women having advanced or ruptured EP. An adnexal mass is palpable in 20% to 50% of these women, and the uterus is slightly enlarged to roughly the size of an 8-week intrauterine gestation in about one third of women. Fever is uncommon.

DIAGNOSTIC MODALITIES

Laboratory Tests

The diagnosis of pregnancy can be reliably determined just 10 days after ovulation using highly sensitive tests for the β subunit of hCG. Although women with EPs generally exhibit lower levels of hCG than women with normal pregnancies of the same gestational age, enzyme-linked immunosorbent assays for hCG have positive results in 90% to 95% cases of EP, with sensitivities approaching 100% when radioimmunoassays are used. The quantification of serum hCG levels is more important than just establishing positivity because quantification allows for the comparison of serial hCG measurements. It is well established that the circulating level of hCG increases by at least 66% every 48 hours in two thirds of women with normal pregnancies, and that such a rise should be appreciable in all women with normal gestations by 72 hours. If this rise is not observed, an abnormal pregnancy is likely. However, the distinction between EP and impending miscarriage cannot be made using this technique alone.

Although a solitary measurement of hCG is insufficient to discern gestational viability or location, several investigators have established that a single determination of the serum progesterone level in the first trimester is strongly predictive of an abnormal gestation when it is less than 15 ng/mL. A value greater than 25 ng/mL suggests a viable intrauterine gestation, with values falling between 15 and 25 ng/mL being indeterminate. After 4 weeks' gestation, the sensitivity and specificity of the serum progesterone level for distinguishing between viable and nonviable pregnancies diminishes with increasing gestational age.

Ultrasonography

In 1981, Kadar and colleagues demonstrated that when serum hCG levels were greater than 6500 mIU/mL and no gestational sac was detected using abdominal ultrasound, virtually all women in their study had EPs. The utility of this finding was limited, however, since 90% of women with EP have hCG levels below this threshold. Intrauterine gestations are not typically appreciable on abdominal ultrasound scans until 5 to 6 weeks' gestation, and the identification of products of conception within the fallopian tube is technically difficult using this imaging modality.

High-resolution vaginal transducers operating in the range of 5.0 to 7.0 MHz now allow for the precise imaging of pelvic structures and the diagnosis of normal pregnancy at earlier gestational ages. Transvaginal ultrasonography allows for the detection of an intrauterine gestation as early as 1 week after missed menses. In an important study by Barnhart and colleagues using transvaginal ultrasonography, the authors demonstrated that if the uterus appears empty at a serum hCG level of 1500 mIU/mL or greater, there is a high likelihood of EP. An intrauterine gestation should always be apparent when the hCG level is 2000 mIU/mL or greater (Third International Standard, formerly First International Reference Preparation) and, except in rare cases of heterotopic pregnancy, should virtually always rule out the presence of EP. A heightened suspicion for heterotopic pregnancy should be maintained for patients who have undergone treatments for infertility using ART. Although technically more challenging, transvaginal ultrasonography is also useful in detecting adnexal masses and has sensitivities and specificities for EP of 81% and 99%, respectively, when a tubal mass is seen. The diagnostic accuracy may be further enhanced by the addition of endovaginal color Doppler flow imaging that suggests an extrauterine placental-type flow pattern, or a greater than 20% discrepancy in tubal blood flow between the adnexa. Routine use of this technique is limited, however, because the equipment is costly and findings require expert interpretation.

A transabdominal scan should be performed first in the patient with a suspected EP to rule out masses that may fall outside of the plane of the vaginal transducer. If the bladder is empty at the time of examination, transvaginal evaluation may be performed first but should not preclude a transabdominal study if the adnexa cannot be fully evaluated. Several case reports describe EPs seen transabdominally that were not appreciated on transvaginal scans, a scenario more likely to occur when pelvic masses such as myomas are present. In patients with suspected EP, several studies have shown that transvaginal sonography provides additional clinical information beyond that obtained via transabdominal scanning alone. During the ultrasonographic examination, the uterine cavity should be evaluated for signs of an early pregnancy such as the double decidual sac sign (Fig. 11-6). The decidual sac sign is created by the inner rim of chorionic villi surrounded by a thin crescent of fluid in the endometrial

Figure 11-6

A, Transvaginal sonogram of an early pregnancy. This sonogram demonstrates the double decidual sac sign. The gestational sac is measured with calipers. The inner ring is formed by the echogenic chorionic villi. The outer ring is the deeper layer of deciduas vera (D). The separating lucent zone is the more superficial decidua vera. B, Sagittal transvaginal sonogram demonstrates the double decidual sac sign, but also the more reliable feature of a yolk sac. (From Levine D: Ectopic pregnancy. In Callen PW: Ultrasonography in Obstetrics and Gynecology, 4th ed. Philadelphia, WB Saunders, 2000, pp 912–934.)

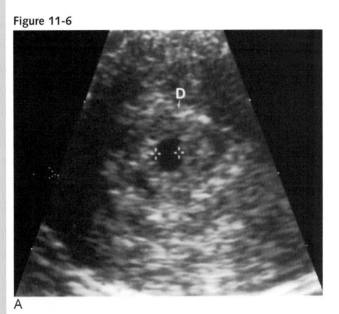

A

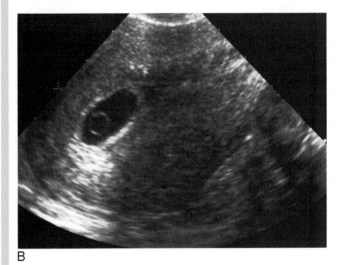

B

cavity, which is itself encircled by the outer echogenic rim of decidua vera. The finding of a yolk sac or embryo further increases the probability of an intrauterine gestation. Because the large majority of EPs are tubal, it is essential to scan above and below both ovaries as well as between the uterus and the ovaries to exclude an adnexal mass. The location of the corpus luteum does not suggest the laterality of the EP. If an adnexal mass is encountered, it should be closely examined for the presence of an echogenic ring, yolk sac, or embryo. The presence or absence of fetal cardiac activity should also be noted. An anechoic simple cyst is unlikely to represent an EP and is more consistent with a corpus luteum cyst. The posterior cul-de-sac should also be examined for free fluid. Complex fluid likely represents blood and is therefore more suggestive of EP. A small amount of fluid is often present in both normal and abnormal pregnancies, but a large amount should increase the examiner's suspicion for hemoperitoneum. The increased sensitivity of transvaginal sonography for hemoperitoneum has rendered routine culdocentesis obsolete.

Sonographic criteria for the diagnosis of EP are shown in Table 11-4. An extrauterine embryo is the sonographic finding most specific for EP; however, most practitioners rely on the more common and sensitive finding of an extraovarian adnexal mass (Fig. 11-7). A pseudogestational sac may be present within the uterus in up to 20% of cases of EP (Fig. 11-8). This small fluid collection is the result of hormonal effects on the endometrium and may be difficult to distinguish from an early intrauterine gestational sac. Features useful in differentiating between a normal early intrauterine pregnancy and a pseudogestational sac are listed in Table 11-5. It is noteworthy that sonographic findings are completely unremarkable in up to 26% of patients with EP.

Quantitative Serum hCG Plus Ultrasonography

Figure 11-9 shows a diagnostic algorithm for the diagnosis of EP without laparoscopy. High-resolution ultrasonography, used in conjunction with ultrasensitive assays for hCG, constitutes the mainstay of modern early diagnosis for EP. Clearly, this approach is most suitable to a woman with symptoms suggestive of an EP who is hemodynamically stable and pre-

Table 11-4

Sonographic Criteria for Diagnosis of Ectopic Pregnancy*

Criterion	Sensitivity (%)	Specificity (%)
Extrauterine gestational sac (with yolk sac or embryo)	8–34	100
Adnexal ring	40–68	100
Complex extraovarian mass	89–100	92–99
Any pelvic fluid	46–75	69–83
Moderate to large amount pelvic fluid	29–63	21–96
Echogenic fluid	56	96
Decidual cast	21	92

*In patients with a positive pregnancy test result and no intrauterine pregnancy.

Figure 11-7

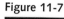

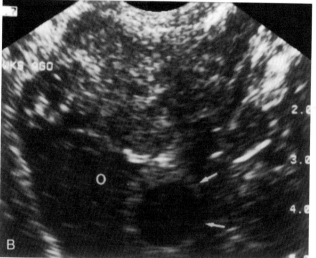

Tubal ring in a patient suspected of harboring an ectopic pregnancy. There is a right tubal ring *(arrows)* adjacent to the ovary (O). This is consistent with ectopic pregnancy. (From Levine D: Ectopic pregnancy. In Callen PW: Ultrasonography in Obstetrics and Gynecology, 4th ed. Philadelphia, WB Saunders, 2000, pp 912–934.)

Figure 11-8

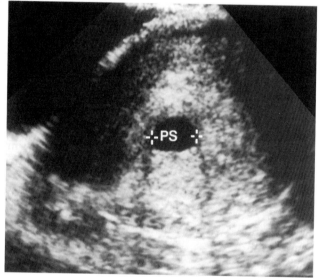

Pseudosac (PS) of ectopic pregnancy. In another patient with ectopic pregnancy, transvaginal scan shows fluid in the mid uterus. It is difficult to determine the location of the fluid with respect to the endometrial cavity because the endometrium is echogenic with enhanced through-transmission. This is a pseudogestational sac in a patient with an ectopic pregnancy. (From Levine D: Ectopic pregnancy. In Callen PW: Ultrasonography in Obstetrics and Gynecology, 4th ed. Philadelphia, WB Saunders, 2000, pp 912–934.)

sents to a facility having both diagnostic modalities readily available. Used together, these techniques have a sensitivity of 97% to 100% and a specificity of 95% to 99% for the diagnosis of EP. Serial measurements of serum hCG to assess the rate of increase, along with ultrasonography, will allow for the accurate diagnosis of EP to be made in the majority of these women before tubal rupture occurs.

Culdocentesis

Culdocentesis is a simple technique for identifying hemoperitoneum that predates high-resolution ultrasonography. A long, spinal-type 16- or 18-gauge needle is passed through the posterior vaginal fornix into

Table 11-5

Differentiating Features of Pseudogestational Sac Versus Normal Early Intrauterine Pregnancy (IUP)

Classic Sonographic Features	Early IUP	Pseudosac
Shape	Round	Ovoid
Location with respect to endometrial cavity	Eccentric	Central
Margins	Well defined	Poorly defined
Decidual reaction	Well defined	Absent
Single or double sac	May show double DSS	Single decidual layer

DSS, decidual sac sign.

Figure 11-9

Tests for suspected ectopic pregnancy (EP). hCG, human chorionic gonadotropin; IUP, intrauterine pregnancy; TVS, transvaginal sonography.

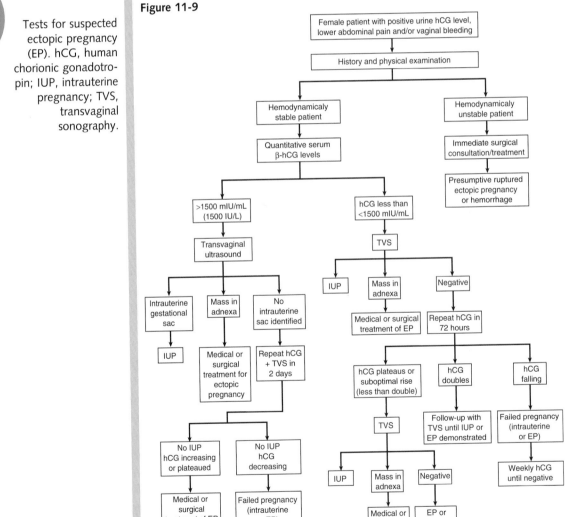

the posterior cul-de-sac and aspiration is performed. In a woman suspected of having an ectopic gestation, the aspiration of nonclotting, bloody fluid has a positive predictive value of about 85% for the presence of EP. A positive finding does not always indicate that tubal rupture has occurred because various degrees of tubal abortion can also cause intraperitoneal bleeding. Aspiration of blood that subsequently clots suggests that the specimen was obtained from a perforated vessel. Many practitioners have now abandoned this invasive technique in favor of transvaginal ultrasonography.

Uterine Curettage

When a nonviable gestation has been diagnosed using measurements of either serum progesterone or hCG, and transvaginal ultrasonography is indeterminate, uterine curettage may expedite the diagnosis of EP. This procedure may be done in an office setting and examination of the tissue performed to determine the presence of gestational tissue. If chorionic villi are identified, EP can be ruled out in most cases. If immediate histologic confirmation is unavailable, serial hCG levels should be obtained. A decrease in serum hCG of 15% or more within 8 to 12 hours after curettage is diagnostic of complete abortion. Some authorities believe that, given the demonstrated accuracy and precision of diagnostic algorithms that use a combination of noninvasive modalities such as high-resolution ultrasonography and sensitive serum biomarkers, uterine curettage is redundant and rarely necessary for diagnosing EP.

271

SURGICAL MANAGEMENT OF TUBAL EP

Surgery has been the gold standard for treatment of tubal EP since Robert Tait successfully performed a salpingectomy for EP in 1884. So-called radical surgery, in which the fallopian tube is entirely removed via laparotomy, remained the only surgical option until the 1950s, when an interest in tubal conservation arose. Stromme reported the first salpingostomy as treatment for EP in 1953.

Laparotomy Versus Laparoscopy

The advent and evolution of advanced endoscopic surgery has allowed for complex surgical procedures to be performed using minimally invasive techniques. For a surgeon having adequate experience in operative laparoscopy and the proper instruments, a laparoscopic approach to the surgical treatment for EP in a patient who is hemodynamically stable appears to be superior to laparotomy. Randomized trials have shown that the laparoscopic approach is associated with significantly less operative blood loss, length of hospitalization, and overall cost than laparotomy, while minimizing the subsequent formation of pelvic adhesions. Postoperative tubal patency and overall pregnancy rates are similar when comparing the laparoscopic and open approaches of surgical treatment of tubal EP. In cases in which the surgeon is not sufficiently skilled to provide rapid laparoscopic surgical treatment to a patient whose clinical condition is deteriorating, laparotomy is warranted and should not be delayed. It should be noted that laparoscopic salpingostomy for EP has been shown by several investigators to be associated with significantly higher rates of treatment failures that result in persistent EP compared with laparotomy.

Radical Surgery

Resection of the involved oviduct (salpingectomy), with or without concomitant oophorectomy or hysterectomy, is 100% effective as a treatment for tubal EP. This procedure may be performed with equal efficacy via laparotomy or laparoscopy, although a laparoscopic approach affords the advantages listed previously. Salpingectomy is currently used less often due a body of evidence supporting more conservative techniques, but it remains clearly indicated in cases of severe tubal damage, uncontrollable tubal hemorrhage, or recurrent EP in the same tube, or when the patient desires surgical sterilization. Some authorities previously advocated resection of the ipsilateral ovary at the time of salpingectomy as a means of minimizing the chance of a subsequent EP. There is no evidence in the literature to support this practice, and it should be abandoned. Unless indicated for technical reasons such as uncontrollable hemorrhage associated with interstitial EP, hysterectomy entails additional morbidity and should not be electively performed at the time of surgery for EP.

Conservative Surgery

As practitioners have developed a greater concern for patients' future fertility, conservation of the affected oviduct at the time of surgery for EP has become increasingly prevalent. This is accomplished using either linear salpingotomy (where the linear incision is sutured closed) or salpingostomy (where the linear incision is left to heal by secondary intention) to treat unruptured ampullary or infundibular tubal EP's. The tube is identified and mobilized, and a 1- to 2-cm linear incision is made using scissors, microelectrode, or laser along the thinnest portion of the tube directly over the bulging gestation. The products of conception are then atraumatically removed using grasping forceps or gentle irrigation or suction, and hemostasis is obtained by way of direct pressure, electrocautery, or defocused laser energy (Fig. 11-10). Aggressive cautery of the placental "bed" within the tube should be avoided to minimize additional damage. The incision may be sutured or left to heal secondarily, although fertility may resume more rapidly for women in whom the incision site is not sutured. Some surgeons elect to use prophylactic injections of a dilute solution of vasopressin at the operative site before undertaking salpingotomy or salpingostomy, but few data exist to strongly support the practice. Caution should be used when administering vasopressin because inadvertent injection into the tubal vasculature can potentially cause acute arterial hypertension, profound bradycardia, and even cardiac arrest.

Laparoscopic salpingostomy has been extensively evaluated and determined to have a clinical efficacy of up to 93%. Approximately 76% of patients who undergo the procedure will demonstrate subsequent tubal patency, and 57% will have intrauterine gestations. The rate of EP after the procedure is around 13%. Because of the narrow lumen and thick

272

Figure 11-10

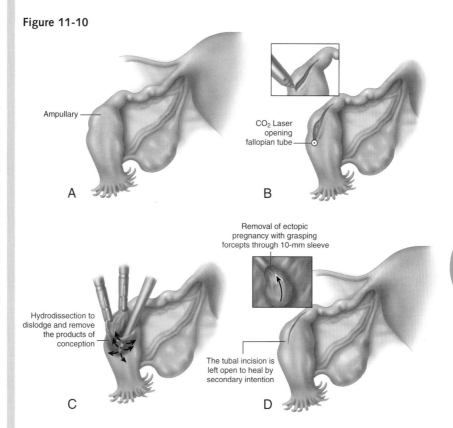

A, An unruptured ampullary pregnancy. B, The pregnancy is revealed by either a CO_2 laser or knife electrode (inset) after a tubal incision is made. C, Products of conception are being separated from the tube. D, Depending on the size of the ectopic pregnancy, the products of conception can be removed through a 5- or 10-mm trocar sleeve (inset). The tubal incision is not sutured and usually heals spontaneously.

Ampullary

CO_2 Laser opening fallopian tube

A   B

Removal of ectopic pregnancy with grasping forceps through 10-mm sleeve

273

Hydrodissection to dislodge and remove the products of conception

The tubal incision is left open to heal by secondary intention

C   D

muscularis of the tubal isthmus, conservative surgical treatment of isthmic EP consists of segmental resection of the affected oviduct. These patients may undergo immediate or delayed tubal reanastomosis. Because there is evidence that term pregnancy rates are significantly decreased in women who undergo segmental resection vs. salpingectomy, segmental tubal resection should be reserved for those patients with isthmic EP in whom salpingostomy is not technically feasible, and the contralateral tube is absent or irreparably damaged.

In a patient with an infundibular or partially extruded fimbrial EP, gentle traction may complete the tubal abortion and resolve bleeding. Brusque digital expression or tubal curettage may increase the risk of subsequent tubal EP and should be avoided.

Persistent EP

Because conservative surgery for tubal EP entails the risk of incomplete removal of trophoblastic tissue, patients must be surveyed closely for persistent ectopic pregnancy (PEP) in the postoperative period. This entity is the most common complication associated with conservative procedures and occurs in 5% to 30% of cases. It is more common when the procedure is performed laparoscopically than when laparotomy is used. A diagnosis of PEP is made when weekly postoperative serum hCG levels plateau or rise and is very likely when the day 7 hCG level is either above 1000 mIU/mL or greater than 15% of the original level. Box 11-1 lists

---

Box 11-1 Factors Favoring PEP After Conservative Surgery

EP size less than 2 cm
EP gestation less than 42 days
Serum hCG greater than 3000 mIU/mL
Implantation of EP medial to site of salpingostomy

---

factors that appear to increase the risk of PEP after conservative surgery. Spandorfer et al. reported that the relative risk of PEP is 3.5 if the day 1 hCG level fails to decline by 50% or more.

Once diagnosed, PEP should be treated promptly to avoid tubal rupture. Treatment options include salpingectomy, repeat salpingostomy, or pharmacotherapy using methotrexate. Surgical management, via either laparoscopy or laparotomy, should be undertaken for a patient with PEP who has persistent abdominal pain. Expectant management may be considered for an asymptomatic patient with PEP in whom hCG levels are not rising. Most patients with PEP can be best served by the administration of methotrexate. A single dose of 50 mg/m^2 has been shown to be highly effective in resolving PEP. One prospective, randomized trial comparing a single dose of methotrexate to placebo given within 24 hours of salpingostomy showed a 90% decrease in the risk of developing PEP in the methotrexate group. The prophylactic use of methotrexate should be strongly considered for patients at high risk of PEP and those for whom close follow-up and hCG monitoring is likely to be difficult.

MEDICAL MANAGEMENT OF TUBAL EP

Multidose Systemic Methotrexate

Tanaka first described the novel use of methotrexate for the treatment of EP in 1982. Since that time, its use has been refined and sufficiently evolved to make methotrexate the primary mode of treatment for unruptured EPs in countless medical centers. Methotrexate is an antineoplastic agent that inactivates dihydrofolate reductase, thereby depleting tetrahydrofolate and inhibiting the *de novo* synthesis of purines and pyrimidines that are critical to DNA synthesis and cell growth. The rapid cell growth of trophoblastic tissue makes it particularly sensitive to the effects of methotrexate, thus forming the basis of pharmacotherapy for EP.

Table 11-6 shows the two principle protocols for methotrexate currently in use as primary treatments for EP. Initially, a multidose regimen consisting of 1 mg/kg given intramuscularly on alternate days for four to five doses, along with the administration of citrovorum factor (reduced folate) on intervening days, was described. This dosing schedule was subsequently refined by ceasing therapy once hCG levels fell at least 15% in 48 hours, or a maximum of four doses was reached, thereby minimizing adverse effects such as stomatitis and liver dysfunction. This regimen has a demonstrated success rate (i.e., no surgical intervention) as high as 94%, with evidence of subsequent tubal patency in 82% and fertility in 66% of those so treated.

Table 11-6

Regimen	Follow-up
Single Dose Methotrexate, 50 mg/m² IM	Assess hCG levels days 4 and 7: If difference ≥15%, assess hCG weekly until undetectable. If difference <15%, repeat methotrexate and resume above. If fetal cardiac activity is present on day 7, repeat methotrexate and resume. Treat surgically if there is a failed response after three doses of methotrexate.
Multiple Dose Methotrexate, 1 mg/kg IM on days 1, 3, 5, and 7 plus Leukovorin, 0.1 mg/kg IM on days 2, 4, 6, and 8	Alternate injections until hCG levels decrease >15% in 48 hours, or until a maximum of four doses of methotrexate has been given. Assess hCG weekly until undetectable. Treat surgically if there is a failed response after four doses methotrexate.

IM, Intramuscularly.

275

Results of this regimen are quite similar to those observed after laparoscopic salpingostomy, with the exception of subsequent EP, which is lower at 7%.

Single-Dose Systemic Methotrexate

Stovall and Ling described their experience with a single-dose systemic methotrexate regimen for EP in 1993. This regimen consisted of a dose of 50 mg/m² without citrovorum. Subsequent studies have shown that this method is associated with a success rate of 87% to 90%, but that repeat doses of methotrexate are necessary in 8% to 10% of patients. A recent systematic review by Barnhart and colleagues included 26 studies of good quality containing 1327 cases of women diagnosed with EP who were treated with methotrexate. This excellent review demonstrated that patients successfully treated using a single-dose regimen had significantly lower mean hCG levels than patients successfully treated using the multidose regimen (2778 ± 2848 versus 5023 ± 5342, P <.001). Furthermore, when consideration of hCG levels and the presence of fetal cardiac activity were factored into the analysis, women treated with a single-dose regimen experienced a significantly higher failure rate (odds ratio, 4.74; 95% CI, 1.77–12.62). Of women in the single-dose group, 14.5% required more than one dose of methotrexate. Although adverse events were rare overall, women receiving single-dose therapy experienced fewer adverse effects than those in the multidose group. These findings suggest that the single-dose regimen may be better suited to women with low serum levels of hCG and without fetal cardiac activity. A Cochrane Systematic Review of the available evidence concludes that the single-dose regimen is "not effective enough to advocate its routine use." Nonetheless, the lower rate of adverse effects, lower overall cost, and convenience for patients and medical practitioners alike has made single-dose methotrexate the preferred treatment regimen for EP in appropriately selected patients.

Patient Selection

The safety and efficacy of medical treatment for EP using methotrexate depends greatly on proper patient selection. Suitable candidates for medical therapy using methotrexate are asymptomatic or mildly symptomatic patients with an unruptured tubal pregnancy sonographically determined to be less than 4 cm, and those who are without clinical or sonographic evidence of active intraperitoneal bleeding (Box 11-2). According to the American College of Obstetricians and Gynecologists, absolute contraindications to treatment with methotrexate include breastfeeding, known or suspected immunodeficiency, alcoholism, blood dyscrasias, peptic ulcer disease, known sensitivity to methotrexate, or active pulmonary, hepatic, or renal disease of any kind (Box 11-3). Tubal masses greater than 3.5 to 4 cm, pretreatment serum hCG levels greater than 5000 mIU/mL, and fetal cardiac activity are all risk factors for treatment failure, particularly using the single-dose regimen, and are considered by some to be relative contraindications to primary methotrexate therapy. All patients should be willing to comply with a plan of close follow-up and to have at their disposal means of transportation necessary to adhere to that plan.

Patient Monitoring

If a patient meets the above criteria and agrees to receive medical therapy blood sampling is obtained for complete blood count, tests of liver and renal function, determination of blood type and Rh factor, and quantitative serum hCG measurement. Single-dose methotrexate is then administered intramuscularly at a dose of 50 mg/m^2, or roughly 1 mg/kg, on designated "day 0." Follow-up determinations of hCG levels are made on day 4 and

---

Box 11-2 Criteria for Receiving Methotrexate Therapy for Ectopic Pregnancy

Absolute
Hemodynamically stable
No evidence of active intraperitoneal bleeding
Ability to adhere to close follow-up monitoring

Relative
Asymptomatic
Ectopic mass < 3.5 to 4 cm
No fetal cardiac activity
Serum hCG < 5000 mIU/mL

Box 11-3 Absolute Contraindications to Methotrexate Therapy for Ectopic Pregnancy

Renal, hematologic, or hepatic disease (including alcoholism)
Pulmonary disease
Peptic ulcer disease
Known or suspected immunodeficiency
Known sensitivity to methotrexate
Breastfeeding

day 7 after administration. It is common to see hCG levels continue to rise after methotrexate administration, often reaching a peak around day 4. This does not suggest treatment failure. When treatment is effective, comparison of these values should demonstrate a decline of serum hCG levels of at least 15% from day 4 to day 7. In the absence of increased pain, weekly determinations of hCG are made until the level is undetectable. The time required for complete resolution of the pregnancy is variable and may take up to 1 month or longer. If the appropriate decline of hCG is not appreciated, or if levels plateau, an additional dose of methotrexate should be given and follow-up resumed as previously described. A maximum of three total doses may be given. For the multidose regimen, the serum hCG level is assessed for a drop from baseline of at least 15% after 48 hours. If a sufficient decrease is not appreciated, therapy is continued up to four total doses and hCG assessed weekly thereafter until it is undetectable.

Patient Counseling

Box 11-4 lists the potential adverse effects associated with methotrexate therapy. The patient should be made aware of these potential adverse effects and instructed to notify the appropriate practitioner or present for urgent evaluation if adverse effects occur. She should be instructed to expect moderate to severe abdominal or pelvic pain, often described as "tearing," beginning 3 to 7 days after therapy and lasting up to 12 hours. Pain lasting longer than 12 hours warrants immediate evaluation. Potential signs and symptoms of tubal rupture such as vaginal bleeding, weakness, dizziness, or syncope should be described, and the patient should be instructed to report the occurrence of any of these symptoms without delay. The patient should be counseled to abstain from sexual intercourse until serum hCG is undetectable, to avoid consumption of alcohol, and to restrict her exposure to sunlight. All nonsteroidal anti-inflammatory agents and folinic acid supplements such as prenatal vitamins should be discontinued.

Patient Safety

No maternal death has ever been reported after the use of methotrexate as primary treatment for EP, but two cases of life-threatening neutropenia with fever and two cases of pneumonitis have been reported. Careful pretreatment screening of patients for hepatic, renal, gastrointestinal, or hematopoietic disease will ensure that associated morbidity remains low. Nonetheless, careful monitoring of patients undergoing this therapy is

Box 11-4   Side Effects of Methotrexate Therapy
Nausea and vomiting
Diarrhea
Dizziness
Gastric distress
Stomatitis
Severe neutropenia (rare)
Alopecia (rare, reversible)
Pneumonitis

crucial for early identification of treatment-related adverse effects, complications, or treatment failure. Patients should be assessed twice weekly and vital signs and blood counts monitored along with serum hCG levels. Bimanual pelvic examinations are limited to avoid iatrogenic tubal rupture, and transvaginal ultrasonography performed only when indicated. Patients for whom close outpatient monitoring is not possible should be hospitalized. Pain that persists beyond 12 hours, a falling hemoglobin or hematocrit level, or signs of hemodynamic instability demand immediate surgical exploration and treatment.

Methotrexate by Direct Injection

Studies have demonstrated that the direct injection of methotrexate into the gestational sac for the treatment of EP is associated with a success rate of 75% to 86%. This method appears to minimize adverse effects compared with systemic methotrexate, but it must be performed either laparoscopically or under ultrasound guidance and requires considerable skill. Because direct injection of methotrexate does not confer a greater likelihood of successful treatment for EP, its use is reserved for special situations.

MEDICAL VERSUS SURGICAL TREATMENT OF TUBAL EP

Efficacy and Safety

Several randomized trials have demonstrated that primary medical treatment using systemic methotrexate is as effective as conservative laparoscopic surgery for the treatment of unruptured tubal EP. A meta-analysis by Morlock and colleagues attributed mean success rates of 87% (range, 75% to 90%) and 91% (range, 72% to 100%) to medical and surgical therapies, respectively. Mean complication rates for medical therapy were 10% for minor and 7% for serious complications. Laparoscopic treatment entailed mean complication rates of 2% intraoperatively and 9% postoperatively. PEP is encountered more often after laparoscopic surgery, occurring in up to 20% of cases, compared with roughly 4% after multidose methotrexate and 8% after single-dose methotrexate. As noted previously, rates of tubal patency and subsequent fertility appear to be similar for both interventions.

Both treatment strategies require close follow-up of patients to confirm pregnancy resolution. However, hCG levels decline to undetectable levels more quickly after laparoscopic surgery, thereby reducing the duration of monitoring after treatment. It appears that most patients prefer primary medical treatment for tubal EP as part of a nonsurgical management strategy. Paradoxically, a study by Nieuwkerk and colleagues suggested that systemic methotrexate therapy had a more negative overall impact on patients' health-related quality of life than did laparoscopic salpingostomy. This finding is possibly due to the stress associated with the persistent risk of rupture and intensive, sometimes prolonged follow-up required of patients receiving medical treatment.

Primary medical treatment with methotrexate for tubal EP appears to provide substantial economic savings compared with laparoscopic treatment. Morlock's decision-analytic model estimated this savings to be $3000 per patient when compared with conservative laparoscopic treatment. A study by Mol and colleagues suggests that this economic savings may be lost when initial serum hCG levels exceed 3000 mIU/mL.

Expectant Management

Several case series describing the expectant management of EP have been reported since the 1950s with success rates that range from 48% to 88%. A review by Yao and colleagues of 10 studies that prospectively examined expectant management in selected patients with EP found an overall success rate of 70%. Most leading authorities agree that candidates for expectant management should be limited to those with an unruptured tubal pregnancy less than 3.5 cm in diameter who are without evidence of active intraperitoneal bleeding and have a declining hCG level of 1000 mIU/mL or less. Because the risk of tubal rupture is present even when hCG levels are declining, it is difficult to recommend the practice of expectant management for cases of known EP when safe, effective treatment modalities are readily available. Expectant management is a reasonable course of action when EP is suspected but the location and viability of a possible early gestation are undetermined.

279

RH SENSITIZATION

All unsensitized, Rh-negative women with an ectopic gestation should receive Rh immunoglobulin at the time of medical or surgical treatment unless the father is known to have an Rh-negative status. A dose of 50 µg is recommended for gestations less than 12 weeks and 300 µg for gestations beyond 12 weeks. The risk of Rh sensitization after EP is believed to range from 0% at 4 weeks' gestation to almost 9% at 12 weeks.

UNCOMMON TYPES OF EP

Interstitial EP

Implantation of the gestation in the portion of the oviduct that traverses the myometrium gives rise to interstitial EP (Fig. 11-11). This type of ectopic gestation accounts for 2% of EPs occurring naturally and 7% of EPs resulting from ART. Interstitial EP may occur after ipsilateral salpingectomy. The anatomic location of interstitial EP favorably accommodates the growing gestation, thereby often delaying both the onset of symptoms and the correct diagnosis. As a result, uterine rupture with massive hemorrhage occurs in up to 20% of these patients when the gestation survives

Figure 11-11

An interstitial pregnancy is recognized as a cornual bulge in the myometrium and serosal surface.

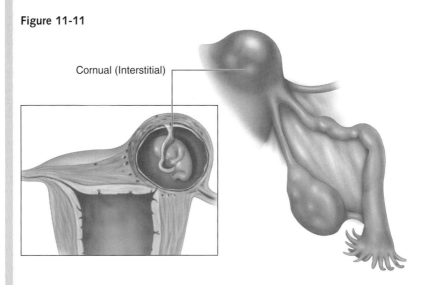

Cornual (Interstitial)

beyond 12 weeks, accounting for the maternal mortality of 2% to 2.5% associated with interstitial EP. Interstitial EP should be suspected in a patient with an asymmetrically enlarged uterus whose sonographic evaluation reveals an eccentrically located gestational sac that appears to be associated with the uterus. The diagnosis can be confirmed by laparoscopy and other diagnoses, such as abdominal, ovarian, or true cornual pregnancy within the horn of a bicornuate uterus, definitively ruled out. Classically, interstitial EP is treated using salpingectomy with or without cornual resection via laparotomy and, more recently, via laparoscopy. If the uterine tissue overlying the gestation is intact and sufficiently hardy, hysteroscopic removal of the pregnancy can be attempted with the aid of direct laparoscopic visualization. Local and systemic methotrexate therapy has also been used successfully to treat interstitial EP. If substantial erosion of the pregnancy into the uterine tissue has occurred, laparotomy affords the best opportunities to achieve rapid control of the profuse hemorrhage that can occur with interstitial EP. If hemorrhage is uncontrollable by conservative means, hysterectomy should be performed without delay.

Abdominal EP

Abdominal EP is quite rare, occurring in only one in 8000 to 25,000 pregnancies Abdominal EP represents 1.4% of all EPs and is associated with a maternal mortality rate of 5.1 per 1000 cases. The vast majority of abdominal EPs implant on the peritoneum secondarily, after either tubal abortion or tubal rupture. Primary abdominal EPs do occur, but the distinction is of little clinical value in directing treatment. In most cases, the growing placenta maintains its attachment to the fallopian tube while progressively extending onto nearby structures such as the posterior aspect of the adnexa, broad ligament, and uterus. The fetus may continue to develop, but overall fetal survival is estimated to be about 10%. Contemporary diagnosis of abdominal EP is greatly facilitated by ultrasonography. Magnetic resonance imaging or computed tomography may be of use when ultrasound findings are suspicious but indeterminate.

Treatment of abdominal EP consists of immediate laparotomy and removal of the fetus to prevent catastrophic hemorrhage. If surgically feasible, the placenta should be completely removed. When the placenta is adherent to vital structures such as bowel and major vessels, no attempt to remove it should be made because massive hemorrhage and significant injury to the patient may result. After delivery of the fetus, the umbilical cord should be ligated as near to the placenta as possible, the abdomen closed, and prophylactic antibiotics initiated. Placental tissue left *in situ* will resorb over time, but abdominal pain and fever may persist for several months during this process and complications related to infection, wound dehiscence, and intestinal obstruction are not uncommon. Systemic methotrexate therapy may hasten the resolution of placental tissue, but its use remains controversial in this setting.

281

Ovarian EP

Ovarian pregnancies are the most common form of abdominal EP. These ectopic gestations tend to present in a manner similar to that of tubal EPs and are associated with early rupture in 30% of cases. Risk factors are uncertain. Often, it is not possible to grossly differentiate between an ovarian EP and a ruptured corpus luteum cyst or other bleeding ovarian neoplasm without histologic confirmation. Treatment has traditionally consisted of resection of the involved ovary, although wedge resection may be used for small gestations. Methotrexate has been used successfully to treat unruptured ovarian EPs.

Cervical EP

The incidence of cervical EP is estimated to be one in 9000 to 18,000 naturally occurring pregnancies, but it is more common after *in vitro* fertilization and embryo transfer. Pisarska and Carson noted that almost 70% of patients with cervical EP have a history of prior uterine dilatation and curettage, 31% of which were performed for the termination of a pregnancy. Painless vaginal bleeding is the presenting complaint in about 90% of these cases, with massive hemorrhage occurring in one third of patients. Abdominal pain is present in only 25% of patients with cervical EP. The cervix may be abnormally large and globular, with a soft consistency. It may appear hyperemic and, in some cases, even cyanotic. Clinical suspicion warrants immediate pelvic ultrasonography, which aids in successful diagnosis in 80% of cases. On ultrasound, the uterus is empty and a gestational sac is seen within the cervical canal below the internal os. Trophoblastic invasion into endocervical tissue is often apparent. Magnetic resonance imaging may prove extremely useful in cases where ultrasound is nondiagnostic.

In the past, hysterectomy was thought to be the only treatment option for cervical EP, which carried a high maternal mortality. The enlarged cervix greatly distorts the surgical anatomy, leading to increased blood loss and making injury to the urinary tract more likely. Today, radical surgical intervention is reserved for those cases in which conservative treatment has failed or in cases of acute, life-threatening hemorrhage. There are numerous reports in the contemporary literature that describe the successful treatment of cervical EP using systemic methotrexate, as well as sonographically guided direct injection of cytotoxic agents. Other reports describe the transcervical evacuation of cervical EP without excessive blood loss after prophylactic angiographic embolization of the uterine arteries. If transcervical evacuation is performed, a 30-mL Foley catheter bulb should be inflated within the cervix to tamponade bleeding, and the vagina should be tightly packed. Overall, the success rate of conservative treatment for cervical EP is around 81%. Nonetheless, a significant number of women with cervical EP will still ultimately require hysterectomy, particularly when the pregnancy advances beyond 18 weeks.

Heterotopic Pregnancy

Heterotopic pregnancy is the simultaneous presence of intrauterine and ectopic gestations. Once mathematically estimated to occur in one in 16,000 to 30,000 pregnancies, the incidence of heterotopic EP in one large series from an institution in the United States was 1 in 8000, with 1 in 70 EPs associated with an intrauterine pregnancy. In this same series, 94% of heterotopic EPs were tubal and 6% were ovarian. The incidence of heterotopic EP is drastically elevated after the use of ART for infertility, accounting for as many as 1% to 3% of all pregnancies arising from *in vitro* fertilization. Tubal disease and the transfer of more than four embryos increase this risk substantially. Because the sensitive modalities of pelvic ultrasonography and serum assays for hCG are of little help in this situation, the diagnosis of heterotopic pregnancy is fraught with pitfalls that are seldom present with solitary extrauterine EPs. Ultrasonography detects only half of tubal heterotopic EPs. The rest are diagnosed at the time of surgery after the onset of symptoms, often due to tubal rupture. As in other types of EP, the most common presenting symptom is lower abdominal pain, found in more than 80% of patients. Heterotopic EP should be suspected in a pregnant woman when the combination of abdominal pain with or without peritoneal irritation, an adnexal mass, and a uterus enlarged to more than 8 weeks' size are present concurrently. The discovery of two corpora lutea and an enlarged, soft uterus on laparotomy or laparoscopy should also alert the clinician to the strong possibility of a heterotopic EP.

The treatment for a heterotopic EP is surgical exploration and removal of the EP using the most appropriate technique. Systemic methotrexate is contraindicated due to the presence of a viable intrauterine gestation. The successful local administration of agents such as methotrexate and potassium chloride has been described. Expectant management is not feasible because hCG levels are not interpretable in this setting.

REPRODUCTIVE PERFORMANCE AFTER EP

After treatment for EP, issues related to future reproductive performance are often foremost among patients' concerns. Considerations in this regard include time to conception after EP, cumulative pregnancy rates, risk of recurrent EP, and live birth rates. These outcomes depend on several variables, both pre-existing and related to the EP, whose effects may be cumulative. Many investigators have sought to better elucidate factors that most strongly predict a woman's reproductive potential after EP. Unfortunately, differences in methodology often preclude direct comparisons of studies in this area. Still, some conclusions can be made.

Between 20% and 60% of women may experience infertility after EP. Several large series and cohort studies have determined the mean rate of intrauterine pregnancy after EP to be between 50% and 80%, with the mean risk of subsequent EP ranging from 10% to 20%. The highest cumulative pregnancy rates are noted by about 36 months after EP. Box 11-5 lists factors that most adversely affect subsequent fertility after treatment for EP. Not surprisingly, both age greater than 35 years and a history of infertility each reduce the probability of future conception after EP by half. Pre-existing tubal damage, either from prior EP, prior episodes of salpingitis, or a history of tubal surgery, detrimentally affects reproductive prognosis to the same degree.

Several investigators have analyzed the effect of treatment type on future fertility according to tubal status. Although there is no clear consensus among experts, conservative surgical and medical treatments for EP appear to enhance future reproductive performance in women with contralateral tubal disease, compared with radical surgery. Fernandez and colleagues, as well as others, have reported no detrimental effect on fertility of salpingectomy for EP when the contralateral tube is healthy. Most studies report similar rates of subsequent EP after radical and conservative surgery. However, rates of intrauterine pregnancies do appear to be higher, and rates of recurrent EP lower after laparoscopic treatment compared with laparotomy. Women treated laparoscopically also appear to conceive sooner after EP than women treated via laparotomy.

Much discussion surrounds the reproductive consequences of tubal rupture that may result from EP. This is because the presence or absence of tubal rupture is itself often the principal determinant of a practitioner's choice of treatment. Patients who experience EP as a result of contraceptive failure rarely have risk factors for infertility and, therefore, tend to have substantially better reproductive outcomes than women who were

---

Box 11-5 Factors Adversely Affecting Fertility After Ectopic Pregnancy

Age > 35 years
History of infertility
Pre-existing tubal damage

not using contraception at the time of their EP. This is particularly true for the IUD. Users of IUDs also tend to be older and often do not seek future pregnancies, typically making their reproductive prognosis of less concern after EP.

KEY POINTS

1. The incidence of ectopic pregnancy (EP) has risen five-fold in the United States since the 1970s.

2. EP accounts for 9% of all pregnancy-related deaths and is the leading cause of maternal death in the first half of pregnancy.

3. Non-white and black women are five times more likely to die from EP than are white women in the United States, making EP the most common cause of maternal death in these groups.

4. Ninety-eight percent of EPs that arise naturally occur in the oviducts; this decreases to 82% after use of assisted reproduction techniques (ART).

5. The use of high-resolution ultrasonography with an ultrasensitive assay for human chorionic gonadotropin (hCG) carries a sensitivity of 97% to 100% and specificity of and 95% to 99% for the diagnosis of EP.

6. Laparoscopic surgical treatment of EP entails less blood loss, shorter hospitalization, and lower overall cost than laparotomy.

7. Laparoscopic linear salpingostomy has a clinical efficacy of up to 93% but entails a higher risk of persistent EP than laparoscopic salpingectomy.

8. Multidose systemic methotrexate for EP has a success rate comparable to that of laparoscopic linear salpingostomy and entails lower rates of subsequent EP.

SUGGESTED READING

Anderson FWJ, Hogan JG, Ansbacher R: Sudden death: Ectopic pregnancy mortality. Obstet Gynecol 6:1218–1223, 2004.

Ankum WM, Mol BW, van der Veen F, Bossuyt PM: Risk factors for ectopic pregnancy: A meta-analysis. Fertil Steril 65:1093–1999, 1996.

Barnhart K, Gosman G, Ashby R, Sammel M: The medical management of ectopic pregnancy: A meta-analysis comparing "single dose" and "multidose" regimens. Obstet Gynecol 4:778–784, 2003.

Barnhart K, Mennuti MT, Ivor B, et al: Prompt diagnosis of ectopic pregnancy in an emergency department setting. Obstet Gynecol 6:1010–1015, 1994.

Breen JL: A 21-year survey of 654 ectopic pregnancies. Am J Obstet Gynecol 106:1004–1019, 1970.

Budowick M, Johnson TRB, Genadry R, et al: The histopathology of the developing tubal ectopic pregnancy. Fertil Steril 34:169–171, 1980.

Buster JE, Pisarska M: Medical management of ectopic pregnancy. Clin Obstet Gynecol 42:23–30, 1999.

Chang J, Elam-Evans LD, Berg CJ, et al: Pregnancy-related mortality surveillance—United States, 1991–1999. MMWR Surveill Sumn 52(2):1–8, 2003.

Ectopic pregnancy—United States, 1990–1992. MMWR 44(3):46–48, 1995.

Ego A, Subtil D, Cosson M, et al: Survival analysis of fertility after ectopic pregnancy. Fertil Steril 75:560–566, 2001.

Hajenius PJ, Mol BWJ, Bossuyt PMM, et al: Interventions for tubal ectopic pregnancy. The Cochrane Database of Systematic Reviews 3, 2004.

Job-Spira N, Fernandez H, Bouyer J, et al: Ruptured tubal ectopic pregnancy: Risk factors and reproductive outcome. Am J Obstet Gynecol 180:938–944, 1999.

Mol BWJ, Ankum WM, Bossuyt PMM, Van der Veen F: Contraception and the risk of ectopic pregnancy: A meta-analysis. Contraception 52:337–341, 1995.

Morlock RJ, Elston Lafata J, Eisenstein D: Cost-effectiveness of single-dose methotrexate compared with laparoscopic treatment of ectopic pregnancy. Obstet Gynecol 95:407–412, 2000.

Peterson HB, Zhisen X, Hughes JM, et al: The risk of ectopic pregnancy after tubal sterilization. N Engl J Med 762–767, 1997.

Rojansky N, Schenker JG: Heterotopic pregnancy and assisted reproduction: An update. J Assist Reprod Genet 13:594–601, 1996.

Society for Assisted Reproductive Technology: American Society for Reproductive Medicine. Assisted reproductive technology in the United States: 2000 results generated from the American Society of Reproductive Medicine/Society for Assisted Reproductive Technology Registry. Fertil Steril 81:1207–1220, 2004

Tulandi T, Saleh A: Surgical management of ectopic pregnancy. Clin Obstet Gynecol 42:31–38, 1999.

Weckstein LN, Boucher AR, Tucker H, et al: Accurate diagnosis of early ectopic pregnancy. Obstet Gynecol 65:393–397, 1985.

12

INFERTILITY: EVALUATION AND TREATMENT

Jeffrey M. Goldberg

DEFINITIONS AND PREVALENCE

Infertility is defined as failure to conceive after 12 months of unprotected intercourse. Of couples trying for pregnancy, 85% succeed within the first year. Therefore, infertility affects 15%, or one of every six to seven couples. *Infertility* is synonymous with *subfertility*. Other commonly used terms are *sterility*, an intrinsic inability to conceive; *fecundity*, the monthly probability of establishing a live birth; and *fecundability*, the probability of conception during one menstrual cycle. *Primary infertility* is the failure to ever establish a pregnancy, whereas *secondary infertility* occurs after a prior pregnancy regardless of the outcome or how long ago it was. Primary and secondary infertility can apply to the individual partners or the couple. It is not a clinically important distinction because it does not affect the evaluation or treatment.

Infertility seems to be on the rise because there are a greater number of couples seeking evaluation and treatment for infertility. This is due to a large population of aging baby boomers in their late 30s and 40s, later marriage, more contraceptive options, and delayed childbearing for career development. There is also a greater awareness and availability of more effective infertility treatment options. Also, infertility no longer carries the same negative social stigma it once did. When matched for age, women are as fertile now as they were in the past few decades, and there is no trend toward increased infertility in developed countries.

PROGNOSTIC FACTORS

The primary factors that influence a couple's chances for success in conceiving a child are the woman's age, duration of infertility, and smoking behavior. Demographic studies over several centuries of populations not using contraception have shown a consistent age-related decline in fertility. The downward slope in the early 30s, accelerates in the mid to late 30s, and plummets after age 40. Pregnancy rates with *in vitro* fertilization (IVF) follow the same pattern (Fig. 12-1). The same IVF database showed that each year after age 40 was significant (Fig. 12-2). A review of 431 initiated IVF cycles in women aged 41 years and older found that no clinical pregnancies occurred in women 45 years and older and no deliveries in women 44 years and older.

The percentage of women not using contraception who remained childless rose with age at marriage: 6% at 20 to 24 years of age, 9% at 25 to 29, 15% at 30 to 34, 30% at 35 to 39, and 64% at 40 to 44. Although it can be argued that this may be due to having older partners and less frequent coitus, studies of donor insemination in women with azoospermic husbands (controlling for male age and timing factors) reported a sharp

Figure 12-1

In vitro fertilization pregnancy rates by woman's age. (From Assisted Reproductive Technology. Centers for Disease Control and Prevention, 2004.)

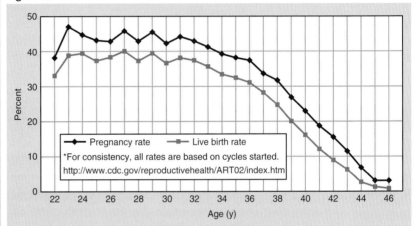

Figure 12-2

In vitro fertilization pregnancy rates by woman's age, 40 years and older. (From Assisted Reproductive Technology. Centers for Disease Control and Prevention, 2004.)

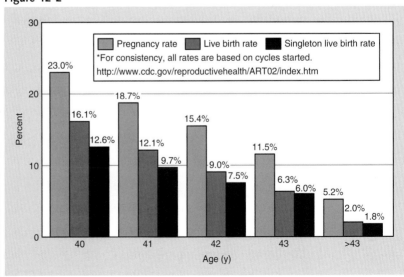

decline in pregnancy rates with increasing female age. A donor insemination program in the Netherlands showed that the probability of having a healthy baby decreased by 3.5% per year after 30 years of age and that a 35-year-old had half the chance of a 25-year-old. With unexplained infertility over 3 years, each year in a woman's age over 30 reduced the outlook for conception by 9%.

Older women have had more time to acquire pelvic inflammatory disease (PID), myomas, endometriosis, and exposure to environmental hazards, all of which may reduce fertility. However, the most significant factor in the age-dependent decrease in fertility is a higher rate of aneuploidy in older oocytes and resulting embryos. This is likely due to abnormalities in the spindle formation leading to unbalanced chromosome segregation in meiosis as well as mitosis in the preimplantation embryo. Karyotypic analysis from spontaneous and elective abortions, amniocenteses, and live and stillborn children show a steady increase in aneuploidy with the woman's age. The spontaneous abortion rate increases from 15% to 20% in young women to approximately 75% in women older than 40 years. The risk for having a child with a genetic anomaly also increases with each advancing year (Table 12-1).

Further evidence that the decline in fertility with age is due to oocyte quality is provided by studies of donor oocyte recipients. When the same cohort of oocytes obtained from one young donor during a specific cycle was evenly distributed between "young" and "old" ovum recipients, there was no difference in pregnancy or live birth rates. Age does not seem to affect the morphology or histologic response of the endometrium-to-steroid stimulation because the capacity to conceive and carry a pregnancy to term when oocyte quality is controlled with donor eggs appears to be independent of uterine aging at least through age 50 As expected, pregnancy wastage directly correlates with the age of the donor. Figure 12-3 demonstrates the live birth rate per embryo transfer by age with the woman's own oocytes or a younger donor's.

A study of fertile couples having coitus on the most fertile day reported clinical pregnancy rates for women aged 19 to 26, 27 to 34, and 35 to 39 years of approximately 50%, 40%, and 30%, respectively, if their partners were the same age. If the male partner was 5 years older the rates were reduced to 45%, 40%, and 15%, respectively, indicating that the age of the male is also a prognostic factor. Although there is no absolute age at which men cannot father a child, most studies suggest a relationship between male age and fertility. However, two studies using a donor oocyte model to control for female age and endometrial receptivity found no effect of men's age on sperm parameters, fertilization, pregnancy, or live birth rates. The American Society of Reproductive Medicine (ASRM) recommends limiting the age of sperm donors to younger than 40.

Duration

The duration of infertility is a significant independent predictor of pregnancy. Figure 12-4 shows the decrease in fecundability within the first year of attempting conception by presumably normal fertile couples. After 3 years

Table 12-1

Risk of Chromosomal Abnormalities by Maternal Age

Maternal Age	Risk for Down Syndrome	Total Risk for Chromosomal Abnormalities
20	1/1,667	1/526
21	1/1,667	1/526
22	1/1,429	1/500
23	1/1,429	1/500
24	1/1,250	1/476
25	1/1,250	1/476
26	1/1,176	1/476
27	1/1,111	1/455
28	1/1,053	1/435
29	1/1,000	1/417
30	1/952	1/385
31	1/909	1/385
32	1/769	1/322
33	1/602	1/286
34	1/485	1/238
35	1/378	1/192
36	1/289	1/156
37	1/224	1/127
38	1/173	1/102
39	1/136	1/83
40	1/106	1/66
41	1/82	1/53
42	1/63	1/42
43	1/49	1/33
44	1/38	1/26
45	1/30	1/21
46	1/23	1/16
47	1/18	1/13
48	1/14	1/10
49	1/11	1/8

American College of Obstetricians and Gynecologists: Technical Bulletin #108, September, 1987.

Figure 12-3

In vitro fertilization pregnancy rates by woman's age with and without donor eggs. (From Assisted Reproductive Technology. Centers for Disease Control and Prevention, 2004.)

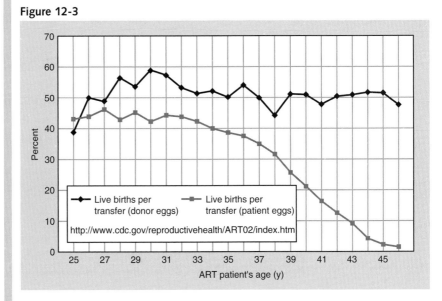

Figure 12-4 Pregnancy rate each month during first year of trying.

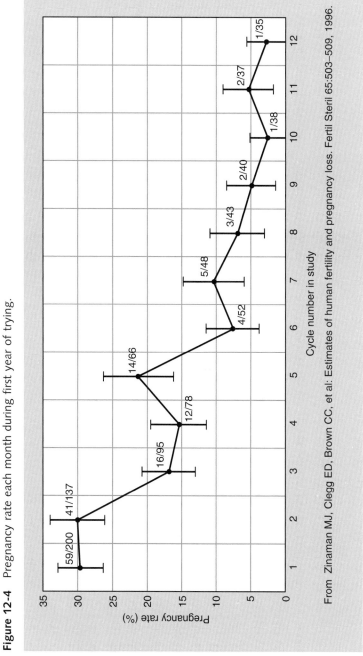

From Zinaman MJ, Clegg ED, Brown CC, et al: Estimates of human fertility and pregnancy loss. Fertil Steril 65:503–509, 1996.

of unexplained infertility, the prospect of pregnancy decreases by 24% each year. Although a couple's age and duration of infertility are nonmodifiable, several behavioral changes can improve their prognosis.

Since the most pregnancies occur with coitus 2 days prior to and including the day of ovulation, couples should be advised to begin trying 3 days before the expected ovulation (Fig. 12-5). A coital frequency of every 1 to 2 days for a week will yield the highest pregnancy rates. Ovulation predictor kits are not recommended for coital timing because they will miss potential fertile days before the luteinizing hormone (LH) surge. Also, some women may not detect the color change and can lose an opportunity to conceive. Couples should be cautioned to avoid the use of vaginal lubricants (K-Y Jelly, Surgilube, petroleum jelly, or saliva) because these can affect sperm function. Women should also refrain from using aspirin and nonsteroidal anti-inflammatory agents around midcycle since their antiprostaglandin action may interfere with the physical release of the oocyte from the follicle at ovulation. Men can be reassured that underwear type (i.e., boxer shorts or briefs) does not appear to affect fertility rates.

Lifestyle Factors

Extremes of weight, strenuous exercise, or emotional stress may compromise fertility when they lead to ovulatory dysfunction. Modifying these factors to enable ovulatory function may restore fertility. It is unknown whether they may have other subtle adverse effects in women with regular cycles. Women with a high body mass index (BMI) had a poorer prognosis with IVF. Another study found no difference in implantation rates with donor oocytes based on BMI, suggesting that excessive weight compromises oocyte quality. Data are lacking regarding the impact of BMI on male fertility.

Figure 12-5

Pregnancy rate by day of coitus.

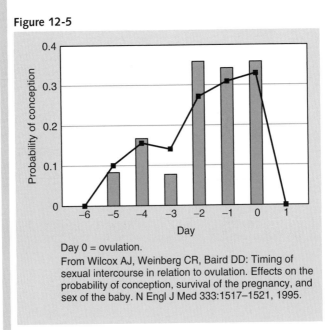

Day 0 = ovulation.
From Wilcox AJ, Weinberg CR, Baird DD: Timing of sexual intercourse in relation to ovulation. Effects on the probability of conception, survival of the pregnancy, and sex of the baby. N Engl J Med 333:1517–1521, 1995.

292

Women engaging in very rigorous exercise regimens may benefit from reducing their level of activity; some studies have suggested that more than 7 hours of aerobic exercise per week may increase the risk of ovulatory factor infertility. Those participating in a moderate exercise program can be encouraged to continue this healthy practice, which may also help to reduce stress. Although it is well known that infertility causes stress, it is unclear whether the converse is true or whether stress reduction improves fertility rates. Patients are encouraged to reduce stress by various means such as psychological counseling, peer support groups, guided imagery, acupuncture, meditation, yoga, or exercise.

The most significant lifestyle modification to facilitate conception is to quit smoking. Smoking increases infertility, spontaneous abortions, and ectopic pregnancies and is associated with low birth weight and intrauterine growth retardation. A meta-analysis of 12 studies with approximately 30,000 women showed smokers had an odds ratio (OR) for infertility of 1.6 (confidence interval [CI], 1.34–1.91). Using that OR and assuming a 25% prevalence of smoking in reproductive age women, up to 13% of female infertility may be caused by smoking. The delay to conception correlated to the number of cigarettes the women smoked. Smokers had a 54% greater chance of not conceiving within 1 year. Women exposed to secondhand smoke were similarly affected.

There is a dose-dependent accelerated follicular depletion with menopause occurring 1 to 4 years earlier in smokers. There is also a higher prevalence of abnormal clomiphene citrate challenge test (CCCT) results in smokers compared with age-matched control subjects. Smoking by either or both partners significantly reduces success in spontaneous and IVF cycles. Women who smoke require higher gonadotropin doses and have lower peak estradiol (E_2) levels, fewer oocytes, higher cycle cancellation and failed fertilization rates, and lower implantation rates. Concentrations of the toxins cadmium and cotinine have been found in follicular fluid during IVF cycles in proportion to the number of cigarettes smoked. Three meta-analyses showed that smokers required nearly twice as many IVF cycles to conceive as nonsmokers.

The data are less consistent regarding the effects of smoking on male fertility. Some studies report a reduction in semen quality whereas others could not confirm it. Sperm concentration, motility, and morphology are often reduced but still within the normal range. A meta-analysis of 27 studies reported a modest reduction in semen quality but not fertility. Another study found that male smokers had a relative risk nearly three times higher for failed IVF cycles with and without intracytoplasmic sperm injection (ICSI).

Smokers are at an increased risk for spontaneous abortions, which may be due to chromosomal anomalies or the vasoconstrictive and antimetabolic properties of nicotine, carbon monoxide, and cyanide leading to placental insufficiency. Smoking may disrupt the meiotic spindle leading to an increased proportion of diploid oocytes and trisomic embryos from meiotic nondisjunction. Men who smoke have a higher percentage of sperm with DNA fragmentation as well as aneuploid sperm, especially disomy Y.

A dose-related risk for ectopic pregnancy has also been shown with women who smoked over a pack a day having an OR of 3.5 (CI, 1.4–8.6). Much of the reduced fecundity with smoking may be reversed within a year of cessation.

The data are not as clear for other lifestyle factors such as alcohol or caffeine. There is no convincing evidence that moderate use of alcohol or caffeine affects male fertility. Several studies have noted that alcohol consumption has a negative impact on the fertility of women. Since no safe level has been determined for fertility or fetal alcohol syndrome, women should be advised to abstain from alcohol when attempting to conceive and during pregnancy. Women who consume more than 250 mg of caffeine daily (>2 cups of coffee) have a higher risk for infertility. More than 500 mg/day was associated with a higher spontaneous abortion rate. Limiting caffeine use to no more than 1 to 2 cups a day is prudent.

EVALUATION

Since *infertility* is defined as failure to conceive within 1 year and 85% of couples will conceive during that time frame, we encourage patients to continue to try on their own for a full year before initiating the evaluation. However, several exceptions to this recommendation can be made. The evaluation of patients with obvious problems such as anovulation, known tubal disease, prior sterilization, or pelvic pain need not be postponed. In women 35 years of age or older, the evaluation should be initiated after they have attempted conception for 6 months. Couples with high anxiety about their infertility after any duration should not be denied attention. The frequency of the etiologic factors is dependent on the study population. The percentages in Table 12-2 add up to over 100% because infertility is frequently multifactorial. Overall, a male factor is present as the sole cause for infertility in approximately 20%, female factors alone account for approximately 40% and the combination of the two compose another 20%. About 20% remain unexplained after a complete evaluation.

It is preferred that both partners are present for the initial consultation. The age of the partners, duration of infertility, and whether they conceived together before are prognostic factors. A standard medical history is obtained including a review of systems, medications taken, prior

Table 12-2

Causes of Infertility

Cause	Incidence
Male	40% to 50%
Ovulatory	15% to 20%
Tubal	15% to 20%
Uterine	5% to 10%
Peritoneal	10% to 15%
Unexplained	15% to 20%

surgeries, and family history. Specific attention should be paid to prior pregnancies established by each partner and their outcomes. Inquire as to when they occurred, how much time was required to conceive, and whether they were spontaneous or the result of treatment. It is important to assess coital frequency, use of lubricants, and whether there are any problems such as erectile dysfunction or dyspareunia. Information regarding prior contraception use and history of sexually transmitted diseases, particularly gonorrhea, chlamydia, and pelvic inflammatory disease should be elicited. It is important to ask about smoking, alcohol, tobacco, and recreational drug use so that they may be strongly discouraged. Other factors such as diet, exercise, and stress as well as occupational exposure to radiation, high temperatures, and chemicals such as organic solvents may contribute to problems with reproduction. *In utero* diethylstilbestrol (DES) exposure is still an issue for women born before the early 1970s.

A careful menstrual history can help determine whether the patient is ovulatory. The menstrual interval should be between 21 and 35 days and not vary by more than 7 days. Patients can usually provide accurate information on timing of their menses with months' or even years' worth of menstrual calendars, basal body temperature charts, and ovulation predictor kits to review. However, the quantity of menstrual blood loss is difficult to assess by history. Very light flow raises concerns about intrauterine adhesions, menorrhagia may be a symptom of myomas, and intermenstrual bleeding could be due to submucosal myomas or endometrial polyps. Although premenstrual molimina such as breast tenderness, bloating, and mood changes are further evidence that the cycles are ovulatory, dysmenorrhea could be a red flag for endometriosis.

In the interest of being complete but not duplicative, the results of prior infertility tests and treatments should be carefully reviewed. Laboratory results, operative reports (and intraoperative photos and/or videos), ovulation induction stimulation sheets, and IVF records must be requisitioned. Hysterosalpingogram (HSG) and ultrasonogram films are always obtained to confirm the radiologists' interpretations.

On physical examination, the patient's height and weight are recorded and body stature is noted. Truncal obesity, buffalo hump, and moon facies are signs of Cushing's syndrome. Abdominal stria and facial erythema support that diagnosis. Other skin changes such as acne or hirsutism should trigger testing for hyperandrogenemia. Acanthosis nigricans is a marker of hyperinsulinemia and appears as thickened hyperpigmented skin usually over the posterior nuchal region buy may also appear in the axilla and groin as well. The thyroid should be palpated and a breast examination performed to assess for galactorrhea. The abdomen is examined for masses or tenderness.

Attention is then turned to the pelvic examination, starting with the external genitalia, looking at the pubic hair distribution pattern (i.e., male or female escutcheon and ruling out herpes and condyloma lesions and clitoromegaly). A speculum examination is performed to check for cervical and vaginal anomalies such as DES-associated changes and cervical stenosis, as well as to rule out infections. A deviated cervix may reflect uterine displacement by endometriosis and/or pelvic adhesions. A Papanicolaou smear is updated as necessary, and cervical cultures for gonorrhea and chlamydia may be obtained based on the patient's age and sexual history. Cervical motion tenderness; uterine size, shape, consistency, and mobility; and adnexal size and tenderness are determined by bimanual examination. Fixed uterine retroversion and tender nodularity in the rectovaginal septum are suspicious for endometriosis. A transvaginal ultrasonogram can be performed in the office to immediately evaluate any abnormal findings.

In recent years, there has been a decreased emphasis on making a specific diagnosis in favor of moving more rapidly toward empiric treatment with superovulation and intrauterine insemination (SO/IUI) or IVF. In a study published in 1994, Guzick et al. performed semen analyses, HSG, postcoital testing, endometrial biopsies, laparoscopy, sperm antibody testing, and cervical cultures for *Mycoplasma hominis* and *Ureaplasma urealyticum* on 64 couples (32 pairs of fertile and infertile couples matched for age and race). At least one abnormal infertility test result was found in 69% of fertile and 84% of infertile couples. Only tubal damage and endometriosis were more common in infertile couples. No significant differences between the groups for the other infertility factors could be demonstrated.

The current basic infertility evaluation includes documentation of ovulation, semen analysis, and an HSG. A brief discussion is warranted to outline the rationale for eliminating tests that have been part of the standard infertility evaluation for many decades. Two tests in particular are the postcoital test and endometrial biopsy.

Postcoital Test

The Sims-Huhner or postcoital test (PCT) was designed to assess the viability of the sperm in the cervical mucus. The quality of preovulatory cervical mucus is described in terms of volume, stretchability (spinnbarkeit), cellularity and drying pattern (ferning), and the number of motile and nonmotile sperm per high power field are determined several hours after coitus. Although the test has been in use for over a century, its timing, technique, and interpretation have never been standardized. The test also suffers from poor reproducibility. Several studies have shown the predictive value of the test to be no better than chance. A study that randomized infertility patients to undergo PCT or no PCT found that the PCT lead to more tests and treatments but had no significant effect on cumulative pregnancy rates at 2 years. The ASRM and the American College of Obstetricians and Gynecologists have stated that there is little scientific rationale for performing a PCT.

Endometrial Biopsy

The concept of inadequate progesterone production resulting in a luteal phase defect (LPD) as a cause of infertility and recurrent miscarriage was proposed in the late 1940s. An endometrial biopsy is obtained in the office with a disposable endometrial sampling device such as the Pipelle in the late luteal phase. A pathologist then "dates" the tissue using a set of histologic criteria based on an idealized 28-day cycle described by

Noyes et al. in 1950. That date is then compared with the patient's menstrual date based on the day of her LH surge or the menses after the biopsy. The tissue should be no more than 2 days behind the menstrual dates.

There has been much controversy regarding the prevalence of LPD and its clinical relevance as a cause of infertility. Studies that have attempted to establish LPD as a cause of infertility have not included a control group of fertile women, and methods to diagnose and treat LPD are largely speculative. There is considerable inter- and intraobserver variability in endometrial biopsy dating as well as an inconsistent expression of LPD in affected women. Additionally, serial endometrial biopsies in normal fertile women have noted LPD in 31% of their cycles. The measurement of luteal-phase progesterone levels is also an inadequate test for diagnosing or excluding LPD. The limitations of the current methods for assessing endometrial receptivity for embryo implantation make it hard to justify their cost and discomfort to the patient.

| **Documentation of Ovulation** | For the majority of patients, the menstrual history is indicative of the presence or absence of ovulatory cycles. Menstrual intervals of 28 ± 7 days not varying by more than 7 days are consistent with normal ovulatory function, especially in the presence of premenstrual molimina and/or dysmenorrhea. A serum progesterone level higher than 3 ng/mL in the luteal phase confirms that ovulation has occurred. A biphasic basal body temperature (BBT) chart, with the temperature in the luteal phase being higher than the follicular phase, is also evidence of ovulation. |

Patients are instructed to take their oral temperature daily before arising with a BBT thermometer. An elevation of approximately 0.5°F usually begins the day after ovulation due to the thermogenic effect of progesterone (when serum levels reach 4 ng/mL). The rise should last 11 to 16 days. A short luteal phase may be due to inadequate progesterone production, which can be supplemented. Although BBT charting is free and without risks, it is not very accurate or reliable and cannot predict ovulation. It is always retrospective. The daily reminder upon awakening that the patient has an infertility problem can increase the psychological stress they are under.

Over-the-counter ovulation predictor kits to detect the midcycle LH surge in the urine are much more accurate and reliable and will predict ovulation within approximately 12 to 36 hours. However, they do not improve pregnancy rates over well-timed intercourse and cost about $30 per kit. Also, some patients may not detect their surge and may miss an opportunity. We recommend the kits for timing IUI but not coitus.

The documentation of normal ovarian function does not reveal anything about the quality of the oocytes or their potential for pregnancy. To this end, several tests have been developed to assess ovarian reserve. The simplest test is a serum follicle-stimulating hormone (FSH) level on cycle day 3. Values greater than 15 mIU/mL are indicative of diminished ovarian reserve and a poor prognosis for pregnancy. Each laboratory test should establish its own threshold levels. An E_2 level should be obtained at the same time since an elevated value may suppress FSH to the normal range. A day 3 E_2 level above 50 pg/mL is also an independent predictor for poor prognosis. A single elevated day 3 FSH connotes a poor prognosis even when values in subsequent cycles are normal. A false-positive elevated day 3 FSH measurement is rare, but false negatives are common.

The CCCT was devised to improve the sensitivity of the day 3 FSH test. The CCCT involves obtaining day 3 FSH and E_2 measurements, administering clomiphene citrate (CC) 100 mg from cycle days 5 through 9, and repeating an FSH measurement on cycle day 10. Approximately 70% of patients with an abnormal CCCT have a normal day 3 FSH level. A study of a general infertility population noted an abnormal CCCT in 10%, and only 5% of those patients had a successful pregnancy. Abnormal CCCT was associated with increasing age; only 3% of women younger than 30 years of age had abnormal results compared with 26% for women older than 39 years. An abnormal CCCT result indicates a poor prognosis for fertility independent of age. Thirty-eight percent of women in the study cohort with unexplained infertility had an abnormal CCCT result.

Ovarian reserve testing is recommended for all infertile women older than 35 years and women younger than 35 years with a single ovary; prior ovarian surgery, chemotherapy, or pelvic radiation therapy; poor response to exogenous gonadotropin treatment; or unexplained infertility, as well as all women before IVF. Women with diminished ovarian reserve undergoing IVF require higher doses of gonadotropins, have a higher cycle cancellation rate, produce fewer oocytes, and have a lower pregnancy rate.

The polycystic ovary syndrome (PCOS) is the most common endocrine disorder in women of reproductive age. The current diagnostic criteria require two of the following three features: anovulation, clinical or laboratory evidence of hyperandrogenemia, or polycystic-appearing ovaries on ultrasonography. The pathogenesis of PCOS is a vicious cycle (Fig. 12-6).

Figure 12-6

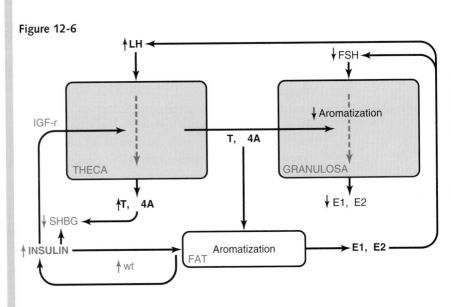

Pathophysiology of polycystic ovary syndrome. LH, Luteinizing hormone; FSH, follicle-stimulating hormone; IGF, insulin-like growth factor; T, testosterone, A, androstenedione E_1, estrone; E_2, estradiol; SHBG, sex hormone binding globulin; wt, weight.

The primary feature is an androgenic microenvironment instead of an estrogenic one within the ovaries. This is due to increased androgen production in the thecal cells and reduced aromatization of those androgens to estrogens within the granulosa cell compartment. The increased androgens decrease hepatic production of sex hormone binding globulin, which leads to a greater proportion of free unbound androgens and estrogens in the circulation. The circulating androgens are aromatized to estrogens in the periphery, especially in fat. These estrogens negatively feed back on the central nervous system to selectively decrease FSH production and increase LH. The increased LH drives the metabolism of androgens from cholesterol in the theca while the reduced FSH limits the capacity of the granulose to aromatize the androgens, and the cycle continues.

Obesity provides more fat for the peripheral aromatization of androgens to estrogens and also contributes to insulin resistance. Patients with insulin resistance develop a compensatory hyperinsulinemia to remain euglycemic. Hyperinsulinemia in turn may lead to further weight gain. It also decreases production of sex hormone binding globulin and facilitates androgen synthesis in the theca cells.

Strategies for restoring ovulatory function include blocking estrogen receptors in the hypothalamus with CC or reducing circulating estrogens by blocking peripheral aromatization with letrozole. Metformin is used to reduce hyperinsulinemia by increasing the sensitivity of the tissues to insulin. Parenteral FSH can be administered to increase aromatization within the granulose cells. Finally, laparoscopic ovarian drilling can be performed to reduce the androgen producing theca cell stroma. These treatments will be discussed later in this chapter.

Semen Analysis

Since 40% to 50% of infertility is attributed, wholly or in part, to the male partner, a male factor should be excluded early in the evaluation with a routine semen analysis. The sample should be obtained by masturbation (without lubricants) into a specimen cup after 2 to 3 days of abstinence and maintained at body temperature during transportation to the laboratory. It should be collected at the laboratory if it will take more than 45 to 60 minutes to transport it there. The test is repeated at least 4 weeks later if the results of the initial study are abnormal. The World Heath Organization established the following normal parameters for the semen analysis (Table 12-3).

Table 12-3

World Health Organization Normal Semen Analysis Parameters

Volume	2 to 5 mL
Concentration	>20 million/mL
Motility	> 50% with forward progression
Morphology (strict criteria)	>15% normal
White blood cells	<1 million/mL

World Health Organization: WHO Laboratory Manual for the Examination of Human Semen and Semen–Cervical Mucus Interaction, 4th ed. Cambridge University Press, Cambridge, UK, 1999.

299

Although men with abnormal semen analysis results have lower fertilization rates and their partners lower spontaneous pregnancy rates with conventional IVF, there is no threshold value below which they cannot establish a pregnancy. Likewise, a normal semen analysis does not rule out sperm dysfunction because a small percentage of men with "normal" semen have very low or no fertilization with IVF. Additionally, semen samples have considerable inherent variability, and there is a high degree of variability between examiners performing the analyses.

In an effort to improve the prognostic value of the semen analysis, Kruger's strict criteria for normal morphology have been applied: higher than 14% is considered normal, 4% to 14% intermediate, and lower than 4% significantly impaired. Men with values lower than 4% typically have severely reduced fertilization with conventional IVF. A recent meta-analysis noted a significant improvement in pregnancy rates with IUI if there were more than 4% normal forms. However, like the standard semen analysis, the result of the Kruger's morphology cannot determine which couple will be unable to conceive. Likewise, at least 25% of men with failed fertilization in IVF have completely normal morphology by strict criteria.

Numerous additional studies of sperm function have been devised in an attempt to improve the predictive value of the semen analysis. These include the hamster zona-free egg penetration test, human hemi-zona assay, hypo-osmotic swelling test, acrosome reaction, and acrosin measurement. These tests lack proven value in distinguishing fertile from infertile men. The success of ICSI for nearly all causes of male infertility has made these tests less relevant.

Hysterosalping-ography

HSG is an x-ray imaging technique in which the uterine cavity and lumina of the fallopian tubes are visualized by injecting contrast material through the cervical canal. The procedure should be performed between the end of menses but before ovulation to reduce the risk of disrupting an early pregnancy or exposing it to radiation. Also, the endometrium is thin during the early follicular phase, which reduces false positives for filling defects or proximal tubal occlusion due to thick mucosal folds. The patients are instructed to take an antiprostaglandin analgesic 30 minutes before the procedure. Antibiotics are not used unless the patient has a history of sexually transmitted infection or the study reveals hydrosalpinges. In those cases, doxycycline is administered orally for 5 days.

It is important to expel all of the air from the cannula to prevent air bubble artifacts that can give the impression of a polyp or myoma. The cervix is cleaned with an antiseptic solution then gently grasped with a single tooth tenaculum on the anterior lip. An acorn tip Jarcho or Rubin's cannula is placed through the external os while applying gentle downward traction on the tenaculum to seal the cervix and straighten the uterine axis. The cannula tip should not go beyond the internal os to prevent uterine perforation or incomplete visualization of a uterine anomaly by placing the tip above a deep septum or bicornuate uterus. Fluoroscopy is initiated and the pelvis is observed for any abnormalities that may affect the interpretation of the study. Contrast media is then injected slowly both for patient comfort as well as to delineate any subtle uterine filling defects that may not be visible after complete filling, particularly with the denser oil-soluble contrast media. If a filling defect is seen, the patient can be rotated to her side to see whether the filling defect moves, confirming is the presence of an air bubble. Only 5 to 10 mL is usually required to complete the study. Water-soluble contrast will be seen to outline loops of bowel immediately, whereas a delayed film is needed 1 to 24 hours later to confirm free spill of oil-soluble media. The patient should be observed for a few minutes after the procedure for signs of a vasovagal reaction, allergic reaction, or bleeding.

Generally, water-soluble contrast media is preferable to oil-soluble contrast because of its improved visualization, rapid absorption, and greater safety. Oil-soluble contrast has the disadvantages of the need for the patient to return for a delayed film, slow absorption over months to years, and the risks of granuloma formation and oil embolism. Proponents of oil-soluble contrast cite studies showing higher postprocedure fertility rates, though others found no difference. The great majority of pregnancies occur within 6 months after the HSG, and patients should attempt to conceive for several cycles after the HSG before initiating more aggressive treatment.

HSG has a very high sensitivity but a low specificity for the diagnosis of uterine cavity abnormalities. If the HSG reveals a normal cavity, no further evaluation is likely to find a pathology that could affect the chance for a normal conception. Sonohysterography (SHG)—ultrasound evaluation after transcervically instilling the uterine cavity with saline—has replaced diagnostic hysteroscopy in delineating intrauterine filling defects noted on HSG. It is quicker to perform and less uncomfortable. SHG is as accurate as hysteroscopy for distinguishing polyps from myomas, but it can demonstrate the extent of the intramyometrial component of submucosal myomas, which can help determine whether they can be removed by operative hysteroscopy. SHG also reveals whether other intramural or subserosal myomas are present as well any ovarian abnormalities.

If HSG suggests tubal patency, tubal blockage is highly unlikely. However, tubal blockage on HSG is not confirmed by laparoscopy in up to 62% of cases, largely due to cornual spasm during the HSG. Laparoscopy is therefore needed to confirm or exclude tubal occlusion noted on HSG. HSG detects pelvic adhesions in approximately half the cases in which they are present. Patients with pelvic pain, abnormalities on pelvic examination or ultrasonography, or risk factors for pelvic adhesions or tubal disease (such as PID or a ruptured appendix) can skip the HSG and proceed directly to laparoscopy because they are significantly more likely to have pelvic pathology requiring laparoscopic treatment.

Laparoscopy

The value of diagnostic laparoscopy in patients with a normal HSG and a lack of risk factors for infertility is debatable. Several studies have noted pelvic pathology in 25% to 60% of these patients. However, the majority of the abnormal findings were minimal to mild endometriosis and peritubal adhesions. There are limited data to support the assumption that treating these conditions improves fertility. One nonrandomized study showed a higher pregnancy rate after adhesiolysis by laparotomy versus expectant management. Two randomized controlled trials of laparoscopic treatment of minimal to mild endometriosis yielded conflicting results.

No test is currently available to diagnose endometriosis preoperatively, but chlamydia antibodies and chlamydial heat shock protein 60 may predict the presence of tubal disease from prior asymptomatic chlamydial salpingitis. Some have suggested using these tests to decide which patients should be offered diagnostic laparoscopy. The trend now is to give women in their 20s and early 30s the choice between diagnostic laparoscopy and controlled ovarian hyperstimulation (COH) with IUI for otherwise unexplained infertility. If pelvic pathology is treated at laparoscopy, the patients are managed expectantly for up to one year. Older women are usually advised to forego laparoscopy and proceed directly to COH/IUI or IVF.

A new technique to assess the peritoneal cavity while avoiding all of the disadvantages of laparoscopy is being evaluated. Transvaginal hydrolaparoscopy involves placing a small scope through the posterior cul-de-sac after filling it with warm saline to float the bowel out of the pelvis. It is performed in the office under local anesthesia with the patient in lithotomy position. Transcervical chromotubation to document tubal patency and office hysteroscopy can be performed concurrently, thereby replacing both HSG and diagnostic laparoscopy. A study reported that it was better tolerated and provided more information than HSG. However, other studies found discordance rates with laparoscopy for endometriosis or peritubal adhesions in 8% to 80% of cases.

TREATMENT

It is difficult to provide patients with meaningful success rates with the various infertility treatments because there is a serious lack of well-designed prospective randomized controlled studies. Also, infertility involves two patients, which doubles the number of variables. The ages of the partners, their lifestyle habits, and the duration of infertility can all influence the chances for success with treatment as discussed above. Surgical modalities and the skill of the surgeon affect the postoperative results.

A general gynecologist can complete the basic infertility evaluation, treat anovulation, and perform surgery to correct specific abnormalities within his or her comfort zone or skill level. Anovulatory patients who do not respond to oral agents for ovulation induction or do not conceive within six ovulatory cycles should be referred to a reproductive endocrinologist for more aggressive treatment. Likewise, patients requiring advanced laparoscopic procedures or microsurgery should be referred, as should patients with unexplained infertility who fail to conceive within four to six cycles of empiric CC therapy. Referral to a reproductive endocrinologist should be expedited for older patients.

Ovulatory Factor

Clomid

CC is a synthetic nonsteroidal estrogen agonist/antagonist. Its mechanism of action is prolonged binding to, and depletion of, the hypothalamic estrogen receptors to block the normal negative feedback of endogenous estrogens on gonadotropin-releasing hormone (GnRH) secretion. This antiestrogen effect increases the GnRH pulse frequency and subsequently FSH and LH secretion. CC also has a direct estrogenic effect on the ovary to sensitize follicular granulosa cells to gonadotropins and up-regulate aromatase activity. CC has a half life of 5 days and can be detected in the feces up to 6 weeks after a single 50-mg dose. However, the pharmacologic effect is brief. It has been the first-line treatment for ovulation induction in women with PCOS or normogonadotropic anovulation. It is not effective for hypoestrogenic patients with hypothalamic amenorrhea or those with significantly elevated FSH levels. Ovulatory rates of 80% are typical, and about half of those patients conceive. Nearly all of the conceptions occur within the first six ovulatory cycles. The multiple pregnancy rate is 5% to 10% and is almost exclusively twins. There is no increase in spontaneous abortions, ectopic pregnancies, or congenital malformations.

CC is administered as a 50-mg tablet daily for 5 days beginning on cycle days 3, 4, or 5. Ovulation usually occurs a week after the last tablet with a range of about 5 to 12 days. Patients are advised to time coitus every 1 to 2 days for a week starting 4 days after the last dose. The infertility evaluation is continued with a semen analysis and HSG after the third ovulatory cycle.

If the patient remains anovulatory, the dose is increased by one 50-mg table each of the 5 days up to 150 mg, though 250 mg may be required in obese patients. Pregnancy rates are lower in women needing higher doses, perhaps due to the antiestrogenic effect on the endometrium. Since there is no benefit to increasing the dose once consistent ovulatory cycles are established, administration of CC is continued at the lowest effective dose for up to six cycles. The fecundity rate beyond six cycles is very low, and there is a slightly increased risk of developing ovarian neoplasms, particularly borderline ovarian tumors, in women who have taken CC for more than 1 year.

Several methods may help women who have failed to ovulate on the maximal dose. Extending the duration from 5 days to up to 10 days may work in some patients. Rarely, patients may develop mature follicles but not have an endogenous LH surge to trigger ovulation. These patients can be followed with pelvic ultrasonography and human chorionic gonadotropin (hCG) administered to serve as a surrogate LH surge when the dominant follicle is 18 to 20 mm in mean diameter. There is no benefit to adding hCG in patients who are already ovulatory on CC alone. Dexamethasone 0.5 mg at bedtime may augment the effect of CC when the serum dehydroepiandrosterone sulfate level is greater than 250 to 300 ng/mL.

Finally, the addition of metformin has a synergistic effect with CC in patients with hyperinsulinemia, and ovulation rates are high in previously CC-resistant patients.

Adverse effects are common but are usually mild. The most common adverse effects are hot flushes, abdominal bloating and discomfort, nausea, headaches, and mood changes. Visual disturbances such as blurred vision or scotoma require immediate discontinuation. Adverse effects spontaneously resolve shortly after CC is stopped. Most of these effects are due to CC's antiestrogenic properties. Also, the antiestrogen effect on the uterus may adversely impact endometrial receptivity by making the endometrium thinner and inducing LPD.

Letrozole

CC has been the mainstay of ovulation induction therapy for more than four decades, but increasing attention is being paid to letrozole. Initial pilot studies with letrozole indicate that it may be as effective at inducing ovulation and pregnancy as CC but without the undesirable antiestrogenic adverse effects. Letrozole is an aromatase inhibitor that blocks the conversion of androgens to estrogens, thus lowering systemic estrogen levels. This serves to reduce the estrogen negative feedback on the hypothalamus without depleting the estrogen receptors. Like CC, letrozole is administered in the early follicular phase to increase FSH and LH secretion at the time of follicle recruitment and development. A 2.5-mg dose is given daily from cycle days 3 through 7. If larger randomized studies confirm the preliminary findings, letrozole may replace CC as the first-line drug of choice for ovulation induction.

Metformin

Hyperinsulinemia is frequently a component of PCOS. It contributes to the hyperandrogenemia and anovulation of PCOS by augmenting LH-induced androgen production in the ovarian thecal cells and by decreasing hepatic sex hormone binding globulin secretion, thereby increasing free unbound androgens. Hyperinsulinemia is typically seen in obese women and may be reversed with weight loss alone, restoring ovulatory function. Patients who remain anovulatory after weight reduction or are unable to lose weight may be treated with metformin. Metformin is a biguanide that has been used for the treatment of type 2 diabetes. It functions to decrease hepatic glucose production, decrease intestinal absorption of glucose, and increase peripheral glucose uptake and utilization by improving insulin sensitivity without inducing hypoglycemia. Serum insulin, testosterone, LH, and low-density lipoproteins are reduced. Metformin is excreted by the kidney, and a normal serum creatinine level should be documented before initiating treatment.

It is available as 500-, 850-, and 1000-mg tablets. The usual starting dose is 500 mg taken with dinner and increasing weekly, or as tolerated, to 500 mg three times daily with meals. Some patients may require the maximum of 2000 mg per day. Diarrhea, nausea and vomiting, flatulence, and abdominal discomfort are common, and about 5% of patients discontinue treatment due to these adverse effects. An extended release form (single daily dosing) is available and may be better tolerated. Another adverse effect is vitamin B_{12} malabsorption in 10% to 30% of patients, though anemia is rare. A complete blood count should be performed annually.

Approximately 50% of patients with PCOS ovulate with metformin. CC is added when ovulation fails to occur after 2 months, resulting in ovulation in 80% to 90%. It is unclear whether metformin or CC should be the first-line treatment for hyperinsulinemic patients with PCOS. In either case, the addition of the other agent after monotherapy failure results in improved ovulatory rates. It is also unclear whether metformin should be continued once pregnancy is established because patients with PCOS are at a greater risk for spontaneous abortion and gestational diabetes. Although metformin has been shown to be safe and effective in treating gestational diabetes, there are no randomized trials to demonstrate that metformin can reduce the incidence of spontaneous abortions or gestational diabetes.

Gonadotropins

Ovulation induction with parenteral gonadotropins is the next step for women who are CC resistant or who fail to conceive after six ovulatory cycles. There are three basic formulations of gonadotropin medications: combined FSH and LH derived from the urine of menopausal women, highly purified urinary FSH, and pure FSH from recombinant DNA technology. They are administered as a daily subcutaneous injection starting on cycle days 3 to 5 after a baseline ultrasonogram is performed to rule out pre-existing ovarian cysts from the prior cycle. The usual starting dose is 75 to 150 IU. The dose is adjusted based on the ovarian response, and a surrogate LH surge is induced with a subcutaneous injection of hCG, 5000 to 10,000 IU, when the lead follicles are about 18 mm in mean diameter. Ovulation occurs 36 to 40 hours later. Several studies have shown that the addition of IUI at ovulation time increases pregnancy rates. IUI is performed by first washing the sperm through a density gradient by centrifugation followed by transcervically placing them at the fundus through a small flexible catheter. Up to 90% of patients will ovulate with controlled ovarian hyperstimulation (COH) and the cycle fecundity rate with COH/IUI approximates that of age-matched fertile couples.

Follicle monitoring with transvaginal ultrasonography and serum estradiol levels is performed 4 and 6 days after the initial dose to ensure optimal dosing of gonadotropins and timing of hCG as well as to reduce the risks of superovulation. The risks of gonadotropin therapy include multiple pregnancy and ovarian hyperstimulation syndrome (OHSS). Multiple pregnancy occurs in approximately 20%, with 15% twins and 5% high-order multiples. Ideally, there should be three to four mature follicles at the time of hCG administration.

If the risk of multiple pregnancy and OHSS is high based on follicle monitoring, there are three courses of action to be considered. The safest option is to cancel the cycle by stopping gonadotropin administration, withholding hCG, and advising the patient to abstain. Alternatively, the patient may wish to continue the cycle and be faced with the prospect OHSS and selective embryo reduction for high-order multiple births. Lastly, the patient may choose to convert to IVF since a good number of mature follicles are available. Aspirating the follicles reduces the risk of OHSS, and limiting the number of embryos transferred to the uterus decreases the risk of high-order multiple births. Additionally, all of the embryos may be electively cryopreserved because pregnancy increases the risk for significant OHSS.

Although the pathogenesis of OHSS is poorly understood, the underlying mechanism appears to be increased vascular permeability with the accumulation of fluid in the third space and an accompanying decrease in the intravascular compartment. In mild to moderate disease, the patients will have enlarged multicystic ovaries and ascites. The severe form of OHSS occurs in approximately 1% of superovulation cycles and may result in massive ascites, hypovolemia, oliguria, hemoconcentration, and hypercoagulability. These patients are at risk for renal failure, cardiac arrhythmias from hyperkalemia, thromboembolism, and adult respiratory distress syndrome. Treatment is supportive because there is no correction for the underlying condition. OHSS is self-limited, with spontaneous resolution usually occurring at the time of menses; however, it may last several weeks if the patient is pregnant. A further discussion of the management of OHSS is beyond the scope of this chapter.

Ovarian Drilling

CC-resistant PCOS patients wishing to avoid the cost, risks, and inconvenience of gonadotropin treatment may consider laparoscopic ovarian drilling. This is the modern equivalent of the ovarian wedge resection originally performed by Stein and Leventhal. The rationale is to reduce the androgen-producing stromal component to restore a normal estrogen to androgen microenvironment within the ovary, which should allow ovulatory function to resume. Postoperatively, serum testosterone and LH levels are lower and FSH levels higher, but insulin levels are not affected. The procedure is performed by inserting a monopolar needle electrode into the ovary and applying current; however, the technique has not been standardized. We make six to 10 punctures per ovary depending on its size, applying 40 watts of coagulation current for 4 seconds per puncture. It is important to avoid the ovarian hilum to prevent troublesome bleeding. There is a theoretical concern of inducing premature ovarian failure with excessive treatment. Although adnexal adhesions do occur with laparoscopic ovarian drilling, they do not seem to compromise fertility.

Approximately 80% will ovulate spontaneously or will become responsive to CC after ovarian drilling, but the duration of the treatment effect is uncertain, with some patients reverting back to their anovulatory status within 6 months. Reported pregnancy rates at 1 year ranged from 54% to 68%. A meta-analysis found no difference in ongoing pregnancy rates between ovarian drilling and gonadotropin treatment for CC-resistant PCOS patients. However, the multiple-pregnancy rate was significantly lower in the drilling group; there was no difference in the miscarriage rate.

Uterine Factor

Myomas are present in 20% to 40% of women of reproductive age and are associated with infertility in 2% to 10%. Myomas may reduce fertility by cornual obstruction, distortion of the tubo-ovarian relationship, interference with sperm pick up from the posterior fornix, inhibition of sperm transport through the uterus, compromise of endometrial blood flow, alteration of uterine fluid, and myometrial irritation with hypercontractility. Myomas that distort the endometrial cavity should be removed, but the management of other intramural or subserosal myomas is more controversial. Although limited data link nondistorting myomas with reduced IVF success rates, routine treatment of these myomas is not universally recommended.

Several different techniques are available for the treatment of myomas; these are discussed in more detail in Chapter 19. The size, number, and location of the myomas determine which treatment is best for the individual patient. Submucosal myomas that are at least 50% intracavitary, as documented by preoperative SHG, may be excised by hysteroscopic myomectomy with a continuous flow resectoscope. Approximately 60% conceive after undergoing this procedure. Conventional abdominal myomectomy results in a cumulative pregnancy rate of 40% to 60% in couples with otherwise unexplained infertility; recurrent pregnancy losses decrease from 40% to 20%. Postoperative adhesions develop in more than 90% after myomectomy, which may be an additional cause of infertility.

Laparoscopic myomectomy is a less invasive outpatient procedure with less postoperative discomfort, a more rapid recovery, and better cosmesis. The myomas are removed from the peritoneal cavity by morcellation and the myometrial defect repaired by laparoscopic suturing. Besides being technically demanding, laparoscopic closure may not be as secure, possibly placing patients at risk for uterine rupture during pregnancy. We limit laparoscopic myomectomy to patients with pedunculated or subserosal lesions, which will not result in a significant myometrial defect. Deeper intramural myomas may be removed by laparoscopic-assisted myomectomy (LAM). This involves excising the myomas laparoscopically then performing a minilaparotomy to remove them and repair the myometrial defect in layers in the standard open fashion. Uterine defect closure after LAM may be more secure than laparoscopic closure, thus reducing the risk for subsequent uterine rupture while still maintaining the advantages of a smaller abdominal incision. The following criteria are recommended for the performance of LAM: uterus up to 16 weeks' size; no more than four myomas, with the largest being 8 cm or smaller; and no cervical or intraligamentous myomas.

Little information is available regarding postprocedure pregnancy rates and outcomes after laparoscopic myolysis or uterine artery embolization. There is concern that reducing uterine blood flow after uterine artery embolization may be deleterious for pregnancy and may increase the risk of premature ovarian failure, particularly in older women. Laparoscopic myolysis and uterine artery embolization are not currently recommended for patients considering future fertility.

Other uterine factors that may be associated with infertility and recurrent pregnancy loss are endometrial polyps and intrauterine adhesions. Both are treated hysteroscopically. The success rates with adhesiolysis are inversely related to the severity of adhesions. The septate uterus carries a high risk for first-trimester spontaneous abortions but does not cause infertility. Hysteroscopic septoplasty restores the term delivery rate to normal. This condition may be distinguished from a bicornuate uterus by evaluating the external fundal contour at laparoscopy or by magnetic resonance imaging. The bicornuate uterus also does not reduce fertility but may lead to preterm delivery or malpresentation. Treatment by a Strassmann metroplasty is indicated only in rare cases of recurrent preterm delivery of previable fetuses. Other anomalies that may impair conception and pregnancy maintenance are adenomyosis and *in utero* DES exposure. Unfortunately, these conditions are not treatable.

Tubal Factor

An estimated 10% to 20% of patients have proximal tubal occlusion on HSG. Causes for proximal tubal occlusion include uterotubal spasm, luminal plugs, salpingitis isthmica nodosa, or fibrosis. If available, selective salpingography can be attempted during the HSG. In this procedure, one fallopian tube is selectively cannulated and injected with contrast. Patency may be restored in up to one third of the tubes. If selective salpingography is unsuccessful, or if proximal tubal occlusion is confirmed at diagnostic laparoscopy, hysteroscopic tubal cannulation may be performed. A 3F catheter with an inner guidewire is directed into the tubal ostium through the operative channel of the hysteroscope while an assistant observes the proximal tube by laparoscopy. Once the obstruction is bypassed, the guidewire is withdrawn and indigo carmine dye is injected to confirm tubal patency. Patency is established about 85% of the time, though approximately one third of these will reocclude. The pregnancy rate after the procedure is 30% to 40% within 6 to 12 cycles with a 5% to 10% ectopic rate. More than 90% of unsuccessfully cannulated tubes have been demonstrated to have fibrosis, chronic salpingitis, or salpingitis isthmica nodosa. Tubal cannulation can be performed under fluoroscopic or even ultrasound guidance if laparoscopy is not otherwise indicated.

Chlamydia trachomatis salpingitis is the most common cause of distal tubal disease, and 50% to 80% of cases are asymptomatic and therefore go untreated. HSG and chlamydia antibody testing both have good sensitivity for predicting tubal disease. Fimbrial phimosis occurring as a result of salpingitis is treated by laparoscopic fimbrioplasty to fully open the distal tube. Hydrosalpinges may be treated by laparoscopic neosalpingostomy. Success rates are determined by the age of the patient and the extent of the tubal damage. Poor prognostic factors are dilated tubes, thick tubal walls, absence of mucosal folds, and dense adhesions. Neosalpingostomy should be reserved for patients with mild disease; some have reported up to an 80% pregnancy rate after this procedure, though success rates of 30% to 50% are more typical, and there is an ectopic rate of about 5%.

More severe hydrosalpinges are better managed by IVF after salpingectomy. Hydrosalpinges reduce the IVF clinical pregnancy rate by 50%. The hydrosalpingeal fluid has been shown to be embryotoxic and to decrease endometrial receptivity by reducing integrins. Performing a salpingectomy before IVF restores the normal success rates. Limited data suggest that salpingostomy has a similar effect; aspirating the hydrosalpinges at the time of the oocyte retrieval is ineffective.

Microsurgical tubal anastomosis after tubal ligation yields high success rates of up to 80% with a slight increase in the risk of ectopic pregnancy. The best results occur in young women who underwent ligation by Falope rings, Hulka or Filshie clips, or Pomeroy partial salpingectomy (as opposed to electrocautery); have a final tubal length of at least 4 cm; have an isthmic-isthmic anastomosis; and have no other infertility factors. A diagnostic laparoscopy is usually performed to ensure that the anastomosis is feasible before undertaking the procedure. The procedure is usually performed on an outpatient basis through a minilaparotomy. A few centers have reported comparable success rates with laparoscopic tubal anastomosis by very experienced laparoscopic surgeons. Adding robotic assistance does not appear to improve success rates.

Endometriosis

The effect of minimal to mild endometriosis and its treatment on infertility is controversial. In one study, endometriosis was 10 times more common, as well as more severe, in women undergoing diagnostic laparoscopy for infertility compared with women undergoing laparoscopic tubal ligation. Women with unexplained infertility or minimal or mild endometriosis had comparable success rates with expectant management for 36 weeks after diagnostic laparoscopy. Two studies reported higher pregnancy rates with COH versus expectant management for patients with minimal to mild endometriosis. The pregnancy rates with treatment were similar to that of women undergoing COH/IUI for unexplained infertility. Minimal to mild endometriosis may just be an incidental finding in women with unexplained infertility. Meta-analyses have shown that there is no improvement in fertility with any medical treatment for any stage of endometriosis.

A Canadian multicenter study randomized patients with minimal to mild endometriosis to laparoscopic treatment or diagnosis only. Cumulative pregnancy rates at 36 months were 30.7% and 17.7%, respectively, a statistically significant difference. A similar multicenter study by an Italian group found no difference between the groups after 1 year of follow-up, 24% versus 29%. A meta-analysis combining these two studies showed a statistically significant increase with surgery (OR, 1.64; 95% CI, 1.05–2.57). No difference was noted when lesions were treated by excision or electrocoagulation. Moderate to severe endometriosis should be treated surgically. Limited data on pregnancy rates after treatment of moderate to severe endometriosis by laparotomy suggest that more severe stages of endometriosis should be surgically treated, with postprocedural pregnancy rates of approximately 60% and 35%, respectively.

The highest pregnancy rates occur within the first year postoperatively. Patients with minimal to mild endometriosis may then be treated with COH/IUI, whereas those with moderate to severe disease should proceed directly to IVF. IVF is more successful than reoperation for persistent or recurrent disease. It is generally recommended that large endometriomas be excised before an IVF cycle is initiated. Some studies suggest that a course of at least 2 months of ovarian suppression with a GnRH agonist may improve IVF pregnancy rates in patients with moderate to severe endometriosis.

Male Factor

Only a small percentage of male infertility has a specifically treatable cause. Hyperprolactinemia and hypothalamic hypogonadism can be treated hormonally; leukocytospermia can be treated with antibiotics. Ejaculatory duct obstruction can be treated by transurethral resection of the obstruction, and vasectomy can be reversed by microsurgical vasovasostomy or vasoepididymostomy. Alternatively, prior vasectomy or other causes of obstructive azoospermia can be treated by microsurgical or percutaneous sperm aspiration for ICSI. IUI can be used for men with ejaculatory dysfunction due to pelvic surgery or diabetes, though IUI is generally of marginal benefit for treating couples with compromised semen quality. Most cases of male factor infertility are now treated by ICSI, which has a high success rate.

The role of antisperm antibodies and varicoceles as a cause of infertility, and the effectiveness of their treatment, have been debated for decades. Some recommend antisperm antibody testing (determining the percentage of the sperm with attached antibodies) when there is isolated low motility, sperm agglutination, unexplained infertility, or before IVF. ICSI should be considered if more than 50% of the sperm are antibody bound. Varicoceles are varicosities of the pampiniform plexus draining the testes (usually on the left) and are present in 15% of the general population and 40% to 80% of infertile men. Insufficient evidence exists that treatment of varicocele in men from couples with otherwise unexplained subfertility improves the spontaneous pregnancy rates. However, it may be offered when the varicocele is palpable, the semen analysis is persistently normal, and the female partner is young and has normal fertility. The varicocele may be treated by surgical ligation or percutaneous fluoroscopic-guided embolization. The full benefit of the procedure may not be realized for up to 1 year.

The majority of male infertility is idiopathic, but recent data suggest that many of these cases are due to genetic abnormalities. The frequency of chromosomal abnormalities that can be observed on karyotypes of peripheral leukocytes is inversely proportional to the sperm count, with less than 1% in normospermic men, approximately 5% in oligospermic men, and 10% to 15% in azoospermic men. Microdeletions of sections of the Y chromosome can be found in 10% to 15% of men with azoospermia or severe oligospermia by using the polymerase chain reaction. Men with nonobstructive azoospermia and severe oligospermia (less than 5 to 10 million sperm/mL) should be informed of the risk that these genetic abnormalities may be transmitted to their offspring, increasing the risks of miscarriage, chromosomal and congenital defects, and male infertility. Karyotyping and Y-chromosome analysis should be suggested before ICSI is performed, and genetic counseling should be offered whenever a genetic abnormality is detected.

For single women or couples in which the male factor for infertility is absolute or in those who decline surgery or IVF, artificial insemination with donor sperm is the only remaining option. Fortunately, it has a high success rate, essentially restoring the normal fecundity rate (assuming the female partner is fertile). The treatment is relatively inexpensive and free of risks. Although studies have shown that success rates are higher with fresh versus frozen semen, nearly all programs use frozen semen exclusively to eliminate the risk of transmitting infections such as syphilis, hepatitis, or HIV. All donors are screened for these diseases. No cases of infection due to donor insemination with frozen semen have been reported.

Insemination is performed the day after the LH surge is detected by an ovulation predictor kit during a spontaneous or CC cycle. Donor insemination may be continued for up to 1 year if the woman is young and ovulatory with a normal HSG. COH can then be added as in the treatment of unexplained infertility. A meta-analysis has shown that success rates are higher with intrauterine as opposed to intracervical insemination.

Unexplained Infertility

Table 12-4 compares the approximate pregnancy rates and cost per cycle for the various treatment options for unexplained infertility. The treatment plan is based primarily on the woman's age and how aggressive the couple wishes to be. Young patients may elect to continue with expectant management for a period of time followed by several cycles of CC, with or without IUI, before progressing to SO/IUI; older women should proceed directly to SO/IUI or IVF.

Expectant Management
Young couples with a normal infertility evaluation should be informed that half of patients trying unsuccessfully for a year will conceive spontaneously in the subsequent year, and 74% will be pregnant within 2 years (a rate normal couples achieve in about 9 months). Many infertility

Table 12-4

Treatments for Unexplained Infertility

	Pregnancy Rate/Cycle	Cost per Cycle ($)
No treatment	1–3%	0
IUI	4–6%	300
CC	4–6%	100
CC + IUI	7–9%	400
hMG	4–10%	2000
hMG + IUI	9–16%	2300
IVF	20–40%	10,000

CC, clomiphene citrate; hMG, human menopausal gonadotropin; IUI, Intrauterine insemination.
Modified from Barbieri RL: Treatment of unexplained infertility, Up-To-Date version 13.1, 2005. Available from: http://www.uptodateonline.com.

patients are anxious and will want to initiate treatment immediately; older couples with fleeting fertility do not have the time to continue trying on their own. As previously noted, the prospect of pregnancy decreases with the duration of infertility.

Clomiphene Citrate With or Without Intrauterine Insemination

CC therapy may correct subtle ovulatory disturbances including LPDs as well as stimulate multifollicular ovulation. A meta-analysis showed a significant improvement in pregnancy rates after CC versus no treatment or placebo in women with unexplained infertility. Although the absolute treatment effect was small, given the low cost and safety, the authors concluded that CC appeared to be a sensible first-line treatment for women with unexplained infertility. However, others have cautioned against the empiric use of CC for these patients because its antiestrogenic effect may paradoxically reduce fertility by compromising endometrial receptivity through the induction of LPDs and reduction of endometrial integrins. One randomized study confirmed lower pregnancy rates in women treated with CC versus expectant management. CC therapy is usually offered to younger patients for up to four cycles. The addition of IUI may further enhance success rates. The IUI is performed the day after the LH surge is detected with an ovulation predictor kit.

Controlled Ovarian Hyperstimulation With Intrauterine Insemination

The use of gonadotropins for COH/IUI in normal ovulatory women with unexplained infertility is exactly the same as for anovulatory women who failed to conceive with CC. COH/IUI may also be used for couples with mild male factor infertility or after laparoscopic treatment of mild to moderate endometriosis, though the success rates for these conditions are approximately half that for unexplained infertility. Some studies have found a correlation between fecundity rates and the total number of motile sperm inseminated, with cutoff values ranging from 1 million to 10 million. Other studies have noted an association between pregnancy rates and the Kruger's morphology. Of all the semen parameters, the percentage of motile sperm after the washing process is most predictive of success. Fecundity rates are approximately doubled with the addition of IUI. Again, female age is an important prognostic factor. COH/IUI has limited usefulness for women older than 40 years, with fewer than 5% having a live birth. The fecundity rate with the first three cycles is significantly higher than with the subsequent three cycles. COH/IUI is therefore limited to three cycles before progressing to IVF.

In Vitro Fertilization

IVF is the only treatment option for couples with severe tubal or male factor infertility and is also the last resort for all other etiologies when lesser treatments have failed. Gonadotropins are administered as for COH but usually at a higher dose in an effort to stimulate more follicles to reach maturation. Several different stimulation protocols have been described, and nearly all include a GnRH agonist or antagonist to reduce the chance of a spontaneous LH surge before oocyte retrieval and to increase the yield of mature oocytes. The patients are monitored as for COH, and hCG is administered once several follicles have reached 18 to 20 mm. Oocyte retrieval is performed approximately 36 hours later via transvaginal ultrasound-guided needle aspiration, usually with the patient under intravenous conscious sedation.

The oocytes are inseminated either with washed sperm or ICSI several hours later, depending on the semen quality. Fertilization status is determined the next morning. The embryos are maintained under carefully controlled culture conditions until they are transferred to the uterus 3 or 5 days after oocyte retrieval at the six- to eight-cell or blastocyst stage, respectively, via a flexible catheter. Performing the embryo transfer under transabdominal ultrasound guidance improves success rates. Luteal support is provided from the time of the transfer until menses or 8 to 10 weeks of gestation with intramuscular progesterone injections, transvaginal progesterone, or serial booster hCG injections, although hCG injections increase the risk for OHSS.

Guidelines for the number of embryos to be transferred are based on the age of the women. Women younger than 38 years should be limited to two embryos, three embryos should be used for women aged 38 to 40 years, and four for women older than 40 years. An additional embryo can be transferred if embryo quality is poor or the couple has had multiple failed attempts. Exceeding the recommended number to transfer does not increase the overall pregnancy rate. Interestingly, it also does not increase the overall multiple-pregnancy rate; however, the high-order multiple-pregnancy rate is significantly increased. Of clinical pregnancies in the United States in 2002, 58% were singleton pregnancies, 29% were twins, and about 7% were triplets or greater. About 6% of pregnancies ended in miscarriage in which the number of fetuses could not be accurately determined. Sixty-five percent of the live births were singleton, about 32% were twins, and almost 4% were triplets or more.

Another reason to limit the number of embryos to replace is that the remaining nontransferred embryos that are developing normally in culture may be cryopreserved for later use. They can be thawed and transferred during a subsequent spontaneous menstrual cycle or after exogenous estrogen and progesterone endometrial priming. Although the pregnancy rate with cryopreserved embryos is substantially less than with fresh embryos (22.7% versus 33.4%), cryopreserved embryos increase the cumulative pregnancy rate per IVF cycle and eliminate the costs, risks, and inconvenience of having to undergo another complete IVF cycle.

The success rates with IVF are determined primarily by the woman's age as previously noted (see Fig. 12-1). The clinical diagnosis does not seem to influence the pregnancy rates except for diminished ovarian reserve, which is a reflection of compromised egg quality (Fig. 12-7). Figure 12-8 shows the attrition from cycle start to live birth. Fourteen percent of the cycles initiated are cancelled before oocyte retrieval due to an inadequate or excessive response to COH. Only 6% of those retrieved have failed fertilization or embryo cleavage with no embryos to transfer.

Figure 12-7

In vitro fertilization birth rate by diagnosis. (Centers for Disease Control and Prevention, 2004. http://www.cdc.gov/reproductivehealth/ART02/index.htm.)

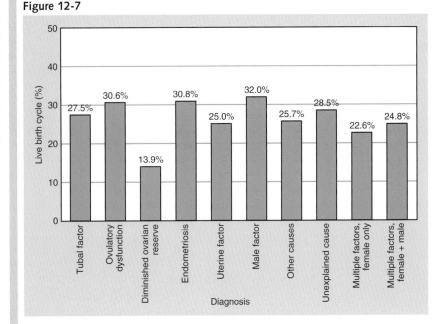

Figure 12-8

Attrition rate from cycle start to live birth. (Centers for Disease Control and Prevention, 2004. http://www.cdc.gov/reproductivehealth/ART02/index.htm.)

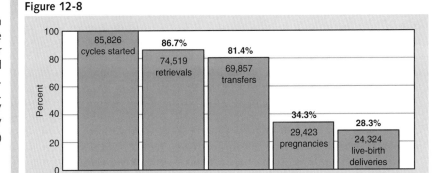

Implantation is the rate-limiting step, with 40.5% of the patients conceiving after embryo transfer. Of those pregnancies, 18% have a nonviable outcome, comparable to spontaneous pregnancies. The most meaningful data for prospective IVF patients are their chance for a live birth per cycle initiated. Clearly, this will be a much lower rate than reporting success as clinical pregnancy per embryo transfer (41% and 26.9%, respectively).

Several other assisted reproductive techniques have been described that are largely of historical interest only. Gamete intrafallopian transfer (GIFT) was popular in the mid to late 1980s when oocyte retrieval was performed laparoscopically and IVF culture techniques were suboptimal. It involved laparoscopic oocyte collection after superovulation and immediate transfimbrial cannulation for placement of several oocytes along with washed sperm into the tubal ampulla. GIFT currently only accounts for a very small percentage of assisted reproductive technique cycles because IVF success rates are higher and the need for laparoscopy is obviated with IVF. The only remaining indication for GIFT is for couples who are opposed to IVF for religious reasons since fertilization occurs *in vivo*.

Hybrids of IVF and GIFT include zygote embryo transfer, pronuclear stage transfer, and tubal embryo transfer; these techniques differ only by the stage of embryo development at the time of transfer. In these procedures, the oocytes are obtained by transvaginal guided needle aspiration and fertilized *in vitro*. The resulting embryos are then transferred into the fallopian tube using the same technique as GIFT. These procedures are only justified now when anatomic anomalies of the vagina or cervix preclude the transcervical embryo replacement.

Gynecologists should be familiar with several ancillary IVF techniques for patient counseling. Assisted hatching is a commonly performed technique, though it is of questionable benefit. It involves thinning a small area of the zona pellucida with an acidic solution via a micropipette or with a laser just before embryo transfer to facilitate embryo hatching from the zona. Other noteworthy techniques are ICSI, ooplasmic or nuclear transfer, and preimplantation genetic diagnosis (PGD).

Intracytoplasmic Sperm Injection

ICSI involves the microinjection of a single sperm into the ooplasma of a mature oocyte after routine COH and oocyte retrieval for IVF. ICSI restores the fertilization rate to normal regardless of the sperm quality, collection method (i.e., ejaculation, microsurgical or percutaneous aspiration, or testicular biopsy), or whether it was fresh or frozen. It normalizes the fertilization rate in couples with unexpected low or non-fertilization with conventional IVF despite a normal semen analysis. Routine use of ICSI for couples with no male factor does not increase pregnancy rates over standard IVF. Congenital malformation rates are not increased with ICSI, but some studies have found a slightly higher rate of genetic abnormalities, particularly sex chromosome anomalies. These are most likely due to abnormalities transmitted from the father rather than to anything intrinsic to the procedure itself. The success of ICSI is the most significant breakthrough in the treatment of infertility since IVF. Before ICSI, men with severely abnormal semen parameters or azoospermia had little to no hope of having their own genetic offspring.

Unfortunately, there is no treatment for compromised oocyte quality for women of advance reproductive age or with diminished ovarian reserve. Two techniques have been proposed in an effort to rejuvenate older oocytes. Ooplasmic transfer involves the injection of ooplasma from a young woman's oocytes into the oocytes of an older woman. The other technique is nuclear (or germinal vesicle) transfer, which places the nucleus from an older oocyte into the enucleated oocyte from a younger woman. Both of these procedures are highly experimental and the safety and efficacy is unknown. Until there is a way to improve oocyte quality, these women are best served by IVF with donor oocytes. As mentioned earlier, the recipient's uterus is not a limiting factor, and the pregnancy, miscarriage, and congenital anomaly rates correlate solely with the age of the donor. Patients may elect to use known or anonymous donors. The donors undergo COH and oocyte retrieval similar to patients using their own oocytes.

Older women who elect to pursue IVF with their own oocytes may add PGD to select only genetically normal embryos to transfer to increase the pregnancy rate and decrease the rate of spontaneous abortions and congenital anomalies due to aneuploidy. Other couples at a greater risk for aneuploidy are those with recurrent pregnancy loss or repeated IVF failures. More than half of all human preimplantation embryos are aneuploidy. Even IVF cycles with normal oocyte donors and no male factor have an aneuploidy rate more than 50%; this could explain the low implantation rates with IVF in general.

Preimplantation genetic diagnosis is performed by extracting a single blastomere or polar body from an eight-cell embryo 3 days after oocyte retrieval using micromanipulation tools similar to ICSI. The cell is then analyzed by fluorescent *in situ* hybridization for several chromosomes, usually 13, 16, 18, 21, 22, X, and Y. Because other chromosomal aneuploidies will not be detected, amniocentesis or chorionic villus biopsy is still recommended. The other concern with PGD is that the embryos are usually transferred 5 days after oocyte retrieval and may not survive in culture that long. A study that randomly assigned patients to PGD or conventional IVF reported that PGD appeared to benefit couples with recurrent pregnancy loss but not repeat IVF failure. PGD is also indicated for couples at risk for having a child with a disease due to a single gene mutation such as cystic fibrosis, Tay-Sachs, sickle cell disease, β-thalassemia, and phenylketonuria. In these cases, the gene of concern is amplified by the polymerase chain reaction for analysis. The role of PGD for older women is inconclusive.

FUTURE

Several exciting techniques are being studied that will revolutionize the treatment of infertility. The first is *in vitro* maturation, which has had initial success in several IVF laboratories. Small antral follicles are retrieved in an unstimulated cycle by transvaginal ultrasound-guided needle aspiration as for conventional IVF. The oocytes are matured and then fertilized *in vitro*. This eliminates the cost, inconvenience, and risk of OHSS with parenteral gonadotropins to induce multiple follicles to mature *in vivo*. This would make it much more feasible for couples to attempt numerous IVF cycles with a greater cumulative success rate.

The second awaited breakthrough is oocyte freezing. Sperm and preimplantation embryos from the pronuclear to the blastocyst stage have been successfully cryopreserved for many years. However, freezing unfertilized oocytes has been a much greater challenge due primarily to the meiotic spindle. Oocyte cryopreservation offers several solutions and new opportunities. Couples undergoing IVF could cryopreserve their extra oocytes, eliminating the ethical dilemma of what to do with unclaimed cryopreserved embryos in the laboratory. This will also enable the creation of donor oocyte banks similar to sperm banks. Currently, recipients must accept the donors that become available, and their menstrual cycles must be synchronized so that the recipient's endometrium is at the appropriate stage to transfer the embryos. With oocyte cryopreservation, couples will be able to select the donor they want from a catalog, donors will not have to travel to the laboratory, and no cycle synchronization will be needed. Also, the cryopreserved oocytes can be quarantined for several months after negative HIV screening to ensure that the donor was not in the process of conversion.

The combination of these two new techniques would eliminate the need for superovulation before oocyte retrieval and should greatly increase the number of women willing to become oocyte donors. Additionally, women in their 20s could cryopreserve their own oocytes, fulfill their career goals, then undergo IVF in their 40s with their young oocytes without compromising their fertility. These techniques could also be applied to women facing the prospect of ovarian failure due to radiation or chemotherapy. Work is also in progress to cryopreserve ovarian tissue for patients facing ovarian failure. The cryopreserved tissue is then reimplanted and oocytes are retrieved for IVF, but there have been no pregnancies to date.

Despite our current progress and promise for the future, many couples will not realize their dreams of having a child. The role of the physician is not only to perform the indicated tests and treatments but to provide for the patients' emotional support and to assist them in achieving closure through adoption or childless living.

KEY POINTS

1. *Infertility* is defined as a year of unprotected coitus without conception and affects approximately 15% of the reproductive-age population.
2. The woman's age, duration of infertility, and smoking are the greatest determinants of fertility potential.
3. Ovarian reserve as measured by the clomiphene citrate challenge test is an independent strong predictor of pregnancy.
4. The basic infertility evaluation consists of documentation of ovulation, semen analysis, and a hysterosalpingogram. Routine postcoital testing and endometrial biopsy are no longer justified.
5. Diagnostic laparoscopy is recommended if the hysterosalpingogram is abnormal or if there is suspicion of pelvic pathology based on pelvic pain, a history of PID, or pelvic surgery. In addition, it may be offered to young women with unexplained infertility.

Continued

KEY POINTS—CONT'D

6. Clomiphene citrate (CC) is the first-line drug for ovulatory factor infertility but may soon be replaced by letrozole. Dexamethasone or metformin can be added to the course of treatment in select women who fail to ovulate with CC alone. CC can also be tried for young women with unexplained infertility for several cycles with or without intrauterine insemination (IUI) before progressing to controlled ovarian hyperstimulation with IUI. Laparoscopic ovarian drilling may also be performed for CC-resistant polycystic ovarian syndrome patients.

7. Gonadotropin therapy may be used for patients whose treatment with CC is unsuccessful or for unexplained infertility. Adding IUI improves the pregnancy rates.

8. Moderate to severe endometriosis should be treated surgically, but the laparoscopic treatment of minimal and mild endometriosis to improve fertility rates is of questionable value.

9. Other surgical procedures for fertility enhancement include myomectomy for fibroids distorting the endometrial cavity, tubal cannulation for cornual occlusion, laparoscopic lysis of adhesions, neosalpingostomy for mild hydrosalpinges and salpingectomy for more severe disease, and tubal anastomosis for sterilization reversal. Submucosal myomas, endometrial polyps, adhesions, and septae can be treated hysteroscopically.

10. The cause of male factor infertility is usually idiopathic and may be due to underlying genetic abnormalities. Most cases require intracytoplasmic sperm injection, which restores the fertilization rate to that of conventional *in vitro* fertilization (IVF) without a male factor. Artificial insemination with donor sperm is also an option.

11. IVF is the only option for couples with severe male or tubal factor infertility. It is also indicated for all other causes of infertility when lesser treatments have failed. The number of embryos transferred should be limited to reduce the rate of high-order multiple pregnancies. Additional embryos can be cryopreserved for later use.

12. The woman's age is the best predictor for success with IVF. Older women and those with diminished ovarian reserve have a poor prognosis and should be encouraged to consider donor oocytes.

13. Couples undergoing IVF who are at increased risk for embryonic aneuploidy, such as those with advanced maternal age, recurrent pregnancy loss, or repeated IVF failures are candidates for preimplantation genetic diagnosis (PGD). Those who are carriers for single gene mutations can have PGD with polymerase chain reaction for the specific gene.

SUGGESTED READING

Adamson GD, Pasta DJ: Surgical treatment of endometriosis-associated infertility: Meta-analysis compared with survival analysis. Am J Obstet Gynecol 171:1488–1505, 1994.

Child TJ, Phillips SJ, Abdul-Jalil AK, et al: A comparison of in vitro maturation and in vitro fertilization for women with polycystic ovaries. Obstet Gynecol 100:665–670, 2002.

Cicinelli E, Matteo M, Causio F, et al: Tolerability of the mini-pan-endoscopic approach (transvaginal hydrolaparoscopy and minihysteroscopy) versus hysterosalpingography in an outpatient infertility investigation. Fertil Steril 76:1048–1051, 2001.

Farquhar C, Vandekerckhove P, Lilford R: Laparoscopic "drilling" by diathermy or laser for ovulation induction in anovulatory polycystic ovary syndrome. Cochrane Database of Syst Rev 2004;p 2.

Fujiwara H, Shibahara H, Hirano Y, et al: Usefulness and prognostic value of transvaginal hydrolaparoscopy in infertility. Fertil Steril 79:186–189, 2004.

Goldberg JM, Falcone T, Attaran M: Sonohysterographic evaluation of uterine abnormalities noted on hysterosalpingography. Hum Reprod 12:2151–2153, 1997.

Griffith CS, Grimes DA: The validity of the postcoital test. Am J Obstet Gynecol 162:615–620, 1990.

Guzick DS, Sullivan MW, Adamson GD, et al: Efficacy of treatment for unexplained infertility. Fertil Steril 70:207–213, 1998.

Hughes EG: The effectiveness of ovulation induction and intrauterine insemination in the treatment of persistent infertility: A meta-analysis. Hum Reprod 12:1865–1872, 1997.

Jacobson TZ, Barlow DH, Koninckx PR, et al: Laparoscopic surgery for subfertility associated with endometriosis. Cochrane Database of Systematic Reviews 2004;p 2.

Larson-Cook KL, Brannian JD, Hansen KA, et al: Relationship between the outcomes of assisted reproductive techniques and sperm DNA fragmentation as measured by the sperm chromatin structure assay. Fertil Steril 80:895–902, 2003.

Lord JM, Flight IHK, Norman RJ: Insulin-sensitising drugs (metformin, troglitazone, rosiglitazone, pioglitazone, D-chiro-inositol) for polycystic ovary. Cochrane Database of Syst Rev 2004;p 2.

Mitwally MFM, Casper RF: Use of an aromatase inhibitor for induction of ovulation in patients with an inadequate response to clomiphene citrate. Fertil Steril 75:305–309, 2001.

Murray MJ, Meyer WR, Zaino RJ, et al: A critical analysis of the accuracy, reproducibility, and clinical utility of histologic endometrial dating in fertile women. Fertil Steril 81:1333–1343, 2004.

Sharara FI, Scott RT, Seifer DB: The detection of diminished ovarian reserve in infertile women. Am J Obstet Gynecol 179:804, 1998.

Silber SJ: Evaluation and treatment of male infertility. Clin Obstet Gynecol 43:854–888, 2000.

Sovino H, Sir-Petermann T, Devoto L: Clomiphene citrate and ovulation induction. Reprod Biomed Online 4:303–310, 2002.

Speroff L, Glass RH, Kase NG: Female infertility. In Speroff L, Glass RH, Kase NG (eds): Clinical Gynecologic Endocrinology and Infertility, 6th ed. Baltimore, MD, Lippincott Williams & Wilkins, 1999, pp 1013–1042.

Tanahatoe SJ, Hompes PG, Lambalk CB: Investigation of the infertile couple: Should diagnostic laparoscopy be performed in the infertility work up programme in patients undergoing intrauterine insemination? Hum Reprod 18:8–11, 2003.

Watson A, Vandekerckhove P, Lilford R, et al: A meta-analysis of the therapeutic role of oil soluble contrast media at hysterosalpingography: A surprising result? Fertil Steril 61:470–477, 1994.

13

ENDOMETRIOSIS AND ADENOMYOSIS

Mohamed A. Bedaiwy and Tommaso Falcone

Introduction

Endometriosis is a benign, chronic gynecologic disorder. Many clinical symptoms attributed to endometriosis are controversial. This stems from the absence of consensus regarding its etiology, pathogenesis, progression, clinical presentation, and treatment.

Endometriosis is defined as the presence and growth of the endometrial glands and stroma in a heterotopic location away from the normal endometrial lining. *Adenomyosis,* on the other hand, is the growth of endometrial glands and stroma into the myometrium to a depth of at least 2.5 mm from the basal layer of the endometrium. It is now established that endometriosis and adenomyosis are two separate entities.

Although the incidence of endometriosis seems to have risen over the past few decades, this increase is largely due to the growing use of laparoscopy in gynecologic practice, which makes it easier to diagnose endometriosis. Most cases of endometriosis are diagnosed during the reproductive years of a woman's life. It has been estimated that endometriosis is discovered in 5% to 15% of laparotomies and laparoscopies performed on women in this age group, in 30% of women with chronic pelvic pain, and in up to 40% of infertile women. Although the etiology of endometriosis is not yet well established, a large number of putative causes have been proposed. These include retrograde menstruation, vascular and lymphatic spread, mesothelial metaplasia, genetic predisposition, immunologic factors, and hormonal influences. Because diagnosis requires direct observation of the endometriotic spots, laparoscopy or laparotomy is needed for a definitive diagnosis. The natural course of the disease is unpredictable. To date, no single noninvasive approach can be used to definitively diagnose the disease. The ectopic endometrial tissue demonstrates cyclicity and is affected by the ovarian hormones. Consequently, it is a disease that most commonly affects women during their reproductive years, although adolescent and postmenopausal endometriosis are recognized subtypes.

Endometriosis has three unique clinicopathologic features. First, although it is a benign disease, it is locally infiltrative, invasive, and widely disseminating. Moreover, it exhibits neoangiogenesis and can affect lymph nodes.

Second, cyclic estrogen and progesterone levels stimulate its growth, whereas continuous levels suppress the disease. Third, women with advanced endometriosis may be asymptomatic, whereas women with mild disease may have debilitating chronic pelvic pain and long-standing resistant infertility.

Etiology

Although the exact etiology of endometriosis is unknown, the following theories are provided to explain independently or together why it occurs in some women and not others (Box 13-1).

Retrograde Menstruation Theory

Sampson's retrograde menstruation theory is probably the most accepted explanation of the disease pathophysiology. It assumes that pelvic endometriosis results from endometrial shed that regurgitates into the peritoneal cavity during menstruation, where it implants. The fact that the ovaries and the pouch of Douglas are the most commonly affected sites lends support to this hypothesis. Further support has been gained from many experiments in primates and clinical observations during laparoscopy. Moreover, endometriosis is frequently found in women with outflow obstruction of the genital tract (e.g., cervical atresia), transverse vaginal septum, and imperforate hymen. Despite its popularity, this theory does not explain why endometriosis does not occur in all women with retrograde menstruation or how endometriosis develops at extrapelvic locations.

Persistence of fibrin matrix could support the initiation of endometriotic lesions in the peritoneal cavity, explaining why some women with retrograde menstruation develop endometriosis while others do not. Hypofibrinolysis associated with the 4G allele of the plasminogen activatory inhibitor-1 gene (PAI-1), was found significantly more often in women with endometriosis compared with controls.

Coelomic Metaplasia Theory

This theory states that endometriosis arises from coelomic epithelial metaplasia. According to this theory, the coelomic epithelium of the peritoneal cavity retains its embryonic feature of multipotentiality and develops into endometriotic tissue. This hypothesis is supported by the ability of the closely similar ovarian surface epithelium to differentiate into several panels of different histologies. This theory provides the only plausible explanation for the development of endometriosis in prepubertal girls,

---

Box 13-1   Theories of Endometriosis

Retrograde menstruation
Coelomic metaplasia
Lymphatic and vascular metastases
Immunologic changes
Genetic predisposition
Iatrogenic dissemination
Direct implantation
Activation of embryonic rests

women with complete müllerian agenesis, and in rare cases, men. As in any metaplastic process, an inducing factor may initiate the process, although it is unclear what this may be. Some have postulated that environmental pollutants such as dioxins are responsible, but this has not been clearly demonstrated.

Lymphatic and Vascular Metastasis Theory

This theory explains rare cases of endometriosis at distant sites, such as the lung, eye, spinal column, forearm, thigh, and nose. Moreover, endometriotic tissue has been recovered from the lymph nodes of patients with the disease. According to this theory, the endometrial tissue is transported via the lymphatic and vascular channels.

Immunologic Theory

The basic premise of this theory is that the immune system is responsible for the pathogenesis of endometriosis. It explains why some women with retrograde menstruation develop endometriosis whereas most others do not. Growing evidence suggests that abnormalities in cell-mediated and humoral components of the immune system in peripheral blood and peritoneal fluid may be the leading etiology. Peritoneal macrophages, which are the predominate cell type in the peritoneal fluid of healthy women and patients with endometriosis, play a central role in the etiopathogenesis of the disease. Macrophages controlled by chemokines secrete numerous growth factors and cytokines that enhance the development of the disease. Vascular endothelial growth factor, tumor necrosis factor α (TNF-α), and interleukin 6 have received much attention. They probably promote angiogenesis, which facilitates the establishment of endometriosis. Other immunologic abnormalities that may be important in the pathophysiology of endometriosis include changes in the secretory products of T lymphocytes and decreased activity of natural killer cells. Support for the immunologic theory is growing to the extent that endometriosis is frequently viewed as an autoimmune disease.

Genetic Theory

Familial predisposition to endometriosis is being increasingly recognized. Simpson and associates demonstrated strong evidence of familial predispositions. First, they reported a seven-fold increase in the incidence of endometriosis in the close relatives of women with the disease compared with healthy control subjects. Second, one tenth of women with advanced disease have a first-degree relative with clinical manifestations of the disease. Third, women who have a family history of endometriosis usually develop the disease at a younger age and have more advanced disease than women whose first-degree relatives are free of the disease. Fourth, many genetic polymorphisms have been reported in patients with endometriosis. Lastly, gene deletions have been detected in women with endometriosis, including increased heterogenicity of chromosome 17 and aneuploidy. Environmental factors such as dioxin exposure are thought to play a role to make these genetic abnormalities manifest.

Direct Implantation Theory

Umbilical endometriotic spots are sometimes discovered in women after a cesarean delivery and laparoscopy, and endometriosis has been reported to develop in episiotomy scars. In these situations, the endometrial glands and stroma may have implanted into these areas during the surgical procedure.

Embryonic Rest Theory

Embryonic rests of the müllerian system in the pelvis are thought to be a precursor for pelvic endometriosis. This is the hypothesis offered to explain deeply infiltrating endometriosis of the cul-de-sac.

In conclusion, no single theory can explain all cases of endometriosis. Endometriosis is most likely caused by multiple factors, including retrograde transport of endometrium, coelomic metaplasia, immunologic perturbations, and a genetic predisposition.

324

Pathology

Anatomic Sites of Endometriosis

The left hemipelvis and ovary are more frequently affected than the right. Ovarian involvement often results in the formation of an endometrioma, a cystic collection of endometriosis. One theory to explain this difference is the left-sided presence of the sigmoid colon, which decreases fluid movement. These findings support the theory that endometriosis is caused by regurgitated endometrial cells. The pelvic peritoneum, posterior cul-de-sac, uterovesical pouch, and the uterosacral, round, and broad ligaments are also common pelvic sites for endometriosis. Pelvic lymph nodes are also involved in up to one third of cases. The cervix, vagina, and vulva are occasionally involved. The rectosigmoid is involved in up to 15% of cases, and it represents a clinical and surgical challenge. Table 13-1 lists the potential sites of endometriosis. Endometriosis can be superficial or deep. Any lesion that penetrates more than 5 mm into the subperitoneal tissues is considered a deep lesion.

Table 13-1

Anatomic Sites of Endometriosis

Common Reproductive Sites	Common Nonreproductive Sites	Uncommon Sites
Ovaries	Sigmoid colon	Umbilicus
Cul-de-sac and rectovaginal septum	Rectum	Cesarean section scar
Pelvic peritoneum	Appendix	Episiotomy scar
Cervix uteri	Bladder[*]	Small bowel
Vagina		Lungs
Fallopian tubes		Kidney
		Sciatic nerve
		Arms
		Nasal mucosa
		Spinal column
		Liver

*Deeper than the peritoneum.

Gross Pathology

The color, shape, and size of endometriotic lesions vary extensively, as do the surrounding inflammatory changes. The lesions can be nonhemorrhagic and subtle. The gross picture of the implant depends on the site, activity, dating of the cycle, and probably the duration of the disease. The lesions exhibit a variety of colors including red, brown, black, white, yellow, pink, or clear vesicle. The color depends mainly on the degree of fibrosis, the size of the implant, and the extent of neoangiogenesis and local hemorrhage. Red lesions are considered to represent the most active phase of the disease.

During the early stages of the disease, the small bleb-like lesions become raised above the surrounding tissues. As the disease progresses, they become larger and deeper in color, eventually turning into the characteristic "powder burn" areas or "chocolate cysts." The older lesions are usually fibrotic, puckered. or retracted from the surrounding tissue. Ovarian endometriomas vary considerably from 1 mm to large chocolate cysts greater than 8 cm in diameter. They are usually associated with periadnexal adhesions and densely adherent to the pelvic sidewalls or broad ligament.

Microscopic Pathology

Histopathologically, endometriosis is diagnosed by the presence of endometrial glands, endometrial stroma, and hemorrhage into the adjacent tissue. The presence of hemosiderin-laden macrophages in the peritoneal fluid or in the vicinity of the implants denotes old lesions. The ectopic endometrial tissue undergoes cyclic changes in response to estrogen and progesterone levels. The endometrial stroma will undergo decidualization upon exposure to high levels of progesterone. A severe inflammatory reaction is usually present due to repeated hemorrhage, which can lead to pressure atrophy of the implants.

Clinical Diagnosis

Symptoms

Many patients with endometriosis are asymptomatic. However, a variety of symptoms characterize endometriosis in symptomatic patients (Table 13-2).

Table 13-2

Symptoms and Signs of Endometriosis

	Symptoms			Signs	
Main	**Menstrual**	**Urinary**	**Rectal**	**Uterus**	**Adnexa**
Chronic pelvic pain	Dysmenorrhea	Suprapubic pain	Dyschezia	Cul-de-sac induration	Ovarian mass
		Dysuria	Constipation	Uterosacral	Fixed
Dyspareunia		Hematuria	Diarrhea	ligament	adnexae
Infertility			Cyclic bleeding per rectum	nodularity	
				Fixed, retroverted	

The classic symptoms of endometriosis are chronic pelvic pain and infertility. Chronic pelvic pain usually presents as secondary dysmenorrhea or dyspareunia. The dysmenorrhea usually begins before the commencement of menstruation. The extent of pelvic pain is not related to the extent of endometriosis in the female pelvis. The pain is believed to be mediated by prostaglandins and cytokines. It varies from a dull ache to severe pelvic pain and is generally present several days before and after the menstrual flow. A study to evaluate the presence of nerve fibers and histopathology of normal peritoneum and endometriosis-harboring peritoneum found that the presence of nerve fibers in peritoneum was not related to endometriosis. Consequently, the severity of endometriosis-related pain is not related to the density of nerve fibers in the peritoneum harboring the endometriotic implants. Deep dyspareunia is a characteristic feature of endometriosis, which is probably due to the immobility of the pelvic organs or involvement of the pelvic ligaments or peritoneum over the posterior fornix.

Infertility is associated with endometriosis. Approximately 15% of women with endometriosis have an associated anovulation. However, other mechanisms have been postulated to explain infertility associated with endometriosis (Boxes 13-2 and 13-3). Interestingly, the peritoneal fluid of patients with endometriosis was found in some studies to have detrimental effects on spermatozoa, oocytes, sperm-egg interaction, and early embryonic development.

Endometriosis involving the gastrointestinal and urinary tracts may be responsible for cyclic abdominal pain, intermittent constipation, diarrhea, dyschezia, urinary frequency, dysuria, and hematuria. Obstructive complications can develop in the gastrointestinal and urinary tracts. In rare

---

Box 13-2 Mechanisms of Endometriosis-Associated Infertility

Ovarian causes
Impaired folliculogenesis
Defective granulosa cell steroidogenesis
Luteinized unruptured follicle syndrome
Reduced oocyte quality
Luteal phase defects

Tubal causes
Tubal distortion
Distal tubal (fimbrial) adhesions
Tubal dysfunction

Immunologic causes
Autoimmunity
Antiendometrial antibody
Antiphospholipid antibody

Local peritoneal factors affecting gametes and early embryos
Cytokines
Prostaglandins
Macrophages

Defective implantation

> **Box 13-3** Possible Negative Effects of Cytokine-Rich Peritoneal Fluid on Gamete Function and Embryonic Development
>
> **Spermatozoa**
> Impairment of acrosome reaction
> Impairment of sperm motility
>
> **Oocyte**
> Impaired folliculogenesis
> Impaired oocyte quality
>
> **Sperm-oocyte interaction impairment**
>
> **Impaired embryonic development**
> Two-cell stage block
> Decreased blastulation

instances, endometriosis causes catamenial hemothorax, bloody pleural fluid, and massive ascites. Premenstrual spotting and menorrhagia are the most common forms of abnormal bleeding in up to 20% of patients with endometriosis.

Signs

A normal pelvic examination is the most frequent clinical finding in patients with endometriosis. However, fixed tender retroversion of the uterus is a classic finding in most patients with advanced endometriosis. In these patients, endometriotic implants can be often palpated over the uterosacral ligaments and in the pouch of Douglas on vaginal examination. The adnexae can be asymmetrically enlarged and tender and are often fixed to the broad ligament or lateral pelvic sidewall. In rare cases, speculum examination demonstrates small areas of endometriosis on the cervix or upper vagina. The signs of endometriosis reach their peak intensity during menstruation. Examination during menses may reveal lesions that may not be felt at other times of the cycle.

Laparoscopic Diagnosis of Endometriosis

Laparoscopy is the standard method for visually identifying endometriotic lesions; this is done under magnification within and outside the pelvis. The gold standard for confirmation of the diagnosis is laparoscopic visualization of endometriosis with its associated scarring and adhesion formation. Biopsy can histopathologically confirm the diagnosis. The extent of the disease should be described systematically according to American Society for Reproductive Medicine (ASRM) classification (Fig. 13-1). In the ASRM system, points are assigned for the severity of endometriosis on the basis of the size and depth of the implants and for the severity of the adhesions. Points are summed, and patients are assigned to one of four stages:

- Stage I: minimal disease, 1 to 5 points
- Stage II: mild disease, 6 to 15 points
- Stage III: moderate disease, 16 to 40 points
- Stage IV: severe disease, more than 40 points

Figure 13-1

American Fertility Society (AFS) scoring system of endometriosis.

Patient's name _____ Date _____

Stage I (Minimal) - 1–5
Stage II (Mild) - 6–15 Laparoscopy _____ Laparotomy _____ Photography _____
Stage III (Moderate) - 16–40 Recommended treatment _____
Stage IV (Severe) - >40
Total _____ Prognosis _____

PERITONEUM	ENDOMETRIOSIS	<1 cm	1–3 cm	>3 cm
	Superficial	1	2	4
	Deep	2	4	6
OVARY	R Superficial	1	2	4
	Deep	4	16	20
	L Superficial	1	2	4
	Deep	4	16	20

	POSTERIOR CULDESAC OBLITERATION	Partial		Complete	
		4		40	

	ADHESIONS	<1/3 Enclosure	1/3–2/3 Enclosure	>2/3 Enclosure
OVARY	R Filmy	1	2	4
	Dense	4	8	16
	L Filmy	1	2	4
	Dense	4	8	16
TUBE	R Filmy	1	2	4
	Dense	4*	8*	16
	L Filmy	1	2	4
	Dense	4*	8*	16

*If the fimbriated end of the fallopian tube is completely enclosed, change the point assignment to 16.

Additional endometrious: _____   Associated pathology: _____
_____   _____
_____   _____
_____   _____

To be used with normal tubes and ovaries

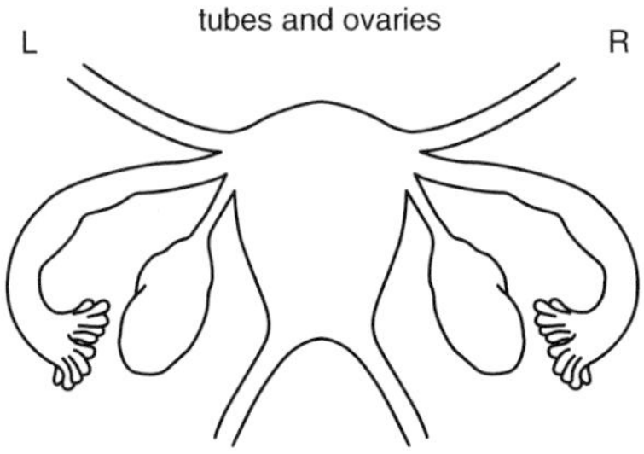

To be used with abnormal tubes and/or ovaries

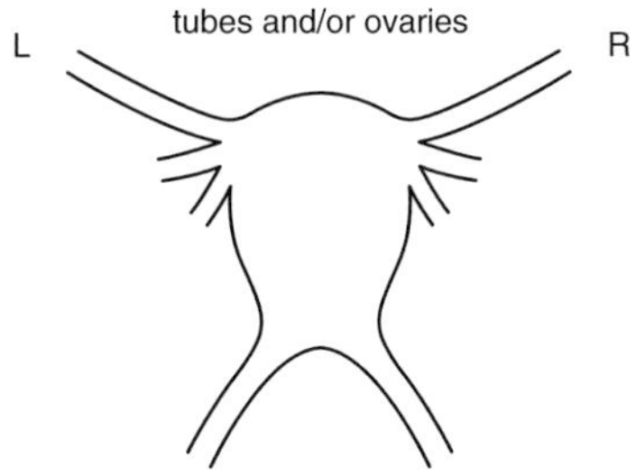

Endometriotic lesions seen at laparoscopy can have different presentations that sometimes occur simultaneously in one lesion (Fig. 13-2). The accuracy of visual identification of endometriosis at laparoscopy depends on the type of lesion. In one study, targeted biopsies were performed for histologic validation, and the laparoscopic findings and diagnosis were compared with the histologic results. The histologic results of the biopsies confirmed the presence of endometriosis in only 84.1% of patients; no evidence of endometriosis was observed in the other 15.9% of patients (false positive). One hundred percent of the "red" lesions, 92% of the "black" lesions, and 31% of the "white" lesions were correctly identified as endometriosis. This study concluded that endometriosis has multiple appearances and that the

Figure 13-2

Varied appearance of lesions in endometriosis on the bladder peritoneum.

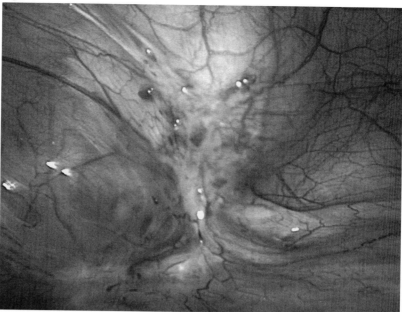

lesions may be confused with non-endometriotic lesions. It is clear that a diagnosis that does not include histology may lead to unnecessary prolonged medical treatment, and operations and may delay the proper treatment measures from being applied. Therefore, meticulous histologic confirmation should be the first step in the laparoscopic diagnosis and treatment of suspected endometriosis.

Imaging for Endometriosis

Ultrasound examination shows no specific signs for endometriosis. However, it can demonstrate the presence of an adnexal mass that could be an endometrioma. Magnetic resonance imaging has not been shown to be superior to transvaginal ultrasonography and should be reserved for exceptional cases.

Serum Markers for Endometriosis

For the past few decades, researchers have been searching for noninvasive methods of diagnosing endometriosis. One method involves measuring serum levels of cancer antigen 125 (CA-125). Levels are elevated in patients with endometriosis and are stage dependent. Despite its low specificity, it stands as the only available clinical marker. It is nonspecific, and levels are increased in the presence of myomas, acute pelvic inflammatory disease, and during the first trimester of pregnancy. It also has a low sensitivity. Consequently, it cannot detect early stages of the disease. Overall, CA-125 does not meet the criteria of an ideal screening or diagnostic test. Moreover, serial CA-125 levels are not cost-effective in following the progression of the disease or the effects of medical intervention.

Differential Diagnosis

Because endometriosis shares some clinical features with malignancy and inflammation, it is important to rule out disorders such as chronic pelvic inflammatory disease, ovarian malignancy, degenerating myomas, hemorrhage/torsion of ovarian cysts, adenomyosis, primary dysmenorrhea, intrinsic bowel disease such as irritable bowel, or intrinsic bladder disease such as interstitial cystitis. Rupture of a large endometrioma can cause signs of an acute abdomen and may mimic ectopic pregnancy, appendicitis, diverticulitis, and a bleeding corpus luteum cyst.

Although uncommon, endometriosis has been associated with malignancy. The criteria for malignant transformation that have been suggested are as follows: (1) the presence of both malignant and benign endometrial tissues in the same organ, (2) cancer arising in the tissue and not invading it from another source, and (3) the presence of tissue resembling endometrial stroma surrounding characteristic glands. It is estimated that cancers arise in approximately 1% of unselected cases when ovarian endometriosis is present. The majority of studies are case reports, small series, and reviews of cases of ovarian carcinoma with associated endometriosis. Recently, 1000 consecutive cases of surgically proven endometriosis were reviewed to evaluate the frequency and types of cancers that were associated with different types of endometriosis. Clear cell and endometrioid carcinomas were the malignancies most commonly seen in ovaries containing endometriosis, whereas clear cell adenocarcinoma and adenosarcoma were most commonly seen in conjunction with extraovarian endometriosis. Endometriosis was more strongly associated with endometrioid and clear cell carcinoma than serous and mucinous tumors.

Management

Management Plan

The main objective in the management of any disease is to prevent its progression or recurrence or, if possible, to eradicate it. These goals are far from being achieved in this puzzling disorder. The current protocols used to manage the disease are all symptom oriented, aimed mainly at treating chronic pelvic pain and infertility. Several randomized clinical trials have demonstrated the efficacy of the surgical treatment of endometriosis for chronic pain and infertility. The treatment plan must be tailored to meet a woman's expectations and her physician's experience. In addition, the patient's age, future reproductive plan, stage of endometriosis, symptom severity, and associated pelvic pathology will influence the treatment plan.

It is desirable—but not always necessary—to establish the nature and extent of endometriosis before therapy via diagnostic laparoscopy. Physicians can start empiric medical therapy with a gonadotropin-releasing hormone (GnRH) agonist without diagnostic laparoscopy once serious pelvic pathology has been excluded, but only in certain patients (e.g., those with chronic pelvic pain). Medical, surgical, or a combined approached could be instituted. Assisted reproductive techniques to overcome endometriosis-associated infertility are frequently needed.

Medical Therapy

The crux of medical treatment is hormone therapy (Table 13-3). Hormones are used to induce amenorrhea, thereby creating an environment that will inhibit growth and promote regression of the disease. Hormone therapy is effective at relieving pain. However, symptoms often recur once therapy is discontinued. Selection of hormone therapy for an individual patient depends on the physician's evaluation of effectiveness, tolerability, cost, and expected patient compliance. There are no major differences between the currently available hormonal therapies regarding their clinical effectiveness in treating chronic pelvic pain. Hormone therapy usually suppresses symptoms and may prevent progression of endometriosis, but it does not provide a long-lasting cure. Hormone therapy for endometriosis-associated pain is effective in two thirds of patients at 1 year. However, a meta-analysis showed that hormone therapy has no value in the management of endometriosis-associated infertility.

Danazol Danazol was once the preferred initial therapy for endometriosis. However, its adverse effect profile has led to decreased use of this drug. Today, GnRH agonists, progestins, and oral contraceptives are used more frequently. Danazol is an orally active mild androgen. It is a synthetic isoxazole derivative of ethisterone (17-alpha-ethinyltestosterone). It creates a hypoestrogenic and hyperandrogenic environment in steroid-sensitive organs. Danazol's side effects are related to its androgenic properties (*see* Table 13-3). It binds to sex hormone binding globulin, which results in a three-fold increase in endogenous free testosterone levels. It may also modulate immunologic functions through an effect on macrophages.

A dose of 800 mg daily produces amenorrhea and inhibits ovulation within 4 to 6 weeks. It leads to estrogen and progesterone levels similar to those of the early follicular phase. Danazol induces atrophy of the endometriotic implants and the endometrium. Generally, patients are instructed to take 400 to 800 mg daily for 6 months. Because the half-life of this oral drug is between 4 and 5 hours, it is recommended to prescribe one tablet four times daily rather than two tablets twice daily. It is metabolized in the liver with cleavage of its isoxazole ring. Danazol has been reported to mildly elevate serum liver enzyme levels in patients with endometriosis, which should be considered when lengthy therapy is needed. A new low-dose regimen has been recently proposed that may decrease the adverse effects.

Danazol produces female pseudohermaphroditism in a developing fetus. Consequently, women should use mechanical contraceptives for the first month of use. Hormonal changes are experienced by 80% of patients taking danazol. The spectrum of adverse effects include menopausal hot flushes, atrophic vaginitis, emotional lability, weight gain, fluid retention, migraine headaches, dizziness, fatigue, depression, oily skin, facial hair, and deepening of the voice, which may not be reversible with discontinuation of therapy (*see* Table 13-3). Up to 10% to 20% discontinue taking the drug because of these adverse effects. Danazol also decreases high-density lipoprotein (HDL) cholesterol levels and elevates low-density lipoprotein (LDL)

Medical Therapy of
Endometriosis

Table 13-3

Medical Therapy	Dose	Adverse Effects
Danazol	600–800 mg daily	Acne, hot flashes, weight gain, muscle cramps, adverse lipid changes ($\downarrow$HDL, $\uparrow$LDL), decreased breast size, hirsutism, irreversible deepening of the voice, breakthrough bleeding, mood changes, and liver damage
Progestins		
Medroxyprogesterone acetate	50–100 mg orally every day	Breakthrough bleeding, weight gain, fluid retention, acne, breast tenderness, headaches, mood changes, muscle cramps, and adverse lipid changes ($\uparrow$LDL, $\downarrow$HDL)
Depo-Provera	150 mg intramuscularly every 3 months	As above
Depo subQ provera 104	104 mg subcutaneously	
Norethindrone acetate	5–15 mg daily	As above
GnRH agonists		
Leuprolide	Depot: 3.75 mg IM every month, or 11.25 mg IM every 3 months OR 0.5–1.0 mg subcutaneously daily	Hot flashes, sleep disturbances, vaginal dryness, joint pain, breakthrough bleeding, headaches, mood change, bone loss ($\downarrow$bone density 5% to 6%) and adverse lipid changes ($\uparrow$LDL, $\downarrow$HDL)
Goserelin	3.6 mg subcutaneously every month OR 10.8 mg subcutaneously every 3 months	As above
Nafarelin	200 μg intranasally twice daily	As above
GnRH agonists with add-back		
	Norethindrone acetate 5–10 mg orally every day	
	Premarin 0.625–1.25 mg + norethindrone acetate 5 mg orally every day	
	Cyclic etidronate 400 mg + calcium 500 mg + norethindrone acetate 2.5 mg orally every day	
Gestrinone	2.5 mg orally twice daily	Acne, hirsutism

HDL, High-density lipoprotein cholesterol; LDL, low-density lipoprotein cholesterol; IM, intramuscularly.

levels. Most important, deaths have been reported from liver failure with prolonged use of this drug.

GnRH Agonists

GnRH agonists are the most commonly used group of drugs for the medical therapy of endometriosis. Prolonged administration of GnRH agonists suppresses gonadotropin secretion and secondarily suppresses endogenous ovarian steroidogenesis. The GnRH agonists bind to receptors for a prolonged time and induce protracted periods of downward regulation. They are 200 times more potent than natural GnRHs. Agonists may be administered via intravenous, intramuscular, subcutaneous, intravaginal, or intranasal routes. Leuprolide acetate (Lupron, parenteral), nafarelin acetate (Synarel, intranasal), and goserelin acetate (Zoladex, subcutaneous implant) are the most commonly used members of this category. The usual doses are provided in Table 13-3.

Chronic use of GnRH agonists produces many endocrine effects. Levels of serum estrone, estradiol, testosterone, and androstenedione decrease significantly. The total serum estrone and estradiol levels and the free serum estradiol concentration are two to three times less than those induced by chronic danazol administration. Unlike danazol, GnRH agonists have neither androgenic side effects nor significant effects on total serum cholesterol, HDL, or LDL levels.

The most common adverse effects of GnRH agonists are hot flashes, vaginal dryness, and insomnia (*see* Table 13-3). A decrease in bone mineral density has been demonstrated in the lumbar spine. However, the bone mineral density appears to recover completely 1 to 2 years after cessation of therapy.

GnRH agonist therapy results in symptomatic relief in up to 90% of patients with endometriosis. The maximal therapeutic effects are seen with endometriotic spots smaller than 1 cm in diameter. A multicenter, double-blind, double-placebo randomized study demonstrated that the therapeutic response to GnRH and danazol was similar. The primary advantage of GnRH agonists over danazol is better patient compliance. Moreover, they produce pseudomenopause without causing androgenic side effects on other steroid-sensitive organs.

GnRH Agonists and Add-Back Therapy

Many clinicians advise the use of "add-back" hormone replacement therapy with chronic GnRH agonist regimens. This reduces vasomotor symptoms, vaginal atrophy, and demineralization of bone. Many randomized series have demonstrated that add-back therapy does not interfere with the agonist's ability to relieve pelvic pain. Add-back therapy has been attempted with progestins and a combination estrogen/progestin in a dose used for hormone replacement therapy. Alternatively, organic bisphosphonates and calcium can be used instead of hormone therapy. Add-back regimens reduce adverse clinical and metabolic side effects associated with hypoestrogenism. Moreover, extended GnRH agonist therapy can be safe for up to 1 year provided that the appropriate add-back preparation is used concomitantly. Norethindrone is the most widely used preparation for add-back therapy. Norethindrone is approved by the FDA for use as add-back therapy with GnRH agonists. Long-term GnRH-agonist down-regulation is safe and effective when combined with HRT add-back for up to 10 years. Furthermore, the low-dose pulsed progestogen, continuous estrogen HRT regimen seems to be safe for use as add-back therapy in terms of bone mineral density.

Oral Contraceptives

For the past three decades, the most commonly used regimen for the treatment of mild/moderate symptoms of endometriosis has been continuous daily combined oral contraceptive pills (COCs). The proven effectiveness, safety, affordability, and availability are probably the main reasons for their widespread use. A 6- to 12-month COC regimen produces amenorrhea and a "pseudopregnancy." Patients are generally instructed to take a single daily monophasic oral contraceptive pill beginning on the third day of their period and to take the tablets continuously until breakthrough bleeding occurs. At that point, the daily dose is doubled to overcome the breakthrough bleeding. After 5 days of a double dose, most patients can return to taking one to two pills per day. The short-term treatment goal is to maintain amenorrhea on the lowest possible dose of the combination used. Discontinuing the COCs, allowing a full flow, and then reinitiating the oral agent can also reduce breakthrough bleeding. Some physicians advise allowing a period to occur every 3 months of continuous use. The adverse effects of COCs include weight gain and breast tenderness, both of which may lead a woman to quit using the pills. However, up to 80% of patients experience symptomatic relief on continuous oral contraceptive therapy, which make them one of the most commonly prescribed medical therapies.

Progestins

Progestins are a possible alternative for women who have a contraindication to or cannot tolerate high doses of estrogen during continuous COC therapy. Medroxyprogesterone (Provera; 30 mg orally per day) or depo-medroxyprogesterone (Depo-Provera; 150 mg intramuscularly every 3 months to a maximum of 200 mg every month) can induce amenorrhea. Subcutaneous medroxyprogesterone acetate (Depo subQ provera 104; Pfizer) was approved by the U.S. Food and Drug Administration (FDA) for the treatment of endometriosis-related pelvic pain. However, both are suitable only in women who have completed their childbearing because injectable medroxyprogesterone can delay the return of fertility. The most prominent side effects associated with medroxyprogesterone are breakthrough spotting or bleeding, which can be treated with low-dose estrogen. Moreover, mood changes, depression, and irritability are also produced by high-dose progestins. Clinical results with progestin-only therapy are similar to those with continuous oral contraceptives.

Antiprogestins

Mifepristone (RU-486) is the only clinically available member of this group. It is known for its use as an abortifacient during the first trimester. Many cohort studies have shown that a dose of 50 to 100 mg/day induces amenorrhea without hypoestrogenism and decreases pain in patients with endometriosis. It is generally well tolerated. However, it has not been used widely for the treatment of endometriosis-associated pain and has not been evaluated in prospective randomized controlled trials.

Gestrinone

Gestrinone has antiestrogen and antiprogesterone effects on the endometrium. It is derived from a 19-nortestosterone steroid nucleus. It acts as an agonist-antagonist on progesterone receptors and an agonist on androgen receptors. It binds weakly to estrogen receptors and induces endometrial atrophy and/or amenorrhea. In a dose of 2.5 mg twice per week, it was shown to be as effective as danazol and GnRH agonists. Its side effects are similar to those of danazol (e.g., acne, hirsutism) and GnRH agonists (e.g., hot flashes). It reduces serum progesterone and sex hormone binding globulin levels but has a small effect on gonadotropins and estradiol. Gestrinone does not negatively affect bone density but has an androgenic effect on serum lipids (decreased HDL, increased LDL). It is available in Europe but not the United States.

GnRH Antagonists

GnRH antagonists block pituitary GnRH receptors, which causes an immediate, dose-dependent decline in gonadotropin secretion and secondarily decreases estrogen production. Theoretically, they are beneficial in the treatment of endometriosis. Animal models have already shown that they suppress endometriotic tissues. However, not enough human data are available to justify their use in clinical practice. In addition, they are expensive and must be delivered via frequent subcutaneous injections.

Nonsteroidal Anti-Inflammatory Drugs

Nonsteroidal anti-inflammatory drugs (NSAIDs) do not treat endometriosis lesions, but they are important in the treatment of endometriosis-associated pain. Because NSAIDs inhibit cyclo-oxygenase, they ameliorate symptoms mediated by prostaglandin synthesis, including dysmenorrhea. The most commonly used NSAIDs are ibuprofen and naproxen. They are equally effective at relieving chronic pelvic pain and dysmenorrhea. Gastric irritation is the most common adverse effect of NSAIDs. Cyclo-oxygenase 2 (COX-2) inhibitors are no more effective at treating dysmenorrhea than naproxen or ibuprofen, but they have a much lower risk of gastric ulceration. The main disadvantage of COX-2 inhibitors is their high cost and possible increased risk of cardiovascular and cerebrovascular events.

Surgical Therapy

Surgery can be used as a primary approach for both chronic pelvic pain and infertility, or when medical therapy fails. It is usually the main treatment for women with moderate or severe endometriosis, especially in those with adhesions and extragenital endometriosis. Surgery is also the primary treatment modality in cases of endometriomas, for which medical therapy has been shown to be ineffective. Unlike medical therapy, surgery has been shown to improve fertility rates in infertile patients.

Surgical Approach

Endometriosis can frequently be treated at the time of diagnostic laparoscopy. Depending on the operative technique chosen, endometriosis can be coagulated, vaporized, or resected. In cases of deeply infiltrating endometriosis, important structures such as the ureters and pelvic sidewall vascular structures must be carefully dissected. Surgical resection provides tissue samples for histologic confirmation of the disease and exclusion of associated malignancy. There are no studies showing that one energy modality is superior to another. Treatment can usually be accomplished using a laparoscopic approach, which is associated with a shorter recovery period and hospital stay than laparotomy. Laparoscopy also reduces the extent of subsequent adhesions.

Sutton and colleagues conducted a prospective, randomized, double-blind controlled trial to assess the efficacy of laser laparoscopic surgery in the treatment of pain associated with minimal, mild, and moderate endometriosis. They included 63 patients with endometriosis-associated chronic pelvic pain. The patients were randomly assigned to undergo laser ablation of the implants plus laparoscopic uterine nerve ablation or diagnostic laparoscopy. Pain symptoms were recorded subjectively and by visual analogue scale. The women and follow-up evaluator were blinded to the treatment modality instituted. Follow-up evaluation was performed at 3 and 6 months after surgery. They found that laser laparoscopy resulted in significant pain relief compared with expectant management 6 months postoperatively. They concluded that operative laparoscopy is an effective treatment for alleviating pain symptoms in women with stages I, II, and III endometriosis. Moreover, the majority of patients who were treated surgically have symptom relief. Less benefit was observed for milder stages of endometriosis. The majority of patients whose pain was initially relieved from surgery remained pain-free 1 year later.

A meta-analysis of two separate randomized clinical trials that evaluated the effect of surgery on stage I and II endometriosis showed a clear beneficial effect on fertility. No randomized trials have been reported for advanced endometriosis, but it is generally believed that fertility is improved after surgery.

Conservative Surgical Interventions

Endometriosis-associated adhesions may be minimal or extensive, filmy or dense, and avascular or vascular. The infiltrative nature of the disease and the associated scarring from endometriosis result in a loss of cleavage planes and tedious, difficult dissections. Special care must be taken not to injure the bladder or bowel during excision of areas that impinge on these structures.

Conservative surgery entails removing all visible endometriotic lesions, preserving ovarian function, and restoring normal pelvic anatomy. In conservative operations, implants are destroyed, endometriomas are removed, and adhesions are lysed; appendectomy and presacral neurectomy may be concurrently performed (Box 13-4). The success of surgical management for fertility depends on how well the surgeon adheres to the principles of microsurgery, which include minimal tissue handling, avoiding tissue desiccation, avoiding hypoxia of the peritoneum, and attempting to restore the normal pelvic anatomy. Laparoscopy has been shown to be as effective as laparotomy in the treatment of ovarian endometriomas. Transvaginal ultrasound-guided aspiration, fenestration, or simple aspiration at laparoscopy are neither proven nor recommended treatments of endometriosis. Maximal surgical effort should be adopted for the excision of the cyst wall and coagulation of the unexcised component. Presacral neurectomy or

---

Box 13-4 Laparoscopic Operative Procedures for Patients with Endometriosis

Adhesiolysis
Excision of peritoneal implants
Ovarian endometriomas: resection, endocoagulation
Genitourinary endometriosis: excision, ureterolysis, resection-reanastomosis, and ureteroneocystomy
Gastrointestinal involvement: simple excision, disc excision and closure, and sigmoidectomy with colorectal anastomosis
Cul-de-sac restoration
Laparoscopic presacral neurectomy
Laparoscopically assisted vaginal hysterectomy and bilateral oophorectomy

---

laparoscopic uterosacral nerve ablation (LUNA) can be performed for intractable endometriosis-associated chronic pelvic pain. However, a recent Cochrane review showed that there is insufficient evidence to recommend the use of LUNA in the management of dysmenorrhea, regardless of the cause. A successful presacral neurectomy relieves only midline pain and does not diminish pain in other areas of the pelvis. Presacral neurectomy was recently found to improve long-term cure rates and quality of life in women treated with conservative laparoscopic surgery for severe dysmenorrhea due to endometriosis.

Definitive Surgical Interventions

In women with advanced disease who have completed childbearing, it is possible to perform a total abdominal hysterectomy with preservation of one or both ovaries. However, a recurrence rate of 30% has been reported, and a second operation involving oophorectomy may be needed. If the ovaries are spared, the need for reoperation increases.

Definitive surgery is indicated for patients with advanced endometriosis who have completed their families and patients with persistent pain after medical and conservative surgery. Definitive surgery involves total abdominal hysterectomy, bilateral salpingo-oophorectomy, and the removal of all visible endometriosis.

Combined Approach

Medical and surgical therapies are often combined for advanced endometriosis. However, the advantages of either preoperative or postoperative medical therapy are debated. It is postulated—but unproven—that preoperative therapy facilitates the subsequent operative procedure. Postoperative medical therapy has been shown in one study to be effective in decreasing recurrence. Others have not supported this conclusion, however.

Decision Making and Selection of Therapy

When deciding on the choice of treatment, the patient's age, symptoms, and future reproductive plans are the most important factors to be considered. Surgical therapy is usually recommended during laparoscopy to establish the diagnosis of the disease. Surgical therapy is the only option after failure of medical therapy. Because patients with endometriosis have many clinical scenarios, many treatment regimens exist. An endometriosis treatment algorithm is provided in Table 13-4.

Table 13-4

Chronic pelvic pain		Infertility	
Investigation: negative Treat with NSAIDS/COCs. If no relief, two options include:		Investigation If HSG and other investigations have normal results, options include:	

Diagnostic
  laparoscopy
	Empiric GnRHa	Diagnostic
		  laparoscopy
			SO+IUI

Endometriosis
  confirmed:
    ↓
	If relief in
	  2 months, treat
	  for 6 months.
		Diagnosis
		  confirmed:
		Treat surgically.	

Treat surgically. ←	If none, scope.	If no pregnancy
		  and early
			If no pregnancy
			  and advanced

If no relief:
Medical suppression
If still no relief,
  options include:
		disease, two
		  options include:
		1. Gonadotropin
			disease:
			IVF-ET

1. Reoperation/
  presacral
  neurectomy, if
  indicated
		+ IUI
		2. IVF-ET	

2. TAH/BSO			
3. Pain management			

If still no relief:
Long-term pain
  treatment
  programs			

NSAIDs, Nonsteroidal anti-inflammatory drugs; COCs, combined oral contraceptives; GnRHa, gonadotropin-releasing hormone agonist; TAH, total abdominal hysterectomy; BSO, bilateral salpingo-oophorectomy; HSG; hysterosalpingogram, IVF/ET, *in vitro* fertilization/embryo transfer; SO, superovulation; IUI, intrauterine insemination.

Management of Endometriosis at Specific Locations

The gastrointestinal tract is the most common site of extrapelvic endometriosis. A wide spectrum of gastrointestinal tract endometriotic lesions exist, ranging from a tiny spot on the serosa of the bowel to obstruction of the rectosigmoid. The rectosigmoid colon and the anterior wall of the rectum are involved in almost all cases of gastrointestinal tract endometriosis. Endometriosis of the appendix is not uncommon, but endometriosis of the small bowel is rare.

Besides fluctuating bowel habits, palpation of a pelvic mass or "rectal shelf" on rectovaginal examination is suggestive of endometriosis. Sigmoidoscopy, colonoscopy, and barium enema do not produce findings that are specific for endometriosis. Normal study results do not rule out endometriosis. A filling defect and the absence of a mucosal lesion with the presence of extramucosal involvement are suggestive of endometriosis. The definitive diagnosis and differentiation of endometriosis from malignancies of the bowel are usually made at the time of surgery.

The treatment of endometriosis of the gastrointestinal tract depends on the extent and severity of symptoms. Hormonal therapy does not appear to have long-term benefit. The importance of preoperative preparation of the bowel is a cornerstone for successful and safe surgery. Surgical procedures include superficial excision, full-thickness excision of the wall, or bowel resection with primary colorectal anastomosis. The latter can be performed entirely by laparoscopy. Although laparoscopic treatment of colorectal endometriosis, even in advanced stages, was shown to be safe, feasible, and effective in nearly all patients, laparotomy is still the most commonly used access for most gynecologists.

Urinary Tract Endometriosis

The urinary tract is involved in 10% of women with endometriosis. In most cases, small endometriotic spots are discovered on the bladder peritoneum and anterior cul-de-sac (*see* Fig. 13-2). The most serious form of urinary endometriosis is ureteral obstruction, which occurs in fewer than 1% of women with advanced pelvic endometriosis. Mural endometriosis and retroperitoneal scarring can lead to ureteral obstruction.

Urinary endometriosis can be treated medically or surgically. Endometriosis of the ureter can be treated by danazol or GnRH agonists. However, surgical therapy is the preferred approach for ureteric endometriosis. The operation requires highly skilled surgeons and urologic consultation. Laparoscopic ureterolysis (Fig. 13-3) and resection of the disease and possibly the ureter with ureteroneocystostomy are the treatments of choice.

Future Treatments

Novel strategies and concepts for the treatment of endometriosis have been recently introduced. The most promising of these new developments are aromatase inhibitors, immune system modulators, and neoangiogenic inhibitors.

339

Figure 13-3

Ureterolysis.

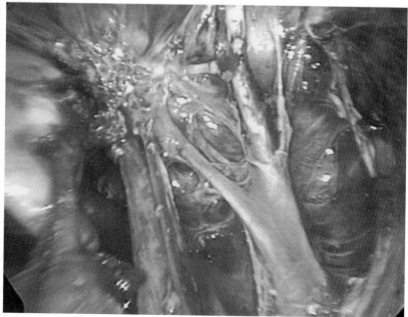

Aromatase Inhibitors

Aromatase converts testosterone and androstenedione to estradiol and estrone. Endometriotic implants express aromatase and consequently generate their own estrogen, which maintains their presence. Animal studies have shown that aromatase inhibitors can effectively eradicate endometriotic implants. Clinical experience with aromatase inhibitors is restricted to case reports. A combination of letrozole and norethindrone acetate has been used to treat 10 patients with the disease. This combination significantly reduced laparoscopically visible and histologically confirmed endometriosis in all patients. Moreover, pain was relieved in nine of 10 patients who were resistant to hormonal therapy. Ailawadi et al. concluded that letrozole should be a candidate for the medical management of endometriosis.

Immune System Modulators

Alterations in the immune system, cytokine secretion, and growth factors are main features of endometriosis. TNF-α seems to play a pivotal role in the modulation of immune system responses, endometrial cell turnover, and cell adhesion. Studies on anti-tumor necrosis factor therapy (pentoxifylline) in animals have shown regression of implants and reversal of surgically induced endometriosis-associated infertility. A small pilot study of pentoxifylline in humans with endometriosis-associated infertility also showed benefit.

One of the most promising areas seems to be the selective blockade of TNF-α activity. In rats with experimental endometriosis, recombinant human TNF-α binding reduced the size of endometriotic-like peritoneal lesions significantly. Similarly, a recent prospective randomized placebo- and drug-controlled study in baboons showed that recombinant human TNF-α binding protein effectively inhibits the development of endometriosis and endometriosis-related adhesions. However, because of the dense adhesive disease, the role of these inhibitors may be limited in patients with advanced endometriosis.

Inhibition of Matrix Metalloproteinases

Suppression of matrix metalloproteinases (MMPs) by progesterone or by a natural MMP inhibitor inhibits the establishment of ectopic lesions of human endometrium in severe combined immune deficiency mice. However, no clinical data are available to support this claim. Currently, a wide variety of MMPs are being evaluated.

Antiangiogenesis Therapy for Endometriosis

Because endometriosis is highly dependent on angiogenesis, an effective therapeutic agent would need to not only prevent endometriosis lesions, but also inhibit the growth of established lesions. Recently, outstanding results have been achieved with Avastin—a humanized anti-vascular endothelial growth factor (VEGF) antibody used in experimental tumor therapy. This approach of neutralizing VEGF provided the first proof that antiangiogenesis is applicable in humans. The major role of VEGF in endometriosis may predict the success of Avastin in endometriosis.

Animal (i.e., mice) models have shown that angiogenesis is a prerequisite for the maintenance and growth of endometriosis and that different kinds of inhibitors of angiogenesis effectively interfere with established endometriosis lesions. However, antiangiogenesis therapy must be tested in humans before it can be deemed safe for clinical use.

Assisted Reproduction and Endometriosis

The use of controlled ovarian hyperstimulation with or without intrauterine insemination may be beneficial for a short course of therapy in patients with endometriosis who have normal pelvic anatomy before more aggressive approaches are used. If controlled ovarian hyperstimulation does not result in a pregnancy, the next step is to turn to more advanced techniques such as conventional *in vitro* fertilization (IVF) or intracytoplasmic sperm injection (ICSI). If initial surgery fails to restore fertility in patients with moderate (stage III) or severe (stage IV) endometriosis-related infertility, IVF with embryo transfer is an effective alternative. Reoperation for asymptomatic patients offers little added benefit. Meta-analyses suggest that patients with endometriosis have a poorer ovarian response and need a higher dose of gonadotropins in IVF or ICSI programs. It remains unclear whether the presence or degree of endometriosis is associated with impaired oocyte quality or the fertilization and implantation rate. The effects of endometriosis surgery on the outcome of subsequent IVF cycles have been studied, and regression analyses have showed that the interval between surgery and oocyte aspiration does not affect implantation rates.

Conclusions

A large number of medical treatments are currently available to treat endometriosis. When deciding on the treatment approach, it is important to consider the patient's preference and to provide appropriate counseling on the risks, adverse effects, and cost. COC pills and NSAIDs are first-line therapy because they are affordable and have mild side effects. If adequate relief is not obtained or if the adverse effects prove intolerable, consideration should be given to the use of progestagens or a GnRH agonist with add-back therapy. If none of these medications prove beneficial or if adverse effects are too pronounced, then surgery is warranted.

ADENOMYOSIS

Introduction

Adenomyosis was believed to be part of endometriosis and was historically referred to as *endometriosis interna*. However, endometriosis and adenomyosis are discovered in the same patient less than 20% of the time. Moreover, endometriosis and adenomyosis are clinically two different entities. The only common feature is the presence of ectopic endometrial glands and stroma. Adenomyosis is derived mostly from aberrant glands of the basal layer of the endometrium. Therefore, these glands are not hormonally responsive and do not undergo the cyclic changes associated with cyclic ovarian hormone production.

Pathogenesis

The exact pathogenesis of adenomyosis remains unknown. Adenomyosis is usually an incidental finding during histopathologic assessment of hysterectomy specimens and autopsy. The barrier between the endometrium and myometrium is broken, and the stroma and glands begin to invade the myometrium along the path of least resistance; this growth is usually adjacent to lymphatic and vascular channels.

Pathology

Gross Pathology

There are two distinctly different pathologic types of adenomyosis:

1. *Diffuse adenomyosis:* There is a diffuse noncapsulated involvement of both anterior and posterior walls of the uterus. The posterior wall is the most commonly affected side.
2. *Focal adenomyosis:* This results in an asymmetric uterus, and the area of adenomyosis may have a pseudocapsule. Diffuse adenomyosis is found in approximately two thirds of cases, and focal adenomyosis is found in one third.

In the first type, the uterus is symmetrically enlarged, usually two to three times its normal size. The cut surface has a spongy appearance and protrudes convexly. The cut surface of a uterus with adenomyosis is darker than the white surface of fibroid. There is no definite capsule around the adenomyosis. It may be associated with both endometrial hyperplasia and endometrial carcinoma. Approximately two thirds of women with adenomyosis have coexistent pelvic pathology—most commonly myomas but also endometriosis, endometrial hyperplasia, and salpingitis isthmica nodosa.

Microscopic Pathology

The standard criterion used in the diagnosis of adenomyosis is the finding of endometrial glands and stroma more than one low-powered field 2.5 mm from the basal layer of the endometrium. On histopathologic examination, endometrial glands and stroma are seen inside the myometrium. The endometrial glands rarely undergo the same cyclic changes as the normal uterine endometrium, despite the fact that both estrogen and progesterone receptors are expressed in tissue samples from adenomyosis.

The glands are either inactive or display a proliferative pattern. There is a lack of inflammatory cells surrounding adenomyotic foci, and bleeding is common in these ectopic areas. Decidual changes might happen during pregnancy or during estrogen-progestin therapy for endometriosis. The surrounding myometrium usually undergoes hyperplasia and hypertrophy of individual muscle fibers. This change in the myometrium produces the globular enlargement of the uterus.

Clinical Diagnosis

Symptoms

Most women with adenomyosis are asymptomatic. Adenomyosis is more prevalent in parous women between the ages of 35 and 50 years. Classically, adenomyosis presented with secondary dysmenorrhea and menorrhagia. Occasionally, the patient complains of dyspareunia, which is midline in location and deep in the pelvis. The severity of pelvic symptoms increases proportionally to the depth of penetration and the total volume of disease in the myometrium.

Signs

On rectovaginal examination, the uterus is bulky and diffusely enlarged, usually two to three times the normal size. Uterine size is typically less than a 14-week gestation. The uterus is globular and tender immediately before and during menstruation.

Imaging

Ultrasound, particularly transvaginal, can help differentiate between adenomyosis and uterine myomas. However, differentiating an adenomyoma from a leiomyoma is sometimes difficult. Magnetic resonance imaging is far more sensitive in differentiating adenomyosis from uterine leiomyoma, especially preoperatively in women who desire future fertility. Attempts have been made to establish the diagnosis preoperatively by transcervical needle biopsy of the myometrium. However, even with multiple needle biopsies, the sensitivity of the test is too low to be of practical clinical value.

343

Management

Medical

Patients with adenomyosis are usually symptomatically treated with GnRH agonists, cyclic hormones, or prostaglandin synthetase inhibitors. However, medical treatment is usually not satisfactory.

Surgical

Endometrial ablation has not been successful in the treatment of menorrhagia associated with adenomyosis. Local resection of focal adenomyosis is sometimes successful. Diffuse adenomyosis had been treated with reductive uterine surgery in cases in which the diagnosis is made at laparotomy for a presumptive leiomyoma. Uterine embolization does not appear to be successful. Hysterectomy is the definitive treatment when the conservative approach fails, although its use is affected by the woman's age, parity, and future reproductive plans. The size of the uterus, degree of prolapse, and presence of associated pelvic pathology determine the choice of abdominal, laparoscopic, or vaginal route for the hysterectomy.

KEY POINTS

Endometriosis

1. Endometriosis is a benign, progressive, recurrent, and locally invasive disease.
2. Retrograde menstruation, coelomic metaplasia, vascular metastasis, immunologic changes, iatrogenic dissemination, and genetic predisposition are the main etiologic theories of endometriosis.
3. The most common cytokine found in the peritoneal fluid is TNF-α.
4. The ovaries are the site most commonly affected by endometriosis. The uterine serosa, the anterior and posterior cul-de-sac, and the uterosacral, round and broad ligaments are also common sites.

Continued

KEY POINTS—CONT'D

5. Grossly, endometriotic lesions can be red, brown, black, white, yellow, pink, or clear vesicles and lesions.
6. Histopathologic confirmation is important to document the diagnosis.
7. Microscopically, endometriosis is characterized by the presence of endometrial glands, stroma, and hemorrhage into the adjacent tissue.
8. Endometriosis is a major cause of cyclic pelvic pain and infertility.
9. Signs of endometriosis include a fixed, occasionally tender, retroverted uterus with scarring and nodularity of the uterosacral ligaments and the pouch of Douglas.
10. Serum CA-125 levels and imaging have poor sensitivity for the diagnosis of nonovarian endometriosis.
11. Medical suppressive therapy is not a useful treatment for endometriosis-associated infertility.
12. GnRH agonists can be used empirically to treat chronic pelvic pain before a diagnostic laparoscopy if investigation has ruled out other disease.
13. Surgical therapy for chronic pelvic pain has been proved to be effective in a randomized controlled trial.
14. Surgical therapy for infertility has been proved to be effective in a randomized controlled trial.

Adenomyosis

15. Adenomyosis is mostly asymptomatic.
16. Menorrhagia is a common symptom of adenomyosis.
17. Surgery is the preferred treatment for adenomyosis.

SUGGESTED READING

Ailawadi RK, Jobanputra S, Kataria M, et al: Treatment of endometriosis and chronic pelvic pain with letrozole and norethindrone acetate: A pilot study. Fertil Steril 81(2):290–296, 2004.

American Fertility Society: Management of endometriosis in the presence of pelvic pain. Fertil Steril 60:952–955, 1993.

American Society for Reproductive Medicine: Revised American Society for Reproductive Medicine classification of endometriosis: 1996. Fertil Steril 67:817–821, 1997.

Bailey HR, Ott MT, Hartendorp P: Aggressive surgical management for advanced colorectal endometriosis. Dis Colon Rectum 37:747–753, 1994.

Barbieri RL: Hormone treatment of endometriosis: the estrogen threshold hypothesis. Am J Obstet Gynecol 166:740–745, 1992.

Bedaiwy MA, Casper RF: Treatment with leuprolide acetate and hormonal add-back for up to 10 years in stage IV endometriosis patients with chronic pelvic pain. Fertil Steril 86(1):220–222, 2006.

Bedaiwy MA, Falcone T: Peritoneal fluid environment in endometriosis: Clinicopathological implications. Minerva Ginecologica 55(4):333–345, 2003.

Bedaiwy MA, Falcone T: Laboratory testing for endometriosis. Clin Chem Acta 340(1–2):41–56, 2004.

Bedaiwy MA, Falcone T, Mascha EJ, Casper RF: Genetic polymorphism in the fibrinolytic system and endometriosis. Obstet Gynecol 108(1):162–168, 2006.

Bedaiwy MA, Falcone T, Sharma RK, et al: Prediction of endometriosis with serum and peritoneal fluid markers: A prospective controlled trial. Hum Reprod 17(2):426–431, 2002.

Bergqvist A: Extragenital endometriosis: A review. Eur J Surg 158:7–12, 1992.

Byun JY, Kim SE, Choi BG, et al: Diffuse and focal adenomyosis: MR imaging findings. Radiographics 19:S161–S170, 1999.

D'Hooghe TM, Bambra CS, Raeymaekers BM, Koninokx PR: Serial laparoscopies over 30 months show that endometriosis in captive baboons (Papio anubis, Papio cynocephalus) is a progressive disease. Fertil Steril 65:645–649, 1996.

Donnez J: Today's treatments: medical, surgical and in partnership. Int J Gynaecol Obstet 64:S5–S13, 1999.

Farquhar C, Sutton C: The evidence for the management of endometriosis. Curr Opin Obstet Gynecol 10:321–332, 1998.

Fedele L, Piazzola E, Raffaelli R, Bianchi S: Bladder endometriosis: Deep infiltrating endometriosis or adenomyosis? Fertil Steril 69:972–975, 1998.

Fong YF, Singh K: Medical treatment of a grossly enlarged adenomyotic uterus with the levonorgestrel-releasing intrauterine system. Contraception 60:173–175, 1999.

García-Velasco JA, Arici A: Chemokines and human reproduction. Fertil Steril 71:983–993, 1999.

Jerby BL, Kessler H, Falcone T, Milsom JW: Laparoscopic management of colorectal endometriosis. Surgical Endoscopy 13(11):1125–1128, 1999.

Leyendecker G: Endometriosis is an entity with extreme pleomorphism. Hum Reprod 15:4–7, 2000.

Ling FWPelvic Pain Study Group: Randomized controlled trial of depot leuprolide in patients with chronic pelvic pain and clinically suspected endometriosis. Obstet Gynecol 93:51–58, 1999.

Mahnke JL, Dawood MY, Huang JC: Vascular endothelial growth factor and interleukin-6 in peritoneal fluid of women with endometriosis. Fertil Steril 73:166–170, 2000.

Mahutte NG: Medical management of endometriosis associated pain. Obstet Gynecol Clin North Am 30 (1):133–135, 2003.

Mahutte NG, Arici A: Endometriosis and assisted reproductive technologies: Are outcomes affected? Current Opin Obstet Gynecol 13(3):275–279, 2001.

Marcoux S, Maheux R, Berube S: Laparoscopic surgery in infertile women with minimal or mild endometriosis. Canadian Collaborative Group on Endometriosis. N Engl J Med 337(4):217–222, 1997.

Mettler L, Schollmeyer T, Lehmann-Willenbrock E, et al: Accuracy of laparoscopic diagnosis of endometriosis. J Soc Laparoendoscopic Surgeons 7(1):15–18, 2003.

Nisolle M, Donnez J: Peritoneal endometriosis, ovarian endometriosis, and adenomyotic nodules of the rectovaginal septum are three different entities. Fertil Steril 68:585–596, 1997.

Olive DL, Pritts EA: Treatment of endometriosis. N Engl J Med 345(4):266–275, 2001.

Outwater EK, Siegleman ES, Van Deerlin V: Adenomyosis: current concepts and imaging considerations. AJR 170:437–441, 1998.

Pagidas K, Falcone T, Hemmings R, Miron P: Comparison of reoperation for moderate (stage III) and severe (stage IV) endometriosis-related infertility with in vitro fertilization–embryo transfer. Fertil Steril 65(4):791–795, 1996.

Proctor ML, Farquhar CM, Sinclair OJ, Johnson NP: Surgical interruption of pelvic nerve pathways for primary and secondary dysmenorrhea. Cochrane Database of Systematic Reviews 4:CD001896, 2004.

Redwine DB: Ovarian endometriosis: A marker for more extensive pelvic and intestinal disease. Fertil Steril 72:310–315, 1999.

Reinhold C, Tafazoli F, Mehio A, et al: Uterine adenomyosis: Endovaginal US and MR imaging features with histopathologic correlation. Radiographics 19:S147–160, 1999.

Ryan IP, Taylor RN: Endometriosis and infertility: New concepts. Obstet Gynecol Surv 52:365–371, 1997.

Shakiba K, Falcone T: Tumour necrosis factor-α blockers: potential limitations in the management of advanced endometriosis? A case report. Hum Reprod 21(9):2417–2420, 2006.

Schenken RS, Guzick DS: Revised endometriosis classification: 1996. Fertil Steril 67:815–816, 1997.

Smith S, Pfeifer SM, Collins JA: Diagnosis and management of female infertility. JAMA 290 (13):1767–1770, 2003.

Stern RC, Dash R, Bentley RC, et al: Malignancy in endometriosis: Frequency and comparison of ovarian and extraovarian types. Int J Gynecol Pathol 20(2): 133–139, 2001.

Surrey ESthe Add-Back Consensus Working Group: Addback therapy and gonadotropin-releasing hormone agonists in the treatment of patients with endometriosis: Can a consensus be reached? Fertil Steril 71:420–424, 1999.

Sutton CJ, Ewen SP, Whitelaw N, Haines P: Prospective, randomized, double-blind, controlled trial of laser laparoscopy in the treatment of pelvic pain associated with minimal, mild, and moderate endometriosis. Fertil Steril 62(4):696–700, 1994.

Takayama K, Zeitoun K, Gunby RT, et al: Treatment of severe postmenopausal endometriosis with an aromatase inhibitor. Fertil Steril 69:709–713, 1998.

Tulandi T, Felemban A, Chen MF: Nerve fibers and histopathology of endometriosis-harboring peritoneum. J Am Assoc of Gynecol Laparosc 8(1):95–98, 2001.

Wheeler JM, Malinak LR: The surgical management of endometriosis. Obstet Gynecol Clin North Am 31:147–156, 1989.

Whiteside JL, Falcone T: Endometriosis-related pelvic pain: What is the evidence? Clin Obstet Gynecol 46(4): 824–830, 2003.

Zondervan KT, Cardon LR, Kennedy SH: The genetic basis of endometriosis. Curr Opin Obstet Gynecol 13(3):309–314, 2001.

Zullo F, Palomba S, Zupi E, et al: Long-term effectiveness of presacral neurectomy for the treatment of severe dysmenorrhea due to endometriosis. J Am Assoc Gynecol Laparosc 11(1):23–28, 2004.

14

ABNORMAL UTERINE BLEEDING

Linda D. Bradley

MENSTRUAL DYSFUNCTION

Dysfunctional uterine bleeding (DUB) is defined as abnormal bleeding in the absence of intracavitary or uterine pathology. Most commonly, DUB is associated with anovulatory menstrual cycles, systemic dysfunction, or medical conditions; it may coexist with intrauterine pathology. It has been estimated that a woman has a 1-in-20 lifetime risk of seeing a doctor for the evaluation of menstrual disturbance. Half of all hysterectomies in the United States are performed to treat abnormal uterine bleeding. Approximately 20% of hysterectomies are performed in women with a normal uterine size.

Most menstrual cycles occur every 21 to 35 days. Normal menstrual flow lasts 3 to 7 days, with the majority of blood loss occurring within the first 3 days. Normal menstrual flow amounts to 35 mL and consists of effluent debris and blood. Patients with menorrhagia lose more than 80 mL of blood with each menstrual cycle and often develop anemia. In general, most normal menstruating women use five to six pads or tampons per day and do not complain of social embarrassment or inconvenience. Approximately 16 mg of iron is lost with each menstrual cycle, and this will rarely result in anemia in women with adequate intake of dietary iron. More than 50% of women who complain of menorrhagia may not actually have heavy menses. Indeed, some patients change their sanitary products more often for hygienic reasons, personal preference, or concern for toxic shock syndrome, than due to heavy flow. Social obligations, sexual activity, hobbies, work, and travel are not interrupted with normal menstrual function.

The following definitions describe menstrual patterns associated with abnormal uterine bleeding:

- *Oligomenorrhea:* Cycle length greater than 35 days
- *Polymenorrhea:* Cycle length less than 21 days
- *Amenorrhea*: Absence of menses for 6 months, or absence of menstrual periods for three normal cycles
- *Menorrhagia:* Heavier and increased flow occurring at regular intervals or loss of more than 80 mL of blood
- *Metrorrhagia:* Irregular episodes of bleeding

- *Menometrorrhagia:* Longer duration of flow occurring at unpredictable intervals
- *Postmenopausal bleeding:* Bleeding that occurs more than 12 months after the last menstrual cycle
- *DUB:* Excessive, erratic, or irregular bleeding not associated with intrauterine pathology

PREVALENCE

Determination of the prevalence of abnormal uterine bleeding is imprecise; however, 9% to 30% of reproductive-aged women have menstrual irregularities requiring medical evaluation. Approximately 15% to 20% of scheduled office gynecologic visits are for evaluation of abnormal uterine bleeding, exceeded only by vaginitis as a chief complaint. Additionally, 25% to 50% of all gynecologic surgical procedures are for the treatment or evaluation of menstrual dysfunction. The majority of menstrual aberrations occur in the menarche or perimenopause.

PATHOPHYSIOLOGY

The hallmark of normal menstrual bleeding is the final result of fluctuations in the hypothalamic-pituitary-adrenal-ovarian axis leading to predictable denudation and sloughing of the endometrium. Hemorrhage followed by prompt hemostasis and repair causes stabilization and regrowth of the endometrium. Physiologically, constant low levels of estrogen prime the endometrium. Normal secretion of progesterone from the corpus luteum stabilizes the endometrium, decreases vascular fragility, and supports the endometrial stroma. Patients with menorrhagia typically have an imbalance of prostaglandin levels and increased fibrinolytic activity.

An intact coagulation pathway is important in regulating menstruation. Menstruation disrupts blood vessels and, in the face of normal hemostasis, the injured blood vessels are rapidly repaired. Restoration of the blood vessel requires successful interaction of platelets and clotting factors. Tissue factors and collagen, located within vessels beneath the endometrium, create a nidus at the site of vessel injury to which platelets adhere, creating a platelet plug that halts bleeding. Simultaneously, exposure of tissue factor activates the clotting cascade, the end point of which is the formation of a fibrin net, which stabilizes the platelet plug or evolving clot. Von Willebrand's factor (VWF) is a large multimeric protein that causes platelets to adhere to sites of blood vessel injury. VWF also protects factor VIII from degradation in the circulation and facilitates fibrin and platelet interactions that result in the formation of a stable clot.

Abnormal uterine bleeding can usually be classified as either *anovulatory* bleeding or *ovulatory* dysfunctional bleeding. Anovulatory DUB is usually due to failure of the corpus luteum to sustain the developing endometrium. Anovulatory bleeding can be episodic or continuous. Patients with anovulatory cycles typically do not experience constitutional premenstrual symptoms. Cycles that vary in length by more than 10 days from one cycle to another are likely anovulatory.

Puberty and the perimenopausal years are typically associated with anovulatory menstrual cycles. The immature hypothalamic-pituitary axis does not develop the necessary hormonal feedback to sustain the endometrium. Likewise, the decline of inhibin levels and rise in follicle-stimulating hormone (FSH) levels reflect the loss of follicular activity and competence as the perimenopausal transition occurs.

Ovulatory dysfunctional bleeding occurs when ovulatory cycles coexist with intracavitary lesions, including polyps, hyperplasia, endometrial cancer, or fibroids, that cause erratic bleeding. Patients who ovulate typically have the following symptoms: breast discomfort, increased mucoid vaginal discharge at mid cycle, premenstrual cramping and bloating, and mood and appetite changes. Tests to confirm ovulatory status are listed in Box 14-1.

SIGNS AND SYMPTOMS

Abnormal bleeding is frustrating for women and is associated with an array of symptoms. Frequent complaints include heavier or prolonged menstrual flow, social embarrassment, diminished quality of life, sexual compromise, and alteration in lifestyle. Pain is not a common presenting symptom unless associated with passage of large blood clots. Incessant menstrual blood loss can be associated with anemia. Typical complaints of anemia include fatigue; unusual food cravings for ice, starch, or dirt (i.e., pica); and headaches. Severe anemia may cause fainting, congestive heart failure, exercise induced fatigue, shortness of breath, and the inability to perform routine activities. DUB is rarely associated with the need for a blood transfusion unless it is a chronic condition. Hemorrhagic shock and death are rare sequelae for DUB.

DIAGNOSIS

Diagnosis of DUB requires a detailed history and review of systems, a thorough physical examination, and appropriate laboratory testing. Eliciting a detailed clinical history will alert the physician to systemic and medical conditions that cause menstrual dysfunction (Box 14-2). Inherited and

Box 14-1   Tests to Confirm Ovulatory Status
Measurement of basal body temperature
Strict menstrual charting
Measurement of serum progesterone concentration
Monitoring urinary luteinizing hormone excretion
Sonographic demonstration of a periovulatory follicle

acquired disorders of coagulation, liver, and renal diseases frequently present with symptoms of abnormal uterine bleeding. A list of questions that are helpful in formulating a differential diagnosis for DUB are listed in Box 14-3.

Box 14-2   Causes of Menstrual Dysfunction

Anatomic
Polyps
Fibroids
Adenomyosis
Cervical (ectropion, cervicitis, eversion)
Endometritis (sexually transmitted diseases, tuberculosis, foreign body)
Ectopic pregnancy
Retained products of conception
Sacculation of cesarean section scar
Endometrial ossification (foreign body) from therapeutic abortion
Endometriosis
Hyperplasia
Malignancy (vulvar, vaginal, cervical, uterine, ovarian, fallopian)
Nongenital (bladder, bowel, rectum)

Endocrine
Thyroid dysfunction
Elevated prolactin (prolactinoma)
Polycystic ovarian disease
Adrenal dysfunction
Hypothalamic/pituitary dysfunction
Estrogen-producing tumors

Hematologic
Anemia
Coagulopathy
Von Willebrand's disease
Platelet disorders
Leukemia

Systemic
Renal impairment
Liver disorders
Obesity
Anorexia
Chronic illness
Rapid fluctuations in weight

Medications
Anticoagulants
Steroids
Herbal and soy products
Antipsychotic agents
Selective serotonin reuptake inhibitors

Miscellaneous
Smoking
Depression
Excessive alcohol intake
Sexually transmitted diseases

Box 14-3 Questions Helpful in Formulating a Differential Diagnosis for DUB

When did the bleeding begin?

What is the pattern of bleeding (i.e., with coitus, amount, duration)?

Is there a family history of bleeding problems, difficulties with bleeding from minor wounds (tooth extraction), nose bleeds, oral bleeding, intestinal bleeding, ecchymosis, petechiae, hemarthroses, soft tissue hemorrhage, hematuria, purpura, hematomas, or easy bleeding after lacerations?

Do you have a new sexual partner?

Is there associated pain, odor, fever, or discharge?

Has there been any change in weight, exercise habits, hirsutism, bruising, acne, hair loss, or eating habits?

Have you had any recent trauma?

Are you using herbal products (e.g., ginseng, ginkgo biloba, soy)?

Are you using any new medications (e.g., SSRIs, antipsychotics, corticosteroids)?

Have you had a recent pregnancy, miscarriage, or therapeutic abortion?

Have you had a recent cesarean section?

SSRIs, Selective serotonin reuptake inhibitors.

The physical examination must be detailed and complete, even in the presence of heavy bleeding. Initially, a thorough inspection of the skin is important, with particular attention made to establish the presence of acanthosis nigricans (seen in women with insulin resistance and anovulation), ecchymosis, or hyperandrogenism (i.e., hirsutism, acne, clitoromegaly, or male pattern baldness). Thyromegaly should be ruled out. A thorough gynecologic examination should be performed, with a systematic evaluation of the vulva, vagina, cervix, uterus, adnexa, bladder, and rectum. Paying special attention to the cervix is important to exclude cervicitis, ectropion, sexually transmitted ulcerations, and cervical polyps. The speculum should be rotated to fully visualize the vaginal fornices and to establish the absence of ulcerations or foreign bodies. The patient should be instructed to empty her bladder to facilitate the evaluation of the adnexae as well as the uterine contour, size, and the presence of uterine tenderness.

The history and physical examination should be used to guide the choice of laboratory studies. Pregnancy testing should always be performed in sexually active women (even those who have had a tubal ligation) and in adolescents (even those who deny sexual activity). In those who have persistent vaginal bleeding after pregnancy, a β-human chorionic gonadotropin should be checked to exclude trophoblastic disease. A Papanicolaou (Pap) smear should be performed as appropriate to rule out cervical causes of bleeding, with biopsy of any visible lesions, even if cytology has negative results. Thyroid-stimulating hormone levels should be evaluated as necessary to exclude hypothyroidism or hyperthyroidism. In addition, prolactin levels should be checked if the patient complains of galactorrhea, oligomenorrhea, or decreased libido. Liver and renal function tests should be checked in women with signs or symptoms of systemic disease. Endometrial biopsy should be performed in women older than 35 years of age, or younger if risk factors for endometrial hyperplasia or malignancy are present. Transvaginal ultrasound (TVUS), saline infusion sonography (SIS), hysteroscopy, or magnetic resonance imaging (MRI) may be used in selected cases (see discussion to follow).

SPECIAL CONSIDERATION: VON WILLEBRAND'S DISEASE

VWF causes platelets to adhere to sites of blood vessel injury, and the lack of this protein causes abnormal bleeding. Von Willebrand's disease (VWD) results from low levels of VWF (type 1), abnormal VWF (type 2), or total absence of VWF (type 3).

VWD is the most common bleeding disorder in women, affecting 1% to 2% of the population and 10% to 35% of women with menorrhagia. A survey of women with VWD revealed that 95% experienced menorrhagia compared with 61% of control subjects, and 59% of women with VWD experienced postpartum hemorrhage versus 21% of control subjects. Other gynecologic aberrations experienced by women with VWF include pain with ovulation, hemorrhagic ovarian cysts, intraoperative bleeding, antepartum bleeding, postpartum hemorrhage, wound complications, and miscarriage. Women with profuse menorrhagia and normal uterine size should be screened for VWD; 13% to 20% of women offered surgical intervention may have the subtle form of type 1 disease.

The spectrum of bleeding in women with VWD ranges from mild bleeding to life-threatening hemorrhage and death. Type 1 disease is usually mild and may escape detection; type 3, accounting for less than 1% of the disease, is severe and life threatening and is diagnosed early in life. The disease is usually inherited in an autosomal-dominant fashion but may occasionally be an acquired disease.

The American College of Obstetricians and Gynecologists (ACOG) recommends testing for VWD in adolescents with severe menorrhagia, in adult women with significant menorrhagia without another apparent cause, and in women undergoing hysterectomy for menorrhagia.

The laboratory workup for VWD is expensive and consists of a panel of tests, including von Willebrand's ristocetin cofactor activity, VWF antigen, factor VIII coagulant activity, ristocetin-induced platelet aggregation, von Willebrand's multimer analysis, and a bleeding time. ACOG suggests that the single best screening test for VWD is von Willebrand ristocetin cofactor activity. More recently, the platelet function analyzer PFA-100 (Dade Behring Inc., Deerfield, IL) has been shown to be both sensitive (90% to 100%) and specific (88% to 95%) in the detection of VWD and platelet function disorders.

Normal hemostasis requires normal collagen and tissue factors—both of which cannot be tested with today's technology. However, the number of platelets is easily detected with a complete blood cell count. Normal prothrombin time and partial thromboplastin time essentially exclude a deficiency of clotting factors (with the rare exception of factor XIII deficiency). Referral to a hemophilia treatment center or a hematologist with an interest in hemostasis and thrombosis is imperative for women with abnormal test results or normal test results but a bleeding history suggestive of VWD.

SPECIAL CATEGORIES OF PATIENTS WITH ABNORMAL UTERINE BLEEDING

Premenarchal Girls

Vaginal bleeding in girls under the age of 9 years deserves special mention. In these patients, sexual abuse should always be considered. Foreign bodies, vulvovaginitis, urologic dysfunction (e.g., urethral prolapse), precocious menstruation, and neoplasm should also be considered in the differential diagnosis.

Adolescents

Anovulatory bleeding contributes to most abnormal vaginal bleeding in adolescents. However, adolescents who require hospitalization, who present with a hemoglobin level less than 10 g/dL, or who require blood transfusion have a risk for coagulopathies approaching 20% to 30%. Specifically, adolescents need evaluation for VWD with ristocetin cofactor assay before initiating hormonal therapy. A rare cause of menorrhagia in this group occurs from congenital or acquired arteriovenous malformation. When traditional surgical approaches aggravate the condition, arteriovenous malformation should be suspected and diagnosed by pelvic arteriography. A list of laboratory tests that should be performed in adolescents with menorrhagia is listed in Box 14-4.

Perimenopause

Perimenopause begins with the first clinical signs of approaching menopause (usually cycle irregularity and vasomotor symptoms) and finishes 1 year after the last menstruation. In North America, the average duration of menopausal transition is 4 years, and its hallmark is menstrual irregularity. Approximately 50% of women will experience menstrual abnormalities by age 45.5 years, 75% of women by age 47.8 years, and 95% by age 50.8 years. Intermittent anovulation during the perimenopause causes recurrent bouts of DUB and associated physical complaints: bloating, cramping, water retention, fatigue, decreased mental clarity, diminished concentration, vaginal dryness, hot flashes, and night sweats. The hormonal milieu is characterized by decreased inhibin levels, variable

Box 14-4 Laboratory Tests in Adolescents with Menorrhagia
Serum HCG
Bleeding time
PT and PTT
CBC with platelets
Ristocetin cofactor assay (VWF)

HCG, Human chorionic gonadotropin; PT, prothrombin time; PTT, partial prothrombin time; CBC, complete blood count; VWF, von Willebrand factor.

estradiol levels, and normal FSH concentrations. Menstrual cycles may be episodically ovulatory and predictable, followed by episodes of erratic menses. This is often frustrating for the patient and physician because the pattern of bleeding changes dramatically.

Seltzer et al. retrospectively reviewed 500 perimenopausal women and categorized bleeding patterns as hypomenorrhea (70%); menorrhagia, metrorrhagia, and/or hypermenorrhea (18%); and sudden cessation of menses (12%). Landgren et al. evaluated 13 women longitudinally with multiple hormonal analyses between 4 and 9 years before menopause and during the year of menopause. They noted an increased frequency of anovulatory cycles characterized by elevated FSH concentrations within 30 cycles of final menstruation. In women with hormonal evidence of ovulatory cycles, FSH did not consistently increase. In addition to menstrual cycle irregularity, there was hormonal heterogeneity.

When evaluating women with perimenopausal menstrual irregularities, pregnancy and cancer must be excluded from the differential diagnosis. Most pregnancies in the perimenopause are unplanned and associated with a high degree of miscarriage and therapeutic abortion. The incidence of uterine cancer ranges from 10 to 40 cases per 100,000 woman-years among women ages 40 to 50 years and increases to 110 cases per 100,000 women aged 70 years.

Oral contraceptive therapy in the perimenopause should be the first line of therapy rather than conventional hormone replacement therapy; traditional doses of postmenopausal hormone replacement therapy do not suppress ovulation or prevent pregnancy. In healthy, nonsmoking women older than 35 years of age, oral contraceptive pills regulate menstrual cycles, decrease vasomotor symptoms, improve bone mineral density, and decrease the need for surgical intervention for DUB. Additionally, endometrial and ovarian cancer rates are reduced in women using oral contraceptive therapy. Generally, oral contraceptives are well tolerated and enhance menstrual health and quality of life for the perimenopausal woman.

Menopausal Bleeding

Menopause is defined as the cessation of menstrual bleeding for 12 months. Approximately 10% of women have reached menopause by age 45 years, 80% of women by age 52 years, and 95% of women by age 55 years. Because bleeding is the most common symptom of endometrial cancer, any bleeding after 12 months of amenorrhea warrants immediate evaluation, no matter how scant or episodic it is. One exception to this rule is in women using sequential hormone therapy, in whom predictable and scheduled bleeding is expected. Endometrial cancer occurs in up to 12.5% of women presenting with postmenopausal bleeding (range, 1% to 25%) and must be excluded from the differential diagnosis. Noncancerous intracavitary lesions including polyps, submucosal fibroids, and endometrial hyperplasia account for 20% to 40% of cases of abnormal uterine bleeding. The differential diagnosis of postmenopausal bleeding is listed in Box 14-5.

Basic laboratory testing in postmenopausal bleeding should include Pap smear, endometrial biopsy, and TVUS. A Pap test should be performed

---

Box 14-5 Differential Diagnosis of Postmenopausal Bleeding

Endometrial atrophy
Uterine polyps
Uterine fibroids
Endometritis
Endometrial hyperplasia
Endometrial cancer
Nongenital sources (e.g., vulvar, vaginal, cervical, fallopian tubes, ovarian, bowel, rectum, bladder)
Anticoagulation therapy
Postradiation therapy

---

because cervical cancer has a bimodal distribution, peaking between ages 35 to 39 and 60 to 64 years. Many insurance companies will only permit Pap smears every 2 to 3 years, and it is possible that many patients with cervical disease may not have been screened for several years. Endometrial biopsy is highly accurate in detecting endometrial cancer when the cancer is global (not focal), involves a greater surface area of the endometrium, and is exophytic. Endometrial biopsy is less invasive and more cost effective than dilation and curettage. However, endometrial biopsy does miss focal lesions such as polyps or fibroids as well as focal disease occurring near the cornua or fundus.

Endometrial Hyperplasia and Endometrial Cancer

Endometrial carcinoma most frequently occurs in the sixth and seventh decades of life, with 75% occurring in women older than age 50 years. Bruchim et al. found that both time since the menopause and endometrial thickness together are predictive of endometrial cancer risk. Specifically, among 95 women with postmenopausal bleeding, the incidence of endometrial cancer increased with the number of years since menopause. No patient had endometrial cancer when the endometrium was less than 5 mm thick, but 18.5% had cancer when the endometrium exceeded 9 mm. The incidence of cancer was 2.5% in women who had been menopausal for 5 years or less but was 21.4% in those who had been menopausal more than 15 years. Evidence suggests that measurement of endometrial thickness by TVUS can accurately discriminate between women at high and low risk of endometrial cancer if a 5-mm endometrial thickness cutoff is used. In a meta-analysis of more than 6000 women with postmenopausal bleeding, the use of a 5-mm cutoff to define abnormal endometrium identified 96% of women with endometrial cancer and 92% of women with any endometrial pathology with false-positive rates of 39% and 10%, respectively. The likelihood of endometrial cancer increases with increasing thickness of the endometrium.

ACOG guidelines recommend endometrial biopsy in women older than 35 years with anovulatory uterine bleeding to rule out endometrial hyperplasia or cancer. Younger patients with bleeding that does not respond to medical therapy or with a history of prolonged unopposed estrogen stimulation resulting from chronic anovulation are also candidates for endometrial sampling. Independent risk factors for endometrial hyperplasia are listed in Box 14-6.

Box 14-6   Independent Risk Factors for Endometrial Hyperplasia

Diabetes
Prolonged steroid use
Obesity
Long history of irregular cycles
Unopposed estrogen therapy
Tamoxifen use
Suspected polycystic ovarian syndrome
Strong family history of ovarian, breast, or colon cancer

CLINICAL TOOLS USED TO EVALUATE THE ENDOMETRIUM

Historically, medical therapy is instituted for 3 months, and when it fails, additional evaluation is warranted. This guideline is appropriate for hemodynamically stable patients with normal laboratory evaluation results. Increasingly, evaluation with imaging is being used more frequently with the initial workup, minimizing unnecessary trials of medical therapy when intracavitary lesions are evident.

Endometrial Biopsy

Endometrial biopsy is generally performed in the office with a Pipelle instrument. The biopsy can be performed quickly, with few complications, and is generally well tolerated by the patient. It has a high sensitivity for detecting endometrial cancer and hyperplasia, but a low sensitivity for detecting other intracavitary lesions including polyps and submucosal fibroids. A meta-analysis of 39 studies reviewing 7914 premenopausal and postmenopausal women with endometrial Pipelle biopsy noted that the detection rate of endometrial cancer was 99.6% in postmenopausal women and 91% in premenopausal women. The detection rate for atypical hyperplasia was 88%, and the specificity was 98% to 100%.

Lesions encompassing a small surface area may be missed. Some studies suggest that the biopsy instrument samples between 10% to 25% of the endometrial cavity. Patients with persistent symptoms despite a normal biopsy and TVUS need further evaluation with SIS or hysteroscopy.

Transvaginal Ultrasound

TVUS is helpful in evaluating women with abnormal uterine bleeding who have a negative endometrial biopsy result or continue to experience abnormal bleeding despite medical therapy. TVUS is most sensitive in detecting disease in patients with postmenopausal bleeding, since a cutoff of 5 mm or less reliably excludes endometrial cancer. In premenopausal women, endometrial thickness varies between the proliferative phase (4 to 8 mm) and the secretory phase (8 to 14 mm), and TVUS should be scheduled between days 4 to 6 of menstrual cycle, when the endometrium is the thinnest. TVUS permits rapid assessment of size, position, and presence of uterine fibroids. The texture of the endometrium can be evaluated for homogeneity or heterogeneity. Adnexal pathology and pelvic tenderness can be assessed. If the uterine size is greater than 12 gestational weeks, then transabdominal scanning is preferred.

Measurement of the endometrial echo in the postmenopausal woman is helpful in determining whether endometrial biopsy or further imaging studies are necessary. Normally, the endometrial echo measures less than 5 mm. Increased endometrial thickness is associated with intrauterine synechiae, endometrial hyperplasia, endometrial polyps, fibroids, and endometrial cancer. When the endometrium is greater than 5 mm, cannot be visualized completely, is indistinct, or is indeterminate, an enhanced view is required with SIS or hysteroscopy. An endometrial echo of less than 5 mm is associated with malignancy in fewer than 0.5% of cases.

Saline Infusion Sonography

SIS infuses saline into the endometrial cavity during TVUS to enhance the image. Many alternate terms have been used to describe this technique: echohysteroscopy, hydrosonography, sonohysterography, sonohysterogram, sonohysterosalpingography, and sonoendovaginal ultrasound. SIS allows the clinician to evaluate the uterus for intracavitary lesions more accurately than TVUS. Causes of increased endometrial thickness can be clearly differentiated with saline infusion. Current indications for SIS are displayed in Box 14-7.

Increasingly, gynecologists are using the more streamlined concept of "one-stop evaluation" for menstrual disorders by combining physical examination, basic laboratory studies, and endometrial imaging (e.g., TVUS or SIS) with endometrial biopsy as indicated. Surgical intervention can be more directly implemented when this evaluation suggests surgical instead of medical therapy.

Hysteroscopy

Hysteroscopy permits full visualization of the endometrial cavity and endocervix and is helpful in diagnosing focal lesions that are missed with endometrial sampling. Thin operative hysteroscopes, with outer diameter sizes ranging from 3 to 5 mm, can be used easily and comfortably in the office. Rapid visual inspection permits accurate diagnosis of atrophy, endometrial hyperplasia, polyps, fibroids, retained products of conception, and endometrial cancer. Directed endometrial biopsies are possible with some

---

Box 14-7 Indications for Saline Infusion Ultrasound

Abnormal bleeding in premenopausal or postmenopausal patients
Evaluation of an endometrium that is thickened, irregular, immeasurable, or poorly defined by conventional transvaginal ultrasound (TVUS)
Irregular endometrial appearance by TVUS in women using tamoxifen
The need to differentiate between sessile and pedunculated masses of the endometrium
Presurgical evaluation of intracavitary fibroids

hysteroscopes. Office hysteroscopy accurately diagnoses many conditions associated with abnormal bleeding. The likelihood of endometrial cancer diagnosis after a negative hysteroscopy result is 0.4% to 0.5%.

Magnetic Resonance Imaging

If conservative medical management of menorrhagia or dysmenorrhea fails to improve a patient's symptoms after evaluation reveals a normal endometrial cavity, MRI may be useful in diagnosing adenomyosis. MRI is also useful in evaluating uterine anomalies, although the increased cost of this procedure over ultrasound rarely justifies its use.

THERAPY

Medical therapy with oral contraceptive pills or progesterone therapy is the hallmark for the treatment anovulatory menstrual cycles. Patients with ovulatory DUB must be evaluated for intracavitary uterine pathology, since hormonal dysfunction is not the likely cause of bleeding. Patients with anatomic causes associated with abnormal bleeding can be treated surgically.

Medical Therapy

DUB due to anovulatory cycles is best treated medically; surgery is suggested when medical therapy fails or is contraindicated. Generally, oral contraceptive pills are the mainstay of therapy. Several medical strategies are also effective in treating this disabling condition, and therapy must be tailored to the individual patient.

Oral Contraceptive Pills

Oral contraceptive pills have many roles in the treatment of menorrhagia and DUB. Combined estrogen-progesterone therapy reduces menstrual blood flow, and estrogen raises levels of both factor VIII and VWF. In patients with mild bleeding, oral contraceptive pills are prescribed in a dose identical to that used for contraception (21 days of hormonally active pills followed by 7 days of placebo, during which time withdrawal bleeding occurs). Care must be taken in counseling the parents of adolescents with DUB that the treatment is being used for its hormonal effects, not as a contraceptive modality.

Nonsteroidal Anti-Inflammatory Drugs

Nonsteroidal anti-inflammatory drugs (NSAIDs) decrease dysmenorrhea rates and menstrual blood loss. Some studies have demonstrated a 30% to 50% reduction in blood loss with proper use. Patients are advised to begin therapy 1 to 2 days before expected menstruation and to continue use throughout the menses. NSAIDs can be combined with oral contraceptive pills if needed. Patients with bleeding disorders and platelet abnormalities should avoid use of all NSAIDs.

Progesterone

Progesterone therapy is effective in women with anovulatory menstrual cycles. It stabilizes the proliferative endometrium and creates a regular sloughing of the endometrium. Cyclic progesterone is useful in women with contraindications to estrogen therapy (i.e., women older than the age of 35 years who smoke, have a history of deep venous vein thrombosis, or have higher-risk cardiovascular factors). Generally, medroxyprogesterone acetate 10 mg for 10 to 14 days each month will induce a regular withdrawal bleed in anovulatory women. This will not, however, provide contraception. Provera, given from days 7 to 21 of the cycle, decreases menstrual blood loss, but may be associated with progestational adverse effects, including bloating, irritability, fatigue, and premenstrual dysphoria.

Long-acting progesterone therapy in the form of medroxyprogesterone acetate (Depo-Provera) induces amenorrhea in the majority of patients. Standard dosing involves Depo-Provera 150 mg given intramuscularly every 3 months. Approximately 80% to 90% of patients completing 12 months' treatment of Depo-Provera will be amenorrheic. Adverse effects include weight gain, irregular bleeding, and depression.

Intravenous Conjugated Equine Estrogen

Profound menorrhagia rapidly responds to high-dose intravenous conjugated equine estrogen, promoting rapid regrowth of endometrial tissue, covering denuded endometrium, stabilizing lysosomal membranes, and stimulating proliferation of endometrial ground substance.

Short-term, high-dose estrogen therapy is used when excessive bleeding occurs in an emergency situation. It successfully stops heavy menstrual bleeding in adolescent and perimenopausal women. Any low-dose 30- to 35-µg ethinyl estradiol products can be used (administered every 6 hours for 5 days) to rapidly stop heavy menstrual bleeding. Once bleeding has stabilized, a single daily maintenance dose will provide regular menstrual cycle and contraception. Low-dose contraception is safe and effective and can be used in women older than 35 years who do not smoke or have a history of thromboembolic disease.

Danazol

Danazol, a weak androgen, creates a hypoestrogenic state and decreases menstrual blood loss by 70% to 80%. A less traditional dosing schedule of 50 to 100 mg daily as well as the conventional 400 to 800 mg daily is helpful. Adverse effects including weight gain, acne, and potential alteration of lipids have been documented.

Gonadotropin-Releasing Hormone

Gonadotropin-releasing hormone (GnRH) therapy creates a hypoestrogenic menopausal-like condition. Cessation of menstruation usually occurs within 3 months of therapy. Menopausal symptoms including hot flashes, night sweats, vaginal dryness, bone loss, poor concentration, insomnia, depression, headaches, and diminished libido may occur with therapy. Compliance is generally good despite these symptoms. Osteoporosis is the biggest risk of prolonged therapy; therefore, treatment is limited to 6 months, unless estrogen "add-back" is instituted. GnRH is a good option for women in the late perimenopausal stage if they have contraindications to other medical therapies; these women may spontaneously transition into menopause while amenorrheic from GnRH therapy. Additionally, intermittent (leuprolide) Lupron Depot therapy in women with uterine fibroids may provide up to 9 months of symptom control (range, 2 to >25 months), decrease uterine volume up to 60%, and allow recovery to normal hemoglobin levels before surgical intervention.

Levonorgestrel Intrauterine Device
The levonorgestrel (Mirena) intrauterine device (IUD) provides another option for DUB therapy. This IUD produces a decline in menstrual blood loss by 65% to 98% within 12 months of use. The device, imbedded with 20 μg of levonorgestrel, causes pseudodecidual changes and amenorrhea with little systemic absorption of progesterone. It is available in the United States; it may have a role for women who have menorrhagia and a normal uterine size and who wish to avoid surgery.

Miscellaneous Agents
Successful medical options for women with anovulatory bleeding and VWD include oral contraceptive therapy (88% success), desmopressin acetate, antifibrinolytic agents, and plasma-derived concentrates rich in the high-molecular-weight multimers of VWF. Obviously, hysterectomy or surgical therapy should not be the first option; rather, medical therapy is paramount for these women. Desmopressin acetate (DDAVP), which is available in concentrated form (1.5 mg/mL; Stimate, Aventis), can be administered intranasally (two sprays for the first 2 to 3 days) during menstruation or intravenously before procedures. DDAVP releases stored VWF from within endothelium and reduces bleeding in patients with type 1 VWD, some forms of type 2 VWD, platelet function disorders, and hemophilia carriage.

Tranexamic acid, an alternative antifibrinolytic, significantly reduces menstrual bleeding. Adverse effects occur in up to one third of patients and include muscle cramps and nausea. This treatment is currently not available in the United States.

Surgical Therapy

The surgical management of abnormal uterine bleeding is reserved for cases in which medical therapy fails or is contraindicated. Treatment modality depends on the etiology of abnormal bleeding as well as the preference of the patient and physician.

Operative Hysteroscopy
Submucosal fibroids and endometrial polyps vary in number, location, and size. Altered endometrial surface area, increased fragility and endometrial vascularity, endometrial irregularities, and abnormal prostaglandin

levels contribute to DUB when patients have submucosal fibroids. Likewise, intracavitary lesions can coexist with anovulatory and ovulatory cycles. Office hysteroscopy and SIS are the most accurate methods to detect intracavitary lesions. Outpatient hysteroscopic myomectomy or polypectomy is quick, safe, and effectively treats symptoms; both are associated with high rates of patient satisfaction.

Myomectomy

Intramural fibroids can also cause disturbances in menstrual flow. Wegienka et al. reported that the risk of heavy bleeding increases as fibroid size increases. The mechanisms of abnormal uterine bleeding in the presence of intramural fibroids are unclear, but they may be attributable to topographic endometrial abnormalities, endometrial glandular atrophy overlying the fibroid, venous congestion, increased endometrial surface area, and alteration of prostaglandin levels.

Treatment options for intramural fibroids are variable. The type of therapy offered is dependent on the patient's desire for pregnancy or her personal wish to preserve the uterus. When fertility is desired, the patient should be counseled for abdominal or laparoscopic myomectomy. The surgical route for myomectomy depends on the number, size, and location of fibroids, as well as the surgical skill of the physician.

Uterine Fibroid Embolization

When pregnancy is not desired and fibroids contribute to heavy menstrual bleeding, the patient can be offered uterine fibroid embolization. Transcutaneous insertion of a catheter through the femoral artery and subsequent occlusion of the uterine artery with embolospheres, polyvinyl acetate (PVA) particles, coils, or Gelfoam causes cessation of blood flow to the fibroid. Shortly thereafter, the fibroid necroses and shrinks in size and volume. Data support up to an 85% to 95% chance of the resolution of menorrhagia-related symptoms.

Hysterectomy

Hysterectomy offers definitive therapy for patients with fibroids who have completed childbearing and do not have a personal desire for uterine preservation. Hysterectomy may be performed vaginally, laparoscopically, or abdominally depending on the number, size, and location of fibroids, as well as the need for concomitant procedures.

Kuppermann et al. randomly assigned 63 women aged 30 to 50 years to undergo hysterectomy or oral medical therapy for abnormal uterine bleeding. After unsuccessful therapy with progesterone or oral contraceptive pills, women who underwent hysterectomy for abnormal uterine bleeding experienced greater symptom improvement in and expressed higher satisfaction with their overall health 6 months after treatment than women assigned to medical therapy. Specifically, women undergoing hysterectomy noted greater improvements in mental health, sexual desire and functioning, sleep, and overall satisfaction with health.

Dilation and Curettage

Dilation and curettage is no longer acceptable as the single surgical treatment for menorrhagia or DUB. It is futile and frivolous in correcting abnormal bleeding, unless intracavitary lesions are totally removed. In the past, this procedure was commonly used to treat menstrual aberrations. However, dilation and curettage is inaccurate due to missed diagnosis, incomplete removal of intracavitary pathology, and a high false-negative rate. Currently, operative hysteroscopy coupled with directed endometrial sampling is the gold standard to evaluate the uterine cavity in the surgical suite. Additionally, full evaluation can be performed in the presence of heavy bleeding, and coexisting intrauterine pathology can be treated when an operative hysteroscope with recirculating inflow/outflow channels is used.

Endometrial Ablation

Endometrial ablation is an outpatient procedure associated with rapid recovery, minimal complications, and high patient satisfaction rates. Second-generation technology relies less on the hysteroscopic expertise of a gynecologist than the preoperative endometrial evaluation to improve surgical success rates. Approximately 12% to 55% of patients who undergo endometrial ablation become amenorrheic, 65% to 70% become hypomenorrheic, and 5% to 19% fail (Table 14-1). Approximately 30% of patients treated by endometrial ablation will require a subsequent surgical procedure. Preoperative patient counseling is critical, and the health care professional should emphasize that the aim of endometrial ablation is a reduction in menstrual bleeding to normal levels or less. Amenorrhea should be considered a bonus and should not be "promised" to the patient.

Endometrial ablation is an alternative to hysterectomy for women with DUB. Traditionally, it has been offered after failed medical therapy in women with a normal uterine cavity, negative laboratory workup results, and completed childbearing. Hysteroscopic and global endometrial ablation procedures destroy the endometrium, preventing regeneration, and thereby alter menstrual flow. This creates an Asherman's syndrome, with resulting hypomenorrhea or amenorrhea.

Management of Acute Moderate to Severe Uterine Bleeding

Patients who present with profound menorrhagia and are hemodynamically unstable should be quickly assessed for the cause of the bleeding. Immediate intervention can be life saving until all diagnostic, laboratory, or culture results are available. Once intravenous lines are placed and aggressive fluid resuscitation has been established, a Foley catheter with a 30-mL balloon can be inserted into the uterus to effectively tamponade the bleeding site until the workup is complete. The balloon is inflated until the bleeding decreases and can remain until the patient is hemodynamically stable (longer than 24 hours). Once the patient is stabilized, the balloon can be deflated slowly over 8 to 12 hours and removed. Some

Table 14-1

Technology	Subjects Treated		Study Success (PBLAC < 75)		Amenorrhea Rates (PBLAC = 0)	
	Thermal (n)	REA (n)	Thermal (%)	REA (%)	Thermal (%)	REA (%)
MEA*	215	107	87	83	55	46
NovaSure†	175	90	78	74	36	32
HTA‡	187	89	68	76	35	47
Cryogen§	193	86	67	73	22	47
ThermaChoice‖,¶	134	126	75	77	14	25

REA, Rollerball endometrial ablation; PBLAC, pictorial blood loss chart; HTA, Hydro ThermAblator Endometrial Ablation System.

Intent-to-treat results as defined by the U.S. Food and Drug Administration.

*Microsulis Microwave Endometrial Ablation (MEA) System, Summary of Safety and Effectiveness Data, PMA P020031, Amendment filing, July 14, 2003. Deputy Director, Office of Device Evaluation, Center for Devices and Radiological Health, U.S. Department of Health and Human Services.

†NovaSure Impedance Controlled Endometrial Ablation System, Summary of Safety and Effectiveness Data, PMA P010013, September 28, 2001. Deputy Director, Office of Device Evaluation, Center for Devices and Radiological Health, U.S. Department of Health and Human Services.

‡BEI Medical Systems Hydro ThermAblator Endometrial Ablation System, Summary of Safety and Effectiveness Data, PMA P000040, April 20 2001. Deputy Director, Office of Device Evaluation, Center for Devices and Radiological Health, U.S. Department of Health and Human Services.

§Cryogen HerOption Uterine Cryoablation Therapy System, Summary of Safety and Effectiveness Data, PMA P000032, April 20, 2001. Deputy Director, Office of Device Evaluation, Center for Devices and Radiological Health, U.S. Department of Health and Human Services.

‖Gynecare ThermaChoice UBT, Summary of Safety and Effectiveness Data, PMA P970021, December 12, 1997. Deputy Director, Office of Device Evaluation, Center for Devices and Radiological Health, U.S. Department of Health and Human Services.

¶Adjusted for the intent-to-treat population—evaluable population.

From Bradley LD: Global endometrial ablation in the presence of fibroids. Cleveland Clinic Foundation Continuing Medical Education Activity, February 2004.

patients experience intense uterine contractions with the inflated balloon, which may require intravenous narcotics or a patient-controlled anesthesia pump.

Emergency hysteroscopy, with a high-flow distention pump, is effective in establishing and treating menorrhagia in critically ill or unstable patients. Fraser noted that the incidence of intracavitary pathology increased as the amount of bleeding increased; 25% of those with a blood loss of less than 60 mL had abnormal findings, compared with 56% of those with moderate menorrhagia (60 to 120 mL blood loss), and 64% of those with severe menorrhagia (>120 mL blood loss). Despite excessive bleeding, clots, debris, and endometrial chips encountered during hysteroscopy can be easily flushed away or removed to aid in the diagnosis and concomitant treatment of the patient.

Women with structural abnormalities, such as polyps or fibroids, should be quickly triaged to operative hysteroscopic resection of focal lesions, whereas women with mild anemia and negative workup results should be treated medically.

OUTCOMES

DUB is usually well categorized after the initial history, physical examination, and laboratory evaluation. Regardless of the patient's age, abnormal uterine bleeding requires a thorough evaluation. Medical management is the hallmark of therapy unless uterine pathology is present. In the case of a menopausal woman with an atrophic endometrium, the patient can be reassured; short-term, low-dose hormone replacement therapy is usually effective in treating the patient's symptoms. Most patients with anovulatory uterine bleeding respond favorably to hormonal manipulation with oral contraceptive therapy or progesterone treatment. For patients who cannot tolerate medical therapy, the levonorgestrel IUD is effective in the treatment of abnormal menstruation. Patients with intrauterine polyps and submucosal fibroids have excellent relief of symptoms after operative hysteroscopy. Women with symptomatic uterine fibroids have a wide array of therapeutic options including medical therapy, myomectomy (abdominal, laparoscopic, or hysteroscopic), hysterectomy, or uterine fibroid embolization. Finally, surgical therapy with endometrial ablation offers 90% success for the treatment of menorrhagia and dysfunctional bleeding in women with a normal uterine cavity and negative workup results who do not desire future fertility. Many therapeutic options are currently available to women with DUB, often obviating the need for hysterectomy.

KEY POINTS

1. A detailed medical history and complete physical examination are necessary in the evaluation of abnormal uterine bleeding.
2. Saline infusion sonography is an integral component in the evaluation of the endometrium in women with an equivocal transvaginal ultrasound.
3. Endometrial ablation should be offered only after a failed trial of medical therapy.
4. Uterine fibroid embolization successfully treats uterine fibroid symptoms including menorrhagia, bulk symptoms, and pain.
5. Consider magnetic resonance imaging if adenomyosis is strongly suspected by clinical history or physical examination.
6. Bleeding diathesis is a common presentation of abnormal uterine bleeding. A von Willebrand's factor panel, bleeding time, and complete blood count with platelet count effectively rules out hematologic causes of abnormal uterine bleeding.
7. The levonorgestrel intrauterine device effectively treats menorrhagia in the majority of women but may be associated with erratic bleeding during the initial months.
8. Office hysteroscopy is an important clinical tool and should be mastered by all gynecologists. It quickly, comfortably, and reliably evaluates the endometrial surface area.

SUGGESTED READING

American College of Obstetricians and Gynecologists: Committee Opinion No. 263. Von Willebrand's disease in gynecologic practice. Obstet Gynecol 98:1185–1186, 2001.

Bettocchi S, Ceci O, Vicino M, et al: Diagnostic inadequacy of dilation and curettage. Fertil Steril 75 (4):803–805, 2001.

Bruchim I, Biron-Shental T, Altaras MM, et al: Combination of endometrial thickness and time since menopause in predicting endometrial cancer in women with postmenopausal bleeding. J Clin Ultrasound 32(5):219–224, 2004.

Carlson KJ, Nichols DH, Schiff I: Indications for hysterectomy. N Engl J Med 328(12):856–860, 1993.

Clark TJ, Voit D, Gupta JK: Accuracy of hysteroscopy in the diagnosis of endometrial cancer and hyperplasia: A systematic quantitative review. JAMA 288:1610–1621, 2002.

Epstein E, Valentin L: Managing women with post-menopausal bleeding. Best Pract Res Clin Obstet Gynecol 18(1):124–143, 2004.

Fraser IS: Hysteroscopy and laparoscopy in women with menorrhagia. Am J Obstet Gynecol 165:1264–1269, 1990.

Goldstein RB, Bree RL, Benson CB: Evaluation of the woman with postmenopausal bleeding. J Ultrasound Med 20:1025–1036, 2001.

Higham JM, Shaw RW: A comparative study of danazol, a regimen of decreasing doses of danazol and norethindrone in the treatment of objectively proven unexplained menorrhagia. Am J Obstet Gynecol 169:1134–1139, 1993.

Hurskainen R, Teperi J, Rissanen P, et al: Quality of life and cost-effectiveness of levonorgestrel-releasing in-trauterine system versus hysterectomy, for treatment of menorrhagia: A randomized trial. Lancet 357:273–277, 2001.

James AH, Lukes AS, Brancazio LR, et al: Use of a new platelet function analyzer to detect von Willebrand

disease in women with menorrhagia. Am J Obstet Gynecol 191:449–455, 2004.

Kupperman R, Varner E, Summit RL: Effect of hysterectomy vs. medical treatment on health-related quality of life and sexual functioning: The medicine or surgery (MS) randomized trial. JAMA 291(12): 1447–1455, 2004.

Landgren BM, Collins A, Csemiczky G, et al: Menopause transition: Annual changes in serum hormonal patterns over the menstrual cycle in women during a nine-year period prior to menopause. J Clin Endocrinol Metab 89:2763–2769, 2004.

Pasqualotto EB, Margossian H, Price LL, Bradley LD: Accuracy of preoperative diagnostic tools and outcome of hysteroscopic management of menstrual dysfunction. J Am Assoc Gynecol Laparoscop 7(2): 201–209, 2000.

Philipp CS, Faiz A, Dowling N, et al: Age and the prevalence of bleeding disorders in women with menorrhagia. Obstet Gynecol 105(1):61–66, 2005.

Seltzer VL, Benjamin R, Deutsch S: Perimenopausal bleeding patterns and pathologic findings. J Am Med Womens Assoc 45:132–134, 1990.

Smith-Bindman S, Kerlikowske K, Feldstein VA, et al: Endovaginal ultrasound to exclude endometrial cancer and other endometrial abnormalities. JAMA 20:1510–1517, 1998.

Walker WJ, Pelage JP: Uterine artery embolization for symptomatic fibroids: Clinical results in 400 women with imaging follow up. BJOG 109:1262–1272, 2002.

Wegienka G, Baird DD, Hertz-Picciotto I, et al: Self-reported heavy bleeding associated with uterine leiomyomata. Obstet Gynecol 101:431–437, 2003.

Widrich T, Bradley L, Mitchinson AR, Collins R: Comparison of saline infusion sonography with office hysteroscopy for the evaluation of the endometrium. Am J Obstet Gynecol 174:1327–1334, 1996.

365

15

MENSTRUAL DISORDERS

Eric R. Sokol, Lawrence Lurvey, and Mikael N. Brisinger

INTRODUCTION

Approximately one third of all outpatient gynecologic visits are undertaken for disorders of menses, making menstrual disorders some of the most common reasons women visit their gynecologists. Menstrual problems can take many forms, including abnormal or irregular bleeding, amenorrhea, dysmenorrhea, premenstrual syndrome, and premenstrual dysphoric disorder. Abnormal bleeding is discussed in detail in Chapter 14, Abnormal Uterine Bleeding, and therefore will not be discussed here. This chapter will begin with a discussion of the normal menstrual cycle, which will provide a basis for understanding problems that can occur when any of the normal physiologic steps of the menstrual cycle become deranged. The specific problems of primary and secondary amenorrhea, polycystic ovarian syndrome, dysmenorrhea, premenstrual disorder, and premenstrual dysphoric syndrome will then be discussed.

NORMAL MENSTRUAL CYCLE

The normal menstrual cycle occurs every 28 ± 7 days, with duration of flow of 2 to 7 days and a loss of less than 80 mL of menstrual blood (Table 15-1). Anything outside of this range is termed *abnormal uterine bleeding*. Menses is highly predictable for most women during their reproductive years.

Physiology of Normal Menstruation

There is a delicate pathway that regulates menstrual bleeding known as the hypothalamic-pituitary-ovarian (HPO) axis (Fig. 15-1). Positive and negative feedback along this pathway results in normal ovulation and menses via the following mechanism:

1. The arcuate nucleus of the hypothalamus generates timed pulses of gonadotropin-releasing hormone (GnRH), which stimulates cells of

Table 15-1

	Normal	Abnormal
Duration	2–7 days	<2 days or >7days
Volume	30–80 mL	>80 mL
Length of cycle	21–35 days	<21 or >35 days

the anterior pituitary gland to produce follicle-stimulating hormone (FSH) and luteinizing hormone (LH).

2. FSH and LH, in turn, stimulate the ovary to release follicles and exert a negative feedback on GnRH.

3. The ovarian follicle secretes estradiol, which has a positive feedback on the anterior pituitary gland. An LH surge ensues, triggering ovulation. The estradiol also makes the endometrium receptive to the ovum released from the follicle, which becomes the corpus luteum.

4. The corpus luteum starts secreting progesterone for about 10 days. The progesterone stops the endometrium from growing and makes it more compact and stable. If a fertilized ovum does not implant into the endometrium, the corpus luteum stops making progesterone.

5. The spiral arterioles that feed the endometrium, which had been stabilized by progesterone, constrict and spasm. The endometrial tissue breaks down between the basalis and spongiosum layer, and menstrual bleeding ensues.

Figure 15-1

Hypothalamic-
pituitary-ovarian
(HPO) axis. GnRH,
Gonadotropin-
releasing hormone;
FSH, follicle-
stimulating hormone;
LH, luteinizing
hormone.

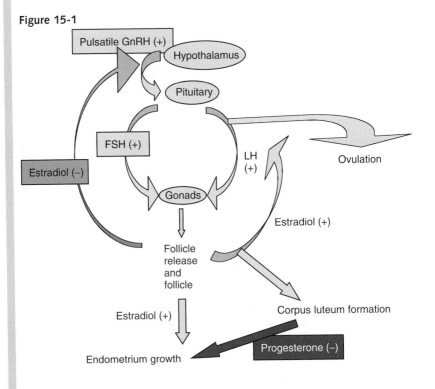

HPO Axis

6. Thrombin is generated in the basal endometrium, which promotes fibrin that activates platelets for hemostasis and cessation of menstruation.

Table 15-2 lists the different prostaglandins involved in the normal menstrual cycle.

PRIMARY AMENORRHEA

Primary amenorrhea is defined as the absence of menstruation by the age of 16 years in the presence of normal growth and secondary sexual characteristics. In contrast, if menstruation has begun but has subsequently ceased for more than three cycles or 6 months, the term *secondary amenorrhea* is used. In general, amenorrhea is caused by a failure of the HPO axis or an absence or obstruction of the end organs such as the uterus or vagina. Causes of amenorrhea can be classified into broad categories depending on the site of dysfunction: hypothalamic and pituitary dysfunction, gonadal dysfunction, and anatomic abnormalities. Box 15-1 lists the most

Table 15-2

Prostaglandins Involved in Menstruation

Prostaglandin	Action
$PGF_{2\alpha}$ and $PGE_{2\alpha}$	Cause uterine contractions
Thromboxane A_2	Promotes vasoconstriction
PGI_2 and $PGE_{2\alpha}$	Promote vasodilatation

$PGF_{2\alpha}$, Prostaglandin $F_{2\alpha}$; $PGE_{2\alpha}$, prostaglandin $E_{2\alpha}$; PGI_2, prostaglandin I_2.

Box 15-1   Common Causes of Amenorrhea
Hypothalamic dysfunction
Functional hypothalamic amenorrhea
Eating disorders
Tumors
Kallmann syndrome
Drugs
Pituitary dysfunction
Adenomas
Sheehan's syndrome
Polycystic ovarian syndrome
Gonadal abnormalities
Turner syndrome
X-chromosome abnormalities
Alkylating chemotherapy
Other causes of premature ovarian failure
Male pseudohermaphroditism
Anatomic abnormalities
Imperforate hymen
Asherman's syndrome

common causes of amenorrhea by category. A thorough history and physical examination coupled with a carefully planned laboratory assessment can elucidate the cause of amenorrhea in most cases.

Hypothalamic and Pituitary Dysfunction

Functional hypothalamic amenorrhea can occur when normal secretion of GnRH from the hypothalamus is disrupted. This is a common cause of amenorrhea and can be caused by physical and emotional stress, which can diminish the normal pulsatile release of GnRH, leading to diminished sex steroid production by the ovaries. The absence of an LH surge leads to anovulation and, ultimately, amenorrhea. Eating disorders can also cause amenorrhea by leading to a loss of body fat and reduced gonadotropin release. Hypothalamic hypogonadism, including functional hypothalamic amenorrhea, accounts for approximately 20% of cases of primary amenorrhea.

A rarer cause of hypothalamic dysfunction is idiopathic hypogonadotropic hypogonadism, which is complete congenital GnRH deficiency. When it is coupled with anosmia, this disorder is called *Kallmann syndrome.*

Hyperprolactinemia can be produced by pituitary tumors and glandular defects and is a rare cause of primary amenorrhea. Many women with hyperprolactinemia will also have galactorrhea, which can aid in the clinical diagnosis.

Anatomic lesions such as tumors can also cause amenorrhea by interrupting the portal system connection between the hypothalamus and the pituitary gland. Examples of such tumors include craniopharyngiomas and hamartomas. Suprasellar tumors often develop before puberty and therefore cause primary amenorrhea. Symptoms such as persistent headaches or other central nervous symptoms coupled with amenorrhea should lead to an evaluation for suprasellar tumors.

Gonadal Dysfunction

Gonadal dysgenesis caused by chromosomal abnormalities is the most common cause of primary amenorrhea in young women, accounting for approximately 50% of cases. The most common of these chromosomal abnormalities is Turner's syndrome, in which a woman is missing an X chromosome (45, X). In women with Turner's syndrome the external genitalia, uterus, and fallopian tubes develop normally until puberty, at which time estrogen-induced maturation fails to occur. The ovaries produce very little estrogen as they are replaced by fibrous tissue, leading to amenorrhea. Spontaneous menstruation and pregnancy can occur in persons who inherit a mosaic karyotype. 46, XX gonadal dysgenesis and 46, XY gonadal dysgenesis are less common causes of primary amenorrhea and ovarian failure.

Polycystic ovarian syndrome (PCOS) is another form of gonadal dysfunction that can cause primary amenorrhea, though women with PCOS often have irregular menstrual cycles or secondary amenorrhea. PCOS is discussed in detail later in this chapter.

Anatomic Abnormalities

Twenty percent of cases of primary amenorrhea are caused by congenital abnormalities of the uterus and vagina. Vaginal agenesis, known as *Mayer-Rokitansky-Küster-Hauser* (MRKH) *syndrome,* is one such example. Persons with MRKH syndrome most commonly have cervical and uterine agenesis, though the uterine development may be variable and the ovaries are normal. These women have normal thelarche, adrenarche, and growth spurt. There is a 50% incidence of associated renal anomalies and a 25% incidence of associated skeletal anomalies. Women with MRKH syndrome often decide to undergo neovaginal construction with progressive vaginal dilators or surgery to facilitate sexual relations.

Other anatomic cause of primary amenorrhea include an imperforate hymen or a transverse vaginal septum. Girls with these conditions will complain of cyclic pelvic pain, eventually resulting in hematocolpos or hematometra. Retrograde menstruation can lead to a hemoperitoneum or severe endometriosis. If the exact outflow obstruction is unclear, imaging, often with magnetic resonance imaging, is helpful. Surgical repair is usually very successful.

Other Causes

A rare cause of primary amenorrhea is complete androgen insensitivity syndrome, in which a person with a 46, XY chromosome develops the phenotypic characteristics of a female because of a defect in the androgen receptor. Other rare causes include 5α-reductase deficiency, 17α-hydroxylase deficiency, vanishing testes syndrome, and systemic diseases such as lupus or Crohn's disease. Because of the intricacies of the diagnosis of primary amenorrhea and the multitude of etiologies, consultation with a specialist in reproductive endocrinology or adolescent medicine is recommended.

Evaluation and Treatment

Although the causes of primary amenorrhea are many, a focused history can guide clinical judgment and lead to appropriate laboratory evaluation. Questions should be geared toward the common causes of primary and secondary amenorrhea because all causes of secondary amenorrhea can cause primary disease. Important questions to ask include whether there is a family history of delayed or absent puberty, how the person's height compares with that of family members (short stature suggests Turner's syndrome), which stages of puberty the person has completed, and whether there were any recent stressors including changes in weight, exercise, or illness. It is also helpful to inquire about symptoms such as headaches or visual changes that would suggest hypothalamic or pituitary disease, whether the patient has noticed galactorrhea, and whether the patient is taking any medications or drugs that could alter hypothalamic gonadotropin secretion.

Physical examination should include an evaluation of pubertal development, breast development by Tanner stage, and genital examination. Ultrasound is useful to evaluate for müllerian anomalies. It is also important to note signs of hirsutism, skin pigmentation, or acne that may suggest etiologies such as PCOS, and to evaluate for signs of

Turner's syndrome such as low hair line, short stature, and widely spaced nipples.

Laboratory evaluation is guided by the findings on the history and physical examination and whether müllerian structures are present (by physical examination or ultrasound). If the uterus is absent, a karyotype and serum testosterone level should be checked to distinguish between such conditions as müllerian agenesis and androgen insensitivity syndrome. If the uterus is present and there is no other lower genital anatomic abnormality, an endocrine evaluation should be performed. One important test is a serum human chorionic gonadotropin (hCG) measurement to exclude pregnancy. A serum FSH test is useful to evaluate for ovarian failure, which would cause the level to be elevated. Other laboratory tests should include serum prolactin and thyrotropin levels, especially if galactorrhea is present. Specific laboratory tests should be geared toward the specific etiologies of primary amenorrhea being sought.

Treatment of primary amenorrhea is dictated by the underlying etiology and often includes counseling, surgery in patients with an anatomic cause, hormone replacement therapy in women with primary ovarian failure, gonadectomy to avert the possibility of gonadal neoplasm in persons with a Y chromosome, and assisted reproductive technologies in those patients desiring fertility. For patients with PCOS, treatment is aimed at achieving the woman's goals, which may include treatment of the hirsutism, menstrual cycling or fertility, and avoiding common sequelae such as obesity, diabetes, and endometrial hyperplasia.

SECONDARY AMENORRHEA

Similar to primary amenorrhea, it is useful to categorize causes of secondary amenorrhea as hypothalamic or pituitary, gonadal, or uterine in nature. Overall, pregnancy is the most common cause of secondary amenorrhea. Other causes include ovarian disease in 40%, hypothalamic dysfunction in 35%, pituitary disease in 19%, uterine disease in 5%, and other causes in 1%. Any evaluation starts with a complete history and a pregnancy test.

Hypothalamic and Pituitary Dysfunction

As in primary amenorrhea, one of the most common causes of secondary amenorrhea is functional hypothalamic amenorrhea. As previously discussed, this condition is characterized by decreased GnRH secretion, resulting in diminished LH pulsatile secretion, anovulation, and amenorrhea. Various factors such as excessive exercise, weight loss, stress, and poor nutrition can interfere with the HPO axis and produce secondary amenorrhea. Although the incidence of obesity in women with amenorrhea is four to five times higher than regularly menstruating women, excessive weight loss with eating disorders such as anorexia nervosa or bulimia is a common finding among women with secondary amenorrhea.

Findings that may suggest these eating disorders include dental decay, odd attitudes toward food, distorted body image, or electrolyte imbalances. In anorexia, peripheral gonadotropin and gonadal steroid levels are low but do increase with weight gain. Estradiol metabolizes the way it does in patients with hyperthyroidism, whereas testosterone metabolizes the way it does in patients with hypothyroidism. Other features of anorexia include low cortisol levels, decreased body temperature, and low triiodothyronine levels. Anorexia is a potentially lethal condition and should be treated in an integrated fashion, preferably by behavioral specialists.

Exercise at a high level can produce secondary amenorrhea; indeed, this is a common finding among professional female athletes. The cause of this is unclear but may relate to decreased energy reserves, lean-to-fat ratio changes, or amount of body fat. The amenorrhea is not solely a function of psychological stress, since young girls training to be professional musicians in one study did not have abnormalities of menses, but those training to be athletes did. Of course, psychogenic stress is a very common cause of secondary amenorrhea. In women under stress, the positive feedback effect of exogenous estrogen on the acute release of gonadotropins is impaired. Low leptin levels in women under emotional stress or stress induced by illness can also lead to decreased LH pulsatility, which can impair menstrual cycling.

Other processes that can impair hypothalamic or pituitary function, leading to secondary amenorrhea, include infiltrative diseases of the hypothalamus (e.g., lymphoma and sarcoidosis) and prolactin-secreting pituitary tumors. The hyperprolactinemia seen in prolactin-secreting tumors and other conditions (such as hypothyroidism) causes suppression of hypothalamic GnRH secretion. Prolactin-secreting tumors are the most common pituitary cause of secondary amenorrhea, accounting for approximately 90% of cases (20% of all cases of secondary amenorrhea).

Gonadal Dysfunction

Ovarian diseases, including ovarian failure and PCOS, are the most common causes of secondary amenorrhea. These conditions disrupt menses by producing a hyperandrogenic state, which causes anovulation and leads to atrophy of the endometrial lining. Ovarian failure occurs with the depletion of ovarian follicles and oocytes, leading to a decrease in the level of circulating estrogens and cessation of menses. When ovarian failure occurs before the age of 40 years, the term *premature ovarian failure* is used. Women who undergo premature ovarian failure should be evaluated for karyotypic abnormalities and autoimmune diseases. The mean age at which menopause occurs in the United States is 52 years.

Uterine Dysfunction

Scarring of the endometrial lining, which can occur after surgical instrumentation of the uterus, is the only uterine cause of secondary amenorrhea. This condition, called *Asherman's syndrome*, prevents the endometrial lining from building up and eventually shedding, leading to a greatly diminished or absent menstrual flow. Women with Asherman's syndrome will often have a history of dilation and curettage for obstetric reasons or a history of uterine infection, and will fail to have menstrual withdrawal bleeding when given an exogenous hormone challenge. The diagnosis of Asherman's syndrome can be confirmed hysteroscopically.

Evaluation and Treatment

Any woman who develops secondary amenorrhea should be evaluated with a pregnancy test because pregnancy is the most common cause of this condition. A serum β subunit hCG measurement is the most sensitive test for this purpose and a sample should be drawn even in women denying sexual activity. Also, a thorough history should include questions about stresses, weight loss, exercise, medications or drugs, menopausal symptoms, galactorrhea, and history of uterine instrumentation or infection. It is important to ask about such symptoms as headaches, visual field changes, and fatigue, which could be signs of hypothalamic or pituitary disease.

Physical examination should proceed as it would for patients being evaluated for primary amenorrhea, including an evaluation of the body mass index, an inspection for signs of systemic illness, and an evaluation of the skin, breasts, and genital tissue for signs of atrophy associated with estrogen deficiency. Also, the breasts should be inspected for galactorrhea. It is also important to note signs of hirsutism, skin pigmentation, or acne, which may suggest etiologies such as PCOS.

Laboratory evaluation is geared toward the most common causes of secondary amenorrhea and should include a serum hCG measurement to rule out pregnancy, a serum FSH to evaluate for ovarian failure, a prolactin level to rule out hyperprolactinemia, and a thyrotropin level to rule out thyroid disease. A testosterone level and serum dehydroepiandrosterone sulfate (DHEA-S) can be checked in patients exhibiting signs of hyperandrogenism (such as can occur with PCOS or androgen-secreting tumors).

As far as treatment goes, amenorrhea is only a symptom. Treatment is aimed at correcting the underlying disorder. For underweight or athletic women, appropriate caloric intake coupled with dietary counseling can be effective in correcting functional hypothalamic amenorrhea. A multidisciplinary approach is most useful for women suspected of having an eating disorder.

If the cause of secondary amenorrhea is hyperprolactinemia, the source of the excess prolactin needs to be corrected. Also, dopamine agonist medications can suppress prolactin levels and lead to a resumption of menstrual cycles. Women with premature ovarian failure should be counseled about the risks and benefits of hormone replacement therapy, and women diagnosed with Asherman's syndrome may benefit from hysteroscopic resection of the uterine scar tissue and prolonged estrogen administration to promote regrowth of the endometrial lining.

Besides attempting to avert long-term sequelae of the disease process, treatment goals can be divided into two categories: to attain fertility or to establish normal menses. For infertility, ovulation-inducing agents are commonly used; these include clomiphene citrate, human menopausal gonadotropin, FSH, and GnRH. These can have good success rates in achieving pregnancy when the cause of the infertility is anovulation or hypo-ovulation. For establishing normal menses, any cyclic estrogen-progesterone combinations given as oral contraceptives will restore menses. Progesterone alone is less useful and may not stimulate the endometrium enough to produce menses. Progesterone can be useful to reassure the patient or to counteract hyperplasia of the endometrium that can result from unopposed estrogen due to anovulation with, for example, obesity. Commonly used agents are medroxyprogesterone at 5 to 10 mg/day for 5 to 10 days to induce menstruation or micronized progesterone as a gel, suppository, capsule, or injection. The treatment for women with PCOS is described below.

POLYCYSTIC OVARIAN SYNDROME

Although there is no universally accepted definition of this much discussed condition, PCOS is marked by hyperandrogenism and chronic anovulation where other causes such as congenital adrenal hyperplasia, hyperprolactinemia, and neoplasm have been excluded. PCOS is classically expressed as hirsutism, irregular menstrual cycles, obesity, and a specific appearance of the ovaries on ultrasound, but these clinical features are variably expressed in patients. A consensus statement at the National Institutes of Health Conference on PCOS identified the following minimal criteria for making the diagnosis:

- Oligo- or anovulation leading to menstrual irregularity
- Clinical or biochemical evidence of hyperandrogenism
- Exclusion of other causes of hyperandrogenism and menstrual irregularity

These diagnostic criteria were subsequently revised by the European Society of Human Reproduction and Embryology/American Society of Reproductive Medicine consensus workshop group. The revised criteria require two of the following three factors to be present to make the diagnosis of PCOS:

- Oligo-ovulation and/or anovulation
- Clinical and/or biochemical evidence of hyperandrogenism
- Polycystic ovaries by ultrasound

PCOS occurs in of 4% to 7% of women and is strongly associated with insulin resistance, which may represent the greatest health risk of this condition since this may raise cardiovascular risk. The obesity and infertility associated with PCOS have obvious adverse affects on health and well-being. To make the diagnosis of PCOS, one should document excess androgens either clinically or biochemically. Free serum testosterone is the most sensitive test to establish the presence of hyperandrogenism. DHEA may be a useful measure of adrenal function and represents a prohormone for testosterone or dihydrotestosterone. Most testosterone (60%) is made by the ovary.

Even though insulin resistance is strongly associated with PCOS, the American Diabetes Association does not recommend screening for diabetes in all women with PCOS, but rather screening selectively based on other risks, including acanthosis nigrans, young age, and fertility considerations. When indicated, women with PCOS should be screened with a 2-hour glucose tolerance test because fasting glucose is a poor predictor in these women. In addition, women with PCOS should be screened for dyslipidemia.

General goals for the treatment of women with PCOS include treatment of hirsutism and other androgenic symptoms, endometrial protection, and treatment of infertility in those desiring pregnancy. Mainstays of treatment for anovulation and amenorrhea with PCOS are exercise and weight control. These have the ancillary benefit of lowering cardiovascular risk as well. Combination oral contraceptives are beneficial because they suppress pituitary LH, suppress ovarian androgen production, and increase circulating sex hormone binding globulin. They also afford a regular period. Combination oral contraceptives are more useful than progestins alone, since progestins may decrease levels of sex hormone binding globulin. For women who want to conceive, drugs that increase insulin sensitivity have been promising. Biguanides such as metformin are used for PCOS and help with both the infertility aspects as well as the hyperinsulinemia. The dose of metformin most often used is 1500 mg/day or 2000 mg in divided doses. In addition to increasing insulin sensitivity, these agents decrease circulating androgens, improve ovulation rates, and improve glucose tolerance. In addition to metformin, clomiphene citrate is used for those attempting conception. Up to 80% of patients with PCOS will ovulate with clomiphene, and up to 50% will conceive within six cycles. The starting dose of 50 mg is sufficient for 50% of the women; the other half can have 100 mg.

Gonadotropins can be used where clomiphene fails. Hirsutism that comes with PCOS is treated with an anti-androgen agent such as spironolactone at 25 to 100 mg twice per day. Other insulin-sensitizing agents such as troglitazone, rosiglitazone, and pioglitazone, and anti-androgen agents such as flutamide and finasteride, although effective, are not commonly used because of concerns about teratogenicity and embryotoxicity.

THERAPEUTIC AMENORRHEA

On occasion, it is desirable to induce amenorrhea. Clinical situations might include a patient with severe anemia due to fibroids who is awaiting surgery or a patient with severe dysmenorrhea. Patients sometimes request an agent to induce amenorrhea due to lifestyle or select events such as a wedding. Many agents are available for this purpose, but the most commonly used are oral contraceptives. Skipping the placebo-pill week and immediately starting the next pack will postpone menses. If done repeatedly, this can result in some breakthrough bleeding that is not physiologically harmful. Longer-term amenorrhea can be brought about with depot medroxyprogesterone acetate (Depo-Provera) injections. This will induce amenorrhea in 50% to 90% of women using it over the course of 1 year. This medication has some unlikable adverse effects such as breakthrough bleeding the first few months as well as increased appetite that often leads to weight gain.

Fewer adverse effects are seen with the progestin-containing intrauterine system (Mirena), which is a cost-effective birth control method as well. GnRH agonists (e.g., Depot-Lupron) are very effective agents to induce amenorrhea, are helpful in the setting of fibroids to control bleeding, and even cause some short-term shrinkage of the fibroid tumors. The recommended duration of use is only 6 months, however, due to concerns about bone loss from low estrogen levels. In general, the adverse effects of GnRH agonists are those of menopause. Danazol is rarely used to induce amenorrhea due to the androgenic side effects it causes. GnRH antagonists such as mifepristone are still being studied for all of their uses and, at this time, would not be recommended as an agent solely to induce amenorrhea.

377

DYSMENORRHEA

Dysmenorrhea is defined as painful menstrual cramps of uterine origin. It is usually divided into the following categories:

- primary dysmenorrhea, when there is no demonstrable pelvic disease; and
- secondary dysmenorrhea, when pelvic disease such as endometriosis, adenomyosis, chronic pelvic inflammatory disease, or uterine fibroids is present.

Primary dysmenorrhea usually starts right after menarche when ovulation is established. Dysmenorrhea is the most common cause of days absent from school in the female adolescent population. If persistent, a careful screen should be done for sexual abuse, endometriosis, or other pelvic pathology, such as an adnexal mass. Secondary dysmenorrhea may arise later in life. Secondary dysmenorrhea is frequently caused by endometriosis (ectopic endometrial tissue). A full description of endometriosis is offered in another chapter, but one of the classic signs is severe pain during menses. The pain usually starts with menstrual flow and continues for up to 72 hours.

Evaluation and Treatment

A complete history for the evaluation of dysmenorrhea should include questions about the specifics of the menstrual cycle, symptoms during menstruation, the severity and location of pain, presence of pelvic pain not related to menstruation, and the impact of symptoms on activities of daily living. Questions should be posed in an attempt to discern between primary and secondary dysmenorrhea and to ascertain whether other processes, such as endometriosis and adenomyosis, are the cause of pain. The physical examination, and in particular, the pelvic exam, may also help discriminate between dysmenorrhea and other pelvic processes that can cause pain. Supportive laboratory testing such as pelvic ultrasonography should be performed if a pelvic mass is suspected.

Dysmenorrhea is usually treated empirically at first. Nonsteroidal anti-inflammatory drugs (NSAIDs) such as ibuprofen or naproxen are the mainstay of treatment. They are most effective if levels are adequate before the release of pain mediators. A good rule of thumb is the "rule of 3s": take three 200-mg ibuprofen, three times a day, starting 3 days before the menses begins. Most NSAIDs are equally effective, although one study shows naproxen to be superior. The most common adverse effects of NSAIDs are nausea, dizziness, and headaches.

There are other lifestyle remedies to consider. Smokers seem to have more dysmenorrhea, and therefore, smoking cessation would be a natural therapy to pursue. Childbirth also seems to reduce the natural course of dysmenorrhea, although for obvious reasons this is difficult to pursue as a separate therapy. High-frequency transcutaneous nerve stimulation can be helpful. Magnesium supplements may reduce pain after 5 to 6 months. Toki-shakuyaku-san (herbal remedy) may reduce pain or decrease the need for NSAIDs after 5 to 6 months of use. Topical heat (about 39°C) may reduce pain as effectively as NSAIDs. Therapeutic amenorrhea is particularly useful for severe dysmenorrhea. A description of methods is given above. Oral contraceptives do not reduce pain, but they can lower the overall amount of bleeding.

Because dysmenorrhea is common, there are a host of popular remedies that have not been proved scientifically. It is unclear how effective the following often-used remedies are: acupuncture, behavioral interventions, oral contraceptives, fish oil, and vitamin B_{12}. Surgical remedies such as laparoscopic uterine nerve ablation are similarly unproven.

PREMENSTRUAL SYNDROME AND PREMENSTRUAL DYSPHORIC DISORDER

Premenstrual syndrome (PMS) is the cyclic somatic and psychological change that occurs during the luteal phase of the ovulatory cycle. More than 75% of women have some of the symptoms of PMS at one time or another during their lives. *The Diagnostic and Statistical Manual of Mental Disorders*, 4th edition, denotes *premenstrual dysphoric disorder* (PMDD) for more severe symptoms that interfere with daily activities and suggests that the term *premenstrual syndrome* be used to describe less severe symptomatology (Box 15-2). More specifically, PMDD is defined as a severe form of PMS in which irritability, internal tension, and anger are prominent. Studies show the prevalence of PMDD to be 3% to 8% among women with regular menstrual cycles.

378

Box 15-2	DSM-IV Criteria for Premenstrual Dysphoric Disorder

Depression (hopelessness; more than just feeling sad or blue)
Anxiety (feeling "keyed up" or "on edge")
Severe mood swings (feeling suddenly sad or extremely sensitive to rejection)
Anger or irritability
Decreased interest in usual activities (e.g., work, school, friends, hobbies)
Difficulty concentrating
Decreased energy
Appetite changes (overeating or cravings for certain foods)
Sleep problems (insomnia, early morning waking, or oversleeping)
Feeling overwhelmed or out of control
Physical symptoms, such as bloating, breast tenderness, or headaches

American Psychiatric Association: DSM-IV, The Diagnostic and Statistical Manual of Mental Disorders, 4th ed. Washington, D.C., American Psychiatric Association, 1999.

The key component in diagnosing PMS/PMDD lies in its cyclic nature. Patients are often "perfectly fine" once menstruation starts or during the week thereafter. Symptoms that persist throughout the entire menstrual cycle are not typically attributed to PMS/PMDD, but rather to something else such as depression, anxiety, or both. It is important to note that PMDD symptoms often sound just like depression, anxiety, or panic disorders. Many researchers advocate using a symptom diary before making a definitive diagnosis, but this might not be practical in a busy clinical setting.

Pathophysiology

No single factor has been considered causative even though many have been suggested, including hormones and blood sugar. However, since symptoms of PMS/PMDD do not occur before menarche or after menopause, there is clearly a link between the rapid fluctuations of hormones in the menstruating woman and the symptomatology. Recent research has found evidence of disturbances of serotonin and endorphin metabolism and the circadian rhythm in women with PMDD. Like patients with PMS/PMDD, depressed patients often have decreased serotoninergic activity. Of note, plasma glucose levels less than 50 mg/dL are rarely seen in patients with PMS, even in those who claim they have "hypoglycemic attacks."

Evaluation and Treatment

The history, physical examination, and laboratory testing should aim to distinguish PMS/PMDD from other medical conditions, such as thyroid disease, and from psychiatric disorders. Strict diagnostic criteria should therefore be used and a symptom diary may be helpful to obtain the correct diagnosis.

First and foremost among the treatment options are lifestyle changes. Increased aerobic exercise is clearly helpful. Dietary changes such as high-carbohydrate foods and frequent meals, which cause a steady intake of tryptophan and in turn increase serotonin synthesis, may also be helpful. Improved sleep, yoga, relaxation, and decreased intake of coffee, alcohol, and cigarettes all have some generalized benefits.

Dietary supplements have received more attention recently A recent study showed that daily supplementation of 1200 mg of calcium carbonate decreased PMS symptoms by 48%, compared with a 30% reduction with placebo. Vitamin B_6 (pyridoxine) supplementation is controversial, there is little evidence to prove its effects, and high doses (over 100 mg/day) can be neurotoxic. Kava is an herbal supplement that has been used to treat general anxiety, but it has recently been shown to be severely hepatotoxic and should be avoided.

Selective serotonin reuptake inhibitors such as fluoxetine are often the first-line treatment for severe PMS/PMDD and have been used successfully to manage both the emotional and somatic symptoms. Adverse effects are mild and frequently transient and include nervousness, insomnia, and nausea. Decreasing the dose can reduce the more troubling side effect of decreased libido.

Fluoxetine is effective even if given only during the luteal phase at 20 mg/day or even in single or intermittent doses. Buspirone, a non-benzodiazepine anxiolytic, has been used with some success in doses of 30 to 60 mg/day during the luteal phase. Side effects include headache, dizziness, and nausea.

Other medications are useful for treating some more specific symptoms that occur with PMS/PMDD. Diuretics such as spironolactone 50 mg/day improve symptoms of bloating and breast tenderness. If diuretics are given in small and intermittent doses, potassium levels do not need to be monitored. NSAIDs help to ease breast tenderness and pelvic pain.

Progesterone vaginal suppositories were the drug of choice for PMS for many years, but these have been found to be no more effective than placebo. Oral and transdermal progesterone are equally ineffective, and since the progesterone levels are already the highest during the PMS phase, giving extra progesterone makes little clinical sense.

GnRH agonists have been discussed elsewhere for the treatment of menstrual disorders. They cause a pseudomenopausal state and are given as an injection or as a nasal spray. Both physical and psychological symptoms improve dramatically once amenorrhea and anovulation occurs, but the adverse effects of hot flashes, decreased libido, and vaginal dryness can be difficult for the patient to undergo. Danazol is similarly effective for PMS, but the androgenic adverse effects are often overwhelming. Bromocriptine decreases the levels of prolactin, which might help breast tenderness, but its common side effects of nausea and hypotension are too great to make it useful as a remedy.

Among the surgical options, hysterectomy with or without bilateral oophorectomy is effective in the treatment of PMS but is considered a last resort. The patient should probably undergo a course of GnRH agonist first to evaluate her response to a postmenopausal state before undergoing surgery, and all medical options should be exhausted.

Remedies that have not been shown to be effective for PMS, but which are still often used, include oral contraceptive pills, synthetic progestins, other dietary supplements or chiropractic treatments.

KEY POINTS

1. *Primary amenorrhea* is defined as the absence of menstruation by the age of 16 years in the presence of normal growth and secondary sexual characteristics.

2. *Secondary amenorrhea* is defined as the absence of menses for more than three cycles or 6 months in a previously menstruating woman.

3. Causes of amenorrhea can be classified into broad categories depending on the site of dysfunction: hypothalamic and pituitary dysfunction, gonadal dysfunction, and anatomic abnormalities.

4. Any woman who develops secondary amenorrhea should be evaluated with a pregnancy test because pregnancy is the most common cause of this condition.

5. Polycystic ovarian syndrome is classically expressed as hirsutism, irregular menstrual cycles, obesity, and a specific appearance of the ovaries on ultrasound.

6. *Dysmenorrhea* is defined as painful menstrual cramps of uterine origin. The term *primary dysmenorrhea* is used when there is no demonstrable pelvic disease, and the term secondary dysmenorrhea is used when pelvic disease is present.

7. Nonsteroidal anti-inflammatory drugs are the first-line treatment of dysmenorrhea.

8. Premenstrual syndrome (PMS) comprises the cyclic physical and behavioral symptoms that occur during the luteal phase of the ovulatory cycle. Premenstrual dysphoric disorder (PMDD) is a severe form of PMS in which irritability, internal tension, and anger are prominent.

9. Selective serotonin reuptake inhibitors such as fluoxetine are the first-line treatment for severe PMS/PMDD.

SUGGESTED READING

American College of Obstetricians and Gynecologists: Management of anovulatory bleeding. ACOG Practice Bulletin, Number 14, March 2000.

APGO Education Series on Women's Health Issues: Clinical Management of Abnormal Uterine Bleeding. Boston, Jespersen and Assoc, May 2002.

Awwad JT, Toth TL, Schiff I: Abnormal uterine bleeding in the perimenopause. Int J Fertil 38:261–269, 1993.

Lahteenmaki P, Haukkamaa M, Puolaka J, et al: Open randomized study of use of levo-norgestrel releasing intrauterine system as alternative to hysterectomy. BMJ 316:1122–1126, 1998.

Lethaby A, Augood C, Duckitt K: Nonsteroidal anti-inflammatory drugs for heavy menstrual bleeding. Cochrane Database System Rev 1:CD000400, 2002.

Lethaby A, Farquhar C, Cooke I: Antifibrinolytics for heavy menstrual bleeding. Cochrane Library 4: CD000249, 2000.

Menorrhagia, Clinical Evidence:. London, BMJ Publishing Group, 2001, pp 1445–1460.

Menorrhagia, Clinical Evidence Concise. London, BMJ Publishing Group, 2004, pp 462–464.

Nichols DH, Sweeney PJ: Ambulatory Gynecology. 2nd ed. Philadelphia, J.B. Lippincott and Co, 1995.

Prentice A: Medical management of menorrhagia. BMJ 319:1343–1345, 1999.

Speroff L, Glass RH, and Kass NG (eds): Clinical Gynecologic Endocrinology and Infertility, 6th ed. Baltimore, MD, Williams and Wilkins, 1999.

Treloar AE, Boynton RE, Behn BG, Brown BV: Variations of the human menstrual cycle through reproductive life. Int J Fertil 12(1 Pt 2):77–126, 1970.

16

MENOPAUSE
Andrea L. Sikon and Holly L. Thacker

DEFINITION/TERMINOLOGY/PHYSIOLOGY

Menopause is the gradual progression to a permanent loss of ovarian follicular function and is retrospectively diagnosed 12 months after the cessation of menses. The average age of menopause onset is 51 years, with approximately 1% of women transitioning before the age of 40 years and 5% after the age of 55 years. Menopause is considered premature when it occurs before the age of 40 years.

With women's life expectancy approaching 80 years, two thirds of the total U.S. population will survive to beyond the age of 85 years. At the end of the millennium, 42 million U.S. women were postmenopausal. The majority of women will spend more than 30% of their lives in the postmenopause years. Despite this increase in life expectancy, the average age of menopause has not changed in centuries.

Most believe that all mammalian females are born with a finite number of ovarian follicles as the primordial follicle oocyte is arrested in the prophase of the first meiotic division. Through the reproductive life span, germ cells are depleted by mostly atresia and, to a lesser degree, ovulation, leading to eventual ovarian failure at menopause. This theory has recently been questioned based on results of mouse studies suggesting that adult ovaries may contain oocytes with the capacity for mitotic division.

During menstrual life, the ovaries make estrogens, androgens, progesterone, and inhibin. The ovarian dominant follicle and corpus luteum produce the most potent of the three human estrogens, 17 β-estradiol (E_2). The peripheral aromatization of androstenedione in adipose and muscle and the metabolism of E_2 produce most of the second most abundant estrogen, estrone (E_1). Small amounts of estrone are also produced by the ovary and adrenal glands. The premenopausal ratio of circulating estradiol to estrone of greater than 1 reverses after menopause, with estrone becoming the dominant circulating estrogen. Estriol (E_3) is the weakest of the three human estrogens. During the childbearing years, the ovary makes inhibin, which inhibits the release of follicle-stimulating hormone (FSH). Inhibin is no longer made in the postmenopausal years, thus allowing for the rises in FSH seen with menopause. Progesterone is produced primarily by the corpus luteum and is the only naturally occurring progestogen. Progesterone opposes estrogen's actions and converts proliferative endometrium into a secretory endometrium in preparation for implantation and pregnancy, with levels decreasing during the menopause transition. Chemically altered, predominantly plant-based progestins are synthetically manufactured to oppose the effects of estrogen in pharmacologic hormone therapy (HT).

Menopause is a defined point in time, with the years preceding the actual onset called the *menopause transition* (or *perimenopause*). Ovarian function usually begins to decline during the mid-30s, accounting for the beginning of menstrual irregularity and decreased fertility. This is due to a decreasing number of ovarian follicles, with the remaining ones likely less sensitive to the stimulatory effects of FSH and luteinizing hormone (LH). Thus, anovulatory cycles occur with increased frequency, causing cycle irregularity. Alternatively, some cycles are associated with the release of several follicles (perhaps accounting for an increased incidence in twins in women in the later reproductive years). During this time of significant hormonal fluctuation, however, pregnancy remains a possibility and should always be considered in the differential diagnoses of secondary amenorrhea.

Although most factors influencing the age of menopause are poorly understood, inherited variations in the estrogen receptor and a dose-dependent association between the quantity and duration of active smoking have been linked to an earlier age of menopause.

DIAGNOSTIC MARKERS

Unfortunately, no reliable biologic marker exists to definitively predict when the menopause transition will occur; however, elevated levels of FSH (30 to 40 mIU/mL) usually signal its beginning. FSH levels are highly variable but peak about 1 year after menopause and decline slightly in the following years, never returning to premenopausal levels (due to loss of ovarian inhibin.) As menses ceases, progesterone and estrogen concentrations also decline. Postmenopausal ovaries continue to make androstenedione and testosterone, which can be peripherally converted to estrone. The adrenals continue to make androgens, predominantly dehydroepiandrosterone sulfate (DHEA-S); however, levels in women decline with age.

Due to their high variability, FSH and estradiol levels cannot reliably diagnose menopause. Instead, a clinical diagnosis is made, taking into consideration age, history, symptoms, date of last menstrual cycle, and a negative pregnancy test result. Knowledge of FSH and estradiol levels may assist in the decision to initiate HT when a woman has had a hysterectomy with uncertain remaining ovarian function, but these may still be variable and difficult to interpret at times. Some have also advocated measuring FSH and estradiol levels to help determine when to transition a woman from hormonal contraceptive (HC) doses to postmenopausal doses of HT; however, these values tend to be unreliable due to the wide fluctuations characteristic of this transitional time.

SYMPTOMS

Estrogen receptors are found throughout the body in variable distributions, thus accounting for the myriad symptoms that can accompany menopause in addition to the cessation of menses and vasomotor symptoms. Receptors for estrogen are found in the urogenital tract, breast, liver, gastrointestinal tract, bone, blood vessels, lungs, and central nervous system. Estrogen's diverse actions are dependent on different receptor types (alpha or beta) found in varying levels in many tissues. An ideal HT drug would have estrogen agonism in the tissues that are the source for symptoms of estrogen deficiency, such as the urogenital system, and would be antagonistic in tissues like the breast and endometrium to avoid deleterious adverse effects.

Menopausal symptoms are widely variable among women in occurrence, frequency, and time of onset. Some women begin to experience menstrual and vasomotor symptoms years before menopause, and others experience little if any accompanying symptoms. No reliable predictors exist to help determine the degree and duration of a woman's symptoms. Women with surgically induced menopause, however, tend to have more intense and longer-lasting symptoms without treatment.

Menstrual Irregularity

Menstrual irregularity is the most common transition symptom, making it difficult to differentiate what constitutes abnormal bleeding that requires further investigation from typical transition changes. Care must be taken to evaluate irregular bleeding because the incidence of endometrial cancer increases with age. Abnormal uterine bleeding is defined in Box 16-1.

Vasomotor Symptoms

Vasomotor symptoms include hot flashes and flushes—sudden, wavelike sensations of intense heat usually starting about the neck and spreading over the body and face, causing a flush followed by perspiration with a chill. Night sweats are hot flashes that occur during the night and are accompanied by drenching sweats. Other vasomotor symptoms include palpitations, skin crawling, and scalp sensations. Although the exact cause of vasomotor symptoms is not entirely understood, it is suspected that some destabilization of the thermoregulatory zone in the hypothalamus occurs during estrogen withdrawal. These vasomotor symptoms can range from minor irritations to a major disruption in quality of life, with approximately 5% to 10% women being severely affected. Although

Box 16-1   Abnormal Uterine Bleeding
Heavier than usual bleeding (blood loss >80 mL), especially with blood clots or anemia
Prolonged bleeding (>7 days)
Frequent menstrual periods (cycle length <21 days)
Bleeding or spotting between menses and/or after sexual intercourse

Box 16-2   Hot Flash Triggers

Warm environment
Stress
Hot/spicy foods
Hot drinks
Alcohol
Caffeine
Medications

unpredictable, active smokers have higher incidences of hot flashes. Hot flash triggers are listed in Box 16-2.

Nonpharmacologic options to treat vasomotor symptoms include deep paced slow diaphragmatic breathing, relaxation therapy, and minimizing potential triggers; these modalities should be suggested to all women experiencing vasomotor symptoms. Currently, the most efficacious and the only U.S. Food and Drug Administration (FDA) approved pharmacologic therapy to treat hot flashes is HT in those without contraindications. Based on smaller studies, a number of alternative agents may also reduce menopausal vasomotor symptoms, including serotonin norepinephrine reuptake inhibitors, selective serotonin reuptake inhibitors, gabapentin (Neurontin), and herbal agents like black cohosh and soy isoflavones. These alternatives are treatment options for those refusing or those with contraindications to HT.

Phytoestrogens have weak estrogen-like effects. The growing interest in the use of phytoestrogens to treat postmenopausal symptoms has led to a number of investigations that have shown conflicting results. However, few clinical trials have evaluated the effects of phytoestrogens on bone mineral density (BMD) or their safety in patients with contraindications to estrogen.

When using HT, the current recommendation is to use the lowest effective dose for symptom control for the shortest time interval with at least yearly clinical reevaluation. Low-dose HCs are an option for reducing symptoms during the perimenopausal time and preventing unwanted pregnancy. The use of continuous pills or the addition of a small dose of estrogen during the placebo week is an option for women who are symptomatic during the placebo week. Seasonale (ethinyl estradiol 0.03 mg/levonorgestrel 0.15 mg) is a 91-day HC regimen based on active pills for 12 weeks with 1 week of placebo versus the conventional 21 days of active pills followed by 7 days of placebo. Intermenstrual bleeding with this prolonged dosing regimen can be a common occurrence, especially within the first few cycles of use. Tables 16-1, 16-2, and 16-3 demonstrate common hormonal therapies used for the treatment of menopausal symptoms.

No evidence-based strategies exist to direct the transition of a patient from HC to HT or how to "wean off" of HT; however, various groups have made general recommendations. The increasing number of variable delivery methods and low-dose formulations available present many therapeutic options. Vasomotor symptoms often recur within 4 days after the cessation of therapy, dependent on the type/route of therapy. Therefore, tapering the dose as well as decreasing the number of days per week HT is taken may be useful in the attempt to discontinue HT therapy.

Many strategies have been reported to help determine when to transition a woman from hormonal contraception to postmenopausal HT. A dose of HC contains four to 10 times the amount of equipotent estrogen in an equivalent HT dose. One course of action is to measure the FSH level on the sixth or seventh day of the placebo week during HC use and switch to HT when the FSH is in the menopausal range (>30 to 40 IU/L); however,

Table 16-1

Major Estrogens in Use

Estrogen	Origin	Medications
Conjugated equine estrogens (CEE)	CEE	Premarin, Prempro, low-dose Prempro, Premphase
Conjugated synthetic estrogens	Synthesized from plant sources	Cenestin, Enjuvia
17 β-estradiol (E$_2$)	Synthesized from plant source	Estrace (micronized oral tablets), Alora, Climara, Estraderm, Vivelle, Vivelle-Dot, Esclim, (transdermal patches), Estrasorb, Estrogel (topical daily application), Vagifem, Estring, (local vaginal application), and Menoring, (vaginal-systemic ring)
17 β-E$_2$ with progestin		Activella (norethindrone acetate), Prefest (norgestimate acetate), CombiPatch (norethindrone acetate), Climara Pro (combined with levonorgestrel)
Ethinyl estradiol	Synthesized estrogen	Femhrt (combined with norethindrone)

Table 16-2

Major Progestogens in Use

Progestogen	Origin	Medications
Medroxyprogesterone acetate	Synthetic 21-carbon derivative of 17-hydroxyprogesterone	Prempro, Premphase, Provera, Cycrin
Norethindrone acetate	Synthetic 19-carbon nortestosterone derivative	Activella, CombiPatch, Femhrt
Norethindrone	Synthetic 19-carbon nortestosterone derivative	Aygestin, Micronor, Nor-QD
Norgestimate	Synthetic 19-carbon nortestosterone derivative	Prefest
Micronized progesterone	Synthesized from yams structurally identical to naturally occurring progesterone	Prometrium
Levonorgestrel	Synthetic 19-carbon nortestosterone derivative	Climara Pro

some postmenopausal women do not exhibit reliably increased levels until HCs are discontinued for a number of weeks to months. Some add estradiol levels in these cases, looking for a fall less than 20 to 30 picograms/mL and an FSH/LH ratio greater than 1 to be diagnostic of menopause. Alternatively, many menopause experts recommend transitioning from HC to HT at the age of 55 years, considered to be an age at which unintentional pregnancy would be unlikely. Caution using HC in women aged 35 years and older should be followed, with avoidance in those women with contraindications (Box 16-3).

Table 16-3

Combination
Hormone
Replacement
Therapeutic Options
Available in the
United States

Product	Estrogen (Dose)	Progestin (Dose)	Delivery Regimen
Activella	Estradiol (1 mg)	NETA (0.5 mg)	Continuous-oral
Femhrt	Ethinyl estradiol (0.005 mg)	NETA (1 mg)	Continuous-oral
Premphase	CEE (0.625 mg)	MPA (5 mg)	Sequential-oral
Prempro	CEE (0.625 mg)	MPA (2.5 or 5 mg)	Continuous-oral
	CEE (0.45 mg)	MPA (1.5 mg)	Continuous-oral
	CEE (0.3 mg)	MPA (1.5 mg)	Continuous-oral
Prefest	Estradiol (1 mg)	NGM (0.09 mg)	Intermittent/ Continuous-oral
CombiPatch	Estradiol (0.05 mg/day)	NETA (0.14 or 0.25 mg/day)	Transdermal
Climara Pro	Estradiol (0.045 mg/day)	Levonorgestrel (0.015 mg/day)	Transdermal

CEE, Conjugated equine estrogens; MPA, medroxyprogesterone acetate; NETA, norethindrone acetate; NGM, norgestimate.

Box 16-3   World Health Organization Guidelines: Relative and Absolute Contraindications to Hormonal Contraception (HC) Use in Women Older Than Age 35 Years

Smokers (>15 cigarettes/day)
Untreated hypertension (i.e., >160 mm Hg systolic, >99 mm Hg diastolic) or with vascular disease
Preexisting cardiovascular/cerebrovascular disease
Current breast cancer
Complicated structural heart disease (e.g., atrial fibrillation, pulmonary hypertension, bacterial endocarditis)
Severe headaches with focal neurologic symptoms
Complications from diabetes
Active thromobembolic disease
Major surgery with prolonged immobilization
Pregnancy/lactation, and less than 6 weeks postpartum
Undiagnosed abnormal genital bleeding
Liver disease (acute viral hepatitis, severe cirrhosis, benign or malignant liver tumors)
Estrogen dependent neoplasias

Atrophic Vaginitis

Atrophic vaginitis is the direct result of estrogen deficiency leading to thinning of the vaginal epithelium, reductions in vaginal blood flow, and decreased lubrication. This can lead to dyspareunia, kraurosis vulvae, and more frequent urinary tract infections. Endogenous estrogen decline causes reductions in epithelial cell glycogen, leading to increased alkalinization of the urogenital areas, thus predisposing to vaginitis and urinary tract infections.

Signs of atrophy on examination begin with an alkaline vaginal pH; an increase of the pH to 6 to 7.5 signifies the loss of the normal acidity of the vagina with falling estradiol levels. Vaginal pH is tested with pH paper. Assessment of the vaginal epithelium on visual inspection is then done for signs of thinning, evidenced by loss of rugae and pale patches, sometimes with petechiae. The periurethral tissue may show the first signs of atrophy because it is the most estrogen-sensitive area. As atrophy worsens, introital stenosis, a narrowed vagina with a small flattened cervix, and a stenotic cervical os can also be found.

Many different types of over-the-counter vaginal moisturizers exist to help to relieve dryness and itching as well as aid in lubrication during intercourse (Box 16-4). In addition, many local delivery systems for vaginal estrogen are available including tablets, rings, and creams (Box 16-5).

Urinary Incontinence

Although many estrogen receptors are found in the female urethra, bladder trigone, and anorectum, the effect of menopause on urinary incontinence is poorly understood after controlling for age. *Incontinence* is defined as the involuntary leakage of urine and includes several different types: stress (SUI), urge (UUI), mixed (stress and urge), overflow, and functional urinary incontinence. Although incontinence can affect women in younger years, the incidence increases with age, affecting approximately 30% to 50% of women in the fifth to sixth decades. Incontinence is not a normal part of aging, and prevalence is likely underestimated due to under-reporting and underdiagnosis.

Box 16-4 Over-the-Counter Nonhormonal Vaginal Moisturizers and Lubricants

Vaginal moisturizers, for daily use to maintain vaginal moisture
Replens
Gyne-Moistrin
Moist Again
RePhresh (lowers vaginal pH)
Silk-E

Personal lubricants, for use at time of intercourse
Astroglide
Condom-Mate Vaginal Suppository
K-Y Jelly
Lubrin vaginal suppository
Today Personal Lubricant

Box 16-5 Local Hormonal Treatment Options

Cream
Estrace (micronized 17 β-estradiol)
Premarin (conjugated equine estrogens)

Vaginal ring
Estring (micronized 17 β-estradiol), changed every 3 months
Femring (local and systemic), changed every 3 months

Vaginal tablet
Vagifem (estradiol hemihydrate), applied to lower third of the vagina daily for
    2 weeks then one tablet intravaginally twice a week

Mixed symptoms of SUI and UUI occur in about 30% of women with incontinence, although one type usually predominates. Although mixed incontinence is the most common form of urinary continence, the prevalence of UUI increases with advancing age, affecting up to 20% of menopausal women. UUI is characterized by detrusor overactivity, causing urine to leak from the bladder with a sense of urgency, often in large amounts with urinary frequency. Usually idiopathic, other potential causes such as infection, tumor, bladder stones, atrophy, or neurologic sources should also be considered.

SUI is common in menopausal women and often occurs while coughing, straining, exercising, or standing. Hormonal changes, aging, prior pelvic surgeries, radiation, childbirth trauma, or neurogenic disorders are contributing factors.

A small subset of women has overflow incontinence, often characterized by frequent dribbling. This occurs when the bladder does not contract normally, resulting in overdistention and leakage when bladder pressure exceeds sphincter pressure. Functional leakage is a result of limitations in the ability to physically reach facilities, most often a result of orthopedic issues or cognitive impairment such as dementia or stroke.

Asking women to keep a urine voiding diary including the time, amount voided, activities surrounding urination, and grading of leakage, urgency, and fluid amounts can help to differentiate the above types. The physical examination should focus on assessing mental status, mobility, neurologic status, and signs of urogenital atrophy or prolapse, sphincter tone, fecal impaction, or masses. After the examination, the initial diagnostic evaluation includes a urinalysis to exclude infection or glucosuria and measuring a postvoid residual by bladder ultrasound or catheterization to determine the completeness of bladder emptying (<50 to 100 mL is normal). More detailed investigations including urodynamics are used in more complicated cases. Serologies for hypercalcemia, hyperglycemia, and kidney function are checked as appropriate.

Attempts to eradicate occult infection and improve reversible causes are the first-line treatments.

Also, some evidence supports the recommendation of pelvic floor exercises first introduced by Dr. Arnold Kegel. When done properly and regularly, significant improvement in symptoms can be noted; both written and verbal instructions should be provided to maximize efficacy. Simple behavioral modifications can also help to reduce symptoms, including scheduled voiding, limiting evening/nocturnal fluid intake, and avoiding exacerbating medications like diuretics. Bladder irritants like tobacco, caffeine, and alcohol should be minimized, and environmental barriers to toileting (e.g., poor mobility, lack of hand rails) should be remedied to lessen functional incontinence.

Topical estrogen may be effective in helping to treat some urinary incontinence symptoms, especially urgency, by reversing vaginal mucosal atrophy and augmenting local support tissues. However, evidence regarding estrogen therapy is mixed, with some studies showing higher rates of incontinence in those taking oral estrogen. An α-adrenergic agonist like pseudoephedrine can be used to treat mild SUI by increasing internal sphincter tone and bladder outflow resistance. A new serotonin and norepinephrine dual-reuptake inhibitor (duloxetine) has been found to be efficacious and safe for use in women with SUI and has also demonstrated efficacy in the treatment of major depressive disorder. Mechanical devices including vaginal inserts like a pessary, periurethral injections (bulking agents), and urethral blockers such as a supersized vaginal tampon can also all be considered for SUI.

The most common medications used for UUI treatment are the anticholinergics oxybutynin (Ditropan) and tolterodine tartrate (Detrol). A newer antimuscarinic/antispasmodic agent, trospium chloride (Sanctura), is also approved for the treatment of overactive bladder symptoms. Treatment options for urinary incontinence are discussed in more detail in Chapter 24, Urinary Incontinence.

Headaches

A link between hormonal fluctuations and migraine flares has been noted, as evidenced in menstrual migraines. Thus, perimenopause can bring about a flare in headaches, with most women experiencing attenuation postmenopausally as hormone levels stabilize.

Effects on Hair/Skin/Nails

Estrogen receptors are abundant in the skin and help to maintain skin collagen and thickness. During the first 5 postmenopausal years, loss of collagen occurs at an exponential rate, with losses of up to 30% declining to approximately 2% in the years thereafter. This loss of collagen accounts for the lessened elasticity and increased laxity causing wrinkling. Androgen hormones also control sebum production and relative increases can be seen in some women, leading to adult-onset acne. The increase in the androgen to estrogen ratio may also partially account for changes in hair and voice during the menopausal transition. Androgens and some progestins can increase hair loss, but estrogen therapy tends to decrease losses.

Androgenic alopecia, more commonly known as *male pattern baldness,* is likely due to increased dihydro-testosterone levels via 5α-reductase conversion or decreasing estrogen levels. Androgenic alopecia is quite common, affecting women at an increased rate of up to 32% by the eighth decade. Androgenic alopecia occurs more commonly in women with a family history of hair loss and can be worsened by androgenic progestins, anabolic steroids, and androgens. Frontal hair is usually preserved, with most loss at the vertex and the temporal areas.

Oral contraceptives containing less androgenic progestins like norgestimate (Ortho Tri-Cyclen) or desogestrel (Desogen, Ortho Cept, Mircette) may help. Evidence exists for the efficacy of minoxidil (Rogaine), the only approved medication for female hair loss. Minoxidil increases hair growth in 3 to 9 months for some women during continued applications. Some recommend spironolactone, although its efficacy is controversial. Finasteride (Propecia) has also been tried to reduce hyperandrogenism with variable results; it can be teratogenic for male fetuses and is not routinely recommended in perimenopausal women. Other antiandrogens like flutamide (Eulexin) have also been studied, but use has been limited by hepatotoxicity.

Hirsutism is an excessive growth of hair in androgen-sensitive skin areas like the chest, abdomen, and face. This is usually also due to ovarian androgen overproduction or inherited peripheral hypersensitivity to normal androgen circulating levels. A review of systems and other signs should always be conducted to exclude rarer causes, such as virilizing tumors or adrenal hyperplasia. Some women also find more fine facial hair appearing on the upper lip and chin, as well as some coarser hair on the chin. Bleaching; removal with waxing, shaving, or laser treatments; and prevention of hair regrowth with topical medications like eflornithine (Vaniqa) may be used to treat the excessive hair growth.

Nutritional deficiencies (including vitamin B_{12}), thyroid dysfunction, systemic lupus erythematosus, and other systemic diseases should also be considered as causes of hirsutism. A thorough medication review for offending agents should also be performed.

Mood and Sleep Changes

The menopausal transition is a time of change that can result in changes in self-esteem, body image, and self concept; however, most women freed from childbearing responsibilities report feeling happier and more fulfilled at this life stage. Multiple mood disturbances have been reported to be associated with the menopausal transition, including irritability, depression, sleep disorders, and memory difficulties. Although up to 10% of women report these symptoms during the transition, a direct link to lowered estrogen levels has not been established. Possible etiologies for mood disturbances may include altered sleep that can arise from night sweats and stressors, exacerbating fatigue, and reducing concentration levels. The fluctuations and unpredictability of symptoms can also induce a sense of loss of control, which can be frustrating and may affect mood.

Women with a history of premenstrual syndrome/premenstrual dysphoric disorder, depression, and more symptomatic menopausal symptoms tend to have a higher incidence of mood-related disturbances in menopause.

Sleep disturbances affect approximately one third to one half of women aged 40 to 54 years. Interference with consistent, high-quality sleep affects multiple systems and can exacerbate comorbidities like mood disorders, fibromyalgia, and migraines. Prolonged or severe symptoms involving three nights or more a week lasting for 1 month should trigger a medical evaluation. A polysomnogram and sleep analysis can be helpful to determine the underlying cause and to exclude sleep-disordered breathing (such as obstructive sleep apnea) that may need further specific intervention.

Memory/ Cognition/ Dementia

Many women report memory and concentration difficulties associated with menopause. Estrogen receptors have been located on cholinergic neurons with neurotropic, antioxidant, and anti-inflammatory effects. This biologic data seemed to support the significant number of observational studies that suggested that HT was partially protective against dementia. However, a recent randomized trial showed an increased risk of dementia in women taking combined conjugated equine estrogens (CEE) and medroxyprogesterone acetate (MPA) without benefit for milder impairments. Several randomized trials of CEE alone in women with pre-existing mild to moderate Alzheimer's disease have shown no significant benefit and a possible worsening at doses of 0.625 mg/day or higher. Due to the limitations of the trials, the true impact of daily CEE/MPA or estrogen therapy in early postmenopause on Alzheimer's disease or dementia remains unclear. Current recommendations suggest that women aged 65 years and older should not be treated with CEE alone or CEE/MPA for the primary prevention of dementia or for cognition benefits.

Sexual Function

Female sexual dysfunction is defined as any disorder affecting any of the phases of the sexual response cycle of desire, arousal, or orgasm. One recent study reported an incidence of sexual dysfunction in 43% of women aged 18 to 59 years. Arguably, some difficulties may be reactionary to other issues, including problematic relationships, comorbidities of self and partner, and easily treatable etiologies like atrophic vaginitis. The first step in the evaluation of sexual dysfunction includes awareness; the physician must ask about a woman's perception of her sexual functioning. Recognizing the tremendous interplay of many organic and psychological features is also a key step in addressing the issue. A thorough history should be obtained detailing any prior abuse; self and partner expectations; relationship, social, and job stresses; as well as details of what part of the sexual relationship is unsatisfactory.

Differentiating between problems with libido, arousal, and orgasm is mandatory, so that further questioning can be more specifically directed. An interview should begin with an assessment of the menstrual cycle, obstetric, gynecologic, and surgical histories, and comorbidities. A decreased libido should prompt an investigation into diagnosed and occult comorbid conditions like depression/anxiety, substance abuse, diabetes, neuropathic etiologies, and thyroid disease. A review of medications and herbal supplements should also be completed to ensure dysfunction is not an iatrogenic side effect. Commonly, women taking antidepressants may have decreased libido as well as a delay in the ability to climax. Questions regarding dyspareunia with any part of relations or decreased sensation should be detailed, as one may uncover a negative feedback cycle of pain or anorgasmia causing diminutions in libido. A focused review of systems should generate a more detailed exploration of any positive symptoms, with a physical examination focusing on the areas in question; the detection of vaginal atrophy, infection, strictures, scarring from prior surgeries or radiation therapy, vaginismus, or levator ani myalgia may help to direct treatment. Fear of incontinence associated with intercourse or orgasm may be an underlying cause of sexual dysfunction and should be identified and treated.

Female sexual dysfunction may be caused by inadequate testosterone levels; an effort has been made to define a true female androgen deficiency syndrome (FDS). The syndrome occurs most commonly after oophorectomy as measurable decreases in bioavailable testosterone occur. This syndrome affects approximately one sixth of all women who have undergone hysterectomy. FDS can only be diagnosed in women with adequate estrogen levels to eliminate the possibility of symptoms being due to estrogen rather than androgen deficiency. Most premenopausal circulating testosterone results from the peripheral conversion of the adrenal androgens DHEA-S and DHEA to androstenedione and then to testosterone and estrone. Testosterone is then aromatized to estradiol or dihydro-testosterone via 5α-reductase. One quarter of circulating testosterone comes from the ovaries. Studies are variable concerning whether there is a consistent decline in testosterone concentrations during menopause. Adrenal androgen levels do not change with menopause itself because postmenopausal ovaries continue to produce androstenedione and testosterone; however, levels decrease with age as metabolism of adrenal androgens is altered. Receptors for androgens are present throughout the body including in the bone, muscle, and brain. To be diagnosed with FDS, symptoms must be clearly present, including a dysphoric mood, alterations in sexual function, and persistent, unexplained fatigue. Free testosterone levels should be at or below the lowest quartile of that considered normal for reproductive age (i.e., 20 to 40 years). Studies are underway to assess the efficacy and safety of various delivery systems of testosterone in women for the treatment of FDS. Estratest, a pill available in two strengths containing 0.625 or 1.25 mg of esterified estrogen with 1.25 or 2.5 mg of methyltestosterone, respectively, may be used for women with refractory hot flashes and FDS. A testosterone patch for women with hypoactive sexual desire disorder who have undergone hysterectomy has been developed. However, it has not yet been approved by the Food and Drug Administration (FDA).

SKELETAL CHANGES

Most bone mass is acquired during the adolescent years, peaking in the second to third decade of life with a subsequent lifelong gradual decline. Menopause may cause an accelerated loss of bone density for the 5 to 7 years that follow in up to 50% of all women.

Osteoporosis

Osteoporosis is a systemic skeletal disease that is characterized by diminished bone strength (i.e., loss of bone density, microarchitecture, and mineralization). Osteoporosis is differentiated from normal losses of aging because it involves an excessive loss of BMD and microarchitecture with consequent altered quality of bone; it results from an imbalance of osteoclastic bone resorption exceeding osteoblastic bone formation. Bones become thin and weak, leading to a progressive loss of their ability to withstand the impact of normal daily activities. Bone fragility increases the risk of fracture from minimal trauma. The World Health Organization defines *osteoporosis* as BMD that is 2.5 standard deviations (SD) or more below the young adult mean value (T-score < -2.5), whereas persons with BMD between 1 and 2.5 SD below average (T-score $= -1$ to -2.5) are said to have osteopenia. Z-scores are sex- and age-matched comparisons of an individual woman's BMD compared with the mean BMD of age-matched women.

Risk Factors

Risk factors for low BMD include advancing age, white or Asian race, family history of osteoporosis in a first-degree relative, thin small bones, early age at menopause/inadequate concentrations of sex hormones, lifelong low calcium intake, low vitamin D intake, smoking, sedentary lifestyle, low body weight (i.e., <127 lb), and excessive alcohol intake. The National Osteoporosis Foundation (NOF) identifies risk factors for hip fracture independent of BMD as prior fragility fracture, family history of osteoporosis or fragility fracture in a first-degree relative, smoking, and body weight under 127 pounds. Advancing age has been identified as an independent risk factor for vertebral fracture, with each decade past the age of 50 years doubling the fracture risk. History of a prior vertebral fracture increases the risk of subsequent vertebral fractures approximately four-fold.

Diagnosis

Dual energy x-ray absorptiometry (DEXA) is the definitive method for quantifying BMD. Central DEXA is the gold standard used to most accurately assess BMD and study treatment impact. Other techniques, like heel ultrasound, measure BMD at peripheral sites and are used for general, simple screening but cannot be used for diagnosis or to follow up treatment response. Many clinicians measure central bone density every 24 months to monitor the effectiveness of treatment and to assess for losses and gains in density. For patients taking glucocorticoid treatment and for those with hyperparathyroidism, more frequent monitoring every 6 to 12 months may be necessary. Indications for BMD testing are displayed in Box 16-6.

The NOF, Medicare, and the U.S. Preventive Services Task Force (USPSTF) recommend BMD testing for all women aged 65 years and older, regardless of ethnicity and risk factors, and for any postmenopausal women younger than 65 years who have one or more additional risk factors for osteoporotic fracture aside from menopause. Identifying women with a loss of height greater than 1.5 inches, kyphosis, or both should also trigger evaluation with a central bone density measurement. Women who are

---

Box 16-6 Indications for Bone Mineral Density Testing

Age 65 years and older in female patient
Prior adult fragility fracture (occurring at or after the age of 40 years)
Family history of fragility fracture
Smokers
Low body weight (<127 lb)
Medical condition or medication use associated with low bone mass
Estrogen-deficient/postmenopausal state in female patient
Discontinuation of estrogen in female patient
Monitoring of treatment with agents to prevent or treat osteoporosis

estrogen deficient and would consider starting treatment or preventive therapy should also be offered BMD screening.

Low T-scores (≤-2.5) are not specific to primary osteoporosis, and other etiologies such as hyperthyroidism, hyperparathyroidism, liver disease, renal disease, and malabsorption syndromes should be investigated. A single low BMD measurement does not equate bone loss—only serial BMD measurements on the same scanner can reveal losses. BMD can predict fracture risk, but many other factors also contribute to this risk, such as bone quality, hip axis length, micro-architectural integrity, and fall risk. A complete assessment with history and physical examination must be completed to make a diagnosis of osteoporosis. When age-matched Z-scores of BMD are low (i.e., ≤-1.5) or when BMD is normal or low in those with a fragility fracture history, secondary causes of osteoporosis should be considered. Up to half of premenopausal women with osteoporosis have secondary causes, most commonly hypoestrogenemia (associated with premenopausal amenorrhea), steroid use, malabsorption from celiac disease, hyperthyroidism, and anticonvulsant use. No evidence-based guidelines exist to define what should constitute an initial secondary evaluation; however, most consider a complete blood count, blood urea nitrogen, creatinine, thyroid-stimulating hormone, calcium, phosphorus, alkaline phosphatase, 25-hydroxyvitamin D, and parathyroid hormone to be part of this investigation. A recent study suggested that all women with osteoporosis undergo an evaluation to exclude celiac disease due to the higher than previously thought prevalence of this disease in the general population, as well as a likely prevalence that is even higher in those with low bone mass. This workup should be tailored and expanded to each specific woman's history (Table 16-4).

Identifying risk factors and bone density measurement by DEXA are currently the best available methods for determining a woman's probability of developing a fracture because bone loss is clinically silent until a fracture occurs. Risk factor considerations in combination with T-scores from DEXA of the lumbar spine and hip are used to select patients for therapy. The NOF recommends initiating therapy for fracture prevention in women with BMD T-scores of ≤-2 SD below the mean in the absence of risk factors and in women with T-scores ≤-1.5 if other risk factors (as listed above) are present. No guidelines exist yet to help determine when to offer pharmacologic therapy to those with low bone mass but with T-scores ≤-1 to -1.4 or for total prevention in those with normal BMD but at high risk by history.

Treatments

Few comparative trials of pharmacologic treatments for low bone mass/osteoporosis exist. Data to assess the potential benefits of combination therapy remain limited.

Hormonal Therapy

HT, best when initiated within the first few years after menopause onset, can improve bone density and decrease the risk of osteoporotic fractures

Table 16-4 Causes of Secondary Osteoporosis

Endocrine and Metabolic Disease	Chronic Diseases	Conditions Causing Nutritional Deficiencies	Hormonal Causes	Medications	Genetic Disorders
Primary hyperparathyroidism	Chronic liver disease	Malabsorption syndromes (e.g., celiac disease)	Early menopause	Glucocorticoids	Homocystinuria
Cushing's syndrome	Hemochromatosis	Vitamin D deficiency	Athletic amenorrhea	Aromatase inhibitors (e.g., Aromasin [exemestane], Femara [letrozole])	Osteogenesis imperfecta
Hyperthyroidism	Multiple myeloma	Calcium deficiency	Pregnancy		Marfan syndrome
Hypophosphatasia	Disseminated carcinomatosis	Gastric and bowel resections	Estrogen deficiency	Excess thyroid hormones	
Chronic renal disease	Rheumatoid arthritis	Alcoholism		Heparin, unfractionated	
Mastocytosis	Ehlers-Danlos syndrome	Anorexia nervosa		Cyclosporine	
Hypercalciuria				GnRH agonists (e.g., Lupron [leuprolide acetate])	
				Chronic Depo-MPA	
				Methotrexate	
				Phenobarbital	
				Phenothiazines	
				Phenytoin	

GnRH, Gonadotropin-releasing hormone; MPA, medroxyprogesterone acetate

by approximately 50% while treating common menopausal symptoms. Estrogen decreases bone resorption by inhibiting cytokine-induced osteoclast activation.

Many clinical studies have used estrogen doses of 0.625 mg/day to prevent osteoporosis, although much lower doses have also been proven to be effective. Increases in spine and hip BMD and decreases in bone turnover markers occurred in elderly postmenopausal women treated with conjugated estrogens (0.625 mg/day) with or without progesterone, plus 1500 mg of calcium and 800 IU vitamin D. A sub-study from the Health, Osteoporosis, Progestin, and Estrogen (HOPE) trial, a large, randomized placebo-controlled trial with low-dose estrogen regimens of 0.3 or 0.45 mg/day, demonstrated similar results. Transdermal estrogen also decreased the risk of new vertebral fractures in women aged 47 to 75 years with established osteoporosis. Menostar is a low-dose transdermal system of unopposed estradiol 0.014 mg/day that is approved by the FDA to prevent osteoporosis in older women; it has been studied in women 60 to 80 years of age. For women with an intact uterus, daily progestin is not required with Menostar due to the very low estradiol dose; however, one should consider administering a progestin for 14 days every 6 to 12 months.

The National Institutes of Health's Women's Health Initiative (WHI) was a large, randomized, placebo-controlled, prospective, preventive trial that was designed to evaluate the long-term use of HT in older postmenopausal women. Major end points included the incidence of cardiovascular disease (CVD), fracture, and invasive breast cancer. The study did not evaluate the risks/benefits of short-term HT use in younger women for the relief of active menopausal symptoms or the effects on quality of life. The WHI was performed, however, in a predominantly older group (mean age, 63 years old) with an underlying inherent increased risk for coronary disease due to increased age. Caution should be used in extrapolating risk to women outside of the realm of those studied (i.e., younger, symptomatic women).

The initial WHI results suggested an increased risk of nonfatal myocardial infarction, stroke, pulmonary embolism, and breast cancer in those taking combined estrogen-progestin therapy (EPT) compared with placebo. Although reductions in colorectal cancer and hip fracture were statistically significant, the reductions did not outweigh the increased overall risk. Breast cancer risk was increased with HT use beyond 5 years of therapy; however, no associated increases in mortality were seen. Women without a uterus taking 0.625 mg/day CEE versus placebo (in the estrogen-only arm of the study) had an increased risk of stroke (12 more cases per 10,000 women each year with estrogen use versus placebo) without an effect on the risk of coronary heart disease. CEE use conferred a decreased risk of bone fractures (six fewer hip fractures per 10,000 women each year with estrogen versus placebo). Interestingly, the effects on breast and colorectal cancer risk observed with combined EPT were not seen with CEE alone. A possible, although statistically insignificant, reduction in breast cancer risk in the CEE-only arm requires further investigation because it showed seven fewer cases of breast cancer per 10,000 women in contrast to eight more cases of breast cancer per 10,000 women in the EPT arm.

HT, even at low doses, can increase BMD and relieve other menopausal symptoms like hot flashes, atrophic vaginitis, sleep disorders, and minor mood disturbances attributed to estrogen deficiency. The concomitant use of progestin with estrogen in women with an intact uterus negates the increased risk of endometrial cancer when estrogen therapy is unopposed; however, since there was no increased risk of breast cancer in the estrogen-only arm of the WHI, there is a trend to use lower or less frequent progestin therapy. Although the findings of the WHI have led to the current recommendation that HT should not be used as primary prevention for CVD, an individualized assessment of the potential risks versus benefits of HT should be reviewed with symptomatic women.

Many medical organizations, including the National Institutes of Health, American College of Obstetrics and Gynecology, and North American Menopause Society, have recommended that the lowest dose of hormones be used with regular reevaluation in those requiring HT. Lower doses have been studied for efficacy but not for long-term outcomes. A recent study of mostly menopausal women showed that most women overestimate the risks and benefits of HT, a finding that is not surprising given the confusing publicity surrounding the WHI, which emphasized relative risk percentages as opposed to absolute risks.

Other Bone Treatment Options

Bisphosphonates
Risedronate sodium (Actonel) and alendronate sodium (Fosamax) are two oral bisphosphonates approved for the prevention and treatment of postmenopausal osteoporosis. Both have been proven to increase spine and hip BMD in a dose-dependent manner and to decrease fracture rates by up to 50% to 60%. Risedronate is also FDA approved for the prevention of glucocorticoid-induced osteoporosis.

The exact mechanism by which oral bisphosphonates improve bone strength is not fully understood. They begin to induce notable increases in BMD within the first year of treatment, making them a feasible treatment for the elderly. The bisphosphonates have a prolonged half-life in bone and therefore the effects on BMD tend to be long lasting. Studies are ongoing to evaluate the best duration of bisphosphonate therapy.

Both once-daily and once-weekly doses are used in the prevention and treatment of osteoporosis in postmenopausal women. Bisphosphonates are generally well tolerated and bone specific and have few drug interactions. They are poorly absorbed, and their major adverse effects are gastrointestinal, thus leading to their difficulty in administration. Specific instruction must be given for the patient to take these drugs with 8 ounces of water on an empty stomach and to remain upright for 30 minutes afterwards. Once-weekly formulations are associated with fewer serious gastrointestinal adverse events compared with daily dosing. Bisphosphonates are not recommended for those with significant renal insufficiency (i.e., creatinine clearance <35 mL/min). Bisphosphonates have equivalent costs for the once-daily as well as once-weekly dosing and are approximately three times as expensive as HT. Studies are investigating the use of an intermittent intravenous bisphosphonate called *zoledronic acid* (Zometa), with results thus far showing increased spine and hip BMD and suppressed markers of bone turnover. This therapy is not yet FDA approved as a treatment for postmenopausal osteoporosis.

Selective Estrogen-Receptor Modulators

Selective estrogen-receptor modulators (SERMs) are nonsteroidal mixed-estrogen agonists and antagonists. Raloxifene (Evista) is the only SERM approved for the prevention and treatment of osteoporosis in postmenopausal women, reducing new vertebral fractures. SERMs exhibit antagonist properties in the breast and partial estrogen agonism in trabecular bone and cardiovascular tissue. Raloxifene has estrogen antagonist properties in the uterus and thus does not increase the risk of endometrial cancer. Several trials are underway to further evaluate the cardiovascular outcomes of SERMs because beneficial effects on serum lipid levels and decreases in homocysteine levels have been suggested. The recommended daily dosage of raloxifene is 60 mg, without regard to meal times. As with estrogen, raloxifene increases the relative risk of venous thromboembolism two- to three-fold. Unfortunately, it brings an increased incidence of vasomotor symptoms and can cause leg cramps, often limiting its use in the immediate postmenopausal years.

Parathyroid Hormone

Injectable parathyroid hormone, teriparatide 1–34 (Forteo), is an anabolic agent in contrast to the existing armamentarium of antiresorptive therapies. Teriparatide stimulates osteoblast-mediated bone formation when given subcutaneously and in intermittent low doses, in contrast to the osteoclastic resorption, which occurs during continuous exposure to high levels of parathyroid hormone in primary hyperparathyroidism. Teriparatide in a dose of 20 µg injected daily increases BMD and decreases the risk of vertebral and nonvertebral fractures in postmenopausal women with at least one vertebral fracture. Teriparatide is most often used in women with osteoporosis at high risk for fracture (i.e., those with a history of osteoporotic fracture or multiple risk factors for fracture) and/or failure or intolerance to other therapies.

Potential adverse effects include transient hypercalcemia/calciuria, orthostatic hypotension, and leg cramps. No adjustment in dosing is required for persons with mild to moderate renal insufficiency (i.e., creatinine clearance 30 to 72 mL/min) nor in patients with a history of congestive heart failure, although no studies have been done with teriparatide use in chronic renal failure or those with significant hepatic impairment. Use of the medicine is approved for up to 2 years of therapy. Contraindications for use include an increased inherent risk of osteosarcoma (such as those with Paget's disease), pediatric and young adults with open epiphyses, and those with a history of radiation therapy to the skeleton. Although a promising and valuable new tool, the current cost of teriparatide remains approximately $600/month. Estrogen or raloxifene can be used concomitantly with teriparatide; however, bisphosphonate use should be stopped during therapy and resumed if tolerated after teriparatide treatment is completed (i.e., after 2 years of parathyroid hormone treatment).

Calcitonin-Salmon Calcitonin-salmon is a hormone available most commonly as a nasal spray that inhibits osteoclast formation, reducing bone resorption. Calcitonin modestly reduces the risk of vertebral fractures at a dose of 200 IU/day over 3 to 5 years in postmenopausal women with a fracture history. Calcitonin is FDA approved for the treatment of osteoporosis in women in the late postmenopausal phase; it is not approved for osteoporosis prevention. Some authors suggest that intranasal use may have a mild analgesic effect in the treatment of compression fractures via unknown mechanisms. Potential adverse effects are local nasal irritation, epistaxis, nausea, and flushing. Because calcitonin is expensive and less effective than other available treatment options, it is usually reserved for patients with intolerance to other agents.

Calcium Supplements Calcium supplements can offset the relative calcium deficiency that many women experience as they age. This deficiency occurs because calcium absorption decreases with age and because many women do not have sufficient calcium intake in their diets. Women should be instructed to maximize their daily dietary intake by eating calcium-rich foods like low-fat dairy products and dark green leafy vegetables. Premenopausal and menopausal women receiving HT should ingest 1000 to 1200 mg/day of calcium. Postmenopausal women who are not undergoing HT should ingest 1500 mg/day. Many formulations of calcium are available. Calcium citrate may be the best type for older women because it does not require gastric acid for absorption and thus can be taken on a full or empty stomach and can be absorbed in the presence of achlorhydria or proton pump inhibitors. Calcium supplementation is contraindicated in persons with a history of hypercalcemia; it is not contraindicated in most of those with a history of nephrolithiasis. Most stones are made of calcium oxalate crystals, and dietary calcium helps to bind intestinal oxalate to form a nonabsorbable complex that is excreted in the feces. If dietary calcium is low, more oxalate can be reabsorbed, thus raising urinary oxalate excretion and predisposing patients to stone formation. Recent studies suggest that a low-calcium diet in such patients promotes a negative calcium skeletal balance and can cause increased renal oxalate excretion, predisposing to increased stone formation. Postmenopausal women with a history of nephrolithiasis should be encouraged to take calcium citrate with meals because it increases urinary citrate, a principal stone inhibitor, and can help to bind intestinal oxalates, thus decreasing urinary levels.

Supplemental Vitamin D Supplemental vitamin D, 600 to 1000 IU/day, is recommended for postmenopausal women, especially those with low levels of sun exposure. A growing number of studies have suggested that the previously recommended daily intake of 200–600 IU/day is suboptimal. Studies also reveal that although values of serum 25-OH D <30 ng/mL are often reported by some labs as "normal," values less than this can cause secondary hyperparathyroidism, and are thus insufficient. Ensuring adequate calcium and vitamin D intake has been shown to likely increase BMD and decrease fracture rates in postmenopausal women. Relative and absolute vitamin D deficiency is an often overlooked cause of low bone mass.

Decrease of Caffeine, Alcohol, and Smoking

Limiting caffeine intake to less than 760 mg/day (the equivalent of three to four cups of coffee) is recommended because higher levels may decrease calcium absorption and increase calciuresis and the relative risk of hip fracture by 20% in older women. Alcohol intake should be limited to less than 2 ounces/day on average; excessive alcohol intake has been shown to decrease BMD in the radius and spine of older women. Smoking cessation should also be encouraged because it is associated with reduced bone mass, perhaps because nicotine alters the hepatic metabolism of estrogen. In addition, regular weight-bearing exercise should be encouraged because it stimulates bone remodeling and helps to maintain BMD; significant declines in BMD and increases in urinary calcium, phosphorus, and serum calcium levels have been demonstrated in healthy adults undergoing periods of bed rest or space travel.

Muscle Strengthening

Muscle strengthening also stimulates the remodeling process and increases mobility and stability, thus minimizing the risk of falls. In longitudinal studies, weight-bearing exercise such as walking and weight lifting with light weights (5 lb) improved bone mass in postmenopausal women.

Hip Protector Pads

Hip protector pads may be worn by women with osteoporosis who are at increased risk for falling. Data suggest that pads worn at the time of a fall significantly decrease the incidence of hip fractures.

CARDIOVASCULAR DISEASE

CVD is the leading cause of death in American women and is particularly prevalent in women of menopausal age. Women often present with atypical symptoms, resulting in delayed or missed diagnoses. Biases from current literature on CVD risks and therapies involving mostly men demand further investigation in female populations; this will help to ensure that current assumptions about the efficacy of therapies for female patients are justified. The first set of evidence-based guidelines for the prevention of CVD in adult women was published in 2004 by a collaborative effort of the American Heart Association with 11 other major associations. The rationale of the guidelines was to classify CVD as a continuum of risk rather than as an absolute present-time diagnosis. Risk is divided into low-, intermediate-, and high-risk groups based on 10-year absolute CVD risks as determined by the Framingham Global Risk Score, which can be calculated using an online tool available at http://www.nhlbi.nih.gov/guidelines/cholesterol/index.htm (Table 16-5).

The evidence for each recommendation was then reviewed and categorized into standardized levels as established by the USPSTF. Table 16-6 and Box 16-7 list current recommendations for CVD risk reduction by risk level.

Table 16-5

10-Year Risk*	Risk Classification
10%	Low
10% to 20%	Intermediate
>20%	High

*Based on the Framingham scoring system.

Recommendation
Classes/Levels of
Evidence as
Established by the
U.S. Preventive
Services Task Force

Table 16-6

Level of Evidence	
I	Intervention is useful and effective
IIa	Weight of evidence/opinion is in favor of usefulness/efficacy
IIb	Usefulness/efficacy is less well established by evidence/opinion

Statins have been shown to lower the relative risk for CVD and related events and have established benefits for postmenopausal women. The updated Adult Treatment Panel/National Cholesterol Education Program III guidelines recommend driving the low-density lipoprotein cholesterol level below 70 mg/dL in high-risk women. High-risk women are those with coronary, cerebral, or peripheral vascular disease; diabetes; or multiple (two or more) risk factors (e.g., smoking, hypertension) that give them a greater than 20% chance of having a heart attack within 10 years.

Antioxidant vitamin supplementation does not have proven benefit for preventing CVD in women and thus should not be routinely recommended for cardioprotection, except for high-risk groups with high homocysteine levels.

Recent recommendations suggest a lower threshold for the treatment of hypertension in the prevention of CVD. The Joint National Committee 7 on the Prevention, Detection, Evaluation, and Treatment of High Blood Pressure published guidelines in May 2003 updating the definition of "normal" blood pressure as <120/80 mm Hg and defining a new category of "pre"-hypertension (i.e., 120–139/80–89 mm Hg).

Newer studies suggest that measurement of a highly sensitive assay of C-reactive protein (hs-CRP) can help predict cardiovascular risk; it is a marker of inflammation directly involved in atherogenesis. The hs-CRP level serves as an independent risk factor for CVD. Presently, its measurement is recommended for those at intermediate risk (10% to 20% CVD risk over 10 years) as determined by traditional factors of comorbidities and social and family history. Although elevated levels can help to establish increased risks, no current treatment strategies are known to directly modify these levels.

Recent evidence suggests that raloxifene may decrease the risk of cardiovascular events in women with an increased baseline risk of CVD; studies are underway to further quantify this risk reduction. As stated above, hormone replacement therapy is no longer recommended solely for the prevention of heart disease.

Box 16-7 Priorities for Prevention in Practice According to Risk Group

High-risk women (>20% risk)
Class I recommendations:
 Smoking cessation
 Physical activity/cardiac rehabilitation
 Diet therapy
 Weight maintenance/reduction
 Blood pressure control
 Lipid control/statin therapy
 Aspirin therapy
 β-Blocker therapy
 ACE inhibitor therapy (ARBs if contraindicated)
 Glycemic control in diabetics
Class IIa recommendation:
 Evaluate/treat for depression
Class IIb recommendations:
 Omega 3 fatty-acid supplementation
 Folic acid supplementation

Intermediate-risk women (10% to 20% risk)
Class I recommendations:
 Smoking cessation
 Physical activity
 Heart-healthy diet
 Weight maintenance/reduction
 Blood pressure control
 Lipid control
Class IIa recommendations:
 Aspirin therapy

Lower-risk women (<10% risk)
Class I recommendations:
 Smoking cessation
 Physical activity
 Heart-healthy diet
 Weight maintenance/reduction
 Treat individual CVD risk factors as indicated

Stroke prevention among women with atrial fibrillation
Class I recommendations:
 High-intermediate risk of stroke
  Warfarin therapy
 Low risk of stroke (<1%/year) or contraindication to warfarin
  Aspirin therapy

ACE, Angiotensin-converting enzyme; ARB, angiotensin receptor blocker.
From Mosca L, Appel L, Benjamin E, et al: Evidence-based guidelines for cardiovascular disease prevention in women. Circulation 109(5):672–693, 2004.

CVD reduction should involve modifying risk factors including blood pressure, lipid, and glycemic control, use of β-blockers or angiotensin-converting enzyme inhibitors, smoking cessation, regular exercise, and aspirin use for moderate- to high-risk women. The Nurses' Health Study showed a clear benefit from dietary and lifestyle modification to exclude habits like smoking, excessive alcohol use, adherence to a healthy low-fat diet rich in fruits, vegetables, and low-fat dairy products, regular exercise, and the maintenance of a normal body mass index (18.5 to 24.9 kg/m^2).

PHYSICAL EXAMINATION

Physical examination of the perimenopausal or postmenopausal woman should be comprehensive and should begin with measurements of height, weight, body mass index, and blood pressure. Attaining an accurately measured height is important because many women may have not been measured in years and would not otherwise note a loss of height. Special attention should be paid to the thyroid, cardiovascular, breast, lymph node, skin, and pelvic examinations. Periodic Papanicolaou (Pap) smears and yearly mammograms should also be performed.

405

Screening

Cancer Screening

Colon cancer screening with fecal occult testing, sigmoidoscopy, or colonoscopy is recommended to start at the age of 50 years, as is yearly mammography. Regular skin surveillance for changes suggestive of melanoma and other malignant changes are also encouraged.

Because the incidence of risk for cervical cancer decreases with age, The American Cancer Society suggests that cervical cancer screening with Pap smears be stopped at the age of 70 years provided that patients have demonstrated three or more documented consecutive, technically satisfactory normal/negative cervical cytology test results or have not had any abnormal test results within the prior 10 years.

The U.S. Preventive Services Task Force recommends the cessation of routine Pap smears for women older than the age of 65 years for cervical cancer screening if they have had adequate recent screening with normal previous Pap smear results and are not otherwise at high risk for cervical cancer (e.g., human immunodeficiency virus infection, high-risk sexual behavior, or coinfection with human papillomavirus and sexually transmitted disease). Cessation of Pap smears is also recommended for women with a prior total hysterectomy for benign disease and for those not considered to be at high risk (i.e., as above and including prior history of invasive cervical cancer or diethylstilbestrol exposure). Table 16-7 lists the most frequent female cancers in the United States in 2004.

Table 16-7

Most Frequent Female Cancers in the United States in Order of Prevalence, 2004. (Adapted from American Cancer Society: Cancer Facts & Figures, 2004.)

Estimated New Cases	Estimated Deaths
1. Breast	1. Lung
2. Lung	2. Breast
3. Colorectal	3. Colorectal
4. Endometrial	4. Ovarian
5. Lymphoma	5. Pancreatic
6. Ovarian	6. Leukemia

Other Screening
Disorders of the thyroid affect up to 20% of women aged 60 years and older. Because the ubiquitous symptoms of hypothyroidism can be difficult to differentiate from many other conditions, including menopause, this disorder should be discerned by laboratory evaluation with a thyroid-stimulating hormone assay. Recommendations for thyroid disease screening vary. The American Thyroid Association suggests starting at the age of 35 years and performing the screening every 5 years thereafter, with annual testing for women aged 60 years and older. The American College of Physicians suggests screening women aged 50 years and older with incidental findings suggestive of thyroid disease, whereas the American College of Obstetricians and Gynecologists suggests screening "high-risk" women, defined as those with autoimmune disease and a family history of thyroid disease, starting at the age of 19 years.

CONCLUSION

In summary, menopause is a time of transition in a woman's life that requires discussion and reassurance because great variability exists in the extent and duration of related symptoms. Most women find this to be a satisfying evolution. Physicians must take a proactive role in health maintenance screening, lifestyle modification, and the diagnosis and treatment of menopause health issues specific to perimenopausal and postmenopausal women.

KEY POINTS

1. Menopause follows a gradual progression to a permanent loss of ovarian follicular function and clinically begins 12 months after the cessation of menses.
2. No reliable biologic marker exists to definitively predict when the onset of menopause will occur.
3. Many symptoms can accompany menopause.
4. Women can experience these symptoms in vastly different ways to variable degrees and duration.
5. Hormonal treatments are the most efficacious and the only FDA-approved treatments for the symptoms of menopause.
6. Nonpharmacologic and nonhormonal treatments exist for most menopausal symptoms, and healthy lifestyle changes should be discussed with all women.
7. Cardiovascular risks increase as women age and accelerated bone mineral density losses occur, particularly within the first 5 to 7 years after the onset of menopause.

SUGGESTED READING

American Association of Clinical Endocrinologists. Available from: http://www.aace.com/pub/pdf/guidelines/menopause.pdf

American College of Obstetricians and Gynecologists, Women's Health Care Physicians: 2003 ACOG practice bulletin Number 50. Osteoporosis. Clinical management guidelines for obstetrician-gynecologists. Obstet Gynecol 103:203–216, 2004.

Anderson G, Limacher M, Assaf A, et al, and the WHI Steering Committee: Effects of conjugated equine estrogen in postmenopausal women with hysterectomy: The Women's Health Initiative randomized controlled trial. JAMA 291(14):1701–1712, 2004.

Chobanian A, and the National High Blood Pressure Education Program Coordinating Committee: Seventh Report of the Joint National Committee on Prevention, Detection, Evaluation, and Treatment of High Blood Pressure (JNC 7). Hypertension 42:1206–1252, 2003. Available from: http://hyper.ahajournals.org/cgi/content/full/42/6/1206

Dawson Hughes B, Bonner F, Gold D, et al: National Osteoporosis Foundation: Physician's Guide to Prevention and Treatment of Osteoporosis. Washington, DC, National Osteoporosis Foundation, 2003, pp 1–13. Available from: http://www.nof.org/physguide/index.htm

Elder J, Thacker HL: Menopause. The Cleveland Clinic Foundation, Cleveland, OH. Available from: http://www.clevelandclinicmeded.com/diseasemanagement

Espeland M, Rapp S, Shumaker S, et al: Conjugated equine estrogens and global cognitive function in postmenopausal women: Women's Health Initiative Memory Study. JAMA 291(24):2959–2968, 2004.

Grundy S, Becker D, Clark L, et al: Third report of the expert panel on detection, evaluation and treatment of high blood cholesterol in adults (Adult Treatment Panel III). Circulation 110:227–239, 2004.

Leib ES, Lewiecki EM, Binkley N, Hamdy RC, and the International Society for Clinical Densitometry: Official positions of the International Society for Clinical Densitometry. J Clin Densitometry 7(1):1–6, 2004.

Mosca L, Appel LJ, Benjamin EJ, et al: Evidence-based guidelines for cardiovascular disease prevention in women. Circulation 109(5):672–693, 2004.

National Heart, Lung, and Blood Institute, National Cholesterol Education Program: Third report of the expert panel on detection, evaluation, and treatment of high blood cholesterol in adults (Adult Treatment Panel III). Available from: http://www.nhlbi.nih.gov/guidelines/cholesterol/index.htm

Rossouw JE, Anderson GL, Prentice RL, et al: Risks and benefits of estrogen plus progestin in healthy postmenopausal women: Principal results from the Women's Health Initiative randomized controlled trial. JAMA 288:321–333, 2002.

Santoro N, Clarkson T, Freedman R, et al: Treatment of menopause-associated vasomotor symptoms: Position statement of The North American Menopause Society (NAMS). Menopause 11:11–33, 2004.

Shifren JL: The role of androgens in female sexual dysfunction. Mayo Clinic Proceedings 79(4 Suppl): S19–S24, 2004.

Shumaker S, Legault C, Kuller L, et al: Conjugated equine estrogens and incidence of probable dementia and mild cognitive impairment in postmenopausal women: Women's Health Initiative Memory Study. JAMA 291(24):2947–2958, 2004.

Sikon A, Thacker HL: Treatment options for menopausal hot flashes. Cleveland Clinic J Med 71 (7):578–582, 2004.

Soules MR, Sherman S, Parrott E, et al: Executive summary: Stages of Reproductive Aging Workshop (STRAW). Fertil Steril 76(5):874–878, 2001.

Stenson WF, Newberry R, Lorinz R, et al: Increased prevalence of celiac disease and need for routine screening among patients with osteoporosis. Arch Intern Med 165:393–399, 2005.

Treatment of menopause-associated vasomotor symptoms: Position statement of The North American Menopause Society. Menopause 11(1):11–33, 2004. Available from: http://www.menopause.org/NR/rdonlyres/4D66CCDC-7F8D-4A16–9BA9–502E14DC7071/0/hotflashes.pdf

U.S. Department of Health and Human Services: Executive summary. Bone health and osteoporosis: A report of the Surgeon General. Rockville, MD, U.S. Department of Health and Human Services, Office of the Surgeon General, 2004.

Utian W, Archer D, Gallager JC, et al: Recommendations for estrogen and progestogen use in peri- and postmenopausal women: October position statement of the North American Menopause Society. Menopause 11:589–600, 2004. Available from: http://www.menopause.org/edumaterials/2004HTreport.pdf

Wright J, Naftolin F, Schneider HP, Sturdee DW: Guidelines for the hormone treatment of women in the menopausal transition and beyond: Position statement by the Executive Committee of the International Menopause Society. Maturitas 48:27–31, 2004.

The Writing Group for the International Society for Clinical Densitometry (ISCD) Position Development Conference: Position statement: Executive summary. J Clin Densitometry 7(1):7–12, 2004.

17

VULVAR EPITHELIAL DISORDERS AND OTHER VULVAR CONDITIONS

Lori A. Boardman and Amy S. Cooper

INTRODUCTION

Vulvar symptoms are common and often chronic, and they can significantly interfere with women's sexual function and sense of well-being. Obtaining expert medical advice to deal with vulvar symptoms can be frustrating because providers often receive scant training in this area of gynecology, and clinicians with a specific interest in this field are rare. The goal of this review is to cover the essentials of vulvar anatomy, to discuss appropriate diagnostic tools, and to provide a structured approach to the evaluation of common vulvar complaints. For our purposes, vulvar complaints will be broadly divided into three categories: pruritus, pain, and palpable masses.

ANATOMY

The labia majora are prominent hair-bearing folds of skin that represent the lateral boundaries of the vulva and meet to form the anterior boundary of the vulva at the mons pubis. The vulva is bounded posteriorly by the fusion of the labia majora at the fourchette. The non–hair-bearing labia minora lie medial to the labia majora and fuse anteriorly to form the prepuce and frenulum of the clitoris. The frenulum represents the anterior portion of the vulvar vestibule, the innermost portion of the vulva. The vestibule is bounded medially by the hymen and laterally by Hart's line, a variably distinct line of demarcation evident at the base of the medial aspect of the each labium minus. Hart's line separates the nonkeratinized squamous epithelium of the vestibule from the keratinized epithelium of the more lateral labia minora. Mucous-producing glands of the vestibule include the paraurethral ducts or Skene's glands, numerous minor vestibular glands, and the major (or Bartholin's) glands. In studying vulvar diseases, it is important to recall that the vulvovaginal region arises from epithelium derived from all three embryologic layers (i.e., endoderm, mesoderm, and ectoderm), a condition that occurs in no other part of the body. Remaining aware of the differences in epithelial and glandular structure, hormonal responsiveness, neural distribution, and immune responses that result from the differences in origin is crucial when assessing vulvar complaints.

HISTORY AND PHYSICAL EXAMINATION

Obtaining a vulvar history can be challenging for several reasons. Women may be uncomfortable discussing this part of their bodies and relatively unaware of the anatomy of this area. If presenting with a specific complaint, patients may be frustrated from prior experiences with providers, experiences that often result in a failure to achieve either a diagnosis or relief of their symptoms. Chronic or recurrent forms of vulvar disease can challenge providers, both from diagnostic and therapeutic standpoints. When taking a history, then, it is important to ask about the onset, duration, location, and nature of vulvar symptoms, as well as any possible precipitating factors.

A history of prior evaluations, previous diagnostic procedures, and all prior treatments (including over-the-counter treatments as well as alternative or complementary therapies) should be elicited. In addition to noting the part of the vulva involved, providers should ascertain whether extragenital sites are involved. Previous events, such as childbirth-related episiotomies or laceration; a history of vulvar laser, cryotherapy, or excisional surgery; or prior treatment for condyloma should be specifically addressed. Finally, a complete medical history and current medication regimen should be obtained before examination.

Patients presenting with vulvar complaints are often quite uncomfortable. If the skin is particularly tender, the patient should be asked to separate the labia herself to decrease any further discomfort. Good lighting is imperative because many changes on the vulva can be subtle. A magnifying lens or colposcope may be useful. The examination should begin with a systematic inspection of the entire vulva, noting any color changes, edema, visible lesions or changes in the architecture of the vulva, vascular changes, and presence and nature of any vaginal discharge. When lesions are present, attention should be paid to documenting the border, size, contour, and color of all visible lesions. Papules should be distinguished from macules and plaques. Changes in pigmentation, ulcers, and erosions should be carefully noted. Each woman should also undergo a speculum examination that includes direct observation for mucopurulent cervicitis and evaluation of vaginal secretions for color, viscosity, and homogeneity. The vaginal walls should be inspected for lesions, erythema, scarring, and the presence or absence of rugal folds.

DIAGNOSTIC TOOLS

Wet Mount and Potassium Hydroxide Preparation

Using microscopy to examine vaginal secretions can be helpful in the evaluation of a patient with a vulvar complaint. Samples should be taken from the lateral vaginal walls in the upper third of the vagina to avoid contamination of the sample with discharge from the cervix. A wet mount (i.e., vaginal secretions diluted with normal saline) and 10% potassium hydroxide (KOH) preparation should be performed. The pH should be checked using pH paper that is sensitive in the 3.5 to 6.0 range, with a pH above 4.5 associated with a variety of vulvovaginal processes, including atrophic vaginitis, bacterial vaginosis, and trichomoniasis. Odor (the "whiff test") should be assessed to confirm the presence of amines after addition of 10% KOH. During microscopy, the provider should comment on the presence and nature of epithelial cells, the presence/absence of lactobacilli, and any potential abnormalities, such as white blood cells, clue cells, hyphae or budding yeast, or trichomonads. The presence of parabasalar cells may also offer information about the estrogen status of the patient. The wet mount and KOH preparation are further discussed in Chapter 22, Genital and Urinary Tract Infections.

Cultures and Serologies

Microscopy, while helpful in diagnosis, can be limited by relatively low sensitivity, particularly with respect to the diagnosis of atypical candidiasis. Although yeast infections caused by *Candida albicans* produce pseudohyphae and blastospores (which can be seen on microscopy), the non-*albicans* species cannot easily be identified under the microscope. Vaginal yeast cultures can aid in the diagnosis of these species and in determining treatment for species that may be resistant to standard antimycotic therapy.

If a sexually transmitted infection is suspected, testing for *Neisseria gonorrhea* and *Chlamydia trachomatis* should be undertaken. Women with ulcerative lesions should be evaluated with dark-field microscopy for *Treponema* species or serologic studies for syphilis as well as a herpes culture. Herpes simplex virus (HSV) serologies can be helpful in cases where active lesions are absent or crusted over or in clinically confusing cases. Culture for *Haemophilus ducreyi* should be performed in settings where chancroid is prevalent. Finally, testing for human immunodeficiency virus (HIV) is indicated in the management of all women who have genital ulcers caused by *Treponema pallidum* or *H. ducreyi* and should be considered for those who have ulcers caused by HSV, as genital ulcerative disease poses an increased risk for HIV infection.

Biopsy

The threshold for biopsy of the vulva should be low. Changes on the vulva are often subtle and can be easily missed. Biopsy of hyperpigmented or exophytic lesions, lesions with changes in vascular patterns, or unresolving lesions should be performed to rule out carcinoma. Skin changes such as thickening, pebbling, hypopigmentation, or thinning of the

411

epithelium indicate a possible dermatologic process, and biopsy will aid in diagnosis and management.

If time allows, eutectic mixture of local anesthetic (EMLA) cream can be placed on the proposed biopsy site approximately 20 to 30 minutes before the procedure. Under sterile conditions, local infiltration of the biopsy site with lidocaine (Xylocaine) or bupivacaine (Marcaine) should then follow. A 3- to 4-mm Keyes punch biopsy should suffice to remove a sample of the suspicious lesion. Care should be taken not to press too deeply into the subcuticular tissue with the Keyes punch because vulvar hematomas have been reported. When sampling ulcerative areas, it is best to biopsy the edge of the ulcer; when sampling hyperpigmented areas, biopsy of the thickest region is recommended. The area can then be sutured or hemostasis can be achieved with Monsel's solution or silver nitrate. If a biopsy was done previously at another institution, it can be helpful to have an expert in dermatopathology review the biopsy if the diagnosis is in question.

Colposcopy

Although the use of the toluidine blue test to distinguish vulvar intraepithelial neoplasia (VIN) from non-neoplastic epithelial disorders of the vulva has been suggested, colposcopic-directed biopsy has largely supplanted this technique. Approximately 5 to 10 minutes before performing vulvar colposcopy, a 3% to 5% acetic acid solution should be applied to the vulva. In cases of extreme inflammation or patient irritation or discomfort, such application should be avoided. The most common abnormalities noted on the vulva in association with VIN are acetowhite epithelium and vascular changes. Biopsy specimens should be taken from any suspicious areas. For patients who are immunocompromised and have known VIN or perianal neoplasia, anal colposcopy should be considered to rule out anal carcinoma.

VULVAR PRURITUS

Dermatitis

The term *dermatitis* (or *eczema*) describes a poorly demarcated, erythematous, and usually itchy rash. Burning can sometimes occur in cases of mucosal involvement. Subtypes are numerous and can be classified as either exogenous (e.g., allergic, irritant, or corticosteroid-induced dermatitis) or endogenous (e.g., atopic or seborrheic dermatitis). Dermatitis is common and has been reported to occur in more than half of patients seen with chronic vulvar symptoms (with atopic dermatitis being by far the most frequently encountered). Irritant or contact dermatitis has been identified in 5% to 26% of women diagnosed with vulvar dermatitis and occurs as a result of exposure to such irritants as semen, condoms, spermicides, and soaps. A frequent irritant is propylene glycol, found in many topical medications.

On examination, clinical signs can be understated and may include poorly defined erythema, scales, fissures, lichenification (i.e., closely set papules), and excoriation. Regardless of the type of dermatitis, the first line of therapy remains topical corticosteroids. Therapy should begin with a mid-potency corticosteroid until symptoms resolve. Application of a weaker corticosteroid, such as 1% hydrocortisone, can then be continued for another 2 to 3 months. In recalcitrant cases, high-potency corticosteroids or tacrolimus may be necessary. Medications with antihistamine and sedative properties, such as diphenhydramine or hydroxyzine, can be added to control nocturnal itching. For exogenous dermatitis, removal of potential irritants or allergens may decrease future recurrences. Those with semen sensitivity (i.e., burning when exposed to ejaculate) may respond to combined treatment with a daily dose of a nonsedating antihistamine such as fexofenadine along with ibuprofen one half hour before intercourse. Incontinent women can also benefit from an application of vitamin A and D petrolatum ointment or similar salve to provide a protective barrier from urine.

Candidiasis

The majority of candidal infections are sporadic, and in nearly 85% of cases are caused by *C. albicans*. Candidal infections are rare before the onset of menarche and peak in the third to fourth decade of life. Although reported rates of infection vary, it is estimated that 75% of sexually active women will experience the symptoms of itching, irritation, soreness, dyspareunia, and dysuria associated with vulvovaginal candidiasis, 45% women will experience two or more vaginal yeast infections, and 5% will suffer from recurrent (i.e., four or more episodes a year) vulvovaginal candidiasis.

A reliable diagnosis cannot be made on the basis of symptoms (none of which are highly sensitive or highly specific) nor the results of physical examination (e.g., erythema, edema, clumpy white discharge, fissures) in the absence of corroborative laboratory data. Direct microscopy, including estimation of the vaginal pH (remains normal at 4.0 to 4.5) and the finding of blastospores, hyphae, or pseudohyphae on saline and 10% KOH preparation tests (sensitivity of 30% to 50% and 65% to 85%, respectively), is necessary to establish the diagnosis. Vaginal cultures are indicated in symptomatic women, with or without corroborative physical findings, with negative microscopy results. Reserving culture for this population will result in treatment of 90% of women who fulfill the criteria for vulvovaginal candidiasis and will limit the use of culture to those women whose yield of positive culture results is greater than the background prevalence of *C. albicans* in asymptomatic women without signs of infection (33% and 10%, respectively).

Treatment choices are dictated by the nature of the infection and the host characteristics. For uncomplicated fungal infections (defined as sporadic or infrequent infections, mild-to-moderate candidiasis, or infections in immunocompetent women), either topical or oral therapy can be initiated. In general, women strongly prefer the latter. For women with complicated disease (defined as severe or recurrent non-*albicans* or candidiasis in women with uncontrolled diabetes, debilitation, immunosuppression, or pregnancy), treatment varies. For severe disease (i.e., extensive vulvar erythema, edema, excoriation, and fissure formation), two options are recommended: a 7- to 14-day course of topical azole or 150 mg of fluconazole in two sequential doses (second dose 72 hours after initial dose).

Women with recurrent vulvovaginal candidiasis present a challenge both in terms of evaluation and treatment. Although testing for diabetes or immunosuppression is often suggested, results are positive in only a minority of these patients. For example, women with recurrent candidiasis should undergo HIV testing only in the presence of other risk factors for HIV infection. Although non-*albicans* species should be suspected and culture is clearly warranted in this population, it should be remembered that repeated vulvovaginitis more commonly occurs with persistent *C. albicans*. For recurrent infection with *C. albicans*, the patient should be treated with the same regimen used for severe disease, and maintenance should follow with either oral medication (weekly fluconazole, 150 mg) or clotrimazole (weekly 500-mg vaginal suppository). In a recent randomized controlled trial of maintenance therapy with fluconazole, women receiving maintenance medication for 6 months, compared with those receiving placebo, were significantly more likely to remain disease-free at both 6 months (91% versus 36%) and at follow-up off of medication 6 months later (43% versus 22%).

Non-*albicans* infections (e.g., *C. glabrata*, *C. parapsilosis*, *C. tropicalis*) do not typically respond to treatment with fluconazole, often as a result of an intrinsic resistance to this medication. Recommended therapy, then, is a 7- to 14-day course of a nonfluconazole azole. If treatment fails, a 2-week course of nightly boric acid vaginal suppositories (600 mg) or nightly 4% flucytosine vaginal cream (requires a compounding pharmacy) can be used. Maintenance therapy consists of a nightly 100,000-unit nystatin vaginal suppository or twice-weekly boric acid vaginal suppositories.

Dermatologic Conditions

Lichen Sclerosus

Lichen sclerosus (LS), a chronic disorder of the skin, is most commonly seen on the vulva, with extragenital lesions reported in between 5% to 20% of patients. Although LS can affect any age group (approximately 9% of cases occurred in prepubertal children in one study of more than 350 women with LS), the mean age of onset occurs in the fifth to sixth decade. Although the exact etiology of this condition is unclear, an autoimmune process or possible genetic link has been proposed. Patients presenting with LS most commonly experience pruritus, followed by irritation, burning, dyspareunia, and tearing. Because LS may be asymptomatic, the prevalence of this condition remains unknown. If, however, an asymptomatic patient with active disease is encountered, she should be treated as described below.

On examination, typical lesions of LS are porcelain-white papules and plaques, often with areas of ecchymosis or purpura. The skin often appears thinned, whitened, and crinkling (hence the description, "cigarette paper" appearance). Although the genital mucosa is largely spared with LS, involvement of the mucocutaneous junctions may lead to introital narrowing. Perianal involvement can create the classic "figure-of-eight" or hourglass shape. Other findings include fusion of the labia minora, phimosis of the clitoral hood, and fissures. LS can affect the entire vulva but most commonly involves the labia majora and minora. Because other vulvar diseases can mimic LS, a biopsy is necessary to confirm the diagnosis. On histology, the squamous epithelium appears thinned, with loss of the rete pegs or epithelial folds. Chronic inflammatory cells appear as an infiltrate located directly beneath the squamous epithelial lining.

The recommended treatment for LS is an ultrapotent topical steroid ointment, such as clobetasol propionate. At present, there are no randomized controlled trials providing clear evidence of superiority for any specific corticosteroid. A regimen for newly diagnosed cases is clobetasol propionate nightly for 4 weeks, followed by use on alternate nights for 4 weeks and, then for ongoing maintenance therapy, twice weekly. If symptoms return, the patient should be instructed to return to the frequency that was previously effective and slowly taper down to the maintenance regimen of twice-weekly use. Because of the potential for significant adverse effects, providers should carefully instruct patients in the use of this medication with the expectation that a 30-g tube should last 12 weeks. Resolution of the hyperkeratosis, ecchymoses, fissuring, and erosions should be expected, although the atrophy and pigmentation changes will remain. Treatment with other topical therapies, including testosterone and progesterone, has inconsistently resulted in improvement in LS, and these are not currently recommended as first-line therapy. Surgery should be reserved exclusively for the treatment of malignancy and postinflammatory sequelae (e.g., release of labial adhesions).

Women with LS are at an increased risk of vulvar cancers, most commonly squamous cell carcinomas (which has not been recorded in extragenital LS). Two studies, each involving more than 200 women with LS, have shown an approximately 5% risk of invasive squamous cell carcinomas. Whether treatment will decrease this long-term risk of malignant change is presently unknown. Follow-up of patients with LS depends on each patient's response to treatment. Initial management should consist of two visits—one at 3 months to assess treatment progress and medication use and a second visit 6 months later to ensure the patient remains confident in her treatment plan and to discuss any residual problems. Annual visits are then recommended for women who have responded to therapy. More frequent follow-up is required for those with poorly controlled disease (e.g., patients who remain symptomatic despite multiple trials of various therapies). Biopsy of any suspicious areas (e.g., persistent ulcers, erosions, erythematous areas) should be undertaken to exclude neoplasia or invasive carcinoma. Finally, a subset of women with LS, despite evidence of clinical improvement, will present with ongoing symptoms of discomfort. This most likely represents neuropathic pain, which should be managed with treatments aimed at removing the neuronal sensitization caused by LS. Such treatments are discussed in the section on vulvar pain syndromes.

Lichen Simplex Chronicus

Vulvar lichen simplex chronicus (LSC), also referred to as *hyperplastic dystrophy* and *squamous cell hyperplasia*, is a common vulvar dermatosis. LSC is a chronic eczematous disease characterized by intense and unrelenting itching and scratching. In vulvar specialty clinics, LSC accounts for 10% to 35% of patients evaluated. Although LSC occurs primarily in mid to late adult life, it can occur in children. The majority of patients will report a history of atopic disease (e.g., hay fever, asthma, childhood eczema). All patients report pruritus, and most will admit to vigorous scratching or rubbing and often report sleep disturbances as a result of their discomfort.

Clinically, LSC appears as one or more erythematous, scaling, lichenified plaques. Various degrees of excoriation are often visible. In long-standing disease, the skin appears thickened and leathery, and areas of hyperpigmentation and hypopigmentation may be present. Biopsy, which may be needed to confirm the diagnosis, reveals marked epithelial thickening (acanthosis) with deepening and widening of the rete ridges into the dermis. Superficial dermal collagenization can be seen directly beneath the epithelium; in the absence of dermal changes, the diagnosis of squamous cell hyperplasia is appropriate.

What LSC represents is an end-stage response to a wide variety of possible initiating processes, including environmental factors (e.g., heat, excessive sweating, irritation from clothing or topically applied products) and dermatologic diseases (e.g., candidiasis, LS). Treatment, therefore, consists of identification and removal of the initiating factor, repair of the skin's barrier layer function, reduction of inflammation, and disruption of the itch-scratch cycle. Vaginal cultures and biopsy of clinically suspicious areas should precede appropriate therapy for underlying disease. Medium- to high-strength topical corticosteroids should be applied nightly until symptoms begin to abate; less frequent use (e.g., alternate nights, then twice weekly) should continue until the condition resolves. Again, medications with antihistamine and sedative properties can be added to control nocturnal itching.

Psoriasis

When psoriasis presents on the vulva, the silver scaling typically seen elsewhere on the body is often lost. The bright erythema and well-defined outline of the disease, however, tend to remain. Although psoriasis is not usually associated with loss of architecture, this can occur. The differential diagnosis includes intertrigo, seborrheic dermatitis, and eczema, although in all of these cases the margins appear less well-defined. When limited to the vulva, local treatment with mid- to high-strength topical corticosteroids, injectable corticosteroids, or topical tacrolimus are helpful in managing the disease.

VULVAR PAIN

Erosive and Ulcerative Diseases

Herpes Simplex Virus

HSV is by far the most common cause of ulcerative genital lesions. Other causes of genital ulcers include syphilis, chancroid, and to a lesser degree in the United States, lymphogranuloma venereum and granuloma inguinale.

HSV, a double-stranded DNA virus, exists as two subtypes: HSV-1 typically causes orolabial lesions and herpes keratitis, whereas HSV-2 primarily infects the anogenital tract. Significant crossover of subtypes does exist, with recent data demonstrating HSV-1 as a cause of anogenital herpes in approximately 20% of current cases. Of the 45 to 60 million people infected with HSV-2, nearly 80% are asymptomatic and therefore unaware of the possibility of sexual transmission.

Genital HSV infections are classified as initial primary, initial nonprimary, recurrent, and asymptomatic. Initial, or first-episode, primary genital herpes is a true primary infection (i.e., the patient will be seronegative for HSV antibodies). The average incubation period after genital acquisition of either HSV subtype is 4 days (range, 2 to 12). Systemic symptoms, such as fever, headache, malaise, and myalgias, are present in two thirds of women with initial primary HSV (compared with 40% of men). The majority of women with a first episode of clinically apparent HSV-2 infection have localized symptoms, including tender, grouped vesicles and bilateral, tender, nonfluctuant inguinal adenopathy. The vesicles are typically confined to the introitus, urethral meatus, or labia and progress into pustules that then erode into exquisitely tender, superficial ulcerations. Crusting of the lesions occurs over the 15 to 20 days before re-epithelialization. Nonprimary infections (acquisition of HSV-2 in persons with prior HSV-1 or, more rarely, the reverse) are infrequently associated with systemic symptoms. The duration of such infections is usually shorter (mean, 9 versus 12 days), with fewer visible lesions and a shorter duration of viral shedding (mean, 7 versus 11 days).

Recurrent genital HSV-2 infection may be symptomatic or, more commonly, asymptomatic. As with nonprimary initial infections, the duration of viral shedding is reduced and lesions are fewer. Nearly half of patients will experience prodromal symptoms (i.e., mild tingling, shooting pains) in the hours or days before the onset of lesions. Recurrences are unfortunately common. In the year after a documented first episode of genital HSV-2 infection, 90% of patients will experience at least one recurrence, 38% will have six or more, and 20% will have 10 or more recurrences. In general, recurrences associated with HSV-1 occur less frequently than with HSV-2. Over time, however, recurrence rates decrease, irrespective of viral type or use of suppressive therapy. Although the risk of transmission increases when genital lesions are present, transmission from asymptomatic shedding, which occurs much more frequently than symptomatic disease, results in transmission in most cases.

Complications associated with HSV infection are numerous. Aseptic meningitis, sacral radiculopathy, and transverse myelitis can affect those with infection, most commonly in cases of primary infection. Neonatal HSV infection, a risk greatest among infants born to mothers with an initial, primary HSV infection near the time of delivery, can result in significant morbidity and mortality. Finally, genital ulcer disease is a well-recognized risk factor for acquisition of HIV.

Viral culture, including two type-specific antibody assays, is the mainstay of diagnosis of HSV infection, but the sensitivity of culture depends on several factors. Approximately 95% of vesicular lesions will grow HSV, compared with 70% of ulcerative lesions and only 30% of crusted lesions. Because viral loads are higher in primary infections, the yield from viral culture is higher in these cases than in recurrences. Type-specific serologic testing for HSV can be useful for diagnosing symptomatic patients with healing lesions and can be used as a screening tool in patients who have risk factors for HSV.

Treatment guidelines for HSV are outlined in Table 17-1. In counseling seropositive patients, it should be mentioned that condom use and antiviral suppressive therapy help reduce transmission to seronegative partners, although the risk of transmission is not completely eliminated. Although several trials suggest that antiviral therapy in the last weeks of pregnancy can help reduce clinically apparent genital HSV disease in the mother, and thus reduce cesarean section rates, vertical transmission can still occur through asymptomatic shedding.

Lichen Planus

Lichen planus (LP), a skin disease most likely related to T-cell autoimmunity, exhibits a wide range of morphologies and in its erosive form can result in significant scarring and pain. Most commonly recognized on the skin or oral mucosa, this condition may affect the lower genital tract. About 1% of the population has oral LP; of women with oral disease, roughly 20% to 25% have genital vulvovaginal disease. Because genital lesions may be asymptomatic and because lesions often go unrecognized during examination, the incidence of genital disease is most likely underestimated.

LP, though most commonly seen in its erosive form, can also present as white epithelium or as red or purple papules. The classic presentation of LP on mucous membranes, including the buccal mucosa, is that of white, reticulate, lacy or fern-like striae (Wickham's striae). On occasion, the skin may appear uniformly white, and thus LP can be confused with LS. The

Table 17-1

Treatment for HSV

Agent	First Episode	Recurrent Genital Herpes, Episodic Treatment	Suppressive Therapy
Acyclovir	200 mg orally 5 times/day for 7–10 days or 400 mg orally 3 times/day for 7–10 days	200 mg orally 5 times/day for 5 days or 800 mg orally twice daily for 5 days	400 mg orally twice daily
Valacyclovir	1000 mg orally twice daily for 7–10 days	500 mg orally twice daily for 3 or 5 days or 1000 mg orally daily for 5 days	500 mg orally once daily (for patients with nine or fewer recurrences/year) or 1000 mg orally once daily
Famciclovir	250 mg orally three times/day for 7–10 days	125 mg orally twice daily for 5 days	250 mg twice daily

pruritic, purple, shiny papules typically associated with LP are rarely found on the genital skin. If present, however, they appear dusky pink in color and without an apparent scale. In erosive LP, deep, painful, erythematous erosions appear in the posterior vestibule and often extend to the labia minora, resulting in agglutination and resorption of the labial architecture. The vaginal epithelium can become inflamed, and erosive patches, if present, are extremely friable. Over time, these eroded surfaces may adhere, resulting in synechiae and, eventually, complete obliteration of the vaginal space. Patients may complain of an increased vaginal discharge, which on examination is filled with white blood cells and immature parabasal and basal epithelial cells. This discharge has often been labeled as desquamative inflammatory vaginitis, but whether this is a type of erosive LP or a distinct type of vaginitis remains controversial.

Biopsy, which reveals a band-like infiltrate of lymphocytes and colloid bodies in the basal layers of the epidermis, may be relatively nonspecific because of the complete loss of the vaginal epithelium. On the other hand, a histologic specimen can help rule out immunobullous diseases such as pemphigoid, pemphigus, and linear immunoglobulin A bullous disease, which may mimic LP. The prognosis for spontaneous remission of vulvovaginal LP is poor. As with LS, women are at increased risk for the development of squamous cell carcinoma of the vulva. Treatment, though not curative, can substantially improve patients' well-being and may preserve the sexual function of affected women. Therapeutic options, shown in small trials to be effective, include topical/systemic corticosteroids, cyclosporin, tacrolimus, psoralen plus ultraviolet A, and topical/systemic retinoids. Vaginal dilators can be useful in keeping the vaginal space patent.

Other Ulcerative Diseases

Behçet's disease is a multisystem, inflammatory disease that occurs with a high prevalence in persons of Mediterranean descent. Behçet's is not a chronic, persistent inflammatory disease, but rather one that consists of recurrent attacks of acute inflammation. Although the etiology is unknown, it appears to be genetically associated with histocompatibility antigens, human leukocyte antigens B51 and DR4. Persons 20 to 40 years of age are most commonly affected, with women and men represented equally. In addition to recurrent oral ulceration, at least two of the following findings must be present to make the diagnosis: (1) recurrent genital ulceration, (2) skin lesions (e.g., erythema nodosum), (3) retinal vasculitis or uveitis, or (4) a positive skin pathergy test. Cardiovascular, pulmonary, and gastrointestinal involvement are the major causes of mortality. Treatment depends on the patient's clinical manifestations. For mucocutaneous involvement, topical corticosteroids, colchicine, and thalidomide have all shown beneficial effects. Patients may benefit from referral to a rheumatologist.

Women can experience combined oral and genital ulcers that do not fulfill the criteria for Behçet's disease. Patients with oral-genital aphthoses present with recurrent superficial, painful, mucosal ulcers. Biopsy does not aid in the diagnosis, and initial management consists of pain relief and treatment of bacterial superinfection. Mid- to high-potency topical corticosteroids can also be helpful. For recalcitrant cases, colchicine and thalidomide can be used. Other processes to be considered in females of any age with recurrent vulvar ulcerations include Crohn's disease (vulvar ulcerations may precede the active intestinal disease by years) and, in girls, leukemia.

Two ulcerative diseases, often seen at the extremes of age, should also be mentioned. Combined symptoms of fever, sore throat, cervical lymphadenopathy, and genital ulcerations may occur with infectious mononucleosis, an Epstein-Barr virus infection. This diagnosis is likely in an adolescent who presents with these findings and a negative herpes culture result. Diagnosis is confirmed with blood smear (atypical lymphocytes) and a positive heterophile antibody test result (e.g., Monospot). Treatment consists of pain relief (e.g., with topical lidocaine) and treatment of bacterial superinfection. Vulvar shingles *(Varicella zoster),* on the other hand, should be included in the differential diagnosis of unexplained vulvar ulcers, rashes, and persistent pain in adults and older persons. Shingles, particularly in older women, can become a neurologic emergency. *V. zoster* virus testing should be performed if HSV test results are negative. Antiviral medications as well as tricyclic antidepressants have been show to reduce the likelihood of persistent postherpetic neuralgia.

Vulvar Pain Syndromes

Vulvodynia and Vestibulitis (Vestibulodynia)

In 2000, the U.S. National Institutes of Health first provided federal funding for research aimed at elucidating the prevalence, epidemiology, and effect of treatment for women with vulvar pain. As a result of such efforts, knowledge and understanding of vulvar pain syndromes has increasingly grown. It was not until 2003 that Harlow and Stewart provided the first estimates of the true prevalence of chronic vulvar pain among American women. Using a population-based cross-sectional sample of nearly 5000 women from Boston area communities, Harlow and Stewart found that 16% of the women surveyed reported histories of chronic vulvar burning, knifelike or sharp pain, or pain on contact that lasted 3 months or longer, and nearly 7% were experiencing such discomfort at the time of participation. Also recently challenged were long-held assumptions about certain patient characteristics associated with vulvar pain. For example, the perception that such pain is uncommon among African American and Hispanic women appears to be unjustified. Indeed, Harlow and Stewart found that Hispanic women were 80% more likely to experience chronic vulvar pain than were white and African American women, whereas white and African American women reported similar lifetime prevalence rates of chronic burning and knifelike pain.

The terminology for vulvar pain has also evolved over time. Patients with vulvodynia tend to fall into different groups based on the location of their pain. The term *generalized vulvodynia* is used to describe involvement of the entire vulva by persistent, chronic pain that is burning, stinging, or irritating in nature, whereas *localized vulvodynia* specifies involvement of only a portion of the vulva, such as the vestibule or clitoris. In both generalized and localized vulvodynia, the pain may be provoked (i.e., triggered by physical contact of a sexual or nonsexual nature), unprovoked, or both. In the case of provoked pain, common triggers include, for example, intromission (resulting in introital dyspareunia), tampon insertion, and the wearing of tight-fitting clothing. Such pain is reproducible on examination of the vestibule with a moistened cotton swab. In both conditions, the pain must be present for a minimum of 3 months to justify diagnosis. Before diagnosing a woman with a vulvar pain syndrome, care must be taken to rule out other possible causes of vulvar discomfort. Biopsy (if warranted by examination) and vaginal cultures can rule out other causes of vulvar burning, stinging, or other painful symptoms.

Proposed triggers for vulvar pain syndromes are numerous and have historically included histories of recurrent vaginal infections such as candidal infections and bacterial vaginosis, use of oral contraceptives, and destructive treatments (for instance, vulvar laser vaporization or exposure to irritant agents such as trichloroacetic acid). Clinical studies do not support the role of past sexual abuse or psychosexual dysfunction as causative agents; however, both depression and anxiety are common with vulvar pain syndromes. Finally, patients with vulvodynia report a higher incidence of irritable bowel syndrome, fibromyalgia, interstitial cystitis, and migraines.

Although a multifactorial process is most likely involved in the development of vulvar pain, the end result appears to be neuropathically mediated pain manifested predominantly as burning. In general, neuropathic pain is believed to result from damage to, and subsequent loss of, peripheral afferent elements, a loss that leads ultimately to changes in the central nervous system. For patients with vestibulitis, the damage has been proposed to result from chronic inflammation. This inflammation then leads to sensitization of first the primary afferents (predominately nociceptors) by inflammatory peptides, prostaglandins, and cytokines, and then the spinal cord. Impulses are transmitted along the afferent sympathetic nerves (primarily C fibers) to the central nervous system, where a reinforcing signal, returned via efferent fibers, sustains the pain loop. The allodynia (i.e., light touch perceived as pain) and hyperalgesia (i.e., excessive response to what should cause slight pain) seen in women with vulvar pain can be explained by this hypothesis.

The evidence for a predominant peripheral process in one form of localized vulvodynia (formerly called vestibulitis), for example, is mixed. Inflammatory infiltrates in vestibular tissue have been seen inconsistently in women both with and without vestibular pain. The presence of histologic inflammation, then, is most likely a nonspecific finding. On the other hand, Foster has documented elevated concentrations of inflammatory cytokines, specifically interleukin-1β and tumor necrosis factor α, in women with vestibulitis. These cytokines promote inflammatory responses and interact with histamine, bradykinin, and substance P to lead to the development of neurogenic inflammation. Structural differences in the vestibular tissue of women affected by vestibulitis compared with unaffected women support Foster's findings. For example, the proliferation of vestibular nerve fibers seen in women diagnosed with this pain disorder provides a morphologic basis for enhanced neuronal firing when pressure is applied to the vestibule. Finally, supporting this hypothesis of a peripheral process in vestibulitis is the observation of the efficacy of surgical skin removal via vestibulectomy, but not perineoplasty (i.e., undercutting of the area without excision of skin and nerve fibers) in relieving pain.

For those women diagnosed with vulvodynia or vestibulitis, treatment recommendations, though numerous, are infrequently evidence based. For example, although tricyclic antidepressants and certain anticonvulsants are mainstays of therapy, data confirming their efficacy in these populations are few. Although anecdotal evidence supports their use, the adverse effects associated with these medications, particularly the sedation and constipation seen with the tricyclic antidepressants, may limit their applicability. In the few published randomized clinical trials among vestibulitis patients, investigators have evaluated a range of modalities including biofeedback, behavioral therapy, surgery, and topical therapy. Bergeron randomly assigned 78 women with vestibulitis to three treatment groups: cognitive behavioral sex therapy, biofeedback, and vestibulectomy. Although participants in all three groups experienced significant improvement in their pain, those undergoing surgery averaged the greatest pain reduction. Differential dropout, however, occurred in the surgery arm, thereby limiting the interpretation of these data. Furthermore, surgical treatment, although highly efficacious, is often seen as an option only after medical and other less invasive therapies have been exhausted.

At present, a number of randomized trials of oral and topical therapy for the treatment of vulvar pain are underway. To date, however, there is only one published randomized placebo-controlled trial of topical therapy for the treatment of vestibulitis. In a study of topical cromolyn sulfate, Nyirjesy found that placebo users, compared with topical cromolyn users, were slightly, though not significantly, more likely to experience resolution of their pain. Although topical cromolyn failed to be of significant benefit, investigators have demonstrated favorable clinical responses using other injectable or topical therapies. In case reports, case series, and small uncontrolled trials of women with vestibulitis, a number of locally administered therapies, including injectable interferon, injectable steroids and lidocaine, topical steroids, topical nitroglycerin, topical lidocaine, and topical capsaicin have shown some efficacy.

The current treatment options for vulvar pain, then, are largely empiric. Types of treatment broadly fall into the following categories: medical therapy, biofeedback and physical therapy, and surgery. Tricyclic antidepressants, the most studied of which is amitriptyline, are started at a dose of 10 to 25 mg and slowly increased until an adequate response is achieved. To minimize anticholinergic adverse effects, the use of secondary amines, such as desipramine, may be preferable. Anticonvulsants, such as gabapentin, can be used either alone or in combination with a tricyclic antidepressant. Gabapentin should be started at a 100- to 300-mg daily dose and gradually increased to three times daily, with most patients achieving a clinical response on a total daily dose of between 900 and 1500 mg. Neither the tricyclic antidepressants nor the anticonvulsants should be abruptly discontinued because significant adverse effects can occur. Topical lidocaine, dosed on an as-needed basis or as a nightly trial for 6 to 8 weeks, can also be used to reduce the discomfort associated with vulvar pain syndromes. Similarly, biofeedback has been shown to be effective in reducing pain and increasing sexual function for women with chronic vulvar pain, and many women prefer these modalities to medical or surgical therapy. Finally, vestibulectomy, associated with clinical cure rates in excess of 80% in a number of trials, is reserved for patients with vestibulitis who have not responded to more conservative therapy, and should be avoided in women with vulvodynia.

PALPABLE MASSES

Human Papillomavirus, Vulvar Condyloma, and VIN

Of the more than 100 human papillomavirus (HPV) subtypes presently identified, at least 35 are specific to the anogenital tract. Current probes for HPV DNA typing allow for identification of half of these anogenital subtypes, including five low-risk and 13 high-risk, or oncogenic, subtypes. At present the routine use of HPV testing in the diagnosis of vulvar HPV-related disease is not recommended. In general, HPV low-risk subtypes 6 and, less commonly, 11 are implicated in the development of genital warts, whereas oncogenic subtype 16 is found in many precancerous VINs, as well as some squamous cell carcinomas of the vulva.

When clinical manifestations of vulvar HPV infection do occur, they often present as bumps or growths on the vulvovaginal or perianal mucosa. Although often asymptomatic, they can cause itching, burning, pain, or bleeding. On examination, condyloma can range in morphologic appearance from flat-topped papules to flesh-colored, dome-shaped papules, keratotic warts, or true condylomata acuminata that have a cauliflower-like appearance. External genital warts tend to occur on the moist surfaces of the vulva, introitus, and perianal area. Distinguishing genital warts from vulvar neoplasia on the basis of appearance alone is not always possible. In general, hyperpigmented, indurated, fixed, or ulcerative lesions, or lesions that do not respond to treatment, should be biopsied because VIN can present as red, white, dark, raised, or eroded lesions. Although the association between smoking and HPV infection is controversial, cigarette smoking has been shown to be a risk factor for both VIN and invasive vulvar carcinoma. Women with vulvar condyloma should undergo routine cervical cancer screening. If cervical warts are found during examination or if vulvar neoplasia is confirmed by biopsy, referral for colposcopic evaluation is indicated. Up to 50% of women with VIN will have antecedent or concomitant lower genital tract neoplasia, usually cervical or vaginal intraepithelial neoplasia. For women with recurrent perianal warts and a history of anoreceptive intercourse, anoscopy is warranted.

Spontaneous regression of genital warts occurs in up to 30% of affected patients. Women at increased risk of developing HPV-related manifestations include those receiving long-term corticosteroid therapy or chronic immunosuppressive treatment, as well as immunosuppressed women with HIV infection and pregnant women. Although neonates are at greater risk of exposure to HPV after vaginal compared with cesarean delivery, the significance of such exposure remains unclear. What is clear is that the majority of such infections in newborns are transient. At present, the data regarding long-term sequelae in infants and children infected with HPV at delivery are inconsistent and do not justify routine cesarean section in women with genital warts.

Topical therapies for genital warts are outlined in Table 17-2. Podofilox and podophyllin are recognized teratogens, and pregnant women should not be exposed to these medications. Clinical trials suggest similar clearance rates, ranging from approximately 20% to more than 80%, for these widely accepted treatment modalities. Local irritation (e.g., pain, burning, and soreness), erythema, edema, and at times, ulceration can result from the use of any of these medications. Careless or excessive use can result in extensive burning of the epithelium, with resultant scar formation. Other outpatient treatment options include cryotherapy and excision or curettage under local anesthesia. Surgical excision or laser vaporization should be reserved for patients with extensive disease.

VIN can occur anywhere on the vulva, perianal skin, and periurethral skin. Lesions may extend into the anal canal, the vagina, or the adjacent thigh and buttock and can take on a variety of appearances (e.g., pigmented, red, white, flat, papular, papillary). Atypical vascular patterns can be identified during colposcopic evaluation, although hyperkeratosis frequently

Table 17-2

Treatment for External Genital Warts

Therapy	Treatment	Application
Patient-applied	Imiquimod 5% cream	Three times weekly for up to 16 weeks
	Podofilox 0.5% solution and gel	Twice daily for 3 days followed by 4 days without therapy; the cycle may be repeated up to four times
Provider-applied	Podophyllin resin 10% to 25% in compound of tincture of benzoin	Carefully applied to the wart and then washed off by the patient between 1 and 4 hours after application
	Trichloroacetic or bichloracetic acid 80% to 90%	First, coat the surrounding normal epithelium with a protective substance (e.g., 5% lidocaine gel); then, use a small cotton-tipped applicator to apply medication to the wart

limits such assessment. VIN is found associated with invasive disease in 2% to 18% of patients, although the risk of malignant transformation is thought to be low (3% to 4%), and the process is slow. In general, increasing rates of VIN 3, as well as invasive vulvar carcinomas, have been reported in women younger than 50 years of age, with the mean age of diagnosis of VIN 3 falling from 50 years (in a series reported before 1975) to 33 years by the mid 1990s. It is also clear that there are two distinct types of VIN: one associated with oncogenic HPV infection (seen more often in younger women, tends to be multicentric and multifocal) and one not related to viral infection (usually found in older women, more likely to be unifocal and unicentric).

Management of VIN depends on multiple factors. For mild neoplasia, observation suffices. For patients with moderate or severe neoplasia, treatment is usually recommended, although observation is initially reasonable for women who have recently completed a course of corticosteroids, who are temporarily immunocompromised, or who are pregnant. Spontaneous regression of untreated VIN 3 has been reported, particularly among young women with multifocal disease. Treatment options include laser vaporization (best used in non–hair-bearing skin; good for clitoral lesions; but higher recurrence rates than with laser excisional therapy), wide local excision (best for localized lesions), or skinning vulvectomy (for widespread multifocal VIN). In a number of recent trials, topical imiquimod, an immune response modifying agent, was shown to be effective in the treatment of VIN 2/3, although properly designed clinical studies are still needed. No matter what treatment modality is chosen, careful and continued surveillance for recurrences will help to decrease the chance of development of invasive disease. Unfortunately, disease recurrence after treatment is not uncommon and has been reported to range from 10% to 50%.

Paget's Disease

Paget's disease of the vulva is a form of intraepithelial neoplasia characterized by adenocarcinomatous cells. In approximately 20% of cases, Paget's disease is associated with an underlying adenocarcinoma in the skin adnexa or Bartholin's gland, and in another 10% to 20% of cases, with a more distant neoplasm (most commonly, of the breast, but also of the urinary or intestinal tract). Most patients are elderly, and their most common complaint is pruritus. Patients typically present with multiple bright red, scaly, eczematoid plaques with a sharply demarcated border, and it is not uncommon for them to have been treated unsuccessfully with topical corticosteroids. Biopsy will confirm the diagnosis; further evaluation to rule out a possible underlying malignancy should include cystoscopy, mammography, colonoscopy, and colposcopy. Referral to a gynecologic oncologist is suggested, and therapy consists of excision with a wide (2 to 3 cm) border. Local recurrence rates exceed 40% in those treated with excision (they are slightly lower with radical vulvectomy), and the prognosis is dictated by the nature of any coexisting adenocarcinoma.

Non–Squamous Cell Malignancies (Melanoma, Carcinoma of Bartholin's Gland, Basal Cell Carcinoma)

Although squamous cell carcinomas account for approximately 80% to 90% of all vulvar malignancies, melanoma, carcinoma of Bartholin's gland, and basal cell carcinoma compose the majority of non–squamous cell malignancies of the vulva. Malignant melanoma of the vulva, which usually presents as an asymptomatic lump, peaks in incidence during the sixth and seventh decades of life. A melanoma may be flat, raised, nodular, or polypoid and is often ulcerated. The color usually ranges from brown to bluish-black, although rarely lesions can be amelanotic. In general, a lesion that changes shape or exhibits atypical features (recall the "ABCD" rule outlined in Box 17-1). In terms of staging, the Breslow technique (tumor thickness) is widely agreed upon to best characterize the clinical behavior of vulvar melanomas, with tumors less than 0.76 mm in thickness having an excellent prognosis. As thickness increases, survival rates drastically decrease. Treatment consists of wide local excision and is best performed by a gynecologic oncologist.

Carcinoma of Bartholin's gland most commonly presents as a deep vulvar mass in the posterior labium majus. Pain, and occasionally bleeding and discharge, may also present with this malignancy, the bulk of which consist of squamous carcinomas and adenocarcinomas. Treatment consists of radical vulvectomy and inguinofemoral lymphadenectomy with adjuvant radiotherapy. Five-year survival rates range from 60% to 80% and depend on the presence of nodal metastases. Approximately 10% of malignant Bartholin's gland tumors are adenoid cystic carcinomas, distinctive both in histology and behavior. Adenoid cystic carcinoma invades and spreads via the perineural spaces; local recurrences are common, although most usually occur years after the initial diagnosis and treatment, and 10-year survival rates approach 60%. Basal cell carcinoma of the vulva, on the other hand, rarely metastasizes and has not been recorded to result in death. This carcinoma typically presents as a nodule or exophytic mass, most commonly found on the anterior portion of the labia majora. Ulceration and excoriation may also be present. Wide local excision is the primary recommended treatment. Inadequate primary excision results in a recurrence rate of about 20%.

Other (Bartholin's Abscess, Hidradenitis Suppurativa)

The most likely diagnosis in a woman with a unilateral, tender, swollen labial mass is an abscess of Bartholin's gland. Such an abscess should occur in the lower third of the introitus between the vestibule and the labia majora. Gonococcal infection has been implicated in a number of cases, although the infection is largely polymicrobial. Although abscesses

Box 17-1 "ABCD" Rule Used to Determine Which Lesions Should Be Biopsied
Asymmetry **B**orders poorly demarcated or jagged **C**olor: Multicolored or black **D**iameter > 6 mm

of Bartholin's gland constitute a relatively frequent finding in the ambulatory setting, agreement as to their most efficacious treatment remains unclear. Currently used treatment modalities include outpatient, less invasive procedures such as needle aspiration with antibiotic coverage, incision (on the mucosal surface of the abscess) and drainage with or without placement of a Word catheter, and more radical surgical therapies such as marsupialization.

Hidradenitis suppurativa, a recurrent skin condition involving the apocrine glands, is characterized by abscesses, sinus tract and fistula formation, and scarring. A disease predominantly of reproductive-aged women of color, hidradenitis can be difficult to treat. Medical management with prolonged courses of antibiotics (e.g., clindamycin), oral contraceptives or Depo-Provera, and/or acitretin can help with early-stage disease, but recurrences often occur, and the disease becomes refractory to conservative management. Surgical therapy, including local incision and drainage and deroofing of sinuses and fistulous tracts, may also help with moderate disease. However, with severe disease, radical excision and healing by secondary intention is the best option to decrease the likelihood of recurrence.

427

KEY POINTS

1. Chronic or recurrent vulvar disease may be challenging for health care providers to diagnose and treat.

2. The threshold for biopsy of the vulva should be low because changes are often subtle and neoplasia needs to be ruled out.

3. Five percent of women will experience recurrent vulvovaginal candidiasis.

4. Clobetasol propionate is the recommended treatment for lichen sclerosus.

5. Lichen simplex chronicus represents an end-stage response to a wide variety of possible initiating processes, including environmental factors and dermatologic diseases. It appears on biopsy as acanthosis, with deepening of the rete ridges into the dermis and superficial dermal collagenization.

6. Eighty percent of the 45 to 60 million people infected with herpes simplex virus type 2 are asymptomatic and therefore unaware of the possibility of sexual transmission.

7. As many as 16% of women have reported a history of chronic vulvar pain.

8. Treatment options for vulvar pain include tricyclic antidepressants, anticonvulsants, biofeedback, and topical analgesics. Vestibulectomy, associated with clinical cure rates in excess of 80%, is reserved for patients with vestibulitis who have not responded to more conservative therapy, and should be avoided in women with vulvodynia.

SUGGESTED READING

Bergeron S, Binik YM, Khalife S, et al: A randomized comparison of group cognitive-behavioral therapy, surface electromyographic biofeedback, and vestibulectomy in the treatment of dyspareunia resulting from vulvar vestibulitis. Pain 91:297–306, 2001.

Boardman LA, Boardman LA: Managing genital herpes simplex virus infections. Women Health Primary Care 3:793–798, 2000.

Boardman LA, Boardman LA: Managing vulvar infections: HPV-related disease and candidiasis. Women Health Primary Care 3:857–862, 2000.

Bornstein J, Heifetz S, Kellner Y, et al: Clobetasol dipropionate 0.05% versus testosterone propionate 2% topical application for severe lichen sclerosus. Am J Obstet Gynecol 178:80–84, 1998.

Bracco GL, Carli P, Sonni L, et al: Clinical and histologic effects of topical treatments of vulval lichen sclerosus: A critical evaluation. J Reprod Med 38:37–40, 1993.

Cardosi RJ, Bomalaski JJ, Hoffman MS: Diagnosis and management of vulvar and vaginal intraepithelial neoplasia. Obstet Gynecol Clin North Am 28:685–702, 2001.

Carli P, Cattaneo A, De Magnis A, et al: Squamous cell carcinoma arising in lichen sclerosus: A longitudinal cohort study. Eur J Cancer Prevention 4:491–495, 1995.

Carlson JA, Ambros R, Malfetano J, et al: Vulvar lichen sclerosus and squamous cell carcinoma: A cohort, case control and investigational study with historical perspective; implications for chronic inflammation and sclerosis in the development of neoplasia. Human Pathol 29:932–948, 1998.

Centers for Disease Control and Prevention: Sexually Transmitted Diseases Treatment Guidelines 2002. MMWR 51:1–80, 2002.

Deitch HR, Huppert J, Hillard PJA: Unusual vulvar ulcerations in young adolescent females. J Pediatr Adolesc Gynecol 17:13–16, 2004.

Edwards L (ed): Genital Dermatology Atlas. New York, Lippincott Williams & Wilkins, 2004.

Foster DC: Vulvar disease. Obstet Gynecol 100:145–163, 2002.

Goetsch MF: Vulvar vestibulitis: Prevalence and historic features in a general gynecologic practice population. Am J Obstet Gynecol 164:1609–1616, 1991.

Harlow BL, Stewart EG: A population-based assessment of chronic unexplained vulvar pain: Have we underestimated the prevalence of vulvodynia? J Am Med Womens Assoc 58:82–88, 2003.

Jones RW: Vulval intraepithelial neoplasia: Current perspectives. Eur J Gynaec Oncol 22:393–402, 2001.

Kimberlin DW, Rouse DJ: Genital herpes. N Engl J Med 350:1970–1977, 2004.

Koutsky LA, Kiviat NB: Genital human papillomavirus. In Holmes KK, Mardh P-A, Sparling PF, et al: Sexually Transmitted Diseases, 3rd ed. New York, McGraw Hill, 1999, pp 347–359.

Lorenz B, Kaufman RH, Kutzner SK: Lichen sclerosus: Therapy with clobetasol propionate. J Reprod Med 43:790–794, 1998.

Lynch PJ: Lichen simplex chronicus (atopic/neurodermatitis) of the anogenital region. Dermatol Ther 17:8–19, 2004.

Moyal-Barracco M, Edwards L: Diagnosis and therapy of anogenital lichen planus. Dermatol Ther 17:38–46, 2004.

Moyal-Barracco M, Lynch PJ: 2003 ISSVD terminology and classification of vulvodynia: A historical perspective. J Reprod Med 49:772–777, 2004.

Neill SM, Tatnall FM, Cox NH: Guidelines for the management of lichen sclerosus. Br J Dermatol 147:640–649, 2002.

Nyirjesy P, Sobel JD, Weitz MV, et al: Cromolyn cream for recalcitrant idiopathic vulvar vestibulitis: results of a placebo controlled study. Sex Transm Inf 77:53–57, 2001.

Oaklander AL, Rissmiller JG: Postherpetic neuralgia after shingles: An under-recognized cause of chronic vulvar pain. Obstet Gynecol 99:625–628, 2002.

Pagano R: Vulvar vestibulitis syndrome: An often unrecognized cause of dyspareunia. Aust NZ J Obstet Gynaecol 39:79–83, 1999.

Parks RW, Parks TG: Pathogenesis, clinical features and management of hidradenitis suppurativa. Ann R Coll Surg Engl 79:83–89, 1997.

Reed BD, Crawford S, Couper M, et al: Pain at the vulvar vestibule: A web-based survey. J Lower Gen Tract Dis 8:48–57, 2004.

Ridley CM, Neill SM (eds): The Vulv, 2 ed. London, Blackwell Science Ltd., 1999.

Rogers RS, Eisen D: Erosive oral lichen planus with genital lesions: The vulvovaginal-gingival syndrome and the peno-gingival syndrome. Dermatol Clin 21:91–98, 2003.

Sakane T, Takeno M, Suzuki N, Inaba G: Behçet's disease. N Engl J Med 341:1284–1291, 1999.

Slade DEM, Powell BW, Mortimer PS: Hidradenitis suppurativa: Pathogenesis and management. Br J Plast Surg 56:451–461, 2003.

Smith YR, Haefner HK: Vulvar lichen sclerosus: Pathophysiology and treatment. Am J Clin Dermatol 5:105–125, 2004.

Sobel JD: Management of patients with recurrent vulvovaginal candidiasis. Drugs 63:1059–1066, 2003.

Sobel JD, Wiesenfeld HC, Martens M, et al: Maintenance fluconazole therapy for recurrent vulvovaginal candidiasis. N Engl J Med 351:876–883, 2004.

Virgili A, Bacilieri S, Corazza M: Managing vulvar lichen simplex chronicus. J Reprod Med 46:343–346, 2001.

Wallace HJ: Lichen sclerosus et atrophicus. Trans St. John's Dermatol Soc 57:9–30, 1971.

Welsh BM, Berzins KN, Cook KA, Fairley CK: Management of common vulval conditions. Med J Aust 178:391–395, 2003.

Wilkinson EJ, Stone IK: Atlas of Vulvar Disease. Baltimore, Williams & Wilkins, 1995.

Wong YW, Powell J, Oxon MA: Lichen sclerosus: A review. Minerva Med 93:950–959, 2002.

18

DIAGNOSIS, WORKUP, AND MANAGEMENT OF PREINVASIVE LESIONS OF THE CERVIX

Pedro F. Escobar, Andres Chiesa-Vottero, and Chad M. Michener

INTRODUCTION

The advent of the Papanicolaou (Pap) smear more than 50 years ago has helped to decrease the rate of invasive cervical cancer by more than 70% in the United States. Unfortunately, nearly 13,000 new cases and more than 4000 deaths occur annually in this country alone, with many more worldwide. Infection with the human papillomavirus (HPV) is thought to be the major cause of nearly a quarter-million cases of cervical dysplasia in the United States each year. Our ability to detect these abnormalities during the natural progression from benign cervical epithelium to mild, moderate, or severe dysplasia and finally to carcinoma *in situ* or frank carcinoma has led to a substantial decrease in morbidity and mortality from cervical cancer. This chapter will focus on imparting an understanding of the various definitions of cervical cancer precursors, the factors involved in dysplastic change, current techniques for diagnosing these changes, and a rational approach to caring for women with preinvasive lesions of the cervix.

THE HISTORY OF CERVICAL CYTOLOGY

In the mid 1920s, Aurel Babes in Romania and George Papanicolaou in New York discovered a link between abnormal cells in the vagina and cervical cancer. They described the abnormalities that eventually led to the development of one of the most successful cancer screening tests in history. Since the 1950s, the Pap smear has been used to screen women for premalignant changes of the cervix. Combining routine Pap smear screening with colposcopic-directed biopsy and therapeutic interventions has led

Figure 18-1

Papanicolaou	I	II		III	IV	V
CIN	Benign	Atypia/ inflammation	CIN 1	CIN 2	CIN 3/ CIS	Carcinoma
Bethesda 2001	Normal	ASC-US	LSIL	HSIL		Carcinoma

Relationship of the Papanicolaou, cervical intraepithelial neoplasia (CIN), and Bethesda systems for cervical cancer precursors. ASC-US, Atypical squamous cells of undetermined significance; LSIL, low-grade squamous intraepithelial lesion; HSIL, high-grade squamous intraepithelial lesion. (Original work by authors, Pedro F. Escobar, Andres Chiesa-Voterro, Chad M. Michener.)

to a significant decrease in the number of women diagnosed with cervical cancer. Conversely, we have seen an increase in the number of cases of cervical dysplasia and other HPV-related diseases during the same period.

The discovery of cervical cancer precursor lesions has also led to an improvement in our understanding of the natural history of abnormalities of the cervix. Histologically, koilocytotic atypia was considered separate from cervical cancer precursors, which were initially subdivided into mild, moderate, and severe dysplasia and carcinoma *in situ* by Reagan et al. in 1953. Generally, when abnormal cells are contained only in the lower third of the epithelium, the lesion was classified as mild. Extension of the abnormal cells into the middle and upper thirds led to a designation of moderate and severe dysplasia, respectively. In 1973, Richart first used the term *cervical intraepithelial neoplasia* (CIN) to describe the differences in cervical abnormalities and divided these into the three categories: CIN 1, 2, and 3. CIN 3 includes both severe dysplasia and carcinoma *in situ* because multiple reports have shown that subdividing these two categories based on histologic examination is poorly reproducible. Clinically, the terms *CIN* and *dysplasia* are often used interchangeably to describe histologic abnormalities of the cervix that have the potential for progression to invasive cancer (Fig. 18-1).

ANATOMY OF THE CERVIX

Embryologically, the endocervix and upper vagina are both covered by the same mucus-secreting columnar epithelium. While *in utero,* the columnar cells in the upper vagina undergo conversion to squamous epithelium termed *metaplasia.* By birth, a distinct junction between the squamous cells and columnar cells is present on the outer portion of the cervix and is known as the *squamocolumnar junction* (SCJ). In response to hormonal stimulation at menarche, further squamous metaplasia occurs, causing movement of the SCJ toward the endocervical canal. During the menopausal years, the SCJ is often in an endocervical location. The region of the cervix that has undergone metaplasia between the initial and current SCJ is known as the *transformation zone;* it is thought to be the area most at risk to the effects of HPV and is a common location for dysplastic changes of the cervix. Destruction or excision of the transformation zone has been the hallmark of treating premalignant diseases of the cervix over the past several decades and will be discussed later in the chapter.

EPIDEMIOLOGY

Before widespread cervical screening, the incidence of invasive cancer of the cervix was more than 30 cases per 100,000 women. Over the last five decades, the incidence decreased to a low of fewer than eight per 100,000 women. However, we have recently begun to see a slight increase in the incidence of invasive cervical cancer, with 9.26 cases per 100,000 women in 2001.

The thought of CIN and cervical cancer representing a continuum rather than separate processes is supported by the incidence rates of various degrees of CIN in different age groups. Based on data from the Surveillance, Epidemiology, and End Results (SEER) Program database, CIN 1–2 is most-common in women aged 25 to 29 years. The prevalence of CIN 3 peaks in the 35- to 39-year-old age group, whereas the peak prevalence of cervical cancer occurs in women older than 50 years. Research has shown that it is the persistence of oncogenic or high-risk HPV subtypes that increases a woman's risk of cervical neoplasia and is necessary for the development of cervical cancer. These findings have led to a strong interest in understanding the biology of HPV infection and finding ways to prevent infection through such mechanisms as HPV vaccines.

RISK FACTORS

Although cervical cancer has long been considered a sexually transmitted disease, only recently has a definite link been made to HPV as a direct cause of cervical cancer and CIN. Previously, researchers tried to find a link between the herpes simplex virus (HSV) and cervical abnormalities. However, the prevalence of HSV infection in patients with cervical cancer was far too low to be a causative agent for the disease. Today, HPV infection is considered necessary, but not sufficient to cause premalignant or malignant changes to the cervical epithelium. In addition, other risk factors such as early age at first coitus, multiple sexual partners, multiparity, and cigarette smoking (Box 18-1) may either simply increase the risk of cervical abnormalities or act as cofactors in addition to infection with HPV.

The Role of HPV

HPV is a 7.8- to 7.9-kDa double-stranded DNA virus that can be sexually transmitted. More than 80 different subtypes of HPV exist; however, only 13 subtypes cause most of the pathology seen in the female genital tract. These subtypes have been subclassified into low-, intermediate-, and high-risk groups based on their association with CIN 3 and cervical cancer (Box 18-2).

Box 18-1	Risk Factors for Cervical Dysplasia and Cancer

Early age of first intercourse
Multiple sexual partners
Partners who have had sex with multiple partners
Multiple pregnancies
History of genital warts
Cigarette smoking
Immunosuppression
   Medications (chronic steroids, immunosuppressants)
   Transplant recipients
   Human immunodeficiency virus infection

Box 18-2	HPV Types and Corresponding Risk of Cancer/High-Grade Dysplasia
High risk	16, 18, 45, and 56
Intermediate risk	31, 33, 35, 39, 51, 52, 58, 59, and 68
Low risk	6, 11, 42, 43, and 44

HPV types 16 and 18 are most closely associated with high-grade dysplasia and cancer. In fact, the presence of HPV 16 or 18 has been shown to increase the relative risk of moderate or severe dysplasia 9- to 16-fold.

The biologic relevance of HPV infection is dependent on cellular interactions beyond simple cellular infection. Typically, HPV enters the cytoplasm of the host and is sequestered in its circular form in particles called *episomes*. Here HPV replication can occur, filling the cellular cytoplasm with viral particles that appear as areas of perinuclear clearing by light microscopy, the process of koilocytosis. Once viral particles enter the nucleus, they can bind to cellular DNA and integrate into the host genome, causing genomic and proteomic alterations.

HPV integration is a process that is biologically necessary but not always sufficient to cause neoplastic transformation. The HPV virus itself is made up of two distinct late regions, L1 and L2, as well as six distinct early regions, E1, E2, and E4 through E7 (Fig. 18-2). L1 and L2 are conserved regions within the HPV genome and are involved in capsid protein production. The E6 and E7 genes are regulators of cell growth and are able to directly transform cells into a malignant phenotype. E6 protein is able to bind to the p53 tumor suppressor protein, leading to degradation

Figure 18-2

Schematic of human papillomavirus type 16 (HPV-16) viral structure. (Original work by authors, Pedro F. Escobar, Andres Chiesa-Voterro, and Chad M. Michener.)

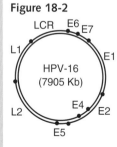

of p53 protein. Removal of p53 from the cell disrupts regulatory control of the cell cycle that typically occurs through p53 modulation of cyclin-dependent kinases. Unchecked cell cycling in the absence of functional p53 protein can lead to undetected genomic abnormalities of the cell and malignant transformation. Similarly, the E7 protein disrupts normal activity of the retinoblastoma gene, *pRb*, by making it unavailable for binding with E2F, a cellular transcription factor. Unbound E2F is able to directly stimulate cell cycling, which goes unchecked by *pRb* (and p53, if E6 is active) due to binding of E7. Again, this can lead to undetected genomic abnormalities and malignant transformation of the cell. E1 is typically involved with DNA replication, whereas E2 is involved in transcriptional regulation of HPV E6 and E7. E2 is a frequent site of DNA integration, allowing disruption of the E6–E7 genes. Disruption of these genes causes abnormal transcriptional control, allowing genetic alterations to go unchecked and aberrant growth to proceed unaltered.

HPV Typing and Correlation with Disease

Testing for the presence of HPV DNA has gone from labor-intensive Southern blotting techniques to rapid HPV identification with the Hybrid Capture II (HC-2) assay (Digene Diagnostics, Gaithersburg, MD). HC-2 employs two separate probes, one for five low-risk subtypes and a second probe for the 13 intermediate- and high-risk HPV subtypes (i.e., 16, 18, 31, 33, 35, 39, 45, 51, 52, 56, 58, 59, and 68). This assay is sensitive to at least 1 pg/mL of HPV DNA correlating to 5000 genomic copies. When compared head-to-head with polymerase chain reaction (PCR) for identification of HPV, HC-2 performed as well or slightly better. Unfortunately, HC-2 does not allow for identification of specific HPV types; it is only a qualitative assessment of the presence of one or more of the 13 intermediate- or high-risk types. HPV typing is used more commonly in the research setting and is currently most often performed using PCR techniques.

Studies that have used HPV typing allowed for the classification of the high-risk versus low-risk viruses, which were discussed previously (*see* Box 18-2). Low-risk HPV types have been identified most commonly in mild dysplasia as well as condyloma acuminata. These lesions have a low risk of progression to cancer and are much less likely to integrate into the host's genome. This means that cellular alterations in E6 and E7 seen after integration of high-risk HPV types usually do not occur. Therefore, the oncogenic potential of these HPV types is essentially nil.

HPV 16 and 18 are the most frequently identified HPV types in high-grade dysplasia and cervical cancer. High-risk HPV has been identified in 93% to 99% of CIN 2 and 3 lesions and in up to 71% of adenocarcinoma *in situ* (AIS). Studies evaluating the presence of HPV in cervical cancer specimens have identified HPV in 90% to 100% of squamous cell carcinomas and 78% to 95% of adenocarcinomas. More than half of all squamous cell carcinomas and one third of the adenocarcinomas of the cervix are associated with HPV 16, whereas HPV 18 is present in approximately 25% of squamous cell cervical cancers. Although HPV 16 and 18 both have the ability to integrate into the host genome and cause oncogenic transformation, HPV 18 has been associated with a higher rate of viral integration. Reports have been published suggesting that HPV 18 is associated with a higher rate of cervical cancer recurrence and may confer a more rapid progression from a normal state to cancer once cells become infected with this HPV subtype. In fact, recent studies have shown a high rate of expression—and more importantly, integration—of HPV 18 in patients with highly aggressive small cell carcinomas of the cervix. Further studies are needed to assess the true natural history of these tumors based on the presence and integration of different HPV types.

Although not all dysplasias or cancers contain HPV, a definite causal relationship between HPV infection and cervical dysplasia or carcinoma has been established. For this reason, HPV testing has recently been added to the cervical cancer screening algorithm for women aged 30 years or older and remains an adjunct to cytologic screening for triaging younger women to colposcopy who have a cytologic diagnosis of atypical squamous cells of undetermined significance (ASC-US).

The FDA has approved a quadravalent vaccine for the prevention of the most common HPV infections causing cervical dysplasia, cervical cancer, and genital warts (types 6, 11, 16, and 18). This vaccine has been shown to be highly immunogenic with more than 99% of those vaccinated producing titers of anti-HPV antibodies to each HPV type. HPV-naïve individuals that were vaccinated had a 90% to 100% reduction in persistent HPV infection or disease after 3 years of follow-up. Immunity with the HPV vaccine appears to persist for more than 4 years, but the absolute duration of immunity has not been defined. Vaccination requires a series of three injections over 6 months and is well tolerated with pain, erythema, and swelling at the injection site as the most common side effects. Current recommendations are to vaccinate all females between the ages of 9 and 26 regardless of prior HPV status. Clinical trials in males and research on therapeutic HPV vaccines are ongoing. The development of these vaccines will probably have the greatest impact on management and prevention of lower genital tract neoplasia since the introduction of the Pap smear.

Other Risk Factors

Cigarette Smoking

The role of cigarette smoking has been evaluated in epidemiologic and *in vitro* studies. Today there is little doubt that cigarette smoking plays a role in the epidemiology of cervical dysplasia and cervical cancers. In fact, women undergoing treatment of HPV-related lesions have higher failure rates than women who do not smoke. Research has shown that highly concentrated levels of nicotine and conitine are present in the cervical mucous of women who smoke. Whether or not these compounds are the biologic culprits for cervical dysplasia in cigarette smokers is not completely understood. However, the poor prognosis associated with the combination of HPV infection and cigarette smoking is undoubtedly a health hazard worth reviewing with patients being seen for abnormalities on their Pap smears.

Herpes Simplex Virus

HSV infection was thought to play a causative role in the etiology of cervical lesions because of a concurrence of this virus in women diagnosed with cervical abnormalities; however, modern studies have shown that many sexually transmitted diseases are found at higher frequency in women with cervical dysplasia or cervical cancer. The association between HSV and cervical dysplasia is too weak to prove HSV as a causative agent for this group of diseases. However, a higher number of sexual partners of the patient and her partner(s) have a direct link to increased risk of HPV infection. Therefore, sexual behavior is probably the common link between HPV, other sexually transmitted diseases, and risk of preinvasive lesions of the cervix.

Immunosuppression

Clearance of HPV infection is partly dependent on an intact host immune system. Patients who are immunosuppressed through acquired (e.g., human immunodeficiency virus infection) or iatrogenic (e.g., chronic steroid use in inflammatory conditions and immunosuppression in patients receiving transplants) means demonstrate higher infection rates with HPV. Additionally, these patients have lower clearance rates of HPV infection/dysplasia and are at higher risk of progression to cancer.

PATHOLOGY OF PREINVASIVE DISEASE OF THE CERVIX

Cervical Intraepithelial Neoplasia

The 2003 World Health Organization Classification of Tumors of the Breast and Female Genital Organs divides CIN, the precursor lesions of cervical squamous cell carcinoma, into three grades: CIN 1, 2, and 3. It acknowledges that the division is subjective, since the histologic features represent a diagnostic continuum. In addition, clinicians were finding that diagnosis and therapy for this group of abnormalities was more complex. The fact that mild dysplasia has a propensity for spontaneous resolution and moderate and severe dysplasia has higher rates of progression led some clinicians and pathologists to question this system.

In 1988, the Bethesda System for cervical cytology was developed with the goal of providing a uniform, reproducible system reflecting the current understanding of cervical neoplasia that provided clinically relevant information to clinicians. This system consolidated the categories of HPV effect, degrees of dysplasia, and grades of CIN to the two tiers of low-grade squamous intraepithelial lesion (LSIL) and high-grade squamous intraepithelial lesion (HSIL). The most recent review and revision of this terminology took place at the Bethesda Workshop in 2001 (Fig. 18-3). Today, approximately 50 million women are being screened in the United States annually. Two million ASC-US and atypical squamous cells that cannot exclude HSIL (ASC-H), 1.25 million LSIL, 300,000 HSIL, and 13,000 cancers are diagnosed using the current system.

Figure 18-3

The 2001 Bethesda System. (With permission from Solomon D, Davey D, Kurman R, et al: Forum Group Members; Bethesda 2001 Workshop: The 2001 Bethesda System: terminology for reporting results of cervical cytology. JAMA 287(16):2114–2119, 2002.)

THE 2001 BETHESDA SYSTEM

Specimen Adequecy
Satisfactory for evaluation *(note presence/absence of endocervical/transformation zone component)*
Unsatisfactory for evaluation . . . *(specify reason)*
  Specimen rejected/not processed *(specify reason)*
  Specimen processed and examined, but unsatisfactory for evaluation of epithelial abnormality because of *(specify reason)*

General Categorization *(optional)*
Negative for intraepithelial lesion or malignancy
Epithelial cell abnormality
Other

Interpretation/Result
Negative for intraepithelial lesion or malignancy
  Organisms
    Trichomonas *vaginalis*
    Fungal organisms morphologically consistent with *Candida* species
    Shift in flora suggestive of bacterial vaginosis
    Bacteria morphologically consistent with *Actinomyces* species
    Cellular changes consistent with herpes simplex virus
  Other nonneoplastic findings *(optional to report; list not comprehensive)*
    Reactive cellular changes associated with
      inflammation (includes typical repair)
      radiation
      intrauterine contraceptive device
    Glandular cells status posthysterectomy
    Atrophy
Epithelial cell abnormalities
  Squamous cells
    Atypical squamous cells (ASC) of undetermined significance (ASC-US)
      cannot exclude HSIL (ASC-H)
    Low-grade squamous intraepithelial lesion (LSIL) encompassing: human papillomavirus/mild dysplasia/cervical intraepithelial neoplasia (CIN) 1
    High-grade squamous intraepithelial lesion (HSIL) encompassing: moderate and severe dysplasia, carcinoma *in situ;*
      CIN 2 and CIN 3
      Squamous cell carcinoma
  Glandular cell
    Atypical glandular cells (AGC) *(specify endocervical, endometrial, or not otherwise specified)*
    Atypical glandular cells, favor neoplastic *(specify endocervical or not otherwise specified)*
    Endocervical adenocarcinoma in situ (AIS)
    Adenocarcinoma
  Other *(list not comprehensive)*
    Endometrial cells in a woman, ≥40 years of age
AUTOMATED REVIEW AND ANCILLARY TESTING *(include as appropriate)*
EDUCATIONAL NOTES AND SUGGESTIONS *(optional)*

The 2001 Bethesda System for Cervical Cytology

The 2001 Bethesda System (TBS) takes into account several factors when results are reported including specimen adequacy, presence or absence of intraepithelial neoplasia, and presence of other cell types within the specimen.

Specimen Adequacy

Specimen adequacy is the most important quality assurance component of TBS. Any specimen with abnormal cells (ASC-US, atypical glandular cells, or worse) is by definition satisfactory for evaluation. Minimum squamous cellularity criteria for conventional Pap smears are approximately 8000 to 12,000 well-preserved and well-visualized cells. For liquid-based cytology (LBC), an estimated minimum of approximately 5000 cells is required. LBC, by virtue of the preparation methodology, presents a more random (and presumably more representative) sampling of the collected cervical material compared with conventional smears. An adequate endocervical/transformation zone (EC/TZ) component requires at least 10 well-preserved endocervical or squamous metaplastic cells. Data on the importance of the EC/TZ component are conflicting.

Negative for Intraepithelial Lesion or Malignancy

Cervical cytology is a screening test used primarily for detection of squamous cell carcinoma of the cervix and its precursors; organisms and other non-neoplastic diagnoses are not the main focus of cervical screening. However, such information may be clinically relevant in certain circumstances. Organisms that may be found during cervical cytology include *Trichomonas vaginalis, Candida* species, bacterial vaginosis, *Actinomyces* species, and HSV. In addition, other nonneoplastic findings include reactive cellular changes associated with inflammation, radiation, and intrauterine contraceptive device.

Endometrial Cells in a Woman 40 Years of Age and Older

Only exfoliated, intact endometrial cells are reported in women aged 40 years or older. Exfoliated endometrial cells are usually derived from a benign process, and only a small proportion of women with this finding have endometrial abnormalities. Endometrial cells have been considered a potential harbinger of endometrial adenocarcinoma when seen in preparations of postmenopausal women or outside the proliferative phase of the menstrual cycle. If the specimen was obtained in the first half of the cycle, the finding correlates with the menstrual history.

Again, cervical cytology is meant to be a screening test for squamous intraepithelial lesions (SIL) and squamous cell carcinoma. It is unreliable for the detection of endometrial lesions and should not be used to evaluate cases of suspected endometrial abnormalities.

Squamous Cell Abnormalities

True squamous cell changes found on Pap smear range from ASC to invasive squamous cell carcinomas. The category of ASC has been the most problematic clinically and is found in approximately 5% of Pap smears. It does not represent a single biologic entity; it subsumes changes that are unrelated to oncogenic HPV infection and neoplasia as well as findings that suggest the possible presence of underlying CIN and, rarely, carcinoma. It is an equivocal category that reflects the inability of pathologists to accurately and reproducibly interpret these specimens.

ASC refers to cytologic changes suggestive of SIL, which are qualitatively or quantitatively insufficient for a definitive interpretation. Designation of ASC requires three essential features (Box 18-3). TBS 2001 divides ASC into two categories: ASC-US and ASC-H.

Atypical Squamous Cells of Undetermined Significance

ASC-US reflects changes that are either suggestive of LSIL or SIL of indeterminate grade. The qualifier "undetermined significance" is added because 10% to 20% of women with ASC-US prove to have an underlying CIN 2 or 3. The percentage of HPV infections among women with ASC-US is strongly correlated with age.

Atypical Squamous Cells Cannot Exclude HSIL

ASC-H is a designation reserved for the minority of cases in which the cytologic changes are suggestive of HSIL. Results from the ASC-US/LSIL Triage Study (ALTS) found that the interpretation of ASC-H was associated with a higher risk of oncogenic HPV DNA detection and a greater risk of underlying CIN 2 or worse (30% to 40%) compared with ASC-US (10% to 15%). The ASC-H category should compose only 5% to 10% of ASC cases.

Squamous Intraepithelial Neoplasia

Conceptually, HPV-associated abnormalities can be divided into transient infections that generally regress over the course of 1 to 2 years and HPV persistence that is associated with an increased risk of developing a cancer precursor or invasive cancer.

At the 1988 Bethesda workshop, the spectrum of SIL was subdivided into two categories based on (1) the desire to use morphologic categories that relate to the biology and clinical management of HPV-associated lesions, and (2) the acknowledged low interobserver and intraobserver reproducibility with conventional three- and four-grade classification systems.

The cytologic distinction between CIN 2 and CIN 3 is poorly reproducible; combining the cytologic correlates of CIN 2 and 3 into a single HSIL category was shown, in the ALTS trial, to have improved reproducibility. Given the variability in interpretation and biologic behavior of "cytologic CIN 2," setting the cytologic threshold for low-grade and high-grade lesions between CIN 1 and CIN 2 is considered appropriate. As a screening test, cervical cytology must emphasize sensitivity.

Even with only two categories of SIL, there is a 10% to 15% interpathologist discrepancy rate between LSIL and HSIL interpretations on cervical cytology slides. Cytology may also be discrepant with histology; 15% to 25% of women with LSIL cytology are found to have histologic CIN 2 or 3 on further evaluation.

Low-Grade Squamous Intraepithelial Lesion

LSIL encompasses HPV, mild dysplasia, and CIN 1. HPV-associated squamous cell changes or cytopathic effects (i.e., koilocytosis) were initially considered to represent a process separate from "true" dysplasia. However, mounting evidence over the past 20 years has established HPV as the main

---

Box 18-3   Criteria for Atypical Squamous Cells

1. Squamous differentiation
2. Increased ratio for nuclear-to-cytoplasmic area
3. Minimal nuclear hyperchromasia, chromatin clumping, irregularity, smudging, or multinucleation

Box 18-4 Criteria for Low-Grade Squamous Intraepithelial Lesion

1. Cell size is usually large overall, with fairly abundant "mature" well-defined cytoplasm.
2. Nuclear enlargement occurs that is more than three times the area of normal intermediate nucleus, resulting in a slightly increased nuclear-to-cytoplasmic ratio.
3. Variable degrees of nuclear hyperchromasia are present, accompanied by variations in nuclear size, number, and shape.
4. Nuclear membranes have a slightly irregular contour, but may be smooth.
5. Perinuclear cavitation ("koilocytosis") consisting of a sharply delineated clear perinuclear zone and a peripheral rim of densely stained cytoplasm. Alternatively, the cytoplasm may appear dense and keratinized; cells with these characteristics must also show nuclear abnormalities.

439

Figure 18-4

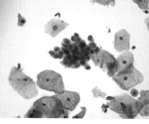 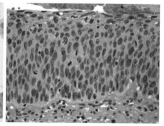

Severe squamous dysplasia of the cervix. Left, High-grade squamous intraepithelial lesion on Papanicolaou smear (liquid-based cytology; magnification, 200×). Right, Cervical biopsy showing cervical intraepithelial neoplasia, grade 3 (hematoxylin and eosin stain; magnification, 200×).

causal factor in the pathogenesis of virtually all cervical cancer precursors and cancers.

Several studies have demonstrated that the morphologic criteria for distinguishing koilocytosis from mild dysplasia or CIN 1 vary among investigators and lack clinical significance. In addition, both lesions share similar HPV types, and their biologic behavior and clinical management are similar, thus supporting a common designation of LSIL. Most CIN 1, especially in young women, represents a self-limited HPV infection.

Criteria for LSIL are listed in Box 18-4.

High-Grade Squamous Intraepithelial Lesion

HSIL (Fig. 18-4) encompasses moderate and severe dysplasia, carcinoma *in situ*, CIN 2, and CIN 3. The criteria for HSIL are detailed in Box 18-5.

Squamous Cell Carcinoma

Although beyond the scope of a cervical dysplasia chapter, a discussion of TBS would not be complete without mentioning squamous cell carcinoma. TBS does not subdivide squamous cell carcinoma. However, for descriptive purposes, nonkeratinizing and keratinizing carcinomas are described separately.

Criteria for keratinizing squamous cell carcinoma include marked variation in cellular size and shape with caudate and spindle cells that frequently contain dense orangeophilic cytoplasm. Nuclei also vary markedly

> **Box 18-5** Criteria for High-Grade Squamous Intraepithelial Lesion
>
> 1. Changes affect smaller and less "mature" cells.
> 2. Overall cell size is variable and ranges from low-grade squamous intraepithelial lesion (LSIL) size to small basal-type cells.
> 3. Nuclear hyperchromasia is accompanied by variations in nuclear size and shape.
> 4. The degree of nuclear enlargement is variable; LSIL size but decreased cytoplasmic area leads to a high nuclear-to-cytoplasmic (N/C) ratio or very high N/C ratio, but actual nuclear size is considerably smaller than that of LSIL.
> 5. The nuclear membrane contour is irregular and frequently demonstrates prominent indentations.

in size, with nuclear membranes that may be irregular in configuration. Numerous dense opaque nuclei are often present. The chromatin pattern is coarsely granular and irregularly distributed with parachromatin clearing. Macronucleoli may be seen and tumor diathesis may be present.

Criteria for nonkeratinizing squamous cell carcinoma include cells disposed singly or in syncytial aggregates with poorly defined cell borders. The cells are frequently smaller than those of many HSIL but display most of the features of HSIL. Nuclei have markedly irregular distribution of coarsely clumped chromatin, and tumor diathesis is often present. In addition, large-cell variant tumors may show prominent macronucleoli and basophilic cytoplasm.

Glandular Cell Abnormalities

Endocervical AIS is considered to be the glandular counterpart of CIN 3 and the precursor to invasive endocervical adenocarcinoma. Similar HPV types have been demonstrated in most invasive endocervical adenocarcinoma and AIS. The cytologic interpretation of AIS correlates with histologic outcomes. However, no low-grade endocervical glandular entity analogous to LSIL has been identified. As noted previously, cervical cytology is primarily a screening test for SIL and squamous cell carcinoma; sensitivity for glandular lesions is limited by problems with both sampling and interpretation.

Atypical Endocervical, Endometrial, or Glandular Cells

TBS interpretation of "atypical endocervical, endometrial or glandular cells" defines an increased level of risk, as opposed to a specific neoplastic precursor entity. It may be used for cases demonstrating some, but not all, of the criteria necessary for AIS or invasive adenocarcinoma. These features include nuclear enlargement, crowding, variation in size, and hyperchromasia. Some non-neoplastic processes that may show atypical cellular changes and may lead to interpretive difficulty include lower uterine segment sampling, tubal metaplasia, repair, endocervical polyps, microglandular hyperplasia, Arias-Stella change, and effects of ionizing radiation. Follow-up of atypical glandular cytologic interpretations shows that high-grade lesions are identified in 10% to 40% of cases and are more often squamous (CIN 2 or 3) than glandular.

The distinction of cytologically benign versus atypical endometrial cells is based primarily on the criterion of increased nuclear size. The presence of atypical endometrial cells, like their cytologically bland counterparts, may be associated with the presence of endometrial polyps, chronic endometritis, an intrauterine device, endometrial hyperplasia, or endometrial carcinoma.

Endocervical AIS

The cytologic interpretation of endocervical AIS (Fig. 18-5) can be difficult and should only be made in cases in which sufficient criteria are present. In problematic cases, the interpretation of "atypical endocervical cells/ glandular cells, favor neoplastic" is justified. Although uncommon, variant forms of AIS exist that may show other morphologic features.

The possibility of coexisting glandular and squamous lesions in the cervix should always be considered when making an interpretation of endocervical AIS. In some studies, up to half of AIS lesions have a coexisting SIL, usually of high grade. Criteria are detailed in Box 18-6.

Adenocarcinoma: Endocervical, Endometrial, Extrauterine, Not Otherwise Specified

441

For endocervical adenocarcinoma, features include abundant abnormal cells, typically with columnar configuration arranged as single cells, two-dimensional sheets, or three-dimensional clusters and syncytial aggregates. Enlarged, pleomorphic nuclei demonstrate irregular chromatin distribution, parachromatin clearing, and nuclear membrane irregularities. Macronucleoli may be present, and a necrotic tumor diathesis may be seen. An invasive adenocarcinoma should be strongly considered in the presence of tumor diathesis, nuclear clearing with uneven distribution of chromatin, or macronucleoli. However, these may be absent.

Figure 18-5

Adenocarcinoma *in situ* (AIS). Left, AIS on Papanicolaou smear (liquid-based cytology; magnification, 400×). Right, AIS on cervical biopsy (hematoxylin and eosin stain; magnification, 100×).

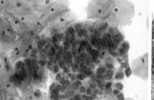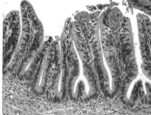

Box 18-6   Criteria for Endocervical Adenocarcinoma *in Situ*

1. Cells appear in sheets, clusters, strips, and rosettes with nuclear crowding and overlap, and loss of honeycomb pattern.
2. Cell clusters have a palisading nuclear arrangement with nuclei and cytoplasmic tags protruding from the periphery ("feathering").
3. Nuclei are enlarged, variably sized, oval or elongated, and stratified.
4. Nuclear hyperchromasia have evenly dispersed, coarsely granular chromatin.
5. Mitoses and apoptotic bodies are commonly seen.
6. Nuclear-to-cytoplasmic ratios are increased.
7. Nucleoli are usually small or inconspicuous.
8. The background is typically clean (no tumor diathesis or inflammatory debris).

For endometrial adenocarcinoma, the features are cells typically occurring singly or in small, tight clusters. Nuclei become larger with increasing grade of the tumor. There is variation in nuclear size and polarity. Nuclei display moderate hyperchromasia, irregular chromatin distribution, and parachromatin clearing in high-grade tumors. Small to prominent nucleoli are present with increasing grade of tumor. Cytoplasm is scant, cyanophilic, and often vacuolated; intracytoplasmic neutrophils are common. A finely granular or "watery" tumor diathesis is variably present. The cytologic findings in endometrial adenocarcinoma are largely dependent on the grade of the tumor. Grade 1 tumors tend to shed few abnormal cells with minimal cytologic atypia; these would usually be interpreted as atypical endometrial cells. High-grade endometrial serous carcinomas morphologically resemble their ovarian counterpart with papillary fragments, large cell size, and prominent nucleoli.

When cells diagnostic of adenocarcinoma occur in association with a clean background or with morphology unusual for tumors of the uterus or cervix, an extrauterine neoplasm should be considered. Sources in the genital tract include the ovaries and fallopian tubes. Although not specific, the presence of papillary clusters and psammoma bodies suggests an ovarian carcinoma. The lack of tumor diathesis is a clue to the noncervical origin of the malignant cells. When diathesis is present, it is usually associated with metastasis to the uterus or vagina.

Other Malignant Neoplasms

Malignant neoplasms, other than squamous and adenocarcinoma, infrequently involve the uterine cervix and may be seen in cervical cytology preparations. These include spindle squamous cell carcinoma, poorly differentiated squamous carcinoma with small cells, small cell undifferentiated carcinoma, carcinoid tumors, malignant mixed mesodermal tumor, sarcomas, and others. Most often, these tumors are uncommon primaries arising in the uterine corpus or adnexa. Metastases to the uterine cervix occur rarely.

SCREENING FOR CERVICAL NEOPLASIA

The trend over the last 50 years in the United States has been a decrease in the number of cervical cancer cases and an increase in the number of cases of preinvasive disease. Most of these changes can be attributed to the successful introduction of the Pap smear for cervical cancer screening. It remains the most successful cancer screening test in terms of cost per woman screened and reduction in the diagnosis of invasive carcinoma. The limitations of screening are mostly due to poor access to screening as seen in developing countries, whereas the success of the screening program is highly dependent on the quality of specimen collection and review.

Cervical Sampling

Sensitivity of the Pap smear is dependent not only on the accurate evaluation of the slides, but also on correct sampling techniques. It is estimated that as many as 50% of false-negative Pap smear results are due to errors in sampling techniques. Early cervicovaginal cytology was obtained by vaginal irrigation with saline and collection of the effluent for cytologic evaluation. Modern Pap smear techniques involve the use of the Ayers spatula, initially made of wood, but now made of plastic to improve release of the cells for fluid-based sampling. A single 360-degree rotation of the spatula allows adequate sampling of the entire exocervix. In addition, the endocervix is sampled using the endocervical brush. The brush allows for more complete sampling than the moistened cotton-tipped applicator that has been used in the past. A single 180-degree rotation of the Cytobrush adequately samples the endocervix. Further rotation may cause undue bleeding, whereas reverse rotation may dislodge cells that were obtained on the original rotation.

In traditional sampling, cells from the spatula are placed on one half of the glass slide then cells from the endocervical brush are rolled onto the other half of the slide. The slide is quickly sprayed with fixative to prevent air-drying artifact that can make evaluation of the slides more difficult (Box 18-7).

The reported sensitivity of traditional Pap smears ranges from 50% to 95% and is dependent on the laboratory being used. When compared with colposcopy and biopsy for confirmation of disease, the Pap smear alone has a sensitivity of approximately 70%. False-negative results typically range from 15% to 50% and can be attributed both to laboratory error as well as poor sampling due to inherent limitations of the test and clinician error.

Liquid-Based Cytology

Today, LBC is used in the majority of centers across the United States. Although fewer cells are screened with LBC, the preparation of the sample allows for easier screening of a more representative population of cells. Two systems are widely used—ThinPrep and SurePath—and both are ap-

443

Box 18-7 Steps for Obtaining a Pap Smear

1. Take Pap smear specimen before performing bimanual examination or collecting other samples.
2. Place spatula firmly against exocervix and rotate 360 degrees.
3. Place endocervical brush into cervical canal and rotate 180 degrees.
4. For traditional cytology:
   a. Smear spatula on one side of the glass slide, then roll brush on the other half.
   b. Hold fixative approximately 10 inches from slide, and spray.
5. For liquid-based cytology:
   a. Place both the spatula and brush into the vial and clean vigorously.
   b. Close lid tightly.
6. If using separate vial for human papillomavirus testing, place brush into endocervical canal, rotate three full turns, place brush into vial, and snap off at score line.

proved by the U.S. Food and Drug Administration (FDA). Studies evaluating ThinPrep have shown that the detection rate of ASC-US or higher is greater than the rates obtained with conventional screening, although the specificity is either similar or slightly lower. It is also likely that the detection rate of LSIL or higher has a greater sensitivity with almost unchanged specificity and that the detection rate of HSIL or higher is greater, as is the absolute sensitivity, with almost unchanged specificity. Another advantage of LBC is the availability of residual material, which potentially can be used for ancillary testing such as detection of oncogenic HPV DNA.

HPV DNA as an Adjunct to Cytologic Screening

A single liquid-based Pap smear carries a false-negative rate of up to 20%. In addition, ASC-US are identified in 3% to 5% of all Pap smears in the United States with an estimated 5% to 10% of these women harboring an underlying high-grade dysplasia. Optimal management of patients with ASC-US smears has yet to be determined. However, studies demonstrate a direct correlation between HPV DNA positivity and severity of cytologic abnormalities such that true high-grade lesions are almost always associated with high-risk HPV subtypes. This led investigators to prospectively evaluate the use of HPV DNA testing (HC-2 assay) as an adjunct to ASC-US and LSIL cytology for deciding which patients should be referred for colposcopy.

The ALTS group in the United States evaluated nearly 3500 women with ASC-US found on Pap smears and concluded that HPV testing is sufficiently sensitive for triaging patients with ASC-US smears to either further follow-up or routine screening. HPV testing was 96% sensitive for identification of CIN 3, with 56% of women going on to colposcopy. A single repeat liquid-based Pap smear with referral for ASC-US or above in the same cohort was only 85% sensitive with a similar number of referrals. A similar study found sensitivities of 89% and 76% for the identification of women with CIN 3 by HPV testing and repeat cytology, respectively. They concluded that HPV testing gives equivalent or better sensitivity for the detection of CIN 3 with less referral to colposcopy than a single repeat ASC-US smear. However, a higher prevalence of HPV DNA in women with LSIL limits the utility of HPV DNA testing as a triage tool for this group of patients. These findings led to the March 2002 FDA approval of HPV testing as an adjunct to cytology for the triage of women with ASC-US smears. We have integrated "reflex" HPV testing into our practice since 1997 and have seen no untoward effects of this change to date.

When Negative Means Negative

Perhaps the most clinically useful aspect of HPV DNA testing is its powerful negative predictive value. Although all studies improved on the sensitivity of LBC, the negative predictive value of HPV testing alone for CIN 3 or cancer is 96% to 99%. A negative HPV test result coupled with negative cytology achieves a negative predictive value of 99.6% or better, giving clinicians and patients confidence that a negative test result really means an absence of significant disease. We take advantage of this predictive power by using HC-2 as a "test of cure" for patients who have undergone loop electrosurgical excision procedure (LEEP) or conization procedures. Several small trials have confirmed that persistence of HPV infection after therapeutic excisional procedures identifies patients at higher risk for recurrent or persistent dysplasia. Our current practice is to follow up with patients who have had persistently positive HPV DNA test results every 6 to 12 months with a lower threshold for return to colposcopy.

HPV DNA for Primary Screening

The excellent performance of HPV DNA testing in the triage of women with mildly abnormal cytology results has led to an interest in combining HPV testing with LBC for primary screening as a "molecular Pap" test. In 4075 previously unselected women in Washington State using combined testing, researchers found sensitivities for the identification of CIN 3 or greater of 61% and 91% for cytology and HPV testing, respectively. Additionally, they found that HPV DNA screening was more sensitive in women younger than 30 years, but significantly more specific in women aged 30 years and older. Women 20 to 24 years old had a higher prevalence of HPV infection (21% versus 5%) and a lower incidence of CIN 3 or greater (3% versus 8%) than women over the age of 35 years, suggesting that HPV infections in younger women are most likely transient and, therefore, less likely to be associated with significant cervical lesions. A large European study confirmed that HPV testing greatly improved sensitivity for the detection of high-grade dysplasia compared with LBC alone (100% versus 81%). However, specificity was only marginally improved by the addition of HPV testing in women older than 30 years. Mass screening in the Shanxi Province of China, where the incidence of cervical cancer is higher and access to health care limited, showed an increase in sensitivity for CIN 2/3 or higher from 94% to 100% with a strong negative predictive value for combination testing.

445

Modern Screening Recommendations

Controversy has arisen regarding the optimal time to begin cervical cancer screening as well the optimal screening interval. Previously, recommendations included initiation of screening 3 years after the first occurrence of intercourse or at the age of 18 years, whichever came first. Recent recommendations from the American College of Obstetricians and Gynecologists include beginning screening 3 years after the age of first intercourse or at the age of 21 years, whichever is earlier. The reason for this change in recommendations stems from a better understanding of the natural history of HPV infection.

HPV infection rates are high in young women, but many of these infections are self-limited and will revert to normal on their own. Additionally, the progression of lesions from mild dysplasia to severe dysplasia or cancer is estimated to be 50 to 60 months (Fig. 18-6). This gives physicians a "window of opportunity" to diagnose and treat significant lesions while not overtreating lesions that are mildly abnormal. With careful follow-up, approximately two thirds of mild dysplasias and half of moderate dysplasias will revert to normal over a period of 12 to 24 months (Table 18-1). We

Figure 18-6

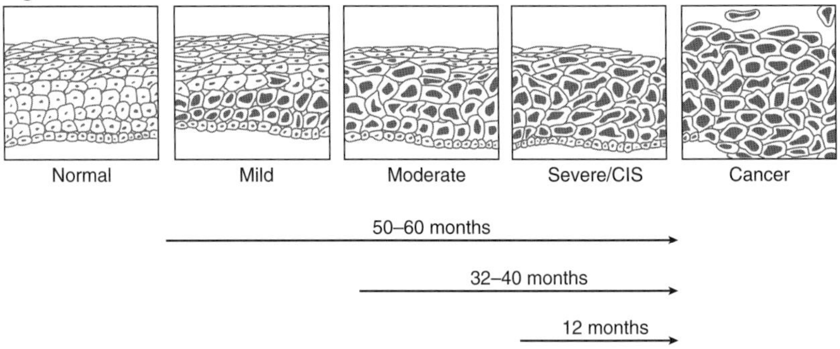

| Normal | Mild | Moderate | Severe/CIS | Cancer |

50–60 months

32–40 months

12 months

Natural progression of cervical dysplasia. Schematic of biopsy specimens showing differences in cellular abnormalities from normal to cancer and time associated with progression to CIN 3/ cancer *(lower arrows)*. CIS, Carcinoma *in situ*. (Original work by authors, Pedro F. Escobar, Andres Chiesa-Voterro, and Chad M. Michener.)

currently practice conservative follow-up of young women with mild to moderate dysplasia, particularly if childbearing is still an issue. Follow-up with repeat combination testing every 6 to 12 months allows us to identify the patients with persistent or progressive disease earlier so that they can have additional testing or therapy.

The timing for ending cervical cancer screening is another controversial issue. Recommendations have been made to discontinue screening in women older than 70 years of age, provided that they have had at least three normal Pap smear results in the previous 10 years. Progression of cervical cancer precursors to invasive carcinoma is slow enough that the risk of developing an invasive cancer after normal smears this late in life is low enough to warrant discontinuation of screening. It should be noted that annual pelvic examination is still recommended to evaluate for new pelvic masses in women in this age group.

Women Older Than 30 Years of Age

A paradigm shift occurred in March 2003, when the FDA approved combination cytologic and HPV testing in all women older than 30 years, an age group in which screening rates are not significantly high. Some authors have proposed that combination testing should be discontinued after the age of 55 years, but current recommendations support continued combination testing for all women older than 30 years of age. Recommendations for cytologic screening are listed in Box 18-8.

The optimal use of HPV testing in women younger than 30 years of age has still not been elucidated. Identification of new high-risk groups based on age, personal history, and possibly additional molecular markers may help to clarify additional groups for whom HPV testing can be used. Until

Table 18-1

Natural History of Preinvasive Cervical Lesions

	Regress	Persist	Progression	
			CIN 3	Cancer
CIN 1	57%	32%	10%	1%
CIN 2	43%	35%	20%	5%
CIN 3	32%	56%	—	12%

> **Box 18-8** Cervical Cancer Screening Guidelines
>
> **Initiation of screening**
> Screening should begin 3 years after first coitus, but no later than the age of 21 years.
> Screening should be performed yearly in women screened only with cytology.
> Women aged 30 years or older should be screened with cytology and HPV testing.
>
> **Screening intervals**
> Women younger than 30 years of age should be screened annually.
> Women aged 30 years and older who are screened with cytology alone and have had three consecutive negative Pap smear results can be screened every 2 to 3 years if they have never had CIN 2 or 3, are not immunocompromised, and were not exposed to diethylstilbestrol *in utero*.
> Women aged 30 years and older undergoing screening with cytology and HPV testing can be screened every 3 years if both test results are negative.
>
> **Discontinuation of screening**
> Women who have undergone hysterectomy and never had CIN 2 or 3 may discontinue annual screening after three consecutive negative Pap smear results are obtained after hysterectomy.
> Women aged 70 years and older who are at low risk may discontinue screening if they have had three negative Pap smear results in the preceding 10 years.

then, HPV testing in women younger than 30 years of age should be reserved as a triage tool for patients with Pap smears indicating the presence of ASC, for follow-up of patients undergoing therapeutic procedures for severe dysplasia, or to identify women with persistence of CIN 1 or 2 requiring additional follow-up.

EVALUATION TECHNIQUES

Visual Inspection with Acetic Acid

Cervical cancer is a major burden to women's health in developing countries. The limited impact of cytology-based cervical cancer screening programs in low-resource settings is now widely recognized. In a policy statement issued by the American College of Obstetricians and Gynecologists, a "single-visit approach" incorporating visual inspection of the cervix with acetic acid (VIA) followed by immediate treatment was considered an acceptable and cost-effective strategy for cervical cancer prevention in low-resource settings. VIA is a simple test that can be performed with the naked eye. During VIA, the health care provider places a vaginal speculum into the vagina and applies dilute (3% to 5%) acetic acid to the cervix. Abnormal tissue temporarily appears white when exposed to acetic acid. The test result is negative if no or only faint acetowhite lesions appear (Fig. 18-7). The test result is interpreted as positive if sharp, distinct, well-defined acetowhite areas with or without raised margins appear with application of acetic acid. A lesion suspicious for

Figure 18-7

Visual inspection with acetic acid—normal cervix.

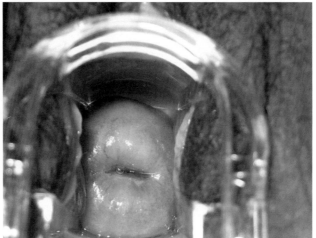

448

cancer will appear as an ulcerative, cauliflower-like growth or as a friable ulcer that bleeds when touched.

Cervicography

Cervicography involves obtaining and evaluating a photographic image of the cervix. The projected photographic image of the cervix simulates colposcopic magnification of approximately 16 times. Studies have shown that the sensitivity and specificity of cervicography for the detection of CIN 2 or 3 range from 54.5% to 90.0% and from 30.0% to 90.2%, respectively. Studies have shown that the sensitivity of conventional cytology smear is low (30% to 87%), and that the addition of cervicography and HPV testing as adjunctive methods improve the detection of cervical disease.

Optical Biopsy Diagnosis

Many components of comprehensive screening and treatment programs practiced in industrialized nations are not feasible for most developing countries. Moreover, an optimal strategy for one particular setting may vary from another due to differences in disease prevalence, health care infrastructure, human and financial resources, and local customs. With this is mind, a noninvasive "optical biopsy," which could provide a point-of-service diagnosis, would be ideal. High-resolution imaging can be obtained with various biophotonic methods such as fluorescence spectroscopy, surface analysis, confocal imaging, and optical coherence tomography, among others. These modalities are based on light-tissue interactions and data processing methods to provide information on morphologic, chemical, and light-scattering changes detected during early tumorigenesis (Fig. 18-8).

Colposcopy

Colposcopy, introduced by Hinselmann in 1925, is part of the standard of care for the proper evaluation of women with abnormal Pap smear results

Figure 18-8

Optical coherence tomography. Left, Normal cervix. Right, Invasive squamous cell carcinoma of the cervix. EP, Epithelium; BM, basement membrane; ST, stroma.

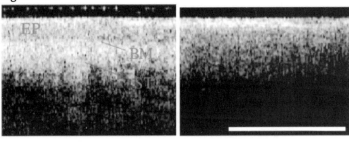

Normal cervix   Invasive cancer

in the United States. A colposcope is a dissecting microscope with various magnification lenses used to examine the cervix, vagina, and vulva. The improved visualization provided by the colposcope allows differentiation of normal and abnormal areas. It also allows accurate biopsies, complete evaluation of the extent of disease, and treatment of abnormal epithelial surface areas. Colposcopy is cost-effective and allows selective rather than routine treatment of precancerous lesions.

The colposcope provides the physician with a low-power setting for a wide view of the entire area and high magnification for diagnosis and aid in biopsy or treatment of precancerous lesions. Binocular viewing is usually done at $13.5\times$ magnification. The intraocular distance can be adjusted before the procedure is begun. Interchangeable magnifications are usually available at $10\times$ and $18\times$. Most colposcopes have working distances of 250 to 350 mm. Complete video, digital camera, and CO_2 surgical laser systems can be easily attached through ocular eyepiece tubes for patient identification, documentation, and treatment. The colposcope also includes a built-in green filter for clear visualization of vascular patterns.

General indications for colposcopy include abnormal screening, positive high-risk HPV DNA in ASC-US triage or HPV test results positive in standard algorithms, suspicious cervical lesions, positive screening results by cervicography or VIA, and history of *in utero* diethylstilbestrol exposure. Contraindications include active or untreated infections, especially sexually transmitted diseases.

Before the examination, the health care provider should obtain a detailed history including allergy to iodine and pregnancy status. The examination is carried out by fully exposing and cleansing the cervix. The initial part of the examination is performed under low power (8 to $10\times$). If a Pap smear is necessary at the time of the colposcopy, it should be obtained at the beginning of the examination. Under low-power magnification, the cervix and vagina are carefully examined with and without the green filter; any discrete, abnormal vascular patterns should be noted at this time. A 3% to 5% solution of acetic acid is applied with a cotton swab to the cervix and upper vagina. The examiner should wait at least 1 to 2 minutes after the acetic acid application before proceeding.

Visual criteria or patterns for identifying atypical areas in the transformation zone that require biopsy include white areas with punctuation (stippling), sharp-bordered lesions with vascular mosaic patterns, acetowhite lesions with sharp borders, or atypical vessels (Table 18-2). There are a variety of instruments that can aid in the inspection of the endocervix, such as narrow and wide specula and skin (iris) hooks. If needed, endocervical curettage can be performed with a Kevorkian curette. This allows histologic evaluation of the endocervical canal. Instruments useful in the performance of colposcopy are displayed in Figure 18-9.

The results are recorded using the standard terminology and form from the American Society for Colposcopy and Cervical Pathology. It is important to strictly document detailed findings. Colposcopy is considered

Visual Patterns on Colposcopy

Table 18-2

Finding	Colposcopic Appearance	Significance
1. Leukoplakia	Thickened white epithelium before acetic acid application, flat, without associated vascular pattern	Usually benign
2. Mosaic	Vascular/capillaries forming a "chicken wire" mosaic pattern	May be normal, but possible neoplasia; caliber and vessel characteristic important
3. Punctation	Red spots associated with AWE mosaic pattern	Inflammation, repair, possible neoplasia
4. Atypical Vessels	Horizontally oriented, non-branching vessels with varied caliber	Seen in cancer and immature metaplasia

AWE, Acetowhite epithelium. May be thin or thick. Thin lesions may be metaplasia or low-grade lesions. Thicker lesions may be moderate or severe dysplasia.

Figure 18-9

Colposcopy instruments and supplies.

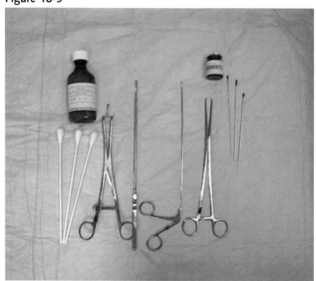

"satisfactory" if (1) 360 degrees of the SCJ is visualized, (2) the entire index lesion is visualized, and (3) cytology, colposcopic impression, and histology are correlated. If biopsy specimens are required, a variety of biopsy forceps of different sizes are available. Figures 18-10, 18-11, and 18-12 display the colposcopic appearance of LSIL, HSIL, and invasive squamous cell carcinoma of the cervix, respectively.

TREATMENT OF INTRAEPITHELIAL LESIONS

Comprehensive screening and treatment programs have led to a dramatic reduction in the incidence of cervical cancer deaths. In the last decade, substantial progress has been made in understanding the origin and path-

451

Figure 18-10

Colposcopy—low-grade squamous intraepithelial lesion.

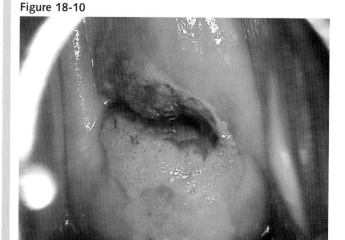

Figure 18-11

Colposcopy—high-grade squamous intraepithelial lesion.

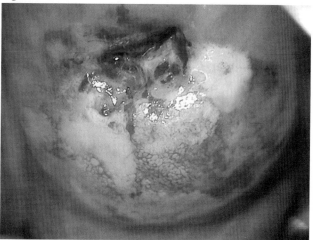

Figure 18-12

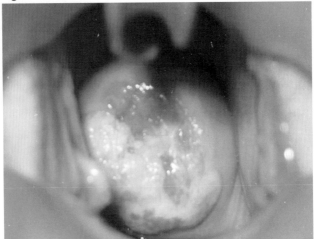

ogenesis of cervical intraepithelial lesions and neoplasia. Several prospective randomized studies provide data concerning different modalities of treatment for intraepithelial lesions as well as the risk of no treatment and/or observation. Overall, cryosurgery, laser vaporization, and LEEP appear to be equally effective for treating premalignant lesions of the cervix (Table 18-3).

Cryosurgery

The proper management of premalignant lesions of the cervix is an important and integral part of any screening program. Understanding the risk of progression to malignant disease is important when making treatment recommendations. Cryosurgery is used to treat several types of cancer and some precancerous or noncancerous conditions. The technology is based on the use of extremely cold temperatures produced by liquid nitrogen (or argon gas) to destroy abnormal tissue (i.e., cryonecrosis). Candidates for cryotherapy of the cervix include patients in whom satisfactory colposcopic examination has been obtained, the lesion has been identified and fully visualized, invasive carcinoma has been ruled out by biopsy, and endocervical curettage has yielded negative results.

Table 18-3

Treatment of
Intraepithelial Lesions

Modality	Diagnosis	Patients (N)	Relapse/Failure Rate (%)	Overall Cure Rate (%)
Cryosurgery	CIN 1	1010	11.5	96.5
	CIN 2/3	1828	*	92.3
Laser	CIN 1	4438	7.7	97.2
	CIN 3	99	9	100
LEEP	CIN 2/3	790	7–9	97–98

*Not stated.
CIN, Cervical intraepithelial neoplasia; LEEP, loop electrosurgical excision procedure.

The procedure is performed in an office setting and requires a cold source—usually liquid nitrous oxide—and cryoprobes of different sizes. The depth and adequacy of the cryonecrosis depends on the type and size of the cryoprobe and the duration and technique of treatment. Generally, a "freeze-thaw-freeze" technique is recommended. In this technique, the index lesion is frozen for a period of several minutes, thawed completely, and then frozen again. Because of the minimally invasive nature of the procedure, complications such as infection and bleeding rarely occur. A common adverse effect of the procedure is cramping and profuse watery discharge (i.e., hydrorrhea).

Laser Vaporization

Laser is an acronym for "light amplification by stimulated emission of radiation." A wide variety of lasers have been developed for medical applications. Lasers can be classified according to their active medium: gas, liquid, or solid. This medium is excited by either an electric current such as direct current or radiofrequency. In gynecologic surgery, the CO_2 laser is the most versatile. Two advantages of laser vaporization for premalignant lesions of the cervix are the increased precision and the decreased thermal damage of the specimen.

Laser vaporization is accomplished with an operative microscope or colposcope fitted with a micromanipulator. The procedure is performed in the outpatient setting and requires a smoke-evacuating system, anodized metal speculums and instruments, and safety goggles. For laser vaporization of the cervix, a laser spot size of 1.5 to 2 mm is required. The usual setting is 15 to 20 W in super-pulse mode with either the micromanipulator or the handheld collimator. The index lesion or area is outlined and a "rapid beam movement" technique is used to reduce thermal tissue conductivity and scarring.

Laser treatment of CIN can achieve both ablative and excisional therapy. The procedure has low morbidity and cure rates ranging from 94% to 98%. The major disadvantages are the need to be trained in laser surgery and the cost of the equipment.

Loop Electrosurgical Excision Procedure

Originally introduced in the United Kingdom as large-loop excision of the transformation zone, LEEP became a popular treatment modality in the United States in the 1990s. Unlike electrocautery or electrocoagulation diathermy, LEEP allows removal or excision of the index lesion rather than destruction, with less bleeding and stenosis. It is performed in an outpatient setting with local anesthetic and has the potential for diagnosis and treatment during a single visit to the office (Box 18-9).

The procedure is usually performed using colposcopic guidance. After the index lesion is identified, the loop-electrode can be tailored to the size and spread of the lesion (Fig. 18-13). Complications such as bleeding and infections are minimal with the LEEP procedure. However, the use of extremely large loop-electrodes for cervical lesions on a flattened ("flush"), scarred cervix may increase the risk of injury to the bladder and rectum. One major advantage of the LEEP procedure is the ability to use colposcopy

453

Box 18-9 Indications for Loop electrosurgical excision procedure or Cold-Knife Conization

1. Discrepancy between Pap smear and directed biopsy results
2. Unsatisfactory colposcopy
3. Abnormal endocervical curettage
4. Biopsy with microinvasive cancer

Figure 18-13

Loop electrosurgical excision procedure— loop sizes.

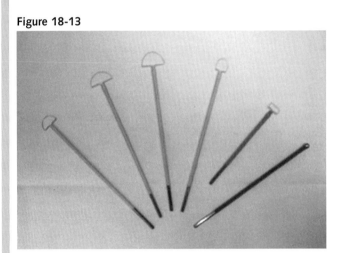

to visualize the lesion during excision and to assess the adequacy of the treatment.

Cold-Knife Conization

The indications for cold-knife conization are similar to those of LEEP (*see* Box 18-9). In cold-knife conization, the index lesion is identified intraoperatively with a colposcope and acetic acid. The lesion is excised with a scalpel and is then properly oriented and marked with a suture to help the pathologist specify the location of any lesions. Monsel's solution (ferrous subsulfate), hemostatic sutures at 3 and 9 o'clock, and Sturmdorf sutures can be used to achieve hemostasis. The major disadvantage of this treatment modality is the requirement of general or regional anesthetic. Cold-knife conization has been mostly replaced by methods discussed previously in this section.

Hysterectomy

Historically, hysterectomy has been the treatment used by American gynecologists for high-grade dysplasia. The trend over the past decade has been to move away from radical treatments such as hysterectomy to more conservative outpatient treatments such cryosurgery and LEEP. The treatment of choice for early microinvasive disease (International Federation of Gynecology and Obstetrics stage IA1) is hysterectomy. The

Figure 18-14

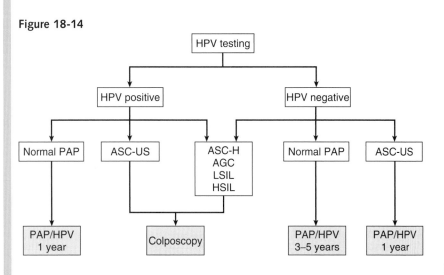

Algorithm for the incorporation of human papillomavirus (HPV) DNA testing into screening programs for women older than 30 years of age. PAP, Papanicolaou smear; ASC-US, atypical squamous cells of undetermined significance; ASC-H, atypical squamous cells that cannot exclude HSIL; AGC, atypical glandular cells; LSIL, low-grade squamous intraepithelial lesion; HSIL, high-grade squamous intraepithelial lesion. (Original work by authors, Pedro F. Escobar, Andres Chiesa-Voterro, and Chad M. Michener.)

Society of Gynecologic Oncologist established the definition of *microinvasion* in 1974 to be "invasion below the basement membrane less than 3 mm without lymphovascular space invasion." The most common indication for hysterectomy in the management of preinvasive cervical disease is in those patients with coexistent gynecologic conditions that warrant hysterectomy. Additionally, hysterectomy may be offered to women with persistent high-grade dysplasia who do not plan to bear (more) children.

CONCLUSIONS

In summary, new technologies have allowed physicians and researchers to develop new algorithms to improve the management of preinvasive cervical disease and to decrease the global burden of cervical cancer. An improved understanding of the natural history of HPV infection has allowed the development of a more conservative approach in younger women with preinvasive disease of the cervix. As science allows us to improve the way we identify and treat malignant precursors, we must continue to translate these changes into clinical practice. The addition of HPV testing to Pap smears for primary screening in women older than 30 years of age is only the latest addition to the clinician's armamentarium. Figure 18-14 gives an algorithm for incorporating HPV DNA screening into the care of women with potentially preinvasive diseases of the uterine cervix. The use of recombinant DNA preventive and therapeutic vaccines will revolutionize the way that we care for women with these diseases.

KEY POINTS

1. Approximately 50 million women are currently being screened with cervical cytology in the United States yearly. Two million atypical squamous cells of undetermined significance and atypical squamous cells that cannot exclude high-grade squamous intraepithelial lesion (HSIL), 1.25 million low-grade squamous intraepithelial lesion (LSIL), 300,000 HSIL, and 13,000 cancers are diagnosed.

2. The spectrum of squamous intraepithelial lesion is subdivided into two categories, LSIL and HSIL. There is a 10% to 15% interpathologist discrepancy rate between LSIL and HSIL. Cytology may also be discrepant with histology; 15% to 25% of women with LSIL are found to have histologic cervical intraepithelial neoplasia (CIN) 2 or CIN 3 upon further evaluation.

3. The precursor lesions of cervical squamous carcinoma are divided into three grades: CIN 1, 2, and 3. Maturation, nuclear abnormalities, and mitosis reach the upper third of the epithelium in CIN 3, the middle third in CIN 2, and the lower third in CIN 1.

4. "Atypical endocervical, endometrial, or glandular cells" defines an increased level of risk, as opposed to a specific neoplastic precursor entity. Follow-up of atypical glandular cytologic interpretations shows that high-grade lesions are identified in 10% to 40% of cases and are most often squamous (CIN 2 or 3).

5. Adenocarcinoma *in situ* is associated with CIN in at least 50% of cases.

6. The Hybrid Capture® II system detects the presence of 13 types of HPV that have been associated with cervical cancer and has been approved for ancillary testing for the management of atypical squamous cells and for primary screening in conjunction with cytology among women 30 years of age and older.

7. Up to 70% of cases of CIN 1 and up to 50% of CIN 2 will regress without treatment.

8. A "single-visit approach," incorporating visual inspection of the cervix with acetic acid followed by immediate treatment, is considered an acceptable and cost-effective strategy for cervical cancer prevention.

9. Colposcopy allows accurate biopsies, complete evaluation of the extent of disease, and treatment of abnormal epithelial surface areas.

10. Overall, cryosurgery, laser vaporization, and loop electrosurgical excision are equally effective for treating premalignant lesions of the cervix.

11. Recombinant DNA technologies have allowed the development of promising new polyvalent preventive and therapeutic vaccines directed against various HPV types.

SUGGESTED READING

Alvarez RD, Helm CW, Edwards RP, et al: Prospective randomized trial of LLETZ versus laser ablation in patients with cervical intraepithelial neoplasia. Gynecol Oncol 52(2):175–179, 1994.

Drezek RA, Richards-Kortum R, Brewer MA, et al: Optical imaging of the cervix. Cancer 8(9 Suppl): 2015–2027, 2003.

Follen M, Meyskens FL Jr, Alvarez RD, et al: Cervical cancer chemoprevention, vaccines, and surrogate endpoint biomarkers. Cancer 8(9 Suppl):2044–2051, 2003.

Kulasingam SL, Hughes JP, Kiviat NB, et al: Evaluation of human papillomavirus testing in primary screening for cervical abnormalities: Comparison of sensitivity, specificity, and frequency of referral. JAMA 288 (14):1749–1757, 2002.

Kulasingam SL, Myers ER: Potential health and economic impact of adding a human papillomavirus vaccine to screening programs. JAMA 290(6):781–789, 2003.

Manos MM, Kinney WK, Hurley LB, et al: Identifying women with cervical neoplasia: Using human papillomavirus DNA testing for equivocal Papanicolaou results. JAMA 281(17):1605–1610, 1999.

Orr JW Jr: Cervical cancer. Surg Oncol Clin N Am 7(2):299–316, 1998.

Slaslow D, Runowicz CD, Solomon D, et al: American Cancer Society Guideline for the Early Detection of Cervical Neoplasia and Cancer. CA Journal [AIS 1] 52:342–362, 2002.

Solomon D, Davey D, Kurman R, et al: The 2001 Bethesda System: Terminology for reporting results of cervical cytology. JAMA 287:2114–2119, 2002.

Solomon D, Nayar R (eds): The Bethesda System for Reporting Cervical Cytology: Definitions, Criteria, and Explanatory Notes. New York, Springer-Verlag, 2004.

Villa LL, Costa RL, Petta CA, et al: Prophylactic quadrivalent human papillomavirus (types 6, 11, 16, and 18) L1 virus-like particle vaccine in young women: A randomised double-blind placebo-controlled multicentre phase II efficacy trial. Lancet Oncol 6(5):271–278, 2005.

Villa LL, Ault KA, Giuliano AR, et al: Immunologic responses following administration of a vaccine targeting human papillomavirus types 6, 11, 16, and 18. Vaccine 24(27–28):5571–5583, 2006.

Waggoner SE: Cervical cancer. Lancet 361:2217–2225, 2003.

Wright TC, Cox JT, Massad LS, et al: 2001 consensus guidelines for the management of women with cervical cytological abnormalities. JAMA 287:2120–2129, 2002.

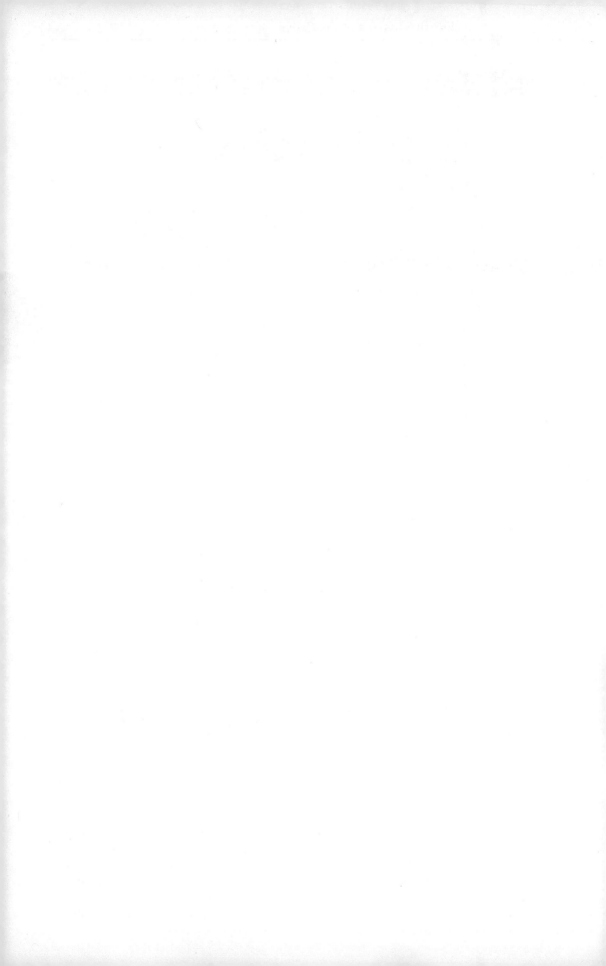

19

LEIOMYOMAS

Linda D. Bradley

INTRODUCTION

Leiomyomas, often referred to as *myomas* or *fibroids,* are the most common benign tumors of the female pelvis. They are composed of benign monoclonal tumors of smooth muscle cells with extracellular collagen and elastin. Each leiomyoma is encased within a noninfiltrating pseudocapsule of connective tissue. Fibroids may be single but are most often multiple, and their sizes range from microscopic to massive. Leiomyomas are classified into subgroups based on their location within the layers of the uterus. Myomas are classified as intramural (within the myometrium), subserosal (found just below the uterine serosa), or submucosal (located just beneath the endometrium) (Fig. 19-1). They may also extend into the broad ligament or become parasitic if they outgrow their blood supply and seek a secondary blood supply by attaching to another organ (such as the omentum).

The pathophysiology of uterine fibroids is poorly understood. Several studies suggest that fibroids arise from a single neoplastic cell within the myometrium. Likely influential factors include genetic predisposition, steroid hormones, vascular abnormalities, and growth factors including platelet-derived growth factors, heparin-binding epithelial growth factors, hepatoma-derived growth factors, and basic fibroblast growth factors.

The reproductive life cycle influences the prevalence and symptomatology of fibroids. For instance, leiomyomas have not been detected in prepubertal girls; however, symptoms heighten during the third and fourth decade of life and usually resolve during menopause. Hormonal responsiveness has been detected *in vitro,* and fibroids have the potential to expand during pregnancy and regress after menopause. Fibroids that begin to grow and develop after menopause should be quickly evaluated and surgically treated due to a higher risk of malignant (sarcomatous) changes.

Prevalence of the disease varies by ethnicity, age, and other factors. Using vaginal probe ultrasonography, 62% of premenopausal women were noted to have occult fibroids. Among Japanese women, fibroids were detected in 10.1% of patients and in 5.4% of Swedish women. African American women have the highest prevalence of fibroids, detection at earlier age, larger and more numerous fibroids, earlier symptomatic presentation, and a higher rate of hysterectomy because of fibroid-related symptoms. Among specimens from women undergoing hysterectomy for any cause, fibroids can be

Figure 19-1

Fibroid types classified by location within the uterine wall. **A,** Intramural and submucosal. **B,** Subserosal. **C** and **D,** Submucosal.

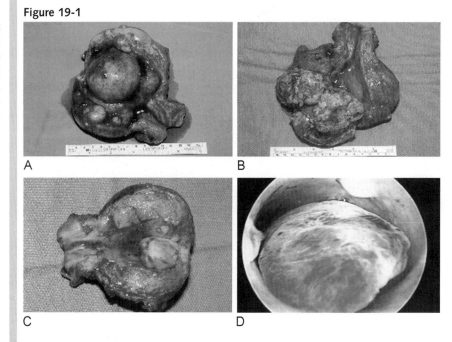

A

B

C

D

detected in 80%. As many as 40% of women have evidence of myomas at autopsy.

CLINICAL MANIFESTATIONS

Most women with fibroids are asymptomatic and require no therapy. Generally, patients who seek medical evaluation have a uterine size of greater than 8 to 10 weeks' gestational size, submucosal fibroids, or an individual fibroid that is greater than 4 cm in diameter. Symptoms classically associated with uterine fibroids include menorrhagia, bulk symptoms, and reproductive dysfunction.

The most common symptom of uterine myomas is abnormal uterine bleeding, with menorrhagia and hypermenorrhea being the classic complaints. The patient typically experiences menses that are predictable but excessively heavy with associated flooding, gushing, clotting, and dysmenorrhea. Evidence suggests that bleeding worsens as uterine size increases. Personal, medical, and financial factors may be adversely affected due to symptomatic fibroids. Social embarrassment, inability to work, alteration of lifestyle, and avoidance of sexual function may be hallmarks of the disease. Iron-deficiency anemia and fatigue are common. Some patients complain of intermittent or chronic watery vaginal discharge, irregular bleeding throughout the month, or postcoital bleeding. The mechanism for abnormal uterine bleeding is poorly elucidated. Theories for the etiology of abnormal uterine bleeding as a result of fibroids are outlined in Box 19-1.

> **Box 19-1** Theories Regarding Origin of Abnormal Uterine Bleeding Secondary to Fibroids
>
> Ulceration over the surface of the fibroid
> Increased surface area of uterine cavity due to intramucosal or submucosal fibroids
> Abnormalities in local venous drainage (congestion and dilation of venous plexus) contributing to venular ectasia
> Increased vascularity of uterus
> Variability in prostaglandin production
> Platelet dysfunction
> Normal uterine contractions are inhibited; decreased expulsion of uterine contractions occurs
> Impaired endometrial hemostasis
> Microscopic or macroscopic abnormalities of the uterine vasculature (more expandable venules)

Additional symptoms, collectively called *bulk symptoms*, include pelvic pressure sometimes radiating to thighs, lower extremities, and the back. Unlike the symmetric enlargement of a pregnant uterus, an irregularly shaped uterus may put pressure on adjacent organs leading to myriad symptoms. The bladder is the most common pelvic viscera involved with anterior and lower uterine fibroids. Urinary frequency, nocturia, and less commonly, urinary retention may occur. Ureteral obstruction, hydronephrosis, and subsequent kidney failure are extremely rare. The bowels are less commonly affected, but constipation, rectal pain, and difficult defection may be encountered. Many patients have worsening bowel symptoms perimenstrually. Dyspareunia, pelvic pain, and infertility may also be involved with uterine fibroids.

Leiomyomata occasionally rapidly enlarge during pregnancy and undergo central avascular necrosis (i.e., red degeneration), resulting in extreme abdominal pain requiring narcotics. Additionally, isolated case reports of sudden hemoperitoneum resulting from spontaneous rupture of a superficial vein coursing over the surface of a subserosal fibroid have been reported. When this occurs, the patient may experience sudden onset of nausea, abdominal pain, hemodynamic instability, and free intraperitoneal blood detected, which can be detected by computed tomography (CT) scan or abdominal ultrasound. Emergent myomectomy (if fertility is desired) or hysterectomy is indicated to treat this rare condition.

EFFECTS ON REPRODUCTIVE FUNCTION

The impact of fibroids on pregnancy and infertility is poorly understood. Luckily, most women with fibroids do not have reproductive problems. However, fibroids have been associated with premature labor and delivery, malpresentation of the fetus, obstructed delivery, postpartum uterine bleeding, more complicated cesarean sections, and early pregnancy-related bleeding. The location of uterine fibroids plays an important role in patients with infertility. Large submucosal fibroids obstructing the endometrial cavity can be associated with poor placentation, poor sperm migration, and blockage of the fallopian tubes. Likewise, intramural fibroids may impinge on the fallopian tubes or distort the endometrial cavity, making pregnancy more difficult. It is important that women experiencing recurrent miscarriages or infertility undergo a thorough evaluation. The effect of fibroids on fertility is discussed in more detail in Chapter 12, Infertility: Evaluation and Treatment.

DIAGNOSIS

History

A detailed history and thorough physical examination should be performed when evaluating a patient for fibroids. If possible, it is helpful to obtain prior medical records, ultrasound reports, and laboratory test results. This information is important to determine rate of fibroid growth and prior symptomatology. If prior surgical procedures have been performed, operative and pathology reports are essential. Patient consent to obtain these records should be sought at the first consultation.

Some patients keep detailed notes or diaries of their menstrual cycles. Use of these menstrual diaries is useful for determining the pattern of bleeding. If monthly diaries are not available, detailed questions about the menstrual cycle and bleeding pattern should be asked. Directed questions regarding the characteristics of the menstrual pattern include frequency, duration, amount of bleeding, flooding, clotting, nighttime changing, embarrassment, and the need to miss scheduled activities. In addition, specific questions should be asked regarding the number of pads or tampons used daily, and if clothing, bedding, or furniture becomes soiled during menstruation. It is important to determine whether sanitary products are saturated at the time of changing because women may change more frequently for hygienic reasons or because of concern about toxic shock syndrome. A list of questions regarding the characteristics of menstrual bleeding is displayed in Box 19-2. Validated questionnaires that measure fibroid symptoms and their impact on quality of life have been developed and are easily administered in an office setting.

Physical Examination

The physical examination should be complete and include inspection of the eyes, hands, and soles of feet for signs of pallor or anemia; palpation of the thyroid gland for nodularity; and inspection of the skin for petechiae, pallor, bruising, or hirsutism. The abdomen should be examined for hepatomegaly, splenomegaly, abdominal, or pelvic masses. The pelvic examination should focus on the presence of vulvar, vaginal, or cervical lesions or foreign bodies that could account for abnormal bleeding. If an abnormal discharge is visible, microscopic examination is essential. A bimanual examination determines the size and contour of the uterus as

Box 19-2	Questions Regarding the Characteristics of the Menstrual Pattern

When did the abnormal uterine bleeding begin?
Do you keep a monthly menstrual diary?
If not, recommend starting menstrual diaries.
Do you have regular menstrual cycles?
What is the number of days of bleeding?
How many total days of bleeding do you have monthly?
Do you have premenstrual spotting or postmenstrual spotting?
What is different about your cycles now?
Do you have menstrual cramping?
When do your cramps begin?
Before bleeding, when passing large blood clots, or throughout the whole period?
Do you have any cravings (i.e., pica)?
For example, ice, starch, dirt, clay, or chalk?
Do you have any other bleeding abnormalities?
Epistaxis?
Easy bruising?
Difficulty in stopping bleeding after small cuts or abrasions?
What medications are you taking?
Blood thinners?
Soy products, red clover, ginseng?
Hormonal preparations?
Oral contraceptive pills?
Depo Provera?
Depo Lupron?
Progesterone IUDs?
Have you ever had any sexually transmitted infections or vaginal infections?
Endometritis or cervicitis?
Trichomoniasis, chlamydia, gonorrhea?

IUD, Intrauterine device.

well as the presence of adnexal or rectal masses. Particular attention should be given to this portion of the examination because much information can be gained regarding uterine contour, bulkiness, or the presence of uterine tenderness.

Diagnostic Studies

Most leiomyomata can be diagnosed clinically and are discovered during routine pelvic examination (if asymptomatic) or during focused evaluation for menorrhagia, dysmenorrhea, or pelvic pressure. The uterus is typically enlarged and has an irregular contour. A number of modalities are available to distinguish symptomatic myomas from other pelvic masses. It is important to note that the presence of leiomyomata does not exclude other pathology, and efforts should be made to thoroughly investigate complaints of abnormal bleeding, pelvic pain, or pelvic pressure.

Ultrasonography

Leiomyomata should be distinguished from other pelvic masses with increased potential for malignancy, such as ovarian tumors. This is usually easily accomplished with transvaginal or abdominal ultrasonography because fibroids appear solid by ultrasound and are usually easily differentiated from adnexal structures. Ultrasound criteria for uterine leiomyomas include uterine enlargement, nodular uterine contour, lack of homogeneity of the myometrium, and focal mass within the myometrium (Fig. 19-2). Most leiomyomas are hypoechoic or heterogeneous compared with normal myometrium, and calcifications may cause posterior shadowing. Degenerating fibroids often appear cystic. If color Doppler imaging is used, marked peripheral and decreased central flow or an avascular core on color Doppler imaging may be noted. Occasionally, other imaging modalities such as CT or magnetic resonance imaging (MRI) are useful, but these techniques are expensive and rarely give more information than is available from simple office ultrasound.

Transvaginal ultrasonography (TVUS) offers improved image quality over abdominal ultrasound for the evaluation of the endometrium. During TVUS, saline can be injected into the endometrial cavity (saline infusion sonography [SIS]) to further delineate submucosal and intracavitary lesions. Saline injected intracervically not only enhances the view of the endometrium and myometrium but also provides an acoustic view that allows for three-dimensional investigation of the uterine cavity and ovaries (Figs. 19-3, 19-4, and 19-5). SIS improves the sensitivity and specificity of TVUS for the detection of endometrial lesions; studies of SIS reveal overall sensitivity of 94% (range, 83% to 100%) and specificity of 85% (range, 72% to 99%) for the detection of endometrial lesions in premenopausal women. Detection of submucosal fibroids has even greater sensitivity (94%; range, 91% to 100%) and specificity (95%; range, 88% to 100%) than TVUS alone.

TVUS and SIS help to determine whether further evaluation with endometrial biopsy or hysteroscopy is needed. They also help to determine the size, location, depth of myometrial penetration, and number of uterine fibroids. This information is useful in planning treatment and helps to determine the hysteroscopic resectability of submucosal fibroids.

Figure 19-2

Transvaginal ultrasound demonstrating a posterior intramural fibroid abutting the endometrium.

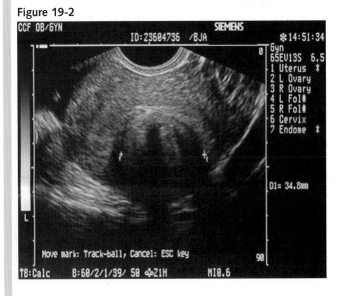

Figure 19-3

Transvaginal ultrasound demonstrating endometrial polyps.

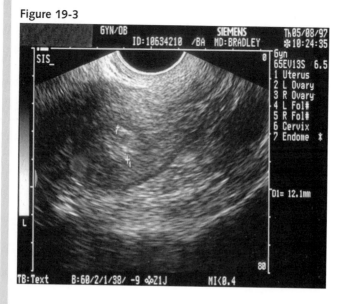

Figure 19-4

Saline infusion sonography demonstrating three endometrial polyps.

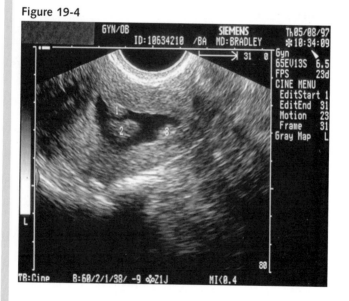

Magnetic Resonance Imaging

MRI is less operator dependent and has greater reproducibility than TVUS. MRI is less able to detect endometrial polyps, but it is more accurate than TVUS and hysteroscopy in the evaluation of exact submucous myoma ingrowth. Additionally, size, number and location of uterine fibroids are better characterized with MRI than ultrasound (Fig. 19-6). Measurements of uterine fibroids are more precise and less subject to inter-rater variability than ultrasound. Adenomyosis—a condition that mimics uterine fibroids, causing diffuse enlargement, tenderness, and bulkiness of the uterus—is best diagnosed with MRI. The disadvantages of MRI include higher costs and limited availability. MRI is contraindicated in women with claustrophobia, pacemakers, defibrillators, or metallic foreign bodies.

Figure 19-5

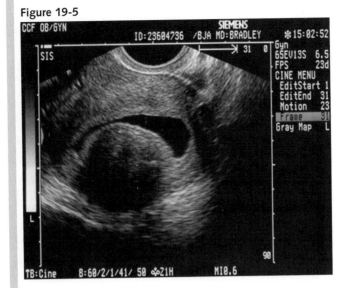

Saline infusion sonography demonstrating a posterior intramural fibroid abutting the endometrium.

Figure 19-6

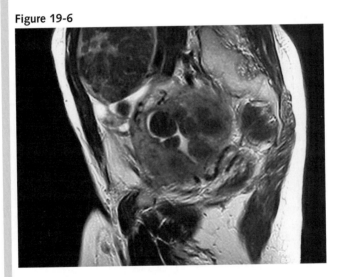

Magnetic resonance image demonstrating two submucosal and multiple intramural fibroids.

Hysterosalpingography

Hysterosalpingography (HSG) involves the transcervical injection of contrast material into the uterine cavity during radiographic imaging (Fig. 19-7). This technique can identify intracavitary lesions and establish tubal patency in cases of infertility. The limitations of HSG include pelvic irradiation and iodinated contrast medium, patient discomfort, and lack of specificity compared with hysteroscopy. Additionally, there is considerable variability in the interpretation and clinical management of patients with abnormal HSG results.

Hysteroscopy

Hysteroscopy has revolutionized the practice of office gynecology. Improved optics and reductions in hysteroscopic diameters have enabled

Figure 19-7

Hysterosalpingogram.

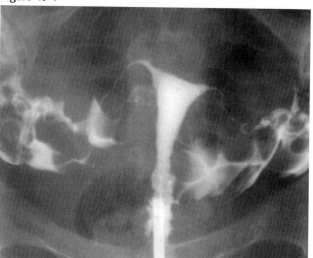

the development of thin operative hysteroscopes with outer diameters ranging from 3 to 5 mm, which can be used comfortably in an office setting.

The advantages of hysteroscopic visualization include immediate office evaluation, direct visualization of the endometrium and endocervix, the ability to detect minute focal endometrial pathology, and the ability to perform directed endometrial biopsies. Traditional "blind" methods of endometrial evaluation (e.g., dilation and curettage, endometrial biopsy) are inadequate for the diagnosis of submucosal fibroids and focal intracavitary lesions; hysteroscopy is particularly useful for identifying focal lesions, which are often missed with endometrial sampling. Hysteroscopy is gaining acceptance as the gold standard for the evaluation of the uterine cavity and the treatment of intracavitary lesions.

Lesions that can be visualized hysteroscopically include submucosal and intramural fibroids, endometrial polyps, synechiae, retained products of conception, foreign bodies, endocervical lesions, endometrial atrophy, endometrial hyperplasia, endometrial cancer, arteriovenous malformations, gestational trophoblastic disease, and pregnancy (Figs. 19-8, 19-9, and 19-10). Infrequently, endometrial gland openings associated with adenomyosis can be seen. Hysteroscopy has a low a false-negative rate (2% to 4%) for detecting endometrial lesions.

Determination of lesion size is not as accurate with hysteroscopy as with TVUS. The eyepiece is focused at infinity, making closer objects appear magnified and further objects appear smaller. This phenomenon can lead to surprises in the operating room, especially when the size of a lesion (particularly submucosal fibroids) is underestimated.

A number of distension media are available for hysteroscopy. Diagnostic hysteroscopic procedures are often performed with carbon dioxide (CO_2) or normal saline. The choice between CO_2 and fluid medium for diagnostic

Figure 19-8

Office hysteroscopy demonstrating a submucosal fibroid.

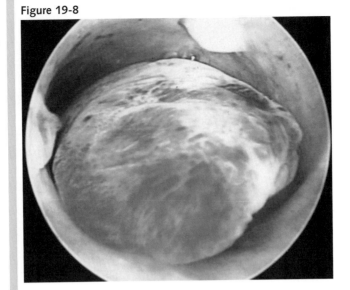

Figure 19-9

Office hysteroscopy demonstrating endometrial polyps.

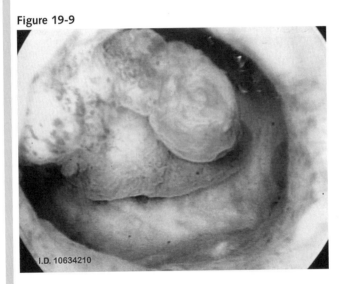

Figure 19-10

Office hysteroscopy demonstrating a hemorrhagic polyp.

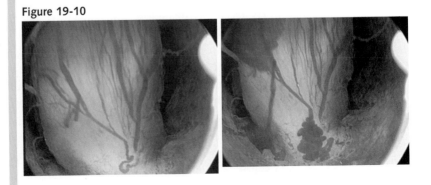

hysteroscopy often is determined by physician preference and the presence of uterine bleeding. Many gynecologists prefer CO_2 for its optical clarity, less mess, and patient comfort during insufflation. Operative procedures should never be performed with CO_2 because of the risk of CO_2 embolism when open venous channels and vascular endometrium are exposed with loop resectoscopy.

Office hysteroscopy is comfortable, quick, and associated with low complication rates. Preprocedural nonsteroidal agents or misoprostol can make the procedure more tolerable, especially in women at risk for cervical stenosis. A low (<1%) complication rate is noted when performed by skilled physicians. Complications include uterine perforation, infections, excessive bleeding, and complications related to the distending medium. These complications are discussed in greater detail in Chapter 30, Endoscopic Approaches to Gynecologic Disease.

The disadvantages of office hysteroscopy include the need for expensive office equipment (e.g., camera, insufflator, hysteroscope, and video equipment), low reimbursement for office procedures, and the cost of the procedure. Despite these disadvantages, hysteroscopy is essential in helping to evaluate patients with an indeterminate or equivocal result from SIS.

469

TREATMENT

Medical Treatments

Treatment of uterine fibroids is generally only necessary when they are symptomatic and symptoms are unresponsive to medical therapies. Therapy is highly dependent on the number, size, location, desire for fertility, and symptoms associated with the fibroids. The closer the fibroids are to the endometrial cavity, the more likely they are to cause earlier symptoms and to require therapy at smaller sizes. Intracavitary, submucosal, and intramural fibroids are more likely to cause menorrhagia and dysmenorrhea, whereas subserosal or pedunculated fibroids may become very large before causing bulk symptoms.

Often, fibroids are present but the patient is asymptomatic. In these cases, patients can be reassured and managed expectantly. In rare cases, asymptomatic large fibroids or intracavitary fibroids can be removed to prevent anticipated problems during pregnancy, although this remains controversial.

Oral Contraceptive Pills and Nonsteroidal Anti-Inflammatory Agents
Mild dysmenorrhea and menorrhagia may be relieved by nonsteroidal anti-inflammatory agents and oral contraceptive pills (OCPs) after other causes of pain and bleeding have been excluded. Therapy should be aimed at the alleviation of specific symptoms. The mechanism of action of low-dose OCPs includes suppression of ovulation, decreased uterine contractions, stabilization of the endometrium, decreased prostaglandin levels, and reduction in menstrual blood flow. A trial of low-dose OCPs is often used in the setting of fibroid-related bleeding, dysmenorrhea, and pelvic pain.

Gonadotropin-Releasing Hormone Agonists

Continued use of a gonadotropin-releasing hormone agonist (GnRH) down-regulates hypothalamic-pituitary gland production and the release of follicle-stimulating and luteinizing hormone, causing a hypoestrogenic state. Additionally, decreased uterine artery blood flow, uterine vessel diameter, and fibroid size have been recorded in women receiving prolonged GnRH agonist therapy. A reduction in mean uterine volume of between 40% and 50% has been documented, with most size reduction occurring within the first 3 months of therapy. Continued GnRH therapy induces amenorrhea in the majority of patients.

For these reasons, GnRH therapy could be considered for late perimenopausal women with fibroid symptoms. Evidence exists that prolonged use of GnRH therapy with add-back estrogen and progesterone can protect against loss of bone density and provide relief of fibroid-related symptoms. Among women with high-risk factors for surgical fibroid therapy, GnRH therapy may provide relief of symptoms until menopause occurs. For anemic patients, combined GnRH therapy and iron are helpful in increasing hemoglobin levels. The addition of GnRH agonists to iron therapy has been shown to improve hemoglobin levels and to decrease transfusion rates more effectively than iron alone. Additionally, surgical route and incision type have been shown to be affected by GnRH therapy. In one study, women who experienced a decrease in uterine volume with GnRH therapy were more likely to have a transverse incision (versus a vertical incision) compared with women not treated with GnRH agonists.

GnRH therapy creates a hypoestrogenic menopausal-like condition. Cessation of menstruation usually occurs within 3 months of therapy. Menopausal symptoms including hot flashes, night sweats, vaginal dryness, bone loss, decreased concentration, and diminished libido may occur with therapy. Compliance is generally good despite these symptoms.

Osteoporosis is the biggest risk of prolonged therapy; therefore, treatment is limited to 6 months, unless estrogen "add-back" is instituted. This is a good option for late perimenopausal women who have significant contraindications for other medical or surgical therapies. Halting menses is a relief, and after therapy, many women spontaneously transition into menopause. Intermittent GnRH (Lupron Depot) therapy provides an average of 9 months of symptom control (range, 2 to 25 months).

Hyaline degeneration and focal necrosis occurs in 1% to 2% of patients being treated for fibroids with GnRH agonists, presumably due to intense vasoconstriction. This may be accompanied by low-grade temperature and fever. Vasospasm may also cause arteriolar sloughing and possible fibroid prolapse. Finally, degeneration may cause the distinct pseudocapsule surrounding the fibroid to be less distinct and more difficult to delineate at the time of surgery.

Surgical Treatments

If requirements for surgical therapy are met, it is important to determine the patient's wishes for future fertility, uterine preservation, and the probable time until menopause. It is also important to preoperatively identify the size, number, location, and depth of intramural extension of uterine fibroids when planning extirpative or hysteroscopic surgery.

Hysterectomy

Over 600,000 hysterectomies are performed annually in the United States, making it the second most common major abdominal operation. Leiomyomas account for 40% of the indications for hysterectomy. By the age of 60 years, almost one third of American women have had a hysterectomy, and the annual rate of hysterectomy was 5.6 per 1000 women in 1997. Inpatient costs exceeded $2 billion in 1997, with outpatient costs likely to be as high.

Historically, hysterectomy has been advocated for women with a uterus greater than 12 weeks' gestational size and in those with rapidly expanding fibroids; however, no data support this idea, and the number of hysterectomies for unjustified reasons is declining. The risk of leiomyosarcoma in women with fibroids is rare (2 to 3/1000). Even among women whose uterine size increases by more than 6 weeks' gestational size in 1 year (rapid growth), the risk of sarcoma is low and is no more common than in women whose uteruses did not enlarge. Unfortunately, no tumor markers or definitive radiographic procedures are available that have a high sensitivity for detecting leiomyosarcoma. For practical purposes, all leiomyomata in premenopausal women are considered benign, and they are considered rarely malignant in postmenopausal women. Therefore, we are still left with the dictum that rapid growth, menorrhagia, systemic symptoms, or weight loss are indications for hysterectomy.

In women who have completed childbearing, hysterectomy offers permanent relief from fibroid symptoms. Additionally, hysterectomy obviates the need for birth control. Multiple studies have demonstrated improved quality of life in those who undergo hysterectomy for fibroid-related symptoms.

Most hysterectomies in the United States are still performed via the abdominal route, followed in number by procedures via vaginal and laparoscopic routes. When performed abdominally and laparoscopically, the cervix is removed in 98% of cases. Vaginal hysterectomy has many distinct advantages over the abdominal approach including less cost, fewer days of hospitalization, less need for postoperative pain medications, quicker return to daily activities, fewer complications, and less operative time. Many factors contribute to the higher rates of the abdominal approach including obsolete guidelines, greater third-party compensation for abdominal surgery, lack of adequate training in vaginal surgery, presumption rather than a confirmation that pathology exists that contraindicates a vaginal approach, and misconceptions that the vaginal approach is less safe.

It is imperative that patients undergoing hysterectomy understand the indications, alternative options, route of surgery, and potential short-term and long-term complications. A decision should be reached by the patient as to whether she wants her ovaries retained or removed. Additionally, a decision should be reached by the patient to determine whether she wants her cervix retained or removed. The route of surgery is most often determined by the surgeon's clinical experience, his or her technical expertise, and potential pathology.

The decision to remove the ovaries should not be taken lightly, especially in women younger than 52 years of age who are still menstruating. If the patient is menstruating normally and has minimal vasomotor symptoms, low risk factors for ovarian cancer, and normal ovarian volume, ovarian conservation can be recommended. Women who are prematurely castrated suffer significantly from menopausal symptoms, ranging from vasomotor symptoms, increased risks of osteoporosis, decreased libido, vaginal dryness, and mood disturbances. Most quality-of-life parameters studied demonstrate an improvement in outcomes after hysterectomy, especially among women who have not been castrated. However, women with psychiatric comorbidities including personality disorders, severe psychosocial problems, and prior psychiatric illness are unlikely to improve after surgery. Also, women who have a strong desire for fertility, prolonged bereavement after previous loss and extreme desire for uterine preservation may have more psychological and emotional discord after hysterectomy. For these reasons, it is imperative to truly understand the patient's preference for surgical procedure and her desire for ovarian conservation, and to have an extensive discussion regarding the benefits and risks of proposed surgical procedure.

Abdominal Myomectomy

Abdominal myomectomy was described in 1845 by Dr. Atlee but did not gain widespread acceptance until the 1930s, when Victor Bonney reported his experience with more than 400 consecutive myomectomies. He is credited with the resurgence of myomectomy as a viable alternative to hysterectomy and with the development of the Bonney clamp, which decreased bleeding associated with myomectomy.

Generally, myomectomy is reserved for women who want to preserve fertility. The goal of myomectomy is to remove all identifiable fibroids with the least alteration to the reproductive tract. The procedure involves incising the myometrium, dissecting the myoma from the surrounding myometrium, and closing the defect in multiple layers with delayed-absorbable suture. This procedure can be completed by laparotomy or laparoscopy (Figs. 19-11 and 19-12).

Risks of abdominal myomectomy include infection, the need for transfusion, and uterine dehiscence during subsequent pregnancy. Women who have had extensive dissection of the uterine wall should be advised to undergo elective cesarean section to decrease the risk of uterine dehiscence, which has been estimated to be about 0.002%. Low-grade fevers are common in the immediate postoperative period in the absence of overt signs of infection. These fevers usually spontaneously resolve and are thought to result from the release of pyrogens or myometrial bleeding. After other causes of fever have been excluded, these patients may be expectantly managed and do not require antibiotics.

Figure 19-11

Abdominal myomectomy. A 6.5-cm submucosal fibroid is visible through the myometrial incision.

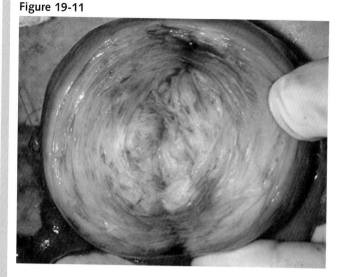

Figure 19-12

Abdominal myomectomy after enucleation of a 6.5-cm submucosal fibroid through the myometrial incision.

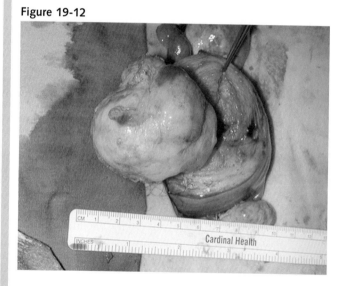

Hysteroscopic Myomectomy

The desire of many women to retain the uterus and return to normal activities quickly prompted the emergence of less invasive technologies for the treatment of symptomatic fibroids. In the early 1980s, the urologic resectoscope was first used to remove intrauterine polyps and fibroids. The development of a continuous-flow resectoscope permitted distension of the uterine cavity with fluid and removal of blood and debris. Further improvements in optics, video recording, and intrauterine distension systems provided additional safety features for operative hysteroscopic procedures.

Operative hysteroscopic myomectomy requires an understanding of fluid management, good hand-eye coordination, sound judgment about when to abandon the hysteroscopic approach, and a thorough preoperative evaluation including a detailed knowledge of the number, size, location, and depth of myometrial involvement of the fibroids.

To perform hysteroscopic myomectomy, the cervix is first dilated with cervical dilators to accommodate an operative hysteroscope (usually 7 to 10 French). Use of a laminaria or misoprostol is recommended to decrease risk of cervical lacerations, to lessen undue force resulting in uterine perforation, and to facilitate dilation. The most common complications associated with operative hysteroscopy are uterine perforation or cervical laceration. Oral or vaginal misoprostol (200 to 400 µg) given 8 to 12 hours before surgery softens the cervix, reduces need for cervical dilation, decreases cervical complications, and reduces operative time in comparison with control subjects. Although misoprostol has several bothersome adverse effects, such as lower abdominal pain and slight vaginal bleeding, few of the associated side effects prevent its use.

The operative hysteroscope should be advanced under direct visualization without undue force. The endocervix, lower uterine segment, and tubal ostia should be visualized at all times. Once the submucosal fibroid has been identified, the wire-loop electrode is advanced in clear view of the surgeon. The electrical wattage generally used with a monopolar current is 60- to 80-W cutting current. As the wire loop is drawn toward the surgeon, small crescent-shaped "chips" or fragments of leiomyoma are created. They can remain free-floating until they interfere with visualization and are then removed with polyp forceps, Corson graspers, or the loop itself. The leiomyoma is shaved until it is flush with the endometrium. The whorled fibrous appearance of the leiomyoma is clearly different from the fascicles of soft underlying myometrium. Intermittently, the intrauterine pressure should be diminished to help enucleate the uterine fibroid. The higher intrauterine pressure created with the fluid pumps may create an artificial or "negative hysteroscopic view" by pushing the leiomyoma into the myometrium. By decreasing the intrauterine pressure, the fibroid bulges into the endometrial cavity, facilitating its complete removal.

Patients generally have minimal postoperative pain after hysteroscopic myomectomy. A serosanguinous discharge for 1 to 4 weeks is typical after the procedure. Mild cramping is easily alleviated with low-dose nonsteroidal anti-inflammatory medications, though a few patients require narcotics for postoperative pain management. Patients typically resume normal activities within 24 to 48 hours after the procedure. Sexual activity can be resumed 1 week postoperatively. If an incomplete resection has occurred, some patients may pass pieces of fibroid tissue several weeks after the procedure.

Patients with fever, malaise, worsening pain, or escalating pain medication requirements should be carefully evaluated for bowel injury, bladder injury, and endometritis. Office evaluation must be undertaken, including thorough abdominal and pelvic examination. Laboratory testing that may be required includes electrolytes, complete blood cell count, sedimentation rate evaluation, ultrasonography, and flat plate radiography of the abdomen (kidneys, ureters, and bladder; upright). Sometimes a CT scan of the pelvis/abdomen may be needed if perforation with bowel or bladder injury is suspected. Complications of hysteroscopic myomectomy are displayed in Box 19-3.

Among women wishing to preserve fertility, some gynecologists empirically prescribe high-dose estrogen to aid in re-epithelization of the endometrium with the aim of decreasing the risk of intrauterine adhesions after hysteroscopic myomectomy. Typically, conjugated estrogen 2.5 to 5 mg daily or estradiol 2 mg twice daily for 25 days, followed by 12 days of progesterone 10 mg, is prescribed. Alternatively, a pediatric catheter inflated with 15 to 20 mL of normal saline or sterile water is inserted for 7 to 10 days to prevent the juxtaposition of the uterine walls. Repeat office hysteroscopy is performed within 7 to 14 days after extensive myomectomy to evaluate the endometrium for synechiae. If detected early, the adhesions are filmy and easily lysed with the distal tip of a hysteroscope. On occasion, repetitive hysteroscopic visualization every 7 to 10 days can be performed until the endometrium is completely healed without evidence of adhesions. Postoperative hysteroscopy is not necessary in women who do not desire fertility or are postmenopausal.

Uterine Fibroid Embolization

Uterine artery embolization historically has been used as a last resort or life-saving procedure in women experiencing hemorrhage due to obstetric and gynecologic conditions. It was first used in the obstetric setting in 1979 to successfully treat a patient with severe postpartum hemorrhage whose condition failed to respond to standard bilateral hypogastric artery ligation. Its role in gynecology, obstetric emergencies, and other cases of intra-abdominal hemorrhage is now well established (Box 19-4).

Box 19-3   Complications of Hysteroscopic Myomectomy

Procedure related: Cervical laceration, uterine perforation, bowel and bladder injury, inability to dilate the cervix, and hemorrhage
Media related: Hyponatremia, gas and air embolism, anaphylaxis, and excessive fluid absorption
Postoperative: Endometritis, lack of symptom resolution, intrauterine synechiae, and unrecognized bowel, bladder, or major blood vessel injury

---

Box 19-4   Indications for Uterine Fibroid Embolization

Severe postpartum hemorrhage
Postabortal bleeding
Abdominal, cervical, and ectopic pregnancy
Gestational trophoblastic disease
Symptomatic leiomyomata
Premyomectomy therapy
Postmyomectomy hemorrhage
Fibroids in postmenopausal patients
Prophylactic use in gynecologic cancer surgery
Bladder cancer
Arteriovenous malformations
Pelvic trauma

Most centers now refer to transcatheter embolization of the uterine vessels as *uterine fibroid embolization* (UFE). Since the performance of prophylactic UFE for uterine fibroids in 1995 by Ravina, the procedure has gained widespread acceptance as a therapeutic option for symptomatic uterine fibroids. Approximately 15,000 UFE procedures are performed annually in the United States, and 50,000 procedures have been performed worldwide.

UFE is a percutaneous angiographic procedure performed by interventional radiology under fluoroscopic guidance. During the procedure, a catheter is threaded through the femoral artery to the uterine artery, which is occluded with polyvinyl alcohol, Embospheres, gel foam, or other particles. This diminishes blood flow to the fibroids and uterus, effectively producing a decline in capillary flow, which enhances clotting and leads to fibroid shrinkage. Rich collateral circulation from the contralateral uterine artery and the ovarian vasculature prevents total tissue necrosis.

For patients whose only options have been operative intervention with myomectomy or hysterectomy, UFE offers preservation of the uterus and the avoidance of major surgery with low complication rates. Ravina originally recommended prophylactic embolization, with the belief that UFE would decrease blood flow to the uterine arteries and thereby minimize blood loss, intraoperative blood transfusions, or conversion to hysterectomy in women scheduled for abdominal myomectomy. In their original series, 11 of 16 patients had resolution of symptoms, three patients had partial resolution, and two patients later required surgical intervention. After a 20-month follow-up period, an overall 20% to 60% reduction in uterine volume occurred. One patient subsequently became pregnant. These dramatic results prompted others to evaluate the benefit of this new minimally invasive procedure for the treatment of fibroids. The success and low complication rate of arterial embolization have encouraged the application of UFE as a nonsurgical alternative to hysterectomy for the management of fibroids. As promising results are consistently reported, the use of this procedure has increased exponentially and become popular among patients.

Advantages of UFE include preservation of uterine function, avoidance of a surgical procedure, short hospital stay, quick return to activities, and low risk of complications (Box 19-5). If the procedure produces unsatisfactory results, myomectomy or hysterectomy remains an option. Contraindications for UFE include the desire for future fertility, acute pelvic inflammatory disease, contrast allergy, coagulation disorders, and associated pathology requiring pelvic surgery. Additionally, patients must have negative results from a recent Papanicolaou smear (<12 months), negative cervical cultures for sexually transmitted infections, and, for those with irregular bleeding or age older than 40 years, an endometrial biopsy result without evidence of hyperplasia or malignancy.

UFE effectively treats all fibroid-related symptoms including bulk symptoms, pain, and bleeding. Qualified interventional radiologists reliably demonstrate an improvement in quality of life, decline in uterine and myometrial volume, improvement in bulk symptoms, and low rates of major

---

Box 19-5 Advantages of Uterine Fibroid Embolization

Avoids major surgery and general anesthesia
No scars
Early ambulation
Shorter hospital stay
Can be offered to women with prior myomectomy
Minimal blood loss
Can be performed in high-risk and markedly anemic patients
Advantageous in patients who have religious prohibitions against blood transfusion
Effectively treats menorrhagia and bulk symptoms and decreases uterine size
Effective in postmenopausal patients with symptomatic fibroids
Potential cost savings

---

complications. Most large case series report 90% improvement in menor-rhagia. Bulk symptoms improve in 80% to 90% of patients, with the average volume of the uterus decreasing by 40% to 60%. Among patients who do not have a decline in uterine size, the majority of patients experience an improvement in bulk or menorrhagia-related symptoms. Most studies are encouraging but offer limited long-term follow-up of patients. Although the long-term success of the procedure remains to be seen, most studies demonstrate durability and excellent outcomes.

Complications from UFE are infrequent; however, gynecologists who evaluate a patient postoperatively must be cognizant of possible minor and major complications. Three categories of complications have been associated with UFE: immediate (related to the technical aspects of the procedure), acute (within 30 days), and long term (greater than 30 days). Approximately 15% to 20% of patients experience postembolization syndrome including fever, pelvic pain, malaise, nausea, and vomiting. Additionally, approximately 15% of those who undergo UFE will require hospitalization. If uterine or fibroid necrosis is not promptly recognized and treated, potentially catastrophic sepsis and poor outcome may occur. Additionally, patients with unrecognized ovarian neoplasms may be untreated or may present with a late diagnosis. Liberal use of imaging, specifically CT scan to rule out abscess formation, should be performed in women complaining of severe pelvic pain after the procedure. Infection, hysterectomy, and need for transfusion are potential complications of UFE. This is particularly important for patients who are Jehovah's Witnesses who may elect UFE as an alternative procedure to laparotomy or hysterectomy with the belief that transfusion will be unnecessary. Boxes 19-6 and 19-7 list procedural and postprocedural complications of UFE.

Future Treatment Modalities

The investigational selective progesterone receptor modulator asoprisnil was recently evaluated in a multicenter phase II study. It induced amenor-rhea or normal menstrual cycles in the majority of women with myoma-induced heavy bleeding. Increased hemoglobin concentration, rapid

Box 19-6	Procedural Complications of Uterine Fibroid Embolization

Groin infection
Groin hematoma
Contrast allergy
Contrast-related renal failure
Arteriovenous malformations
Pseudoaneurysm
Misembolization of abdominal vessels
Radiation exposure

Box 19-7	Postprocedural Complications of Uterine Fibroid Embolization

Postembolization syndrome
Ischemic necrosis with prolonged purulent drainage
Endometritis/pyometrium
Transcervical expulsion of uterine fibroids
Premature ovarian failure
Anorgasmia
Sepsis
Death

suppression of duration and intensity of bleeding (by week 4), reduction in fibroid size, and endometrial vascular suppression were identified in endometrial biopsies. As a selective progesterone receptor modulator, asoprisnil has an agonist/antagonist effect on progesterone receptors, with a high degree of tissue selectivity as well as antiproliferative effects on the endometrium without suppressing ovarian function. With further studies underway, it holds the promise of becoming an excellent medical therapy for uterine fibroids.

Recently, interferon-α has been shown to inhibit growth factors that stimulate proliferation of cells. Additionally, techniques that inhibit DNA synthesis may one day lead to definitive therapy of leiomyomata. Numerous nonsurgical approaches to the treatment of symptomatic and asymptomatic patients with uterine fibroids will likely be possible in the future.

CONCLUSIONS

Patients now have an array of options available for the treatment of symptomatic uterine fibroids. Since most fibroids are benign, patients and physicians should never feel rushed into making a therapeutic decision. Patients with symptomatic fibroids should seek a compassionate and well-trained gynecologist who is knowledgeable about all fibroid options.

The physician should have a thorough understanding of the patient's reproductive needs and personal desires. Choice of therapy depends on the reproductive desires of the patient, her age, the size and number of fibroids, and the patient's desire to maintain the uterus.

Sometimes, expectant management and reassurance are all that are needed in perimenopausal or minimally symptomatic women. Some fibroid-related complaints can be simply treated with nonsteroidal medications, low-dose OCPs, or GnRH therapy. If medical measures fail to treat fibroid-related symptoms, many surgical and minimally invasive techniques are available for the treatment of fibroids. Hysterectomy always solves fibroid-related bleeding and bulk symptoms, with prospective studies indicating improved quality of life and excellent symptom relief. Myomectomy should be considered in women wishing to preserve their fertility. This can be accomplished by laparotomy, laparoscopy, and hysteroscopy. Additionally, UFE is a viable option for women not desiring pregnancy or who want nonsurgical intervention. Women should understand all available options, including the short- and long-term outcomes associated with each treatment modality.

479

KEY POINTS

1. No medical or surgical therapy is indicated for asymptomatic leiomyomata.

2. Abnormal uterine bleeding is the most common clinical presentation for uterine fibroids, followed by bulk symptoms and subfertility.

3. The mechanism for fibroid-related abnormal bleeding is not well understood but most likely includes increased surface area, platelet dysfunction, prostaglandin aberrations, and ulceration over surfaces of the myoma.

4. Endometrial biopsy and dilation and curettage alone inadequately detect or treat leiomyomata and should be performed with hysteroscopy for the most accurate diagnosis.

5. Office hysteroscopy is quick, well tolerated, and provides rapid diagnosis of intracavitary lesions such as submucosal fibroids, endometrial polyps, hyperplasia, and endometrial cancer.

6. Saline infusion sonography has a high sensitivity in detecting intracavitary lesions and can determine the number and depth of myometrial penetration of leiomyomata.

7. Magnetic resonance imaging is the gold standard for the detection of adenomyosis.

8. Close attention to fluid management is imperative in women undergoing hysteroscopic myomectomy.

9. Uterine fibroid embolization successfully treats menorrhagia in 85% to 90% of patients, bulk symptoms in 80% to 90%, and has greater than 90% clinical success in treated patients.

SUGGESTED READING

American College of Obstetricians and Gynecologists: Quality Improvement in Women's Health Care, revised ed. Washington, DC, ACOG, 2000.

Barrington JW, Arunkalaivanan AS, Abdel-Fattah M: Comparison between the levonorgestrel intrauterine system (LNG-IUS) and thermal balloon ablation in the treatment of menorrhagia. Eur J Obstet Gynecol Reprod Biol 108:72–74, 2003.

Bettocchi S, Ceci O, Vicino M, et al: Diagnostic inadequacy of dilation and curettage. Fertil Steril 75(4):803–805, 2001.

Bradley L, Widrich T: State-of-the-art flexible hysteroscopy for office gynecologic evaluation. J Am Assoc Gynecol Laparosc 2(3):263–267, 1995.

Bradley LD, Falcone T, Magen A: Radiographic imaging techniques for the diagnosis of abnormal uterine bleeding. Obstet Gynecol Clin North Amer 27(2):245–276, 2000.

Brown SE, Coddington CC, Schnorr J, et al: Evaluation of outpatient hysteroscopy, saline infusion hysterosonography, and hysterosalpingography in infertile women: A prospective, randomized study. Fertil Steril 74(5):1029–1034, 2000.

Buttram VC Jr, Reiter RC: Uterine leiomyomata: Etiology, symptomatology, and management. Fertil Steril 36:433–445, 1981.

Carlson KJ, Miller BA, Fowler FJ Jr: The Maine Women's Health Study: II. Outcomes of nonsurgical management of leiomyomas, abnormal bleeding, and chronic pelvic pain. Obstet Gynecol 83:566–572, 1994.

Cicinelli E, Romano F, Anastasio PS, et al: Transabdominal sonohysterography, transvaginal sonography, and hysteroscopy in the evaluation of submucous myomas. Obstet Gynecol 85:42–47, 1995.

Coccia ME, Becattini C, Bracco GL, et al: Intraoperative ultrasound guidance for operative hysteroscopy. J Reprod Med 45:413–418, 2000.

Dueholm M, Lundorf E, Hansen E, et al: Evaluation of the uterine cavity with magnetic resonance imaging, transvaginal sonography, hysterosonographic examination, and diagnostic hysteroscopy. Fertil Steril 76(2):350–357, 2001.

Emanuel MH, Verdel MJ, Wamsteker K: A prospective comparison of transvaginal ultrasonography and diagnostic hysteroscopy in the evaluation of patients with abnormal uterine bleeding: Clinical implications. Am J Obstet Gynecol 172:547–552, 1995.

Indman PD: Use of Carbosprost to facilitate hysteroscopic resection of submucous myomas. J Am Assoc Gynecol Laparoscop 11(1):68–72, 2004.

Jansen FW, Vredevoogd CB, Ulzen K, et al: Complications of hysteroscopy: A prospective, multicenter study. Obstet Gynecol 96:266–270, 2000.

Khaund A, Moss JG, McMillan N, Lumsden MA: Evaluation of the effect of uterine artery embolisation on menstrual blood loss and uterine volume. BJOG 111(7):700–705, 2004.

Kovac SR: Transvaginal hysterectomy: Rationale and surgical approach. Obstet Gynecol 103:1321–1325, 2004.

Mihm LM, Quick VA, Brumfield JA: The accuracy of endometrial biopsy and saline sonohysterography in the determination of the cause of abnormal uterine bleeding. Am J Obstet Gynecol 186:858–863, 2002.

Mueller GC, Gemmete JJ, Carlos RC: Diagnostic imaging and vascular embolization for uterine leiomyomas. Semin Reprod Med 22(2):131–142, 2004.

Payne JF, Haney AF: Serious complications of uterine artery embolization for conservative treatment of fibroids. Fertil Steril 79(1):128–131, 2003.

Preutthipan S, Herabutya Y: Vaginal misoprostol for cervical priming before operative hysteroscopy: A randomized controlled trial. Obstet Gynecol 96:890–894, 2000.

Pron G, Bennett J, Common A, et al: The Ontario uterine fibroid embolization trial: Part 2. Uterine fibroid reduction and symptom relief after uterine artery embolization for fibroids. Fertil Steril 79 (1):120–127, 2003.

Propst AM, Liberman RF, Harlow BL, Ginsburg ES: Complications of hysteroscopic surgery: Predicting patients at risk. Obstet Gynecol 96:517–520, 2000.

Ravina JH, Herbreteau D, Ciraru-Vigneron N, et al: Arterial embolization to treat uterine myomata. Lancet 346:671–672, 1995.

Spies JB, Ascher SA, Roth AR, et al: Uterine artery embolization for leiomyomata. Obstet Gynecol 98 (1):29–34, 2001.

Thomas JA, Leyland N, Durand N, Windrim RD: The use of oral misoprostol as a cervical ripening agent in operative hysteroscopy: A double-blind, placebo-controlled trial. Am J Obstet Gynecol 186:876–879, 2002.

Walker WJ, Pelage JP: Uterine artery embolisation for symptomatic fibroids: Clinical results in 400 women with imaging follow up. BJOG 109(11):1262–1272, 2002.

Wegienka G, Baird DD, Hertz-Picciotto I, et al: Self-reported heavy bleeding associated with uterine leiomyomata. Obstet Gynecol 101:431–437, 2003.

Widrich T, Bradley L, Mitchinson AR, Collins R: Comparison of saline infusion sonography with office hysteroscopy for the evaluation of the endometrium. Am J Obstet Gynecol 174:1327–1334, 1996.

20

DISORDERS OF THE FALLOPIAN TUBE AND OVARY

Renee T. Page and S. Gene McNeeley

Gynecologic conditions presenting as a pelvic mass range from simple physiologic ovarian cysts to cancer of the ovary, fallopian tube, and uterus. Conditions that present as an adnexal mass can also involve a wide range of organ systems. The likelihood of a pelvic or adnexal mass being malignant or nongynecologic in origin varies with age. This chapter primarily reviews the evaluation and management of benign pelvic masses of gynecologic origin.

PELVIC MASS IN THE NEWBORN AND CHILDREN

Abdominal and pelvic masses are rare in newborns. Ovarian tumors in the newborns account for fewer than 5% of intra-abdominal tumors. The ovarian follicular cyst is the most common ovarian cyst; it can be diagnosed by prenatal ultrasound or may present as a palpable asymptomatic mass in the newborn after delivery. The ovarian cyst is due to stimulation of the fetal ovary by maternal gonadotropins or persistent hypothalamic pituitary activity. Physical examination usually reveals a small mobile cyst, which is confirmed by ultrasound. Observation is recommended as the most appropriate means of treatment, and the ovarian cyst should regress during the first 2 months of life. Ovarian torsion rarely complicates a simple ovarian cyst of the newborn.

Ovarian tumors account for approximately 1% of intra-abdominal tumors in children. The most common malignancies diagnosed in the pediatric population include neuroblastoma, Wilms' tumor, lymphoma, hepatoblastoma, and germ cell tumors (Box 20-1). The vast majority of ovarian neoplasms diagnosed in children are germ cell tumors and are usually benign. The mature cystic teratoma is the most common benign germ cell tumor.

In contrast to women of reproductive age, epithelial tumors are extremely uncommon in childhood. When present, the majority are benign serous cystadenomas and mucinous cystadenomas. Abdominal pain is the presenting symptom in the majority of children with ovarian masses. Other symptoms include poor appetite, urinary symptoms, and rarely,

---

Box 20-1   Causes of Pelvic Mass in Children

Ovarian
Follicular cyst
Benign cystic teratoma
Dysgerminoma
Wilms' tumor

Neuroblastoma

Burkitt's lymphoma

Gastrointestinal

Musculoskeletal

---

weight loss. Ovarian neoplasms of germ cell origin may produce estrogen or testosterone, resulting in precocious development or masculinization. Torsion is more likely to be seen in children with benign masses.

Since physiologic ovarian cysts are the most common ovarian lesions seen in the pediatric age group, observation is the preferred management for simple ovarian cysts confirmed by ultrasound. A palpable abdominal mass, any solid ovarian mass, or any cystic ovarian lesion larger than 10 cm should be considered neoplastic, necessitating surgical intervention.

PELVIC MASS IN ADOLESCENTS

From the beginning of menarche to age 20 years is an age group in which pelvic masses become more frequently encountered and more problematic. Although ovarian neoplasms and cysts account for the majority of pelvic masses in adolescents, disorders of the fallopian tube are also frequently encountered (Box 20-2). Sexual activity usually begins during adolescence, placing the woman at risk for sexually transmitted infections and two

---

Box 20-2   Adnexal Masses in Adolescents

Obstructive
Transverse vaginal septum
Blind uterine horn

Ovarian
Functional cyst
Hemorrhagic corpus luteum
Germ cell tumors
Other ovarian neoplasm

Fallopian tube
Paratubal cyst
Ectopic pregnancy
Pyosalpinx/hydrosalpinx
Tubo-ovarian abscess

Appendiceal abscess

---

important complications: pelvic inflammatory disease with tubo-ovarian abscess and ectopic pregnancy. The latter is discussed in detail in Chapter 11, Ectopic Pregnancy.

Congenital Obstructive Lesions

Persons with congenital obstructive lesions present with complaints of cyclic abdominal and pelvic pain, primary amenorrhea, oligomenorrhagia, and dysmenorrhea. Hematocolpos is present on gynecologic examination in the presence of an imperforate hymen. The transverse vaginal septum presents with similar symptoms and is differentiated from imperforate hymen by the presence of a hymeneal ring distal to the site of obstruction. A patient with a blind uterine horn presents with cyclic menstrual bleeding and severe cyclic pelvic pain. A pelvic mass may be palpable on examination. Approximately one third of patients will have concomitant urinary tract abnormalities including pelvic kidney, renal agenesis, horseshoe kidney, or other abnormalities of the collecting system. An intravenous pyelogram allows for a thorough evaluation of the urinary tract. Pelvic ultrasound may detect a blind uterine horn, although the abnormality is often discovered inadvertently at the time of diagnostic laparoscopy for pelvic pain. Excision of the imperforate hymen or transverse septum and excision of the blind uterine horn result in prompt resolution of symptoms.

Ovarian Masses

Adnexal masses often present with abdominal complaints that can mimic other diseases in adolescents—particularly, appendicitis. Acute onset of pain associated with nausea and vomiting are the most common symptoms of ovarian cysts. Ovarian cysts account for one fifth as many admissions as appendicitis in young women. Physical findings for both appendicitis and ovarian cysts include lower abdominal tenderness, rebound tenderness, and adnexal tenderness on bimanual examination. A complete blood count and pregnancy test should be performed. In addition to pelvic ultrasound, computed tomography (CT) scan or magnetic resonance imaging can provide important information regarding nongynecologic causes of abdominal and pelvic pain.

Functional Ovarian Cysts

The majority of ovarian masses in adolescents consist of functional cysts. Follicular cysts are the most common cystic mass encountered. Follicular cysts are believed to arise from gonadotropin effect on the ovary, and persistent cysts result from either failure of the dominant follicle to rupture or the failure of an immature follicle to undergo atresia. Follicular cysts are filled with clear fluid and usually measure less than 3 cm in diameter. Persistent follicular cysts can easily exceed 5 to 8 cm in diameter. The cysts are usually asymptomatic and are discovered during a routine pelvic examination or ultrasound of the pelvis for other reasons. The initial management of a suspected follicular cyst is observation for 4 to 8 weeks. A persistent ovarian cyst requires further evaluation to exclude an ovarian neoplasm. Oral contraceptives have been recommended to suppress ovarian function in expectation of more prompt clinical improvement and resolution of the cyst. However, randomized clinical trials have failed to prove benefit compared with observation alone. Nonsteroidal anti-inflammatory agents can be prescribed for pain.

Corpus luteum cysts measure 3 to 10 cm or more in diameter (Fig. 20-1). The cyst cavity may be filled with clear fluid or blood due to hemorrhage into the corpus luteum cyst (Fig. 20-2). Occasionally, a corpus luteum cyst can be associated with intra-abdominal hemorrhage presenting as a surgical abdomen, similar to that encountered with ovarian torsion and ruptured ectopic pregnancy or endometrioma. A serum human chorionic gonadotropin evaluation and pelvic ultrasound scan should be performed. The presence of a significant hemoperitoneum requires operative intervention. Ovarian cystectomy or fenestration of the ovarian capsule during laparoscopy is the treatment of choice. In patients with mild symptoms and the presence of a small hemoperitoneum, observation alone is appropriate.

Theca lutein cysts are the least common functional cysts and arise from excessive stimulation of the ovaries by endogenous or exogenous gonadotropins. Molar pregnancies and choriocarcinoma are associated with theca lutein cysts in approximately 50% and 10% of patients, respectively.

Figure 20-1

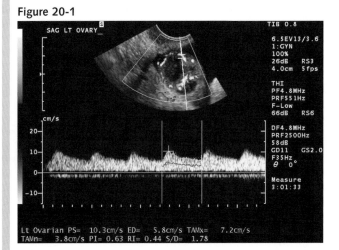

Corpus luteum. Sagittal transvaginal image shows a hypoechoic complex cystic corpus luteum with characteristic circumferential low impedance arterial pattern on Doppler image. (Ultrasound courtesy of Samuel Johnson, MD.)

Figure 20-2

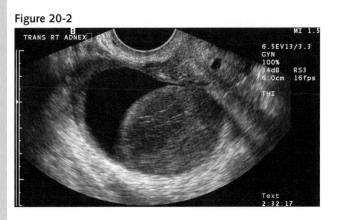

Hemorrhagic cyst. Transvaginal sonographic image demonstrates a thin-walled complex cyst with well-demarcated geographic area of clot within an otherwise anechoic cyst. (Ultrasound courtesy of Samuel Johnson, MD.)

Bilateral ovarian enlargement is present, and the ovaries may exceed 20 cm in diameter. Stromal edema, multiple follicular cysts, and corpus luteum cysts are present. Lower abdominal discomfort is the most common symptom. Hyperstimulation syndrome resulting from exogenous gonadotropin therapy results in weight gain and ascites. More severe findings include pleural effusion, electrolyte imbalance, hypokalemia, and hypotension. The preferred management is observation. Hyperstimulation syndrome can be life threatening, often requiring hospitalization and careful fluid and electrolyte management. Ovarian torsion and intra-abdominal hemorrhage have been reported with theca lutein cyst, which can be managed by laparoscopy or laparotomy.

Ovarian Neoplasms

Neoplastic masses begin to occur more frequently during adolescence, and the majority of these neoplastic lesions (approximately 60%) are germ cell tumors. Epithelial tumors account for approximately 20% of neoplastic lesions in adolescents. Malignant ovarian tumors account for approximately 5% of ovarian masses in adolescents. Ovarian neoplasms often present with abdominal complaints that can mimic other diseases. Ultrasound, including Doppler flow studies, will characterize the cyst appearance and content and may help determine whether torsion is present. It is important to note that torsion may be intermittent, and positive blood flow on a Doppler study does not exclude the possibility of torsion. Indications for operation include the presence of a cystic mass greater than 10 cm in diameter or a persistent cystic mass previously managed conservatively. Although laparoscopic drainage of follicular cysts has a very low recurrence rate, recurrence rates of 30% to 40% have been reported for other benign cysts that had been drained surgically. If there is any suspicion of malignancy, cystectomy or oophorectomy should be performed. Ovarian conservation should be performed when possible.

Adnexal Masses Associated With Infection

Adolescents have the highest incidence of sexually transmitted infections, including those caused by *Neisseria gonorrhoeae* and *Chlamydia trachomatis*. Unrecognized or untreated cervical infections may result in pelvic inflammatory disease. The most common inflammatory disorders of the fallopian tube resulting in a mass are pyosalpinx and tubo-ovarian abscess (Fig. 20-3). The prevalence of pyosalpinx is unknown, although tubo-ovarian abscess occurs in approximately 15% of women developing pelvic inflammatory disease and approximately 40% of women hospitalized for treatment of pelvic inflammatory disease. Common symptoms of pelvic inflammatory disease are nonspecific and include lower abdominal pain, fever, abnormal bleeding, and vaginal discharge. Physical findings include cervical motion tenderness, uterine and adnexal tenderness, and the presence of a palpable mass on pelvic examination. Abnormal laboratory findings include leukocytosis and elevated erythrocyte sedimentation rate or C-reactive protein level. Approximately 20% of women with pelvic inflammatory disease will test positive for chlamydia, 40% will test positive for gonorrhea, and 10% will test positive for both. Since all masses are not palpable and many women

Figure 20-3

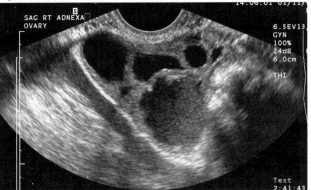

Tubo-ovarian abscess. Transvaginal sonographic image shows a multi-compartmentalized complex cystic adnexal mass consisting of thick irregular walls and septa and echogenic fluid with a gradient effect (fluid/debris level). (Ultrasound courtesy of Samuel Johnson, MD.)

with acute pelvic inflammatory disease will not tolerate a pelvic examination, a transvaginal and transabdominal ultrasound will confirm the presence of pyosalpinx or tubo-ovarian abscess.

Approximately 90% of women hospitalized for the treatment of pelvic inflammatory disease respond to the parenteral cefoxitin, 2 g every 6 hours, plus doxycycline, 100 mg every 12 hours. Evidence suggests that initial therapy of suspected or confirmed tubo-ovarian abscess consisting of ampicillin (2 g every 6 hours) plus clindamycin (900 mg every 8 hours) and gentamicin (1 mg/kg every 8 hours) is more effective than cefoxitin plus doxycycline and is associated with shorter duration of hospitalization and fewer surgical interventions. Unilateral tubo-ovarian abscess is seen in approximately 50% of patients with tubo-ovarian abscess. The presence of an intrauterine contraceptive device is not predictive of unilateral tubo-ovarian abscess.

Before the ready availability of broad-spectrum antibiotics, surgical intervention primarily consisted of total abdominal hysterectomy and bilateral salpingo-oophorectomy. As an alternative to hysterectomy, colpotomy drainage of the abscess offers a conservative alternative for those whose conditions fail to respond to parenteral antibiotic therapy. Although this is helpful in many patients, unrecognized bowel injury and the need for emergency surgery may occur. Recently, ultrasound-guided transvaginal drainage of pelvic abscesses has been shown to be safe, associated with fewer complications, and possibly resulting in more rapid clinical improvement compared with antibiotic therapy alone. CT-guided drainage has also been shown to be effective in draining pelvic abscesses, although it needs to be performed by an experienced interventional radiologist. Laparoscopic drainage of the abscess or pyosalpinx offers a minimally invasive alternative to laparotomy for women whose conditions fail to respond to parenteral therapy, but its utility may be limited by extensive adhesive disease in women with acute tubo-ovarian abscess. Laparotomy is usually reserved for patients whose conditions do not respond to medical therapy (Box 20-3). Since unilateral abscesses are common, conservative surgery is recommended, especially in young

> **Box 20-3** Indications for Laparotomy or Laparoscopy in Women with Tubo-Ovarian and Pelvic Abscess
>
> Suspicion of rupture
> Uncertain diagnosis
> Failed medical therapy
> Recurrent or chronic pelvic inflammatory disease
> Postmenopausal pelvic abscess

women of low parity. Total abdominal hysterectomy with bilateral salpingo-oophorectomy is definitive therapy.

PELVIC MASS IN REPRODUCTIVE-AGE WOMEN

Women with pelvic masses often require surgical intervention. The masses are most often benign and can be removed by the practicing obstetrician-gynecologist. Since cancer rates are more prevalent as women age, a careful history and physical examination is necessary. Important symptoms include abdominal pain, nausea, early satiety, bloating, and increasing abdominal girth. Bimanual pelvic examination is helpful but has limitations for evaluating the adnexa, especially in patients with characteristics such as obesity, significant uterine enlargement, and abdominal scars, all of which limit the accurate palpation of the adnexa. A thorough abdominal examination and careful assessment of regional lymph nodes is necessary. Transvaginal ultrasound is useful to determine high-risk characteristics of the cyst (e.g., large size, complexity, septations, or excrescences). Cancer antigen 125 (CA-125) can be checked in those women with suspicious-appearing ovarian lesions, although it has not been shown to be useful as a screening tool in premenopausal women. In postmenopausal women with a pelvic mass, a CA-125 measurement may be helpful in predicting a higher likelihood of malignancy. However, up to 50% of early stage cancers and 20% to 25% of advanced cancers are associated with normal values. CT scan with contrast will assist in detecting metastatic disease if suspicion is high. Tumor markers should be obtained as needed to assist in managing other pelvic and intra-abdominal neoplasms.

When a gynecologic malignancy is diagnosed, a formal staging procedure is required to achieve optimal outcome. Numerous studies have documented better outcomes for patients with ovarian cancer initially managed by a gynecologic oncologist. Optimal surgical resection and proper staging during the primary operation are important for predicting long-term survival of women with ovarian cancer. Proposed guidelines for referral of a patient with a pelvic mass are listed in Box 20-4. When used with other clinical information, the guidelines are a helpful tool in deciding whether referral to a gynecologic oncologist is appropriate.

It is commonly believed that benign and malignant ovarian neoplasms are asymptomatic. Although the majority of ovarian neoplasms are

---

Box 20-4   Guidelines for Referral of a Newly Diagnosed Pelvic Mass

Premenopausal (<50 years old)
CA-125 > 200 U/mL
Ascites
Evidence of abdominal or distant metastasis
Family history of one or more relatives with ovarian or breast cancer

Postmenopausal (≥ 50 years old)
CA-125 > 35 U/mL
Ascites
Evidence of abdominal or distant metastasis
Family history of one or more relatives with ovarian or breast cancer

---

CA-125, Cancer antigen 125.

diagnosed incidentally, up to 70% of women diagnosed with ovarian cancer recall having symptoms of 3 months' or longer duration. Common symptoms include abdominal pain or other constitutional symptoms. Persistent symptoms such as abdominal pain, indigestion, increasing abdominal girth, urinary frequency, constipation, or unexplained weight loss should be investigated and ovarian cancer and other intra-abdominal tumors excluded.

Although most masses arise from the genital tract, nongynecologic causes of pelvic masses are encountered more frequently with increasing age (Box 20-5). As with adolescents, functional ovarian cysts and ectopic pregnancy continue to be important causes of adnexal masses and should

---

Box 20-5   Nongynecologic Causes of Pelvic Masses in Reproductive-Age Women

Gastrointestinal
Rectosigmoid carcinoma
Cecal carcinoma
Appendiceal abscess
Sigmoid diverticulitis
Inflammatory bowel disease

Urinary tract
Neoplasm
Pelvic kidney
Bladder stone

Retroperitoneal tumors
Lymphoma
Anterior meningocele
Neurofibroma
Extramedullary hematopoiesis

Peritoneal inclusion cyst
Vascular
Iliac aneurysm
Arteriovenous fistula

Metastatic cancer
Breast
Gastrointestinal

be managed appropriately. As the list of potential causes for adnexal masses expands, the evaluation of the adnexal mass becomes more extensive. These include selective use of tumor markers, CT scan with and without contrast, colonoscopy, and other tests deemed appropriate. Benign cysts are usually unilateral, mobile, cystic, and on examination, smooth. In contrast, malignant ovarian neoplasms are more likely to be bilateral with both solid and cystic components, irregular to palpation. At time of surgery, ascites, nodularity with areas of hemorrhage, and necrosis are more likely to be present.

In general, indications for surgical intervention include a solid mass at any age or a simple cystic mass that persists after 6 to 8 weeks of observation. It has been recommended that any cystic mass in a postmenopausal woman be removed; however, the vast majority of simple cysts 5 cm in diameter or smaller are benign. Close observation with serial ultrasound examinations is an option in properly selected postmenopausal women with small, simple ovarian cysts.

489

Ovarian Neoplasms

Eighty percent of ovarian neoplasms are benign. The most common ovarian neoplasm encountered in women of reproductive age is the benign cystic teratoma, which accounts for approximately one third of all ovarian neoplasms (Fig. 20-4). Bilateral teratomas are encountered in approximately 15% of cases. Cystic teratomas are composed of cells from all three germ layers. Products of the skin appendages account for the majority of the neoplasm, including hair and sebaceous material. Other common histologic findings include skin, cartilage, bone, muscle, and mucosa of the respiratory and gastrointestinal tract. Neural tissue is also present. Endocrine abnormalities associated with benign cystic teratomas include hyperthyroidism with struma ovarii, carcinoid syndrome, and autoimmune hemolytic anemia. Benign ovarian neoplasms frequently seen in women of reproductive age are noted in Box 20-6.

Figure 20-4

Teratoma. Transvaginal sonographic image demonstrates a central markedly hyperechoic and attenuating ovarian mass with poor posterior wall definition (i.e., "tip-of-the-iceberg" sign). (Ultrasound courtesy of Samuel Johnson, MD.)

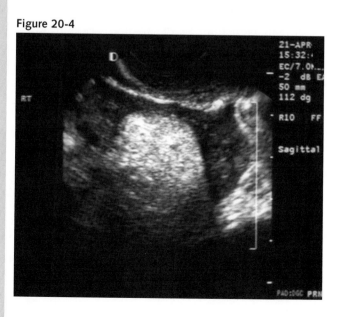

Box 20-6 Benign Ovarian Neoplasms in Women of Reproductive Age
Germ cell
Benign cystic teratoma
Epithelial
Mucinous cystadenoma
Serous cystadenoma
Stromal
Brenner tumor
Fibroma
Thecoma

Torsion of the ovary is an uncommon but important cause of pelvic pain in children, adolescents, and women of reproductive age. Fallopian tube torsion usually accompanies the ovarian torsion. Ovarian hyperstimulation syndrome and the presence of a functional cyst or mature teratoma are important risk factors for ovarian torsion. Clinical features include sudden onset of severe colicky pelvic pain, nausea, and vomiting. Due to the nonspecific nature of these symptoms, there is frequently a delay in diagnosis. Physical examination may reveal a tender palpable abdominal or pelvic mass. Transvaginal and transabdominal ultrasound including Doppler flow studies are most useful in diagnosing ovarian torsion. As stated above, blood flow may be present on Doppler ultrasound if torsion is intermittent. Laparoscopy is the procedure of choice for the diagnosis and management of ovarian torsion. Whenever possible, untwisting of the adnexa with or without fixation to the pelvic sidewall should be performed. Despite delays in diagnosis, evidence suggests relatively high ovarian salvage rates of necrotic-appearing ovarian mass. In the presence of a mature cystic teratoma or other benign neoplasm, cystectomy should be performed. Ovarian torsion is rarely associated with gynecologic malignancy.

Cystic teratomas may rupture as a consequence of torsion or spontaneously in fewer than 1% of patients. Peritonitis is a well-described complication of cyst rupture and may occur in up to 10% of those with rupture. Ascites and Meigs' syndrome may be associated with struma ovarii. Malignant transformation is rare. Squamous cell carcinoma accounts for 80% of carcinomas arising in a cystic teratoma, followed by adenocarcinoma in 7% to 10% of cases.

The most common benign epithelial tumor is the serous cystadenoma, accounting for more than 25% of all benign ovarian tumors. They account for approximately 50% of serous tumors. The cysts may be unilocular or multiloculated and are bilateral in 15% to 20% of cases. Mucinous tumors account for approximately 15% of all ovarian tumors, and 75% of mucinous tumors are benign. Mucinous cystadenomas are more likely to be unilateral and can be massive, filling the entire abdomen. Benign mucinous tumors are more likely to be multiloculated and contain thick viscous fluid. Brenner tumors have been reported to occur with mucinous tumors. Ovarian cystectomy or oophorectomy is performed based on the size of the mass and the age and reproductive needs of the woman.

Benign solid tumors in the ovary consist of fibromas, thecomas, and Brenner tumors. Typically these tumors are small, and often they are discovered incidentally at the time of surgery for other gynecologic reasons. Meigs' syndrome (i.e., ascites and hydrothorax) has been reported with these benign neoplasms.

Endometrioma

Endometriosis is a progressive disease discussed in greater detail in Chapter 13, Endometriosis and Adenomyosis. Many patients with endometriosis are asymptomatic and small endometriomas involving the ovarian surface are not palpable on pelvic examination. Larger cysts filled with old blood range in size and can be 20 cm or more in diameter (Fig. 20-5). Symptomatic patients with endometriomas have symptoms similar to those of women with endometriosis involving other pelvic structures. Acute pain due to rupture of an endometrioma is a common presentation. Physical findings include lower abdominal and ovarian tenderness on pelvic examination. With advanced endometriosis, the pelvic organs may feel "fixed." Endometriomas usually do not respond to medical therapy. Surgical management reflects the patient's age and future reproductive plans. Two randomized studies of the laparoscopic management of ovarian endometrioma of greater than 3cm diameter revealed that, compared with laparoscopic cautery of the endometrioma, laparoscopic excision of the cyst wall was associated with a reduced rate of recurrence, reduced requirement for further surgery, and a reduced recurrence rate of dysmenorrhea, dyspareunia, and nonmenstrual pelvic pain. It was also associated with a subsequent increased rate of spontaneous pregnancy in women who had documented prior subfertility.

491

Ovarian Remnant Syndrome

Ovarian remnant syndrome has been increasingly recognized as a cause of pelvic pain after extirpative surgery. Adhesive disease due to endometriosis and pelvic inflammatory disease obscures surgical planes, and even experienced surgeons may inadvertently leave viable ovarian tissue *in situ*. The

Figure 20-5

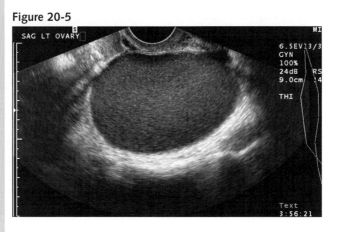

Endometrioma. Transvaginal sonographic image of the left ovary show a homogenous complex cystic mass with a thin smooth wall and increased through transmission. (Ultrasound courtesy of Samuel Johnson, MD.)

most common symptom is chronic pelvic pain, which may be accompanied by a retroperitoneal cystic mass. The ovarian remnant can be excised via laparotomy or laparoscopy. However, only a skilled surgeon or laparoscopist should perform this. The ureter must be identified and dissected from the remnant. Retroperitoneal resection of a remnant ovary is safe and provides relief of pelvic pain. Ovarian cancer has been reported to arise in an ovarian remnant.

Leiomyomas

Leiomyomas of the uterus are the most common gynecologic neoplasm, occurring in approximately 10% of white women and 30% to 40% of African American women older than 35 years of age. Most leiomyomas are asymptomatic and confined to the body of the uterus. The most common symptoms include enlarging pelvic-abdominal mass, pain, and bleeding. Pedunculated, parasitic, and broad ligament myomas present as firm palpable adnexal masses and are easily mistaken for an ovarian or tubal neoplasm. Pedunculated myomas may be accompanied by acute pelvic pain due to torsion similar to that seen with ovarian torsion. An ultrasound scan may reveal a solid mass or a cystic adnexal mass due to cystic degeneration (Figs. 20-6 and 20-7). A pedunculated myoma becomes parasitic as it outgrows its uterine blood supply and obtains a secondary blood supply from other organs such as the omentum or mesentery. Ascites and hydrothorax have been reported in association with a pedunculated myoma (i.e., pseudo-Meigs' syndrome). A broad ligament myoma may be mistaken for a solid adnexal neoplasm. Hydroureter is a common complication of broad ligament myomas.

Disseminated peritoneal leiomyomatosis is a rare condition that occurs primarily in premenopausal women. It is characterized by numerous nodules of benign smooth muscle proliferations and usually mimics the macroscopic appearance of peritoneal carcinomatosis. Careful histologic examination is required because the peritoneal implants resemble other malignancies.

Laparoscopy is effective for removing pedunculated myomas (see Fig. 20-7). Laparotomy may be required for larger pedunculated, broad

Figure 20-6

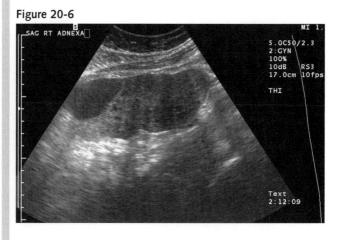

Cystic fibroid. Sagittal transabdominal sonographic image of the right adnexal demonstrates a predominantly solid hypoechoic mass with cystic area of degeneration anteriorly. (Ultrasound courtesy of Samuel Johnson, MD.)

Figure 20-7

Intraoperative appearance of cystic degeneration in pedunculated myoma.

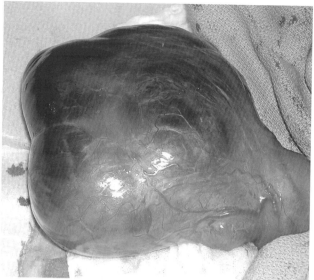

ligament, and parasitic myomas. Careful dissection and identification of the ureter as it courses through the pelvis is paramount in the surgical management of these myomas.

Leiomyosarcoma is a rare genital cancer. Malignant degeneration has been reported in approximately 0.5% of patients with myomas. It is unknown whether the myomas undergo sarcomatous transformation or whether the sarcoma arises spontaneously. Rapid growth of a previously diagnosed myoma or growth of a postmenopausal myoma should raise suspicion for sarcoma or other gynecologic malignancy.

Peritoneal Inclusion Cysts

Peritoneal inclusion cysts (Fig. 20-8) are usually a consequence of prior gynecologic or other intra-abdominal surgery. Ultrasound findings include thin septae with anechoic fluid. Most are asymptomatic and do not require

Figure 20-8

Inclusion cyst. Transvaginal sonographic image of an amorphous anechoic fluid collection with internal septa partially surrounding an ovary that is enlarged by a hemorrhagic cyst. (Ultrasound courtesy of Samuel Johnson, MD.)

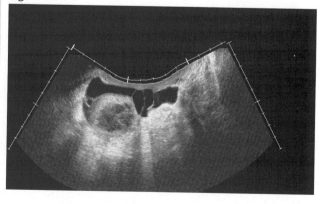

intervention. Symptomatic cysts can be drained by percutaneous or transvaginal aspiration aided by ultrasound or CT scan.

ADNEXAL MASS OF PERIMENOPAUSAL AND POSTMENOPAUSAL WOMEN

The majority of ovarian cancer is diagnosed in women older than 50 years of age. One in every 70 women will develop ovarian cancer, and two thirds of these cancers are stage III or IV at the time of diagnosis (Fig. 20-9). Serous cystadenocarcinoma is the most common ovarian cancer diagnosed in this age group. Although the prevalence of cancer increases dramatically, benign gynecologic conditions such as endometriosis and fibroids less frequently require surgical intervention in this age group. The evaluation and management of an adnexal mass in persons of this age group are similar to that previously described. With the greater likelihood of gynecologic cancer, referral to a gynecologic oncologist is more likely. Laparotomy and removal of the adnexa has been the standard approach to managing ovarian masses in perimenopausal and postmenopausal women. Laparoscopy is becoming more widely accepted as a treatment modality in this setting. Preoperative evaluation must exclude metastatic disease.

Other nongynecologic cancers occur more frequently in this age group as well. Approximately 1% of referrals for gynecologic cancers may have a tumor of nongynecologic gastrointestinal origin. Abdominal pain is the most common symptom, and an adnexal mass is usually present. Colon cancer is the most common gastrointestinal malignancy presenting as an adnexal mass in postmenopausal women. In addition to gynecologic and gastrointestinal cancer, cancer metastasizing to the ovary occurs more frequently, predominantly from the breast and stomach.

Figure 20-9

Ovarian malignancy. Transvaginal sonographic image demonstrates a complex cystic mass with multiple irregular solid mural nodules. (Ultrasound courtesy of Samuel Johnson, MD.)

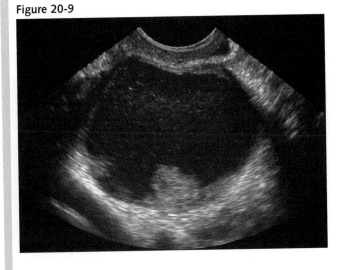

Postmenopausal Pelvic Abscess

The clinical characteristics of postmenopausal women with pelvic abscess are distinctly different from those of younger women, in whom community-acquired tubo-ovarian abscess usually represents end-stage disease of acute or chronic salpingitis. In postmenopausal women with this condition, a history of pelvic inflammatory disease is frequently absent. Symptoms are often vague and nonspecific. Most women have moderate to severe pelvic pain and may give a history of recent endometrial instrumentation. Only one third of women will have a history of fever. Bowel symptoms such as diarrhea or crampy abdominal pain are common. The medical history may be significant for diverticulitis or inflammatory bowel disease. Underlying gynecologic malignancy is reported in 25% to 44% of menopausal women with pelvic abscess. These cancers include carcinomas in the cervix, uterus, ovary, and fallopian tubes. Colon cancer is the most common gastrointestinal neoplasm causing pelvic abscess.

Postmenopausal women respond less quickly to medical therapy compared with younger women with tubo-ovarian abscess. Management consists of broad-spectrum antibiotic therapy and a thorough evaluation to exclude the presence of underlying gynecologic and nongynecologic cancer or other causes of intra-abdominal sepsis. Failure to respond to antibiotic therapy should prompt surgical intervention. Total abdominal hysterectomy and bilateral salpingo-oophorectomy are usually required. Common intraoperative complications include rupture of the abscess and bowel injury.

CONCLUSION

In summary, adnexal masses arise from multiple organ systems, although primarily from the ovary and fallopian tube. Symptoms are usually nonspecific. Therefore, it is imperative that a thorough history and physical examination are supplemented with appropriate laboratory and radiologic tests. Most adnexal masses can be managed by a practicing obstetrician-gynecologist. Women with masses suspicious for ovarian cancer should be referred to a gynecologist for further evaluation and management.

SUGGESTED READING

ACOG Committee Opinion No. 280: The role of the generalist obstetrician-gynecologist in the early detection of ovarian cancer. Obstet Gynecol 100:1413–1416, 2002.

Berlanda N, Ferrari MM, Mezzopane R, et al: Impact of a multiparameter, ultrasound-based triage on surgical management of adnexal masses. Ultrasound Obstet Gynecol 20:181–185, 2002.

Bromley B, Goodman H, Benacerraf BR: Comparison between sonographic morphology and Doppler

waveform for the diagnosis of ovarian malignancy. Obstet Gynecol 83(3):434–437, 1994.

Canis M, Pouly JL, Wattiez A, et al: Laparoscopic management of adnexal masses suspicious at ultrasound. Obstet Gynecol 89(5):679–683, 1997.

Dottino PR, Levine DA, Ripley DL, et al: Laparoscopic management of adnexal masses in premenopausal and postmenopausal women. Obstet Gynecol 93(2): 223–228, 1999.

Exacoustos C, Romanini ME, Rinaldo D, et al: Preoperative sonographic features of borderline tumors. Ultrasound Obstet Gynecol 25:50–59, 2005.

Heaton FC, Ledger WJ: Postmenopausal tuboovarian abscess. Obstet Gynecol 47(1):90–94, 1976.

Hulka JF, Hulka CA: Preoperative sonographic evaluation and laparoscopic management of persistent adnexal masses: A 1994 review. Journal of Am Assn of Gyn Lapar 1(3):197–205, 1994.

Im SS, Gordon AN, Buttin BM, et al: Validation of referral guidelines for women with pelvic masses. Obstet Gynecol 105(1):35–41, 2005.

Kurjak A, Schulman H, Sosic A: Transvaginal ultrasound, color flow, and Doppler waveform of the postmenopausal adnexal mass. Obstet Gynecol 80(6):917–921, 1992.

Lerner JP, Timor-Tritsch IE, Tederman A, et al: Transvaginal ultrasonographic characterization of ovarian masses with an improved, weighted scoring system. Am J Obstet Gynecol 170(1):81–85, 1994.

Manaffee SA, Elkins TE: Pelvic mass. In Ransom SB, McNeeley Jr. SG (eds): Gynecology for the Primary Care Provider. Philadelphia, W.B. Saunders, 1997, pp 113–124.

McNeeley SG, Hendrix SL, Mazzoni MM, et al: Medically sound, cost-effective treatment for pelvic inflammatory disease and tuboovarian abscess. Am J Obstet Gynecol 178(6):1272–1278, 1998.

Padilla LA, Radosevich DM, Milad MP: Accuracy of the pelvic exam in detecting adnexal masses. Obstet Gynecol 96(4):593–598, 2000.

Roman LD, Muderspach LI, Stein SM, et al: Pelvic examination, tumor marker level, and gray scale and Doppler sonography in the prediction of pelvic cancer. Obstet Gynecol 89(4):493–500, 1997.

Sassone AM, Timor-Tritch IE, Artner A, et al: Transvaginal sonography characterization of ovarian disease: Evaluation of a new scoring system to predict ovarian malignancy. Obstet Gynecol 78:70–76, 1991.

21

CONDITIONS OF THE FEMALE BREAST

Susan H. Lee and Stephen S. Falkenberry

INTRODUCTION

Obstetrician-gynecologists are considered specialists in women's health and are regarded by many women as their primary health care provider. In fact, most women will initially see their obstetrician-gynecologist for complaints of the breast. A breast examination is also a routine part of an annual gynecologic or first obstetric visit.

Although approximately 90% of all symptoms of the breast are related to benign breast disease, breast cancer remains the most common female malignancy, accounting for 32% of all cancers, and is second only to lung cancer in incidence. It is imperative that obstetrician-gynecologists have a current and thorough knowledge of benign breast disease and its treatments, appropriate assessments for evaluating women who present with breast abnormalities, risk factors, screening guidelines, and current treatment options for breast cancer. This chapter will review benign and malignant breast disease, including diagnosis, evaluation, and treatment.

BREAST ANATOMY

Embryology

The mammary glands arise from the primitive milk streak at approximately 5 weeks' gestation. The paired milk lines are ventral bands of ectoderm that extend from the axilla to the groin. The milk streak normally regresses so that mammary development proceeds on the thorax. Subsequent to milk streak regression, the epithelial breast buds differentiate into modified sweat glands. During the third trimester of gestation, canalization of the epithelium with duct formation occurs; during this stage of development, the nipple areolar complex forms and becomes pigmented. During puberty, under the influence of follicle-stimulating hormone and luteinizing hormone, the increase in ovarian estrogenesis leads to development and maturation of the female breast.

Anatomy of the Adult Breast

The anatomic extent of the breast is defined by the second and sixth ribs vertically and the sternal edge and midaxillary lines horizontally, with extension into the axilla (i.e., axillary tail of Spence). Approximately 90% of the blood supply to the breast occurs via the internal mammary and lateral thoracic arteries, with minor contributions from the thoracodorsal, intercostal, subscapular, and thoracoacromial arteries.

Lymphatic drainage of the breast is unidirectional and centrifugal with 97% and 3% of the lymphatics draining toward the axillary lymph nodes and the internal mammary lymph node, respectively. The axillary lymph nodes are divided into levels based on their relationship to the pectoralis minor muscle. Level 1 lymph nodes lie lateral to, level 2 posterior to, and level 3 medial to the pectoralis minor muscle. The internal mammary lymph nodes lie along the sternum in the intercostal spaces.

Nerves

The important nerves to consider relative to the treatment of breast cancer, which are often encountered in the performance of axillary lymphadenectomy, are as follows:

1. The long thoracic nerve courses along and innervates the serratus anterior muscle. Injury to this nerve results in scapular "winging."
2. The thoracodorsal nerve passes posterior to the axillary vessels and joins the thoracodorsal vessels coursing along the anterior surface and innervating the latissimus dorsi muscle. Injury to this nerve usually results in minor motor weakness of internal rotation and abduction of the arm.
3. The intercostal brachial nerve passes from medial to lateral, inferior to the axillary vessels. Injury to this nerve results in partial or full anesthesia to the medial arm ("pocketbook anesthesia").
4. The medial and lateral pectoral nerves, anatomically located opposite to their names, innervate the pectoralis major and minor muscles. Injury to these nerves results in weakness and atrophy of the pectoralis muscles.

Microscopic Anatomy

The mature female breast is composed of 15 to 20 lobes, each drained by a collecting duct, terminating at the nipple. The duct system is the functional unit of the breast, allowing transportation of milk produced in the glandular lobules. The terminal duct lobular unit (TDLU) is composed of the lobule, ductules within the lobule (acini), and short segments of terminal duct. Most malignancies arise in the TDLU.

With aging, and most noticeably after menopause, the breasts become less dense mammographically and softer to palpation due to fatty replacement of the breast parenchyma. Additionally, weakening of the suspensory ligaments of Cooper result in varying degrees of ptosis, especially after lactation.

BENIGN DISEASES OF THE BREAST

Fibrocystic Changes

Fibrocystic changes (FCC) is a nonspecific term referring to one or more benign physiologic changes and pathologic abnormalities. It is the most common condition of the breast; approximately one third of all women between 20 to 50 years old have findings on physical examination of FCC. Thirty to sixty percent of biopsy or autopsy specimens have shown histologic changes consistent with FCC of the breast, even in asymptomatic women. These changes may be nonproliferative, proliferative without atypia, or proliferative with atypia and can include cysts, fibrosis, metaplasia, papillomatosis, adenosis, and hyperplasia. Symptoms of FCC vary and include mastalgia (especially before and during menses), increased breast nodularity, or cyst formations. The development of FCC has been attributed to several unconfirmed factors, including hyperestrogenic states caused by ovarian dysfunction, progesterone deficiency, high prolactin secretion, high follicle-stimulating hormone–to–luteinizing hormone ratios, and low androgen levels. Symptoms of FCC decrease after menopause, and only about 10% of postmenopausal women are symptomatic.

499

Essentials of Diagnosis: Mastalgia

The most common symptom of FCC is mastalgia, which can be cyclical or noncyclical. Women who are premenopausal or nulliparous or were a young age at first parity are more likely to have cyclical mastalgia. Cysts and sclerosing adenosis may present as mastalgia, breast lumps, or mammographic abnormalities.

Treatment

The treatment of FCC is aimed at reassurance and palliation of symptoms by possibly correcting the various endocrine imbalances blamed for its etiology. Eighty to ninety percent of patients will decline treatment after reassurance that they do not have cancer. Because the most common presentation is mastalgia, most treatments are directed at this symptom:

1. Abstinence from certain medications (e.g., histamine and β-blockers, theophyllines) and methylxanthines (e.g., caffeine) has not proved to be beneficial according to randomized controlled trials. The same can be said for avoiding high-fat foods and high-tyramine-content foods, such as red wine.
2. Evening administration of primrose oil (3 g/day for 4 to 6 months), which contains gamma linolenic acid, a precursor of prostaglandin E_1, was effective in 45% and 30% of patients with cyclical and noncyclical mastalgia, respectively. It is used as first-line therapy due to minimal adverse effects (fewer than 2% of patients will have mild gastrointestinal discomfort) and low cost. However, the onset of action may take 4 to 6 weeks, and treatment is usually 4 to 6 pills a day for 3 to 6 months.

3. Oral contraceptives have demonstrated improvement in 50% of patients. The adverse effects of other hormones usually preclude their use unless symptoms are severe.

4. Bromocriptine suppresses prolactin secretion and has been shown to be effective in 20% of patients with noncyclical and 47% of patients with cyclical mastalgia. However, the use of bromocriptine is not currently recommended due to its potential serious adverse effects of seizures, strokes, and deaths, as well as intolerable symptoms of headaches, nausea, vomiting, and dizziness.

5. With tamoxifen, 90% of patients with cyclical and 56% of patients with noncyclical mastalgia have reduction in their symptoms. Adverse effects include symptoms of hot flashes, vaginal discharge, and increase in cataracts, thromboembolic events, and uterine cancer. Tamoxifen is indicated only for severe pain that is unresponsive to conservative treatment, and when pregnancy is contraindicated.

6. Danazol (100 mg twice a day for 2 months; more than 6 months' duration not recommended because of adverse effects), a testosterone derivative, is the only medication approved by the US Food and Drug Administration for mastalgia. Its mechanism of action is unknown. Seventy percent of patients with cyclical mastalgia and 31% of patients with noncyclical mastalgia find relief after danazol therapy. Its adverse effects include menstrual irregularities, hirsutism, muscle cramps, depression, dyspareunia, acne, voice changes, and weight gain. It is contraindicated in women with thromboembolic disease, and pregnancy should be avoided.

7. Luteinizing hormone–releasing agonists such as leuprolide acetate are used in acute severe cases of mastalgia with an 80% response rate; however, they significantly affect bone mass and are expensive.

8. Vitamins, diuretics, and progesterone have not been proved to be beneficial in randomized controlled trials.

Before medical treatment, other etiologies for mastalgia such as costochondritis, previous trauma, and activity-induced muscular pain must be ruled out. For patients who are refractory to pharmaceutical management, psychiatric evaluation and a trial of antidepressants should be considered. Breast pain with associated bloody nipple discharge, breast mass, or infection requires further evaluation.

Treatment of breast cysts depends on characteristics and symptoms. Reassurance is usually all that is required for small, simple asymptomatic cysts. Palpable or tender gross simple cysts may resolve with aspiration or may be excised if they are recurrent. The aspirate should not be sent for cytology unless there is an associated mass or the fluid is bloody. Asymptomatic, simple-appearing cysts that are documented on an ultrasound scan may be followed up with clinical examinations as long as they remain stable and the patient does not desire treatment. An ultrasound every 6 months for a year to document no change or resolution may be considered. A septated cyst can also be followed up with an ultrasound scan in a similar manner. An excisional biopsy is recommended for complex cysts or those associated with a solid lesion to rule out malignancy. Sclerosing adenosis, presenting as a mass or mammographic abnormality, also requires a biopsy for definitive diagnosis.

Cancer Association

FCCs are not associated with an increase in the risk of developing breast carcinoma unless there are proliferative changes, especially with atypia. Intraductal hyperplasia and sclerosing adenosis confer a slight increase in risk (1.5 to 2.0 times the relative risk), whereas intraductal hyperplasia with atypia (ADH) confers a moderate risk (4 to 5 times the relative risk). The relative risk is doubled in the presence of a family history positive for breast cancer in a first-degree relative. In patients with ADH on core biopsy, there is a 20% to 25% chance of ductal carcinoma *in situ* (DCIS) or invasive cancer in the surrounding tissue, and an excisional biopsy is recommended. Ten percent of women with ADH diagnosed on a breast biopsy specimen will develop invasive breast carcinoma over the subsequent 10 to 15 years. Tamoxifen for 5 years may also be considered for chemoprevention in patients with ADH if the 5-year risk is greater than 1.7 based on calculation with the Gail Model (Box 21-1) The risks involved with use of tamoxifen should be considered and reviewed with the patient to assist in the decision whether to initiate therapy.

Fibroadenoma

Fibroadenoma is the most common palpable mass in women younger than 30 years of age. Autopsy studies have found fibroadenomata in up to 25% of normal breasts. Fibroadenoma is a solid lesion composed of benign epithelial and mesenchymal elements (biphasic tumor) and originates in the TDLU. These lesions typically develop in teenagers and young reproductive-aged women. A multiplicity of lesions is seen in 10% to 15% of cases. Fibroadenomata probably develop in response to estrogenic stimulation of susceptible breast tissue. Studies have shown that women with fibroadenomata have higher than normal levels of plasma estradiol and lower than normal levels of plasma progesterone. There is evidence that the use of oral contraceptives before the age of 20 years may increase the risk of development of fibroadenomata. Although not considered a precursor lesion itself, studies have suggested that fibroadenomata may be a long-term risk factor for the development of breast cancer in

---

Box 21-1 Gail Model Risk Assessment Tool*

Race: white/Non–African American versus African American
Age (valid only for women older than 34 years of age)
Age at first menses
Age at first live birth
Number of first-degree relatives with breast cancer
Number of previous biopsies
If previous biopsies, presence of atypia

*Numbers are put into a Gail Model calculator, and that gives the 5-year and lifetime risk scores.

women with a family history of breast cancer or with fibroadenomata associated with ADH. The reported relative risks of breast cancer range from 1.6 to 3.1.

Diagnosis and Management

In most cases, fibroadenomata present as solitary palpable lumps or as non-palpable mammographic densities. As with any palpable or mammographic lesion, histologic or cytologic diagnosis is imperative. This can be accomplished with excision, core biopsy (usually under ultrasound guidance), or fine-needle aspiration cytology, depending on the circumstances and patient preference. Follow-up without confirmation of diagnosis in women younger than 20 to 25 years of age who have classic clinical and ultrasound findings of fibroadenomata depends on the size of the lesion, clinical symptoms, and the comfort level of the patient. The size limit of lesions that can be observed is controversial (2 versus 3 cm). In women older than 25 years of age, fine-needle cytology should be definitively consistent with the diagnosis of fibroadenoma; otherwise, histology is essential. In women who choose conservative follow-up over excision, fibroadenomata usually remain stable and 30% will experience regression in 5 years; however, they may also grow or become symptomatic, especially during pregnancy. Continued growth is an indication for excision to rule out the possibility of a more ominous lesion, such as phyllodes tumor, the sometimes malignant counterpart to fibroadenomata.

Breast Infections

The most common infectious processes in the breast are lactational mastitis and nonlactational subareolar abscesses.

Lactational Mastitis

Lactational mastitis is a bacterial infection, usually caused by *Staphylococcus aureus* or *Streptococcus* species, resulting from entry of oral flora from a nursing infant into the ductal system due to breaks in the surface epithelium. Infection initially manifests as painful erythema in a wedge-shaped distribution, usually in one breast. Fever, malaise, and leukocytosis are common. When recognized early, treatment with appropriate penicillins or cephalosporins usually results in prompt resolution. Clindamycin may be considered in patients who have severe allergies to penicillin. Continued pumping/feeding with the affected breast and warm compresses are also recommended. In untreated and sometimes treated cases, mastitis will progress to abscess formation, which is usually polymicrobial in etiology. Ultrasound and clinical examination are diagnostic, and successful treatment requires aspiration of the exudate (if amenable) or incision and drainage with appropriate broad-spectrum antibiotics to include gram-negative and anaerobic coverage.

Nonlactational (Subareolar) Abscess

Subareolar abscess in nonlactating women is the result of obliteration of the ductal lumen by squamous metaplasia, resulting in distension of the ducts by keratinous material with subsequent bacterial infection. Studies have demonstrated an association between ductal squamous metaplasia and cigarette smoking. Women with nonlactational abscesses present with a painful, erythematous breast, usually with an underlying area of induration, most commonly at the areolar edge. The abscess will spontaneously drain, forming a sinus at the areolar edge in most cases. The treatment is primarily incision and drainage with antibiotics. When the acute infection has resolved, the involved ductal system should be excised. Even with aggressive management and surgical excision, there is a 30% to 50% risk of recurrence, requiring removal of the nipple areolar complex by partial (central) mastectomy.

Nipple Discharge

Nipple discharge is a common and usually benign symptom. Nipple discharge is easily categorized by careful history and physical examination. Although numerous classification systems have been described, abnormal discharge from one or both nipples can be grouped into one of two categories:

1. Normal end-organ (breast) response to abnormal endocrine signals (e.g., galactorrhea)
2. Functional and/or structural abnormalities of the end organ

Galactorrhea

Galactorrhea is the inappropriate production of milk more than 1 year after weaning. The discharge is milky white in character, originates from multiple duct orifices, and is usually bilateral. Although causes of galactorrhea are numerous, they share a common feature—an absolute or relative increase in prolactin, leading to milk production. The most common cause of galactorrhea is medication-induced hyperprolactinemia (Box 21-2). More serious causes of hyperprolactinemia are prolactin-producing pituitary adenomas and hypothyroidism, both of which require therapy. In the absence of a prolactinoma or thyroid dysfunction, galactorrhea is not a life-threatening condition, though it may be associated with amenorrhea, infertility, and osteoporosis.

Box 21-2   Medications Associated With Galactorrhea
Opiates
Oral contraceptives
Tricyclic antidepressants
Methyldopa
Metoclopramide
Phenothiazines
Cimetidine
Calcium channel blockers
Prochlorperazine
Butyrophenones
Amphetamines

In the evaluation of galactorrhea, the history should focus on reproductive history including menstrual history, medication intake, symptoms suggestive of thyroid disease, and neurologic symptoms (especially changes in visual fields and headaches). Physical examination reveals multiductal, often bilateral, milky white discharge without other palpable findings.

Mammographic and ultrasound imaging are unrevealing. Clinical galactorrhea should be evaluated with a serum prolactin level and thyroid function studies. Although hyperprolactinemia is diagnostic of galactorrhea, galactorrhea can occur in the setting of a normal serum prolactin level (relative hyperprolactinemia). A normal serum prolactin level rules out a pituitary adenoma. Abnormal serum prolactin levels should be confirmed with fasting serum levels. If the hyperprolactinemia persists, magnetic resonance imaging (MRI) of the pituitary gland is appropriate, though microadenomas are rarely visible if the serum level is less than 100 ng/mL. Pituitary prolactinomas and hypothyroidism should be treated, but the decision to treat hyperprolactinemia in the absence of these specific diagnoses should be based on symptomatology, reproductive considerations, and perceived risk of long-term sequelae such as osteoporosis. Both pituitary adenomas and other nonthyroid causes of hyperprolactinemia are treated with dopamine agonists such as bromocriptine and cabergoline. Most micro- and small macroadenomas of the pituitary can be managed successfully with medical therapy, with surgical resection reserved for refractory cases.

End-Organ Lesions

Several conditions of the breast may result in nipple discharge. FCCs often cause a clear to yellow discharge, usually from multiple duct orifices, and may be spontaneous or provoked. Ductal ectasia is a benign condition characterized by structural weakening of the fibromuscular ductal wall, resulting in ductal dilation. There is an accumulation of ductal fluid, which is usually dark green and easily grossly mistaken for blood. Standard occult blood testing can distinguish sanguineous discharge from the dark green discharge associated with ductal ectasia. The most common cause of bloody nipple discharge is a benign intraductal papilloma. Although occasionally visible on mammogram or ultrasound, intraductal papilloma usually is diagnosed upon excision of the affected duct. Approximately 15% to 20% of cases of unilateral, uniductal, and spontaneous bloody discharge are associated with DCIS or invasive cancer, and duct excision should be performed.

In summary, women with clinical galactorrhea should undergo appropriate endocrinologic and imaging evaluation as previously described. Women with bilateral discharge not consistent with galactorrhea should be offered reassurance after performing appropriate physical and mammographic examination. In women with spontaneous, unilateral, uniductal, and especially bloody discharge, duct excision is recommended.

Fat Necrosis

Although fat necrosis is extremely rare, the presentation can mimic scirrhous or inflammatory breast carcinoma or a breast abscess. Fat necrosis is the result of trauma to the breast that may appear clinically as a retraction of breast tissue, tenderness, erythema, or a mass. The "trauma" to breast tissue may be caused by injury or can appear as a sequela to surgery. Radiation therapy for carcinoma may also exacerbate the formation of fat necrosis. Mammographic appearance varies with the stage of development of fat necrosis. In it early stages, it may present as nonspecific microcalcifications requiring a biopsy to rule out a malignancy. In the later stages, it may present as cysts with thick, possibly calcified walls specific to fat necrosis, or as a nonspecific irregular spiculated scar requiring a biopsy. Histologic examination reveals foreign body–type giant cells and foamy histiocytes with possible inflammatory cells surrounding lipid-filled small cysts with fibrosis in later stages.

If there is reliable history of previous trauma, observation for a finite period of time may be an option. Without resolution, biopsy must be performed for definitive diagnosis. If the only finding is a lipid-filled cyst with fibrous capsule calcification typical for fat necrosis, aspiration or continued observation can be considered. If there are also other findings such as a spiculated lesion or indeterminate microcalcifications, the possibility of fat necrosis and an adjacent malignancy must be entertained.

Malformation of the Breasts

Failure of the embryonic lines to regress results in ectopic breast tissue appearing as supernumerary nipples or accessory breast tissue, usually in the axillary, abdominal, or groin region. Locations outside of the milk line are very rare. The incidence of supernumerary nipples is 5% to 6% and 1% to 2% in the Asian and white population, respectively. In rare instances, there are associated renal and limb deformities. Supernumerary breast tissue most commonly occurs in the axilla. It may be unnoticed until pregnancy and lactation, when it responds to hormonal changes and becomes engorged and tender. Milk may be expressed if there is an associated nipple. The tissue usually regresses after parturition; if persistent, it may be surgically removed after the woman is finished with her childbearing. This ectopic breast tissue is susceptible to both benign and malignant changes that can occur in normally located breast tissue.

Other developmental abnormalities include failure of milk line development or its complete regression. These conditions are usually unilateral, are very rare, and may be associated with a congenital syndrome such as Poland's syndrome (i.e., congenital absence of the breast, pectoralis major muscle and upper limp deformities). The occurrence of bilateral precocious breast development or failure of breast development in puberty may be due to a systemic disorder. Ovarian tumors may produce precocious development and pituitary tumors and chromosome abnormalities (Turner's syndrome), and adrenal hyperplasia may cause lack of development.

The etiology of unilateral or bilateral hypertrophy of the breasts is unknown. Hypertrophy of the breasts usually occurs in puberty and occasionally with pregnancy and lactation. Medical treatment is ineffective, and surgical reduction mammoplasty with or without antihormonal therapy (e.g., danazol, tamoxifen) or bilateral mastectomy with reconstruction in extreme cases may be necessary. Minor asymmetry of the breasts is common, and usually reassurance is all that is required. With a large degree of asymmetry, surgery may be considered. Benign and malignant conditions must be considered if the onset of asymmetry is acute.

BREAST CANCER

According to the American Cancer Society's 2006 estimates, the numbers of women diagnosed with invasive and *in situ* (DCIS) breast cancer are 212,920 and 61,980, respectively. The lifetime risk of developing breast cancer is approximately 1 in 7, though this number assumes survival to the age of 85 years. Breast cancer is the third leading cause of cancer deaths (15% of all cancer deaths), and in 2006, it is estimated that 40,907 women will die from the disease. The increase in screening mammograms has been credited for the decreasing incidence of breast cancer deaths since 1990. Although the incidence of breast cancer has been decreasing in the past few years, the prevalence has been increasing as the baby boomer population enters menopause and survival for this malignancy improves. Also, as women delay their childbearing, more cases of pregnancy-associated breast cancer can be expected. Risk factors for breast cancer are listed in Box 21-3. It is important to note that oral contraceptives have not been proved to increase the risk of breast cancer.

Clinical Detection

In most cases, breast cancer presents as an asymptomatic mass or as a mammographic finding. Symptoms attributable to breast cancer such as skin ulceration, erythema, discharge, and pain are usually indicative of locally advanced disease. All palpable masses should be evaluated with appropriate imaging or biopsy studies to determine the nature of the mass.

Box 21-3   Risk Factors for Breast Cancer

Female sex
Increasing age (peaks at 70 to 80 years)
Past medical history of breast cancer
Family history (especially first-degree relatives)
BRCA1 or *BRCA2* gene mutation
Previous breast biopsies (especially proliferative changes with atypia)
Nulliparity
Delayed primiparity (older than 30 to 35 years old)
Early menarche (younger than 12 years old)
Late menopause (older than 55 years old)
Cyclical hormone replacement therapy (Women's Health Initiative study)
Previous radiation for Hodgkin's lymphoma
Higher socioeconomic status
Obesity (postmenopausal)
High alcohol consumption (more than 2 to 3 drinks/day)
Sedentary lifestyle (possible risk factor)

In the evaluation of a palpable mass, the single most important objective is to determine whether a mass is solid or cystic. With the exception of a classic fibroadenoma in women younger than the age of 20 to 25 years, solid masses require cytologic or histologic evaluation.

Early Detection

The presentation of breast cancer has changed due to the implementation of widespread screening mammography. Because of earlier stages at diagnosis and more diagnoses of DCIS, the prognosis has been improving. According to the Surveillance, Epidemiology, and End Results Program, the 5-year overall survival rate for breast cancer had increased from 75% in 1974–1976 to 86% in 1992–1998.

Several studies have supported a reduction of breast cancer mortality with regular screening mammograms. A trial of seven counties in Sweden demonstrated a decrease of 44% in death rates after a national screening program had been in effect for 10 years. In a meta-analysis of eight randomized trials, for women older than 50 years of offered mammography versus the control group, there was a 22% decrease in breast cancer mortality after 14 years of observation. In women between the ages of 40 and 49 years, there was a 20% decrease in breast cancer mortality, but these results were not evident until 11 years after the start of program. These numbers may be even greater because of improved technologic advances in mammography, including computer-assisted digital mammography, after these studies were done.

Although regular screening via mammogram is advocated for women 40 years of age and older, the recommended interval of screening varies by different organizations. The American Cancer Society, the American College of Radiology, the National Comprehensive Cancer Network, and the American Medical Women's Association recommend that women older than 40 years of age be offered annual screening mammography. The National Cancer Institute and the U.S. Preventive Services Task Force recommend mammogram screening every 1 to 2 years for all women older than 40 years old. The American College of Obstetrics and Gynecology recommends screening mammograms every 1 to 2 years for women aged 40 to 49 years and then annually starting at 50 years of age. Due to the limited studies on screening mammograms in women older than 74 years, there is no general consensus beyond this age. If a woman is healthy with minimal comorbidities, screening should be continued. According to the Cancer Genetics Studies Consortium, women with *BRCA1* or *BRCA2* mutations should be screened annually by mammography and biannually with clinical breast examinations beginning at 25 to 35 years of age. Women with a significant family history of breast cancer should be screened starting an age 10 years younger than the age at which the affected relative was diagnosed.

The Breast Imaging Reporting and Data System atlas (BIRADS) is set up by the American College of Radiology to standardize breast imaging reports including mammography, ultrasound, and MRI (Table 21-1). For BIRADS categories 4 and 5, if the histologic findings of the core biopsy

Table 21-1

BIRADS Category	Indication	Malignancy Risk	Follow-Up
0	Inconclusive	N/A	Additional imaging
1	Normal finding	N/A	Routine screening
2	Benign finding	N/A	Routine screening
3	Probable benign finding	<2.5%	Short-interval follow-up imaging (i.e., 6 months)
4	Indeterminate, suspicious finding	25% to 50%	Aspiration or biopsy (R/O malignancy)
5	High suspicion for malignancy	75% to 90%	Aspiration or biopsy (R/O malignancy)

R/O, Rule out.

are benign and there is concordance with the radiologic findings, patients can be followed up with a 6-month or annual radiologic examination, depending on the results. If a core biopsy cannot be performed due to technical difficulty or type of lesion (i.e., radial scar), if malignant or atypical cells are identified, or if the pathology results are inconclusive or discordant with the radiologic presentation, surgical excision is required.

There is no evidence thus far from randomized controlled trials supporting screening with ultrasound alone in women aged 40 years and older. Ultrasound can be used as an adjunct to screening mammography in this age group, but not as its replacement. Mammogram sensitivity is decreased with increased breast density, and the ultrasound can be used additionally in patients with dense breasts. Also, ultrasound has not been advocated as a screening tool in the general population because of a lack of standardization and an inability to identify microcalcifications (a possible sign of early breast cancer). In women younger than 40 years, the ultrasound scan can be used as the initial imaging test. On ultrasound, it is possible to differentiate a simple cyst from a complex cyst or solid lesion and to characterize the likelihood of malignancy. Solid or complex cystic lesions identified on ultrasound should be considered for biopsy. If the pathology is benign and concordant with the sonogram appearance, these patients may be followed up without surgical excision.

MRI can also be useful for acquiring additional information, but there is no evidence supporting its use for primary screening. The sensitivity of MRI is higher than mammograms for invasive carcinoma, but the specificity is lower and a biopsy is necessary to determine a lesion's benign or malignant nature. The sensitivity of MRI for DCIS is also lower because of its limited ability to detect microcalcifications, thus limiting its usefulness for initial screenings. MRI may be a useful adjunct for patients with previous breast surgeries, implants, dense breasts with a diagnosed cancer, or multicentric breast cancers or for women who are carriers of the *BRCA* mutation.

Although there are several ongoing randomized controlled trials to determine the efficacy of other screening modalities, mammography is currently the best screening tool. However, it is important to remember that approximately 10% of all breast cancers, especially lobular carcinoma, are not seen on mammography. The role of ductal lavage is controversial and investigational and currently should not be used in routine screening.

Annual physical examinations by a medical provider should be part of breast cancer screening. There are no definitive data on the benefit of breast self-examination, but it is recommended monthly, a week after menses, if the woman is comfortable performing it.

Pathology

Approximately 80% to 85% of malignant breast tumors are ductal adenocarcinomas. The term *not otherwise specified* (NOS) distinguishes the most common type of ductal carcinoma from other relatively uncommon ductal lesions such as tubular, medullary, and mucinous carcinomas. Due to mammographic screening, DCIS—the preinvasive counterpart to ductal carcinoma—has increased from 2% to 3% of all currently diagnosed breast cancers in mammographically screened women in the prescreening era to approximately 20% to 25%.

509

Invasive lobular carcinoma, characterized microscopically by cordlike stromal infiltration (i.e., "Indian filing"), accounts for approximately 10% to 15% of invasive carcinomas. Both ductal and lobular carcinomas arise in the TDLU. Invasive ductal and lobular carcinomas are similar in biologic behavior, and the prognosis and treatment are the same when matched for prognostic features such as tumor size, lymph node status, hormone receptor status, and vascular space involvement. Relative to ductal carcinomas, lobular carcinomas are more difficult to assess with regard to tumor size. Both mammography and clinical examination often underestimate the extent of lobular carcinomas due to the infiltrative pattern of growth seen on histology. The less common ductal carcinomas such as mucinous, medullary, tubular, and papillary carcinomas demonstrate a lower tendency to metastasize to regional nodes or distant sites than the more common NOS and lobular counterparts.

Parenchymal, vascular, lymphoid, and metastatic lesions of the breast compose fewer than 5% of breast malignancies and are beyond the scope of this review.

DCIS is a precursor to invasive ductal carcinoma, and therefore, treatment is aimed at removing the lesion and minimizing the risk of recurrence. When recurrences do occur, 50% of them are invasive.

Lobular carcinoma *in situ* (LCIS) is a peculiar lesion, in most cases representing a marker for abnormal breast epithelial proliferation. In addition, it presents a higher than normal risk for subsequent development of ductal and lobular breast cancer (both ipsilateral and contralateral). Recent evidence suggests that LCIS is indeed a precursor to invasive lobular carcinoma in more cases than previously recognized. The risk of developing breast cancer in either breast, regardless of the side of LCIS, is 1% to 1.5% per year, or a 20% to 30% lifetime risk. At this time, treatment is usually directed toward evaluating the lesion by excision to rule out coexisting invasion. If the lesion is localized without an adjacent invasive component or DCIS, observation with routine screening is recommended. If a patient has additional strong risk factors or desires surgical management, bilateral simple mastectomies with immediate reconstruction is the operation of choice. Tamoxifen has been shown to be of limited value in reducing the risk of invasive breast cancer in women with LCIS.

When a histologic diagnosis of cancer is made, further evaluation and management should be directed toward achieving the following objectives:

1. Determination of the extent of disease (i.e., staging)
2. Surgical excision of the cancer, when possible, with lumpectomy or mastectomy
3. Completion of locoregional treatment with radiation when indicated
4. Systemic therapy, when indicated, to address risk of known or distant disease (adjuvant treatment)
5. Surveillance for evidence of locoregional or distant recurrence
6. Reduction of risk of new breast primary cancers (prevention)

Staging

Breast cancer stage is determined by the combination of tumor size, nodal status, and presence or absence of distant metastases (TNM) (Table 21-2). In January 2003, the staging criteria were changed, especially with regard to regional lymph nodes. The number of positive axillary lymph nodes, as well as metastasis to the intramammary lymph nodes and the ipsilateral infraclavicular and supraclavicular lymph nodes, were taken into account. Compared with the previous staging criteria, the new criteria would upstage patients from stage II to III, thus removing higher-risk patients from stage II and improving the prognosis of stage III patients. This difference must be kept in mind when considering treatment because current stage II and III patients may not be the same as similarly staged patients when the efficacy of the treatments was studied. Also, the overall survival for stages II and III would be improved based on the new staging system.

Treatment

Surgical Treatment

The objectives of surgery are both therapeutic and diagnostic. They include the following:

1. Complete removal of the primary tumor with cosmetically acceptable results
2. Evaluation and possible removal of axillary lymph nodes for prognosis and locoregional control

The decision to perform breast-conservation surgery (i.e., wide local excision, partial mastectomy, or lumpectomy) or mastectomy is based on the following:

1. Patient preference
2. Tumor size relative to breast size

Table 21-2

Current Breast
Cancer Staging with
Tumor Size, Regional
Nodal Status, and
Distant Metastasis
(TNM)

Stage	TNM Criteria	TNM Description
0	T_{is} N0 M0	Noninvasive cancer, negative nodes, no distant metastasis
I	T1 N0 M0	Tumor ≤2 cm, negative nodes, no metastasis
IIA	T0–T1 N1 M0	Tumor ≤2 cm, positive 1–3 axillary node(s) or microscopic intramammary node, no distant metastasis
	T2 N0 M0	Tumor >2 but <5 cm, negative nodes, no distant metastasis
IIB	T2 N1 M0	Tumor >2 but <5 cm, positive 1–3 axillary node(s) or microscopic intramammary node, no distant metastasis
	T3 N0 M0	Tumor >5 cm, negative nodes, no distant metastasis
IIIA	T0–2 N2 M0	Tumor <5 cm, positive 4–9 axillary node(s) or clinically positive intramammary nodes without axillary metastasis, no distant metastasis
	T3 N1–2 M0	Tumor >5 cm, positive 1–9 axillary nodes or microscopic intramammary nodes or clinically positive intramammary nodes without axillary metastasis, no distant metastasis
IIIB	T4 N0–2 M0	Tumor of any size with extension to the chest wall (excluding pectoralis muscle) or skin involvement, edema (peau d'orange), skin ulceration, satellite nodules and/or inflammatory breast carcinoma, positive 1–9 axillary nodes or microscopic intramammary nodes or clinically positive intramammary nodes without axillary metastasis, no distant metastasis
IIIC	Any T N3 M0	Any tumor, positive ≤10 axillary lymph nodes or infraclavicular lymph nodes or clinically apparent ipsilateral internal mammary lymph nodes with 1–3 positive axillary lymph nodes or >3 axillary lymph nodes with only microscopic internal mammary lymph nodes or ipsilateral supraclavicular lymph nodes, no distant metastasis
IV	Any T Any N M1	Any tumor, any node, distant metastasis

is, *In situ*.

3. Focality of lesion
4. Medical eligibility or feasibility of radiation therapy in the postoperative setting

With neoadjuvant chemotherapy, women with locally advanced disease may be rendered eligible for breast-conservation surgery. Women with multicentric disease (involving more than one quadrant) usually require mastectomy.

Surgical Technique
Lumpectomy (i.e., partial mastectomy) entails the removal of the entire breast lesion with negative margins. The definition of negative margins

for invasive cancer is controversial and varies from one cell layer to 2 mm. With DCIS, larger margins of 2 mm to 1 cm are preferable. In cases of invasive breast cancer or DCIS with microinvasion, this is combined with axillary lymph node evaluation, usually a sentinel lymph node biopsy (SLNB). When mastectomy is performed for DCIS, an SLNB should be performed to address the possibility of finding invasive disease on final pathologic evaluation.

SLNB is a technique that allows selective identification and removal of the first-line axillary (sentinel) lymph nodes draining the tumor site in the breast. This is accomplished by injecting a combination of radiocolloid (technetium-99) and vital blue dyes such as isosulfan blue or methylene blue into the breast lesion or subareolar area of the breast and removing the lymph nodes demonstrating radiocolloid or blue dye uptake. A collimated gamma counter is used to identify the radiocolloid containing lymph nodes. The procedure is an outpatient operation, is usually done with the patient under local anesthesia with sedation, and theoretically carries a negligible risk of postoperative lymphedema. In experienced hands, the sentinel lymph node can be identified in 96% of cases, and studies have shown false-negative rates of 2% to 4% with no apparent increase in the risk of axillary recurrence relative to axillary lymphadenectomy. Removal of any suspicious-appearing lymph nodes at the time of SLNB is imperative to minimize the risk of false negativity. A lymph node may be falsely negative if tumor infiltration prevents uptake of the radioactive colloid or dye. If the SLNB is positive intraoperatively on touch preparation cytology or frozen-section histology, a full axillary lymph node dissection can be performed. If the results are negative, or if no intraoperative evaluation is performed, the final pathology will determine whether an axillary dissection is indicated. Occasionally, in patients of advanced age and multiple comorbidities, no further axillary dissection is performed.

Mastectomy entails the removal of the entire breast with the underlying pectoralis fascia. The pectoral muscles and nerves are preserved. When combined with axillary lymphadenectomy, the procedure is termed *modified radical mastectomy*. Radical mastectomy includes removal of the underlying pectoralis muscle and is, for the most part, a procedure of historical interest only. Immediate reconstruction with subpectoral implants, latissimus dorsi, or rectus abdominis myocutaneous flaps can be performed in patients who desire this option and especially in cases where the extent of disease (i.e., tumor size, lymph node status) does not suggest the need for postmastectomy radiation.

Systemic Therapy

Systemic therapy is used in the treatment of breast cancer for the following reasons: (1) to treat the possibility of occult metastatic disease (adjuvant therapy), (2) to treat known metastatic disease, and (3) to treat primary tumors before surgery is performed (i.e., neoadjuvant systemic therapy). The current systemic therapy options include cytotoxic chemotherapy, hormonal therapy, and agents such as the antibody to the growth factor Her-2/*neu*, trastuzumab.

Chemotherapy

Cytotoxic chemotherapy is a well-documented, effective therapy for the treatment of women at risk for systemic relapse. Most women younger than 60 years of age with primary tumors greater than 1 cm in diameter or with lymph node involvement should be considered for cytotoxic chemotherapy, in addition to hormonal therapy in cases of estrogen receptor positivity. Women older than 60 years of age with lymph node involvement or with tumors greater than 1 cm in diameter and hormone receptor negativity or tumors greater than 2 cm and hormone receptor positivity are also candidates for cytotoxic chemotherapy. Currently, the most active chemotherapy regimen in the adjuvant treatment of breast cancer is a combination of doxorubicin (Adriamycin) and cyclophosphamide (AC). Other commonly used regimens include taxanes such as paclitaxel, docetaxel, and a combination of cyclophosphamide, methotrexate, and 5-fluorouracil (CMF). Other drugs are currently being investigated in both the adjuvant and metastatic settings, including carboplatinum, gemcitabine, vinorelbine, capecitabine, and other antimetabolites. The choice of chemotherapy regimen should be based on the patient's overall medical condition and certain primary tumor characteristics. For instance, women whose tumors overexpress Her-2/*neu* have been shown to have a greater benefit from AC than CMF. The cardiotoxicity of doxorubicin is a limiting factor in patients with comorbid cardiac conditions. The addition of a taxane to AC has been shown in studies to decrease the risk of systemic relapse in patients treated in the adjuvant setting and is recommended in lymph node–positive patients. Early trials from the National Surgical Adjuvant Breast and Bowel Project showed no improvement in survival with the addition of chemotherapy to hormonal therapy in women older than 60 years with estrogen receptor–positive tumors 2 cm in diameter or smaller with negative lymph nodes. In this group, the value of cytotoxic chemotherapy is debatable. Although the relative benefit of chemotherapy in reducing the risk of systemic relapse, and therefore breast cancer mortality, is similar across prognostic subgroups, the absolute benefit will vary depending on the risk of relapse before adjuvant treatment. Most studies have shown an approximately 30% reduction in systemic relapse and mortality with the addition of systemic chemotherapy, particularly in women younger than 60 years of age with tumors greater than 1 cm in diameter.

Common adverse effects of chemotherapy include alopecia, nausea, myelosuppression, mucositis, and risk of second hematologic malignancies. As previously mentioned, doxorubicin carries the additional risk of cardiotoxicity.

Her-2/*neu* protein mediates growth, differentiation, and survival of cells. Between 20% and 30% of breast cancers are positive for Her-2/*neu* neu tumor marker overexpression, and the cancers tend to be more aggressive with a poorer prognosis. The results of the Herceptin Adjuvant (HERA) trial and the NSABP-31/ N9831 trials demonstrated a statistically significant increase in disease-free survival (DFS) of 8.4% after 2 years and 18% after 4 years. Based on these studies, Herceptin is recommended when the tumor is positive for Her-2/*neu* and is greater than 1 cm in diameter (regardless of lymph node metastases) or less than 1 cm in diameter with a positive lymph node. Herceptin also carries the risk of cardiotoxicity and is administered for 6 months to 1 year.

Hormonal Therapy

Approximately 80% of all breast cancers are positive for estrogen and progesterone receptors, thereby allowing for the systemic treatment of breast cancer with hormonal therapy. Tamoxifen is a selective estrogen receptor modulator and acts as an estrogen receptor antagonist in the breast and as an agonist in the uterus and bone. Studies of tamoxifen therapy for 5 years have demonstrated a 50% reduction in local breast recurrence, 30% decrease in mortality, and prevention of new breast cancer development. The risks of endometrial cancer and thromboembolic events due to hypercoagulability are increased two to four times with tamoxifen but occur in fewer than 1% of women taking the medication. Taking tamoxifen may also increase cataracts, but the most common adverse effects are hot flashes, vaginal discharge, and irregular menses. A benefit of tamoxifen therapy is preservation and possible increase in bone marrow density, thus decreasing the risk of osteoporosis. Pregnancy is not recommended during tamoxifen therapy, and contraception is advised. Tamoxifen may be offered to both premenopausal and postmenopausal women with hormone receptor positive tumors.

The major source of estrogen in postmenopausal women is the adrenal gland, with peripheral conversion of adrenal androgens to estrogens in adipose tissue and muscle. Aromatase completes the conversion of androgen to estrogens. Aromatase inhibitors block this enzyme and prevent estrogen production. Currently, anastrazole and letrozole are the most commonly used third-generation aromatase inhibitors. The 5-year update on the Arimidex or Tamoxifen Alone or in Combination trial showed that anastrozole significantly prolonged disease-free survival and time-to-recurrence and significantly reduced distant metastases and contralateral breast cancers when compared to tamoxifen in postmenopausal women with early-stage, hormone receptor–positive disease. The treatment period with aromatase inhibitors is also 5 years. This advantage of anastrazole over tamoxifen may be shown to be greater as the study continues. Unlike tamoxifen, anastrazole has significantly less increased risk of endometrial cancer and much less risk of hypercoagulability. However, it increases the risk of bone loss and fractures and can only be used in postmenopausal women. Supplementation with minerals, vitamins, and medication and close monitoring of bone density are recommended due to the risk for osteoporosis. Also, the lack of data on long-term safety and efficacy of anastrazole must be considered.

Neoadjuvant Chemotherapy

Neoadjuvant chemotherapy (also known as *preoperative* or *induction chemotherapy*) is used in patients to decrease the size of the tumor to allow for breast conservation surgery or to allow for surgery of locally advanced tumors (stage III) that are otherwise inoperable. Patients with stage III breast cancer are considered to have locally advanced breast cancer and have a high incidence of local recurrence with mastectomy alone. In addition to surgery, radiotherapy, chemotherapy, and hormonal therapy (if applicable) are used. With the advent of neoadjuvant chemotherapy, those patients with larger operable cancers may have the option of breast conservation surgery, and those patients with larger inoperable tumors without metastases may be rendered operable depending on response to treatment. There have even been reports of complete clinical remission in 10% to 20% of patients, and of these, one third have shown complete pathologic response.

Response to neoadjuvant chemotherapy is an important prognostic indicator of disease-free survival and overall survival. In studies, it decreased the size of the tumor by more than 50% in 80% to 90% of patients and demonstrated an 80% to 90% clinical nodal response. Approximately 45% of patients will be candidates for lumpectomy after neoadjuvant chemotherapy. It also allows for an evaluation of tumor response to chemotherapy and a change to alternative regimens if the first-line chemotherapy is ineffective. Complete response to neoadjuvant chemotherapy is a prognostic indicator of disease-free survival and overall survival. However, it impedes the ability to evaluate the original size of the tumor (especially if there is complete response) and preoperative axillary node status. Sentinel lymph node biopsy may be performed prior to the initiation of the chemotherapy for axillary staging. During the course of treatment, if there is excellent response, a clip should be placed to delineate the original location of the tumor. Survival has been demonstrated to be equal between neoadjuvant and adjuvant chemotherapy. Hormonal therapy alone as neoadjuvant therapy in receptor-positive locally advanced breast cancer is still investigational, but thus far studies have demonstrated better response with the addition of chemotherapy.

Radiation Therapy
Radiation therapy is an important treatment modality in reducing the risk of locoregional recurrence. It is given after the primary tumor is removed with satisfactory margins by lumpectomy. Adjuvant radiotherapy is not indicated after a mastectomy unless the tumor is greater than 5 cm in diameter or there are more than three positive lymph nodes. A boost dose can be given for positive margins after a mastectomy. Although the overall survival advantage of radiation therapy is small, adjuvant radiation therapy after breast conservation surgery reduces the risk of local recurrence by 60% to 65% over 10 years post-treatment. Traditionally, post–breast conservation surgery radiotherapy has consisted of whole breast teletherapy to a dose of approximately 5000 Gy with an additional 1000 to 1500 Gy boost to the tumor bed in cases of close margins or large primary tumor size. The supraclavicular nodes are included in the treatment field when multiple axillary lymph nodes are involved or in cases where inadequate or no axillary evaluation is performed.

An alternative to whole breast radiation currently being evaluated is accelerated or more limited tumor bed radiation therapy (partial breast irradiation). The rationale behind this approach is to limit the area of breast tissue treated, thereby preserving the option of future breast conservation and radiation in the event of recurrence or a new ipsilateral primary tumor, to shorten the duration of treatment, and possibly to minimize the toxicity to lung, heart, and breast skin. This can be accomplished through brachytherapy after-loading catheters, brachytherapy balloons (such as MammoSite), or limited teletherapy. Use of the MammoSite balloon has been increasing due to ease in placement and administration of radiation, and only 5 days of treatment versus 7 weeks in conventional therapy. Currently, there is a national trial being conducted to determine its long-term outcome.

Prognosis

The most important prognostic indicators in breast cancer are nodal status and tumor size. Without systemic therapy, a patient with negative lymph nodes has a 5-year recurrence risk of 20%, whereas with more than four positive nodes, the risk of recurrence is 55% to 80%, regardless of tumor size. The larger the tumor size, the higher the likelihood of nodal metastases. A tumor less than 1 cm in diameter has a 10% to 20% risk of axillary nodal metastases, and a tumor 2 to 3 cm in size has a 30% to 57% risk. Tumor grade, hormone receptor and histologic subtype status, and Her-2/*neu* status are other predictive factors of outcome. The lower the tumor grade and the higher the hormone receptor positivity, the better the prognosis. Good response to neoadjuvant chemotherapy is also thought to be a positive prognostic indicator. Survival is inversely proportional to clinical stage and has been increasing annually since 1989. Overall, patients with stage I cancer have a 10-year survival of 78%. Patients with stage I cancer and tumors less than 1 cm in diameter (T1a, T1b) have long-term survival greater than 90%. Patients with stage IV disease have a 5-year survival rate of approximately 10%.

Post-Treatment Follow-Up

The goals of post-treatment follow-up are as follows:

1. To monitor for disease recurrence, both locoregional and distant
2. To detect post-treatment adverse sequelae such as lymphedema, breast edema, breast contraction, or sequelae to chemotherapy, radiation therapy, or both
3. To assess other health and quality-of-life issues related to breast cancer diagnosis and treatment such as chronic fatigue, osteoporosis, sexual dysfunction, body image issues, depression, and reproductive or menopausal dysfunction
4. To enable early detection and prevention of new breast primary cancers

Although studies have failed to determine survival advantage for routine diagnostic studies aimed at detecting distant disease, detection of locoregional disease with clinical examination and radiologic screening is useful and makes possible the detection of treatable and curable recurrences. For this reason, women with breast cancer should be seen for clinical examination every 3 months during the first 2 to 3 years after treatment, after which the interval may be increased to every 4 to 6 months, depending on the disease status. Ipsilateral mammography is usually performed every 6 months for 1 to 2 years after breast conservation surgery and annually thereafter along with contralateral annual mammography. Routine studies such as tumor markers, chest radiography, computed tomography, and bone scanning are not recommended by the American Society of Clinical Oncology, and testing should be based on specific signs or symptoms.

Pregnancy-Associated Breast Cancer

Approximately 3% of breast cancers are diagnosed in pregnant women, complicating one in 3000 pregnancies. Pregnancy-associated breast cancer is almost always diagnosed as a clinical lesion, since pregnant women usually do not undergo mammographic screening during pregnancy. Relative to nonpregnant age-matched control subjects, pregnant women have significantly larger tumors and a higher incidence of lymph node metastasis. Because of this, prognosis is poorer in pregnancy-associated breast cancer. When pregnant and nonpregnant women are matched for known prognostic factors such as tumor size, lymph node status, vascular space involvement, and hormone receptor status, there is no difference in outcome. It is apparent that pregnancy itself does not adversely influence outcome; rather, more advanced disease at diagnosis explains differences in prognosis. Possible explanations for pregnant women presenting with more advanced disease are as follows:

1. Pregnant women do not undergo screening mammography.
2. Pregnancy-related breast changes make detection of palpable masses difficult.
3. There is a reluctance to perform diagnostic imaging and biopsy during pregnancy.
4. Delay in diagnosis may result from attributing palpable findings to pregnancy changes such as "blocked milk duct."

The lesson to be learned from these observations is that, as in nonpregnant women, palpable masses require appropriate evaluation without delay. Ultrasound and MRI are safe diagnostic modalities in pregnancy, and low-dose digital mammography with abdominal shielding poses minimal risk to the developing fetus, especially after organogenesis is complete.

The treatment of breast cancer in pregnancy is very similar to that in the nonpregnant woman. Breast conservation surgery and mastectomy can be performed safely during pregnancy, and chemotherapeutic agents such as doxorubicin and cyclophosphamide are well tolerated after the first trimester, with no reported increase is neonatal morbidity attributable directly to the chemotherapeutic agents.

Radiation therapy and radiocolloid injection for SLNB is contraindicated in pregnancy. Radiation effect on the fetus is dependent on gestational age. During preimplantation to 2 weeks' gestation, there is an "all or none" phenomenon resulting in death or no effect. During organogenesis, the radiation effects may be teratogenic. After the first trimester to birth, microcephaly, mental and physical developmental delays, and ocular lesions may occur. Hormonal therapy also should not be administered during gestation. With careful multidisciplinary planning, a favorable outcome can be anticipated.

Hereditary Breast Cancer

There will be a positive family history in approximately 15% to 20% of all patients with breast cancer, but a germline mutation can be identified in only 5% to 10%. The number of affected relatives, the relationship of the relatives to the patient, and the age at which these relatives were diagnosed influence breast cancer risk. The most prevalent germline mutations identified in breast cancer are *BRCA1* and *BRCA2*. They are increased in Ashkenazi Jews, French Canadians, and Icelanders.

BRCA1 composes 20% to 40% of familial breast cancers and is associated with a lifetime breast cancer risk of 50% to 85% and a second primary breast cancer of 40% to 60%. The gene is autosomal dominant and is located on chromosome 17. The breast cancers are usually hormone receptor–negative, carrying a less favorable prognosis. However, there is an increased risk for medullary breast cancer, which carries a favorable prognosis. There is a 16% to 44% lifetime risk for ovarian cancer and increases in risk for prostate and male breast cancer. There is a possible small increase in risk for melanoma and colon cancer.

BRCA2 composes 10% to 30% of familial breast cancers and also carries a 50% to 85% risk for breast cancer. There is also a 50% increase in risk for contralateral breast cancer by the age of 70 years. It is autosomal dominant and is located on chromosome 13. The breast cancers are usually hormone receptor positive, and the onset is later in age than *BRCA1* breast cancers. There is a 10% to 20% lifetime risk of ovarian cancer. It carries a greater risk of male breast cancer than *BRCA1*, with a 6.3% risk for male breast cancer by the age of 70 years (in the general population, this risk is less than 1%). Prostate, laryngeal, and pancreatic cancer and melanoma may also be associated with this gene mutation.

Genetic counseling and testing should be considered in patients who appear to be at an increased risk for carrying one of these germline mutations. If possible, it is most efficacious to test the family member affected with the breast cancer. It is important to consider the ethical, social, and legal implications of genetic susceptibility testing before any genetic workup. Patients who test positive as carriers of *BRCA1* or *BRCA2* gene mutations must be closely screened at a younger age. They may be screened annually by mammography and clinical breast examinations beginning at 25 to 35 years of age or starting at an age 10 years younger than the age at which the affected relative was diagnosed. Although there is no definitive consensus, annual MRI screening can be performed and staggered with the mammograms so that testing is done every 6 months. Bilateral prophylactic mastectomies may decrease the risk of breast cancer by 90%. In addition, bilateral prophylactic oophorectomies can be performed to decrease the risk of breast cancer by 25% to 50% and to decrease the risk of ovarian cancer by 99%. However, there is a persistent

1% risk of peritoneal cancer. It is imperative to remove the entire tubo-ovarian complex to decrease the risk of ovarian cancer. Chemoprevention with tamoxifen may confer a 50% reduction in risk pending a positive hormone receptor status. Other germline mutations less frequently associated with breast cancer are Li-Fraumeni syndrome, Cowden disease, Peutz-Jeghers syndrome, ataxia-telangiectasia, and hereditary nonpolyposis colorectal cancer.

Future Directions

Hope for major improvements in breast cancer morbidity and mortality over currently available treatment modalities rests on several possibilities. These include the following:

1. Better identification of women at risk is needed, with application of primary preventive strategies to these women. Currently, *BRCA1*, *BRCA2*, and, to a lesser extent, *p53* mutation detection allows identification of women at high risk for developing the 5% to 10% of cases attributable to these tumor-suppressor gene mutations. Unfortunately, the other 90% to 95% of cases are not explained by these mutations, and therefore, identification of other genetic predispositions holds great promise.

2. Improved screening tools such as digital mammography, high-resolution ultrasound, and breast MRI may lead to earlier diagnosis and improved outcomes.

3. Improvements are needed in the identification of women most likely to benefit from adjuvant therapy by distinguishing tumors at high and low risk of systemic relapse through genetic and biomolecular profiling (i.e., proteonomics). Currently, most women who receive chemotherapy, hormonal therapy, or both do not benefit from their treatment, yet they suffer the adverse effects of treatment. The majority of these women's conditions are destined not to recur. Accurate categorization of tumors would allow low-risk women to avoid the toxicity of treatment and allow high-risk women higher-intensity treatment. A tumor assay, Oncotype Dx, was in introduced in 1994, and it is predictive of the magnitude of benefit for chemotherapy in patients with estrogen receptor–positive, node-negative tumors. A Recurrence Score is calculated based upon a 21 gene panel, and a patient is placed in a low-, intermediate-, or high-risk category for the likelihood of recurrence within 10 years. Chemotherapy recommendations can then made depending on the Recurrence Score. Further long term followup is pending, but for patients fitting the criteria who are borderline candidates for chemotherapy or are uncertain about receiving chemotherapy, this assay may be helpful.

4. Novel treatments such as biomodulators, vaccines, and genetic therapies should be developed.

For now, the most important step is to improve compliance with recommended screening guidelines and to identify high-risk women to the extent that our current understanding permits.

KEY POINTS

1. Although the lifetime risk for breast cancer is one in seven, 90% of all patients' complaints are due to benign etiologies.

2. No palpable mass is unequivocally benign on clinical examination alone; therefore, all palpable masses require radiographic and, in some cases, cytologic or histologic evaluation.

3. The treatment for fibrocystic changes is aimed at the symptom(s) (usually mastalgia) and there is no increased risk of breast cancer unless there are proliferative changes, especially atypia.

4. Nipple discharge can be categorized according to history and physical examination findings. Thyroid disease and pituitary adenoma should be excluded in cases of galactorrhea. Malignant ductal lesions should be excluded in cases of spontaneous uniductal, unilateral discharge.

5. Fat necrosis is rare, may mimic malignancy on clinical examination and mammogram, and usually requires a pathology diagnosis.

6. Screening mammography is the best radiologic modality for breast cancer detection (not as accurate for lobular breast cancer) and has been credited with the decreasing mortality of breast cancer through early detection.

7. Currently, the majority of women with breast cancer are candidates for breast conservation surgery, either primarily or after neoadjuvant chemotherapy, without compromising survival.

8. Sentinel lymph node biopsy is a safe and effective alternative to standard axillary lymphadenectomy in women with invasive breast cancer and clinically normal axillary lymph nodes.

9. Chemotherapy should be considered for positive lymph node(s) and/or a tumor larger than 1 cm in diameter. Hormonal therapy is given if the estrogen and/or progesterone receptors are positive.

10. Adjuvant radiotherapy is given postlumpectomy after full excision of the tumor with negative margins and after any indicated chemotherapy. It is given after mastectomy if the tumor is larger than 5 cm in diameter or if there are more than three positive lymph nodes.

11. The evaluation of palpable abnormalities in pregnancy should not be delayed, and appropriate evaluation with ultrasound, mammography, and magnetic resonance imaging is safe. Breast biopsy is a safe procedure and can be performed with the patient under local anesthesia during pregnancy.

12. When corrected for stage and other prognostic factors, pregnancy-related breast cancers are similar to nonpregnancy cancers with regard to prognosis.

13. Five to ten percent of patients with breast cancer will have a germline mutation, usually *BRCA1* or *BRCA2*, but 15% to 20% will have a positive family history.

SUGGESTED READING

Bruzzi P, Green SB, Byar DP, et al: Estimating the population attributable risk for multiple risk factors using case-control data. Am J Epidemiol 122:904–914, 1985.

Falkenberry SS: Breast cancer in pregnancy. Obstet Gynecol Clin North Amer 29(1):225–232, 2002.

Falkenberry SS: In Gershenson D (ed): Surgical Procedures in the Diagnosis and Treatment of Breast Cancer: Operative Techniques in Gynecologic Surgery. vol 5:. Philadelphia, W.B. Saunders Company, 2000, pp 138–154.

Falkenberry SS: Nipple Discharge. Obstet Gynecol Clin North Amer 29(1):21–29, 2002.

Humphrey LL, Helfand M, Chan BKS, et al: Breast screening: A summary of the evidence for the U.S. Preventative Services Task Force. Ann Int Med 137:347–360, 2002.

Marchbanks PA, McDonald JA, Wilson H, et al: Oral contraceptives and the risk of breast cancer. N Engl J Med 346:2025–2032, 2002.

National Comprehensive Cancer Network, Inc: Practice Guidelines in Oncology vol 1. Jenkintown, PA, National Comprehensive Cancer Network, 2007.

Tavassoli FA: Pathology of the Breast, 2nd ed. Norwalk, CT, Appleton & Lange 1999.

Writing Group for the Women's Health Initiative Investigators: Risks and benefits of estrogen plus progestin in healthy postmenopausal women. JAMA 288:321–333, 2002.

521

22

GENITAL AND URINARY TRACT INFECTIONS

Paul K. Tulikangas and Megan O. Schimpf

INTRODUCTION

The female genitourinary tract is a continuous system, and organisms infecting one organ often infect adjacent organs. Although it is often separated into the upper and lower genitourinary tracts for descriptive purposes, its continuity must be kept in mind to understand the pathophysiology and natural history of genitourinary infections. This chapter will provide an overview of infections of the entire female genitourinary tract.

INFECTIONS OF THE VULVA

Patients with vulvar infections often present with nonspecific complaints of burning, itching, pain, dyspareunia, or a combination of these and are frequently seen by multiple health care professionals before an adequate diagnosis is made. Careful evaluation of the vulva must be undertaken by someone with a thorough understanding of the differential diagnosis for vulvar irritation. Patients with vulvar complaints must be evaluated in the office, not just treated for presumed candidal infections over the telephone.

Parasitic Vulvar Infections

The skin of the vulva is frequently a site of parasitic infestation. The two most common parasitic vulvar infections are pediculosis pubis and scabies. Both are caused by sexual contact or contact with contaminated clothes or bedding. According to the National Institutes of Health, approximately 3 million people in the United States are infected with pediculosis pubis annually. Although the incidence of scabies is difficult to determine, epidemics appear to cycle at approximately 10- to 30-year intervals. Pediculosis pubis is the most contagious sexually transmitted disease (STD), with over 90% of sexual contacts becoming infected after a single exposure.

Pediculosis pubis is caused by infestation with the crab louse, *Pthirus pubis*, which uses claws on its legs to attach to the skin at the base of the pubic hair, on which female lice lay eggs (i.e., nits). Eggs hatch within 5 to 10 days and develop into adult, egg-laying lice over a period of

10 days. Pale brown insects or their eggs can often be seen at the base of the hair shaft. The predominant clinical symptom is constant itching in the vulvar area, which is caused by allergic sensitization to the crab louse. Diagnosis can be made by examining scrapings under the microscope and visualizing the crablike louse. Pediculosis pubis is treated with permethrin 1% cream, applied to the affected areas and washed off after 10 minutes. Lindane 1% shampoo is an alternative but should not be used in children or in women who are pregnant or lactating.

Scabies is caused by the parasite *Sarcoptes scabiei*. These parasites typically burrow under the skin, where they deposit their ova. Unlike infestations with the crab louse, scabies is widespread over the body and causes diffuse itching. The most common manifestation of scabies is pruritic, papular lesions on the fingers or in the interdigital webs. Burrows are often visible on the wrists and elbows. Similar to pediculosis pubis, diagnosis can be made by microscopic examination of a skin scraping. Scabies is treated with permethrin 5% cream, which must be applied over the entire body from the neck down and then washed off in 8 to 14 hours. Alternative treatments include lindane 1% cream or oral ivermectin. After treatment, bedding and clothing should be decontaminated. Consideration should be given to treating anyone who has come into close contact with the patient.

Genital Warts

Genital warts are caused by members of the papilloma virus family. At least 30 types of human papilloma virus (HPV) have been discovered. Types 6 and 11 most often cause genital warts. Other types commonly present in the anogenital region, particularly types 16, 18, 31, 33, and 35, are associated with cervical neoplasia and will be covered in greater detail elsewhere. Patients with genital warts can be infected with multiple types of HPV.

Genital warts typically present as exophytic lesions on the posterior fourchette and labia. They can spread to the labia, perineum, perianal area, and vaginal or cervical areas. Small condylomata are often asymptomatic, whereas larger condylomata are usually painless but bleed easily.

Treatment is directed toward relief of symptoms from the exophytic lesions and induction of an immune response (Box 22-1). Although many treatments are effective in relieving the symptoms of condyloma, no therapy has been shown to eradicate HPV. Patients should be counseled about this before therapy and encouraged to use condoms.

Box 22-1   Recommended Treatment Regimens for External Genital Warts

Patient applied (one of the following):
Podofilox 0.5% solution or gel
Imiquimod 5% cream

Provider administered (one of the following):
Cryotherapy with liquid nitrogen or cryoprobe
Podophyllin resin 10% to 25%
Trichloroacetic acid or bichloroacetic acid 80% to 90%
Surgical removal

Centers of Disease Control and Prevention: Workowski KA, Berman SM: Sexually transmitted diseases treatment guidelines, 2006. MMWR 55:1–94, 2006.

ULCERATIVE GENITAL DISEASE

In the United States, the most common causes of genital ulcers in young, sexually active people are genital herpes, syphilis, and chancroid. There is, however, a long differential diagnosis of genital ulcers worldwide, and a careful travel and sexual history should be taken as part of the clinical examination.

Genital Herpes Infections

At least 50 million people in the United States are infected with the genital herpes simplex virus (HSV). Genital herpes is caused by viral infection with a double-stranded DNA virus that may cause latent or persistent infections. It is transmitted by either genital or oral-genital contact. Two types of HSV have been identified: types 1 (HSV-1) and 2 (HSV-2). Most recurrent cases of genital herpes are caused by HSV-2.

Many patients with genital HSV are unaware they are infected. However, primary infections tend to be the most symptomatic with the formation of blisters, which eventually form tender vesicles that develop into pustules. Dysuria, fever, headaches, myalgias, and rarely, aseptic meningitis can occur. Recurrent episodes occur in most infected women but the symptoms tend to be less severe.

Genital herpes infection is diagnosed by the pathognomonic appearance of vesicles that do not follow a neural distribution grouped together on an erythematous base. HSV can be isolated in cell cultures from the mucocutaneous lesions associated with a herpes outbreak. It is difficult, however, to isolate the virus from these lesions once they start to heal. HSV antibodies develop several weeks after infection, and serologic testing for these antibodies is available. This can determine whether a genital herpes infection is caused by HSV-1 or HSV-2 and can be helpful in counseling patients regarding recurrences.

Management of genital herpes should include counseling regarding sexual and perinatal transmission, the natural history of the disease, and types of therapy available. Oral antiviral medications are available to treat first clinical episodes and recurrent episodes and to serve as daily suppressive therapy (Box 22-2). Antiviral medications have been effective in reducing morbidity and decreasing the number of recurrences associated with HSV infections.

Syphilis

Unlike many other genital ulcerative conditions, syphilis can be a systemic disease and may present subtly at different stages. Although the incidence is decreasing across the United States, urban centers still have relatively high rates of syphilis.

Syphilis is caused by the spirochete *Treponema pallidum*. Transmission occurs through contact with infected mucocutaneous lesions, which are rare after the first year of untreated disease. Nonetheless, exposed contacts should still be evaluated. Syphilis can be transmitted vertically, so all pregnant women should be offered screening.

Primary syphilis is classically described as the first symptomatic episode of syphilis, which usually presents as a single painless ulcer or chancre at the site of infection, appearing approximately 3 weeks to 3 months after exposure.

525

Box 22-2 Recommended Treatment Regimens for Genital Herpes

First clinical episode of genital herpes (one of the following):
Acyclovir 400 mg taken orally three times a day for 7–10 days
Acyclovir 200 mg taken orally five times a day for 7–10 days
Valacyclovir 1 g taken orally twice a day for 7–10 days
Famciclovir 250 mg taken orally three times a day for 7–10 days

Episodic therapy for recurrent genital herpes (one of the following):
Acyclovir 800 mg taken orally twice a day for 5 days
Acyclovir 400 mg taken orally three times a day for 5 days
Acyclovir 800 mg taken orally three times a day for 2 days
Valacyclovir 500 mg taken orally twice a day for 3 days
Valacyclovir 1000 mg taken orally once a day for 5 days
Famciclovir 125 mg taken orally twice a day for 5 days
Famciclovir 1000 mg taken orally twice a day for 1 day

Suppressive therapy for recurrent genital herpes (one of the following):
Acyclovir 400 mg taken orally twice a day
Valacyclovir 500–1000 mg taken orally once a day
Famciclovir 250 mg taken orally twice a day

Centers for Disease Control and Prevention; Workowski KA, Berman SM: Sexually transmitted diseases treatment guidelines, 2006. MMWR 55:1–94, 2006.

Secondary syphilis includes skin changes such as a rash or multiple mucocutaneous lesions, joint pain, and lymphadenopathy. *Latent syphilis* is defined as the period after infection with *T. pallidum* when patients are seroreactive but have no other signs or symptoms of the disease. *Tertiary syphilis* presents with more severe systemic symptoms, including cardiac, ophthalmic, and auditory disease as well as gumma lesions. Any patients with advanced disease, including neurologic symptoms, gummas, ophthalmic disease, human immunodeficiency virus (HIV) infection, or failure of treatment, should be evaluated for neurosyphilis using examination of cerebral spinal fluid.

Presumptive diagnosis of syphilis can be made on the basis of serologic test results. This is initiated with either the Venereal Disease Research Laboratory or rapid plasma reagin test. Results from both of these nontreponemal tests may be negative at the time of initial presentation of a patient with syphilis, depending on the length of time since exposure. If the results of either are positive, a treponemal test such as the fluorescent treponemal antibody absorption test (FTA-ABS) should be performed for confirmation because several conditions can cause false-positive results on the first-line nontreponemal tests. Results of the FTA-ABS remain positive for life, even after successful therapy. Darkfield microscopy or direct fluorescent antibody staining of lesion exudates or tissue should be viewed as the diagnostic gold standard, but may not be available in clinical practice.

The most effective therapy for primary and secondary syphilis is benzathine penicillin G, 2.4 million units given intramuscularly in one dose. Both tertiary and neurosyphilis require longer regimens of therapy. Oral penicillin is not adequate. Patients diagnosed with syphilis with documented allergies to penicillin should be progressively desensitized and then treated, especially during pregnancy. Some penicillin-allergic patients have been treated with doxycycline or tetracycline, and some studies indicate that ceftriaxone or azithromycin may also be effective. All treated patients should be serologically retested at 3 and 6 months because treatment failures occur with all regimens.

Before the initiation of therapy, patients should be warned about the possibility of the Jarisch-Herxheimer reaction, an acute febrile illness with flulike symptoms seen in the first 24 hours after the initiation of treatment. Treatment is supportive.

Chancroid

Chancroid is an ulcerative genital condition caused by *Haemophilus ducreyi*. Transmission rates have been increasing in the United States, and chancroid has emerged as a major risk factor for HIV transmission in Africa. Patients typically present with a painful genital ulcer with or without painful lymphadenopathy, which is present in up to one half of cases. The ulcer is typically deep, painful, friable, and often purulent.

527

Definitive diagnosis can be made from a Gram stain of the base of the ulcerative lesion, which typically shows gram-negative bacilli in chains of clusters. Diagnosis may also be made with specialized cultures, but these are not widely available.

Treatment is curative and prevents transmission. Recommended treatment regimens vary based on regional antibiotic sensitivity patterns and are displayed in Box 22-3. Sexual contacts should be treated regardless of symptoms.

Lymphogranuloma Venereum

Lymphogranuloma venereum presents clinically as tender lymphadenopathy in the inguinal or femoral areas (called *buboes*), typically unilaterally. Some patients present with a single painless ulceration at the site of inoculation, but often this has resolved by the time patients are seen. Women and homosexual men may also develop proctocolitis or perianal inflammation. If untreated, patients can develop perineal scarring and fistulas. This disease is rare in the United States.

Lymphogranuloma venereum is caused by the obligate intracellular *Chlamydia trachomatis* serotypes L1, L2, or L3. Diagnosis is made by identification of *C. trachomatis* organisms from infected tissue by polymerase chain reaction testing or culture.

Box 22-3 Recommended Treatment Regimens for Chancroid*

One of the following:
Azithromycin 1 g taken orally in a single dose
Ceftriaxone 250 mg given intramuscularly in a single dose
Ciprofloxacin 500 mg taken orally twice a day for 3 days
Erythromycin base 500 mg taken orally three times per day for 7 days

---

*Ciprofloxacin is contraindicated for pregnant and lactating women. Azithromycin and ceftriaxone offer the advantage of single-dose therapy. Worldwide, several isolates with intermediate resistance to either ciproflaxin or erythromycin have been reported.
Centers for Disease Control and Prevention; Workowski KA, Berman SM: Sexually transmitted diseases treatment guidelines, 2006. MMWR 55:1–94, 2006.

The recommended treatment regimen is doxycycline 100 mg taken orally twice daily for 3 weeks. An alternative regimen is erythromycin 500 mg four times daily for 3 weeks. In some cases, buboes need to be aspirated or drained to prevent inguinal ulcerations and scarring. Although some clinicians have used azithromycin, especially in pregnant women, no data are available to support its effectiveness. All recent sexual partners should be tested.

Granuloma Inguinale

Granuloma inguinale, also known as *donovanosis*, is caused by *Klebsiella granulomatis*, a gram-negative intracellular bacterium. It presents with painless, indurated, ulcerative lesions in the genital, perineal, or inguinal areas without lymphadenopathy. The lesions are classically vascular and can bleed easily on contact, although some are sclerotic, necrotic, or hypertrophic. Granuloma inguinale is more common in developing countries than in the United States.

Diagnosis is made by histologic identification of Donovan bodies (i.e., bipolar staining rods within monocytes) from a biopsy specimen taken from the ulcer base. Chancroid may be confused with granuloma inguinale and should always be ruled out before diagnosis is made.

Treatment is with either doxycycline 100 mg twice daily for 3 weeks, trimethoprim-sulfamethoxazole (Bactrim DS) twice daily for at least 3 weeks, or azithromycin 1 g orally once per week for 3 weeks or until all lesions have healed. Additional therapy with gentamicin can be added if improvement is not seen in the first few days of therapy. Relapses have been seen 6 to 18 months after effective therapy. Sexual partners should be evaluated.

Tuberculosis

Tuberculosis, which is caused by *Mycobacterium tuberculosis*, can infect the genitourinary tract. Genital disease is a rare result of tuberculosis in the United States but is more prevalent in developing countries. Approximately 8% to 15% of patients with extrapulmonary tuberculosis experience genitourinary complications. Tuberculosis infections are acquired by inhalation of aerosolized droplets. Genitourinary tuberculosis is usually caused by metastatic spread of the organism through the bloodstream and lymphatic system.

The kidney is the most common site of infection in the genitourinary tract. Tuberculosis can cause calcified granulomas with sloughing of lesions into the collecting system, abscesses, calyceal strictures, and secondary hypertension. Tuberculosis may extend from the kidney into the ureter, where it can cause ureteritis, with strictures and destruction of the ureter. Tuberculosis that involves the bladder may result in ulcers, fibrosis, and ureteral stricture. Tuberculosis can also affect the female genital tract, resulting in chronic endometritis, tubal scarring, and infertility.

Evaluation for tuberculosis usually involves intradermal injection of a purified derivative of tuberculin. The site is examined after 48 to 72 hours; a positive reaction consists of an indurated area surrounded by erythema. Cutpoints for a positive test result have been defined by the Centers for Disease Control and Prevention but are beyond the scope of this chapter. Confirmation of diagnosis can then be made using acid-fast staining

528

and chest x-ray. If tubercular endometritis is suspected, a culture of endometrial biopsy tissue or menstrual blood can be obtained. Hysterosalpingographic changes for tuberculosis include sacculations, sinus formations, and "pipe-stem" fallopian tubes.

Treatment for tuberculosis includes multidrug combination regimens and should involve an infectious disease specialist. Surgical therapy is indicated if medical therapy fails.

VAGINITIS

The normal vaginal discharge contains secretions from glands adjacent to the vagina, vaginal transudate, cervical secretions, and the normal bacterial flora. The most common normal bacterial flora is lactobacillus, an aerobic gram-positive rod. Lactobacilli secrete hydrogen peroxide and convert sugars to lactic acid, which maintain a vaginal pH of 3.8 to 4.2.

Vaginal infections typically present as either an abnormal discharge or vaginal irritation. All vaginal complaints should be evaluated by a wet mount preparation, a vaginal pH test, and appropriate cervical cultures. Wet mount examination is performed by checking vaginal pH with phenaphthazine paper, then placing a drop of the vaginal discharge on two slides with a drop of saline. A drop of 10% potassium hydroxide (KOH) is added to one of the slides, and the examiner "whiffs" (i.e., smells) the KOH slide for the presence of a fishy (amine) odor. The saline sample is then examined under the microscope for the presence of clue cells, yeast, and motile trichomonads. Clue cells are vaginal epithelial cells covered in bacteria and have a granular appearance under the microscope.

Bacterial Vaginosis

Bacterial vaginosis (BV) is caused by an overgrowth of anaerobic bacteria, replacing the normal lactobacilli and causing an increase in vaginal pH. BV is typically polymicrobial but is usually associated with an overgrowth of *Gardnerella vaginalis* and *Mycoplasma hominis*. Other organisms commonly involved include *Mobiluncus* species, *Prevotella* species, *Porphyromonas* species, *Bacteroides* species, and *Peptostreptococcus* species. Although cultures for *G. vaginalis* have positive results in almost all cases of BV, *G. vaginalis* may be detected in 50% to 60% of healthy asymptomatic women.

Patients with BV are at increased risk for urinary tract infections (UTIs), pelvic inflammatory disease (PID), and vaginal cuff cellulitis at the time of hysterectomy. Pregnant women with BV are at increased risk for preterm labor and preterm premature rupture of membranes.

Although BV is more common in women with multiple sexual partners, it is not considered an STD because it is also found in celibate women; treatment of male partners does not prevent recurrences. BV may be asymptomatic or may present with a thin, homogenous vaginal discharge and a musty odor. BV is diagnosed by means of wet mount examination. Amsel's criteria for the diagnosis of BV by wet mount examination are listed in Box 22-4.

529

Box 22-4 Amsel's Criteria for the Diagnosis of Bacterial Vaginosis

Three of four of the following are necessary for diagnosis:
1. Thin, homogenous, white vaginal discharge
2. Clue cells (>20%)
3. Positive results of "whiff test"—a fishy odor when 10% KOH is applied to the discharge
4. Vaginal pH >4.5

Centers for Disease Control and Prevention; Workowski KA, Berman SM: Sexually transmitted diseases treatment guidelines, 2006. MMWR 55:1–94, 2006.

Treatment regimens for BV include oral metronidazole, 500 mg taken twice daily for 7 days; metronidazole gel 0.75%, one applicator administered intravaginally daily for 5 days; or clindamycin cream 2%, one applicator administered intravaginally at bedtime for 7 days.

Vulvovaginal Candidiasis

Vulvovaginal candidiasis (VVC) is a local yeast infection typically caused by *Candida albicans*. Non-*albicans* species have also been associated with VVC, including *C. glabrata*, *C. tropicalis*, and *C. parapsilosis*. Non-*albicans* infections are thought to be more resistant to topical imidazole and triazole therapies.

Patients with VVC typically present with vulvar or vaginal pruritus and burning, with or without dysuria. A thick white floccular discharge (like cottage cheese) is often noted. Many yeast infections are associated with systemic antibiotic use, diabetes mellitus, and immunosuppression. Diagnosis is made by physical examination in combination with the presence of hyphae or blastospores on KOH preparation. Candida vaginitis is associated with a normal vaginal pH. A small number of women may develop chronic recurrent VVC with persistent irritation, pruritus, or burning. Diagnosis in these women should be made by microscopy and fungal culture. It is important to note that many women with chronic irritative symptoms who assume they have chronic VVC actually have chronic atopic dermatitis or atrophic vulvovaginitis.

Box 22-5 outlines the topical therapies for VVC. In addition to these topical regimens, a one-time dose of fluconazole 150 mg has been effective in the treatment of uncomplicated VVC. Recurrent cases may respond to a second dose of fluconazole 72 hours after the first dose or a 7- to 14-day course of the topical regimens. In rare cases, boric acid gelatin capsules or nystatin vaginal suppositories may be helpful.

Trichomoniasis

Trichomoniasis is caused by the anaerobic protozoan *Trichomonas vaginalis*. Trichomoniasis is almost exclusively transmitted sexually. However, trichomonads can survive up to 45 minutes on clothing, towels, toilet seats, and bath water, and they can be transmitted through these fomites. The infection is common, infecting more than 180 million women worldwide and 2 to 3 million American women annually.

Women with trichomoniasis may be asymptomatic or may present with vaginal discharge, vulvar pruritus (25%), and dysuria (20%). Examination typically demonstrates a diffuse, malodorous, frothy discharge. Additionally,

---

Box 22-5   Recommended Treatments for Vulvovaginal Candidiasis

One of the following:

Butoconazole 2% cream 5 g administered intravaginally for 3 days

Butoconazole 2% cream 5 g (Butoconazole 1–sustained release), single intravaginal application

Clotrimazole 1% cream 5 g administered intravaginally for 7 to 14 days

Clotrimazole 100 mg vaginal tablet, one tablet per day for 7 days

Clotrimazole 100 mg vaginal tablet, two tablets for 3 days

Miconazole 2% cream 5 g administered intravaginally for 7 days

Miconazole 100 mg vaginal suppository, one suppository per day for 7 days

Miconazole 200 mg vaginal suppository, one suppository per day for 3 days

Miconazole 1200 mg vaginal suppository, taken once

Nystatin 100,000-unit vaginal tablet, one tablet per day for 14 days

Tioconazole 6.5% ointment 5 g intravaginally in a single application

Terconazole 0.4% cream 5 g administered intravaginally for 7 days

Terconazole 0.8% cream 5 g intravaginally for 3 days

Terconazole 80 mg vaginal suppository, one suppository per day for 3 days

Fluconazole 150 mg oral tablet, one tablet in a single dose

Centers for Disease Control and Prevention; Workowski KA, Berman SM: Sexually transmitted diseases treatment guidelines, 2006. MMWR 55:1–94, 2006.

erythema of the vagina and punctate hemorrhage of the cervix (i.e., "strawberry cervix") may be present in up to 10% of cases. Live, motile trichomonads are seen on the wet mount preparation with increased numbers of white blood cells, a vaginal pH of 5 to 7, and a positive whiff test result. Diagnosis can also be made by culture.

Trichomoniasis is treated with metronidazole 2 g administered orally in a single dose. An alternative regimen is metronidazole 500 mg given twice daily for 7 days. Partners should be treated in all cases, and women should be screened for the presence of other sexually transmitted infections, including HIV, syphilis, and hepatitis B. Topical treatments are not effective for trichomoniasis.

CERVICITIS

Chlamydia

Chlamydial cervicitis is a sexually transmitted infection caused by *Chlamydia trachomatis*, an obligate intracellular organism. *Chlamydia trachomatis* causes an estimated 3 million new sexually transmitted infections in the United States each year. Studies indicate that 75% to 90% of women and 50% to 90% of men with a chlamydial infection are asymptomatic. Common symptoms in females with chlamydia include mucopurulent cervicitis, urethral syndrome, inflammation of Bartholin's glands, and endomyometritis. Up to 40% of PID in the United States is caused by *C. trachomatis*. Finally, chlamydia may result in Fitz-Hugh-Curtis perihepatitis syndrome and infertility.

Because many people infected with chlamydia are asymptomatic, screening at-risk populations is important. All sexually active adolescents and women aged 20 to 25 years should be screened for chlamydia. Any women with a new sexual partner or multiple sexual partners should also be screened. It is critical that sexual partners are also referred for treatment because reinfection is common. Rescreening is recommended 3 to 4 months after treatment. If chlamydial cervicitis is detected and treated, morbidities such as PID, infertility, and chronic pelvic pain can be prevented. Chlamydia may be diagnosed by cervical culture, although rapid, accurate culture results may be difficult to obtain. For this reason, other diagnostic modalities have been developed, including direct fluorescent antibody testing, enzyme immunoassay, and polymerase chain reaction for the fluorescence of chlamydial nucleic acids. Treatment regimens for chlamydial cervicitis are outlined in Box 22-6.

Gonorrhea

Gonococcal infections are caused by the gram-negative diplococcus *Neisseria gonorrhoeae*. Like chlamydial infections, they are often asymptomatic in women and, if untreated, can lead to PID.

Disseminated gonococcal infection can develop from gonococcal bacteremia and often leads to petechial skin lesions on the extremities and joint involvement. Rare cases of endocarditis and meningitis can also be seen. Treatment of these severe sequelae usually involves inpatient intravenous antibiotics.

Selective media can be used to culture *N. gonorrhoeae*. However, a DNA probe is the most common form of testing. Because 10% to 30% of patients infected with *N. gonorrhoeae* will be coinfected with *C. trachomatis*, hlamydia should also undergo screening for *N. gonorrhoeae*. Many practitioners recommend dual therapy for both organisms unless chlamydia infection can be absolutely ruled out. Treatment regimens for uncomplicated gonococcal infections are listed in Box 22-7. Sexual partners should be treated to prevent reinfection and spread of these STDs.

UPPER GENITAL TRACT INFECTIONS

Endometritis

Endometritis, or inflammation of the lining of the uterus, can be either chronic or acute. The most common nonobstetric etiologies for acute endometritis are PID and recent gynecologic procedures. Common bacterial

---

Box 22-6 Treatment Regimens for Chlamydial Cervicitis

Recommended regimens (one of the following):
Azithromycin 1 g taken orally in a single dose
Doxycycline 100 mg taken orally twice daily for 7 days

Alternative regimens (one of the following):
Erythromycin base 500 mg four times daily for 7 days
Erythromycin ethylsuccinate 800 mg four times daily for 7 days
Ofloxacin 300 mg twice daily for 7 days
Levofloxacin 500 mg taken orally once a day for 7 days

Treatment in pregnancy (one of the following):
Azithromycin 1 g taken orally in a single dose
Amoxicillin 500 mg three times daily for 7 days

Centers for Disease Control and Prevention; Workowski KA, Berman SM: Sexually transmitted diseases treatment guidelines, 2006. MMWR 55:1–94, 2006.

> **Box 22-7** Recommended Treatment Regimens for Uncomplicated Gonococcal Cervicitis
>
> **One of the following:**
> Cefixime 400 mg taken orally in a single dose
> Ceftriaxone 125 mg administered intramuscularly in a single dose
> Ciprofloxacin 500 mg taken orally in a single dose*
> Ofloxacin 400 mg taken orally in a single dose*
> Levofloxacin 250 mg taken orally in a single dose*
>
> **Plus**
> Treatment for chlamydia if chlamydial infection is not ruled out

*Quinolones should not be used for infections in men having sex with men (MSM) or in those with a history of recent foreign travel, infections acquired in California or Hawaii, or infections acquired in other areas with increased quinolone-resistant *N. gonorrhoeae* (QRNG) prevalence. Centers for Disease Control and Prevention; Workowski KA, Berman SM: Sexually transmitted diseases treatment guidelines, 2006. MMWR 55:1–94, 2006.

infections include *C. trachomatis* and *N. gonorrhoeae*, along with tuberculosis in developing countries.

Chronic endometritis can be linked to a number of precipitating factors, including long-standing infection, foreign bodies including pedunculated fibroids and intrauterine devices, and recent radiation therapy. Patients present with symptoms of abnormal uterine bleeding, vague pelvic pain, or both. Diagnosis can be confirmed by endometrial biopsy and, in some cases, an endometrial culture. The diagnosis of chronic endometritis can be made with plasma cells on biopsy. The term *endomyometritis* is used when the infection affects the myometrium as well as the endometrium.

Because postoperative endometritis is a relatively rare complication, the American College of Obstetricians and Gynecologists does not recommend routine antibiotic prophylaxis for minor transvaginal procedures unless a woman has had previous pelvic infections or is undergoing surgical pregnancy termination. Patients with either of these characteristics should receive 3 days of postoperative therapy with doxycycline.

Acute endometritis is treated similarly to PID (*see* below). Chronic endometritis can be treated with 10 days of doxycycline.

Pelvic Inflammatory Disease

PID encompasses a spectrum of acute infections of the female genital tract, including cervicitis, endometritis, endomyometritis, parametritis, salpingitis, and tubo-ovarian abscesses (TOAs). It is the most frequent gynecologic reason for emergency department visits in the United States. When considering PID as a diagnosis, it is important to exclude other causes of abdominal pain in women.

Adolescents and women with a previous diagnosis of PID are at highest risk. A careful sexual history for new or multiple partners should be taken. Barrier contraception is protective, preventing up to 50% of endocervical gonococcal and chlamydial infections. The relationship between oral contraceptive use and PID is unclear.

The most common causes of PID are sexually transmitted organisms ascending from the vagina and cervix, including *C. trachomatis* and

N. gonorrhoeae. Fifteen percent of women with either endocervical chlamydia or gonorrhea go on to develop PID, and each organism accounts for one third of all PID cases in the United States. Most infections are polymicrobial and may include common vaginal flora such as streptococci, *Gardnerella vaginalis,* and anaerobes.

Frequent signs and symptoms of PID include abdominal pain or tenderness, adnexal tenderness, and cervical motion tenderness on pelvic examination, which are the minimum diagnostic criteria. Additional signs that favor PID include fever involving a temperature above 101°F (>38.3°C), mucopurulent cervical discharge, irregular vaginal bleeding, recent onset of symptoms (within the previous 48 hours), white blood cells on microscopic examination of vaginal discharge, elevated erythrocyte sedimentation rate, elevated C-reactive protein concentration, and cervical cultures with positive results for *C. trachomatis* and *N. gonorrhoeae.* Fitz-Hugh-Curtis syndrome, in which "violin-string" adhesions are seen near the liver on laparoscopy, was initially described in women with *N. gonorrhoeae* infections but is now linked to any widespread infection throughout the abdomen. It affects up to one third of patients with PID and may present acutely with right upper quadrant pain.

Diagnosis is sometimes difficult; no single sign or symptom is both sensitive and specific for the diagnosis of PID, and it is important for clinicians to maintain a low threshold to treat. Pelvic ultrasound, endometrial biopsy, and operative laparoscopy can be helpful in making a definitive diagnosis.

Long-term sequelae of PID can be devastating in the absence of prompt, effective treatment. Women who have had even one episode of PID are at higher risk for tubal factor infertility, ectopic pregnancy, recurrent PID, and chronic pain. A significant number of these women will never have been formally diagnosed with PID.

Given the usual polymicrobial nature of PID, antibiotic regimens cover a broad spectrum of pathogens. Treatment should be initiated with a presumptive, clinical diagnosis while culture results are pending. As previously stated, a low threshold should be maintained, and sexually active young women with a combination of lower abdominal pain, adnexal, and cervical motion tenderness should be treated with empiric therapy. Most women can be treated as outpatients. Box 22-8 outlines the oral antibiotic regimens available for treatment of PID. If a patient does not improve after 72 hours of outpatient treatment, hospitalization for parenteral therapy should be considered. At that time, further imaging and other diagnostic tests can be ordered if needed.

Hospitalization is reserved for patients with severe, systemic disease, uncertain diagnoses possibly requiring operative intervention (for example, appendicitis), pregnancy, failure to improve with or to tolerate oral therapy, high fever, persistent nausea and vomiting, or TOA. Some clinicians also advocate treating young, nulligravid patients and those likely to be noncompliant as outpatients with parenteral therapy. Intravenous therapy (Box 22-9) should be continued for 24 to 48 hours after significant clinical improvement before discharge home with a prescribed oral

---

Box 22-8 Outpatient Pelvic Inflammatory Disease Therapy

Regimen A
Ofloxacin 400 mg taken orally twice daily for 14 days*
or
Levofloxacin 500 mg taken orally once daily for 14 days*
with or without
Metronidazole 500 mg taken orally twice daily for 14 days

Regimen B
Ceftriaxone 250 mg administered intramuscularly in a single dose
plus
Doxycycline 100 mg taken orally twice a day for 14 days
with or without
Metronidazole 500 mg taken orally twice a day for 14 days
or
Cefoxitin 2 g administered intramuscularly in a single dose and Probenecid,
    1g orally administered concurrently in a single dose
plus
Doxycycline 100 mg taken orally twice a day for 14 days
with or without
Metronidazole 500 mg taken orally twice a day for 14 days
or
Other parenteral third-generation cephalosporin (e.g., ceftizoxime or cefotaxime)
plus
Doxycycline 100 mg taken orally twice a day for 14 days
with or without
Metronidazole 500 mg taken orally twice a day for 14 days

---

*Quinolones should not be used in persons with a history of recent foreign travel or partners' travel, infections acquired in California or Hawaii, or infections acquired in other areas with increased quinolone-resistant *N. gonorrhoeae* (QRNG) prevalence.
Centers for Disease Control and Prevention; Workowski KA, Berman SM: Sexually transmitted diseases treatment guidelines, 2006. MMWR 55:1–94, 2006.

therapy. Sexual partners of women with PID in the 60 days before diagnosis should be examined and treated.

Tubo-Ovarian Abscess

TOA can be a serious complication of PID, but it can also occur in association with diverticular disease or appendicitis or after pelvic surgery. TOA formation follows agglutination of neighboring pelvic organs (e.g., bowel, ovaries, and fallopian tubes), forming a palpable mass. These are usually polymicrobial abscesses that form pockets of purulent material encased by necrotic tissue and fibrin. Abscesses formed by acute PID contain a mixture of anaerobes and facultative or aerobic organisms.

Imaging helps makes the diagnosis of TOA apart from PID. Ultrasound is preferable, although a computed tomography (CT) scan may help rule out other diagnoses such as appendicitis.

A patient with a TOA should be admitted for parenteral antibiotic therapy with a broad-spectrum regimen that adequately covers anaerobic bacteria. Appropriate regimens include clindamycin plus an aminoglycoside, ofloxacin with metronidazole, or ampicillin/sulbactam with doxycycline.

Box 22-9   Parenteral PID Therapy

Regimen A
Cefotetan 2 g administered intravenously every 12 hours plus doxycycline 100 mg administered orally or intravenously every 12 hours

or

Cefoxitin 2 g administered intravenously every 6 hours plus doxycycline 100 mg administered orally or intravenously every 12 hours

Regimen B
Clindamycin 900 mg administered intravenously every 8 hours plus gentamicin 2 mg/kg of body weight administered intravenously or intramuscularly as a loading dose, then 1.5 mg/kg of body weight every 8 hours or single-daily dosing

Alternative regimens
Ofloxacin 400 mg administered intravenously every 12 hours*
with or without
Metronidazole 500 mg administered intravenously every 8 hours
or
Levofloxacin 500 mg administered intravenously daily*
with or without
Metronidazole 500 mg administered intravenously every 8 hours
or
Ampicillin/sulbactam 3 g administered intravenously every 6 hours plus doxycycline 100 mg administered orally or intravenously every 12 hours

*Quinolones should not be used in persons with a history of recent foreign travel or partners' travel, infections acquired in California or Hawaii, or infections acquired in other areas with increased quinolone-resistant *N. gonorrhoeae* (QRNG) prevalence.
Centers for Disease Control and Prevention; Workowski KA, Berman SM: Sexually transmitted diseases treatment guidelines, 2006. MMWR 55:1–94, 2006.

Patients should be carefully monitored for signs of sepsis or worsening infection. Administration of oral antibiotics should be continued for 10 to 14 days after improvement is seen with parenteral antibiotics, and soon after discharge patients should be seen for outpatient follow-up. Up to 75% of patients with TOA will respond to antibiotic therapy alone.

If abscesses do not respond to antibiotic therapy within 48 to 72 hours, surgical drainage is imperative. Some authors have reported success with percutaneous aspiration under ultrasound or CT guidance. If this fails or is deemed inappropriate, abscess drainage can be attempted laparoscopically or by laparotomy. In reproductive-aged women, every effort should be made to preserve ovarian and uterine function if childbearing has not been completed.

Human Immunodeficiency Virus

HIV is an RNA retrovirus that causes acquired immunodeficiency syndrome (AIDS) by attacking the cells of the immune system (helper [CD4] lymphocytes and monocytes). Infection of these cells leads to an eventual breakdown of the immune system, making the patient susceptible to opportunistic infections such as tuberculosis and *Pneumocystis carinii* pneumonia. The virus may also directly attack the central nervous system (causing the AIDS-dementia complex) and the gastrointestinal tract (causing malabsorption and diarrhea).

HIV is spread by the inoculation of blood via a contaminated needle or blood product, intimate sexual contact, or perinatal transmission. Over the past decade, heterosexual transmission of HIV has become increasingly important, with more than 40% of cases occurring after heterosexual transmission or intravenous drug use. Currently, more than 20% of persons infected with HIV are women.

Diagnosis of HIV infection is usually made using HIV type 1 antibody tests such as enzyme-linked immunosorbent assay, and then confirming positive results with Western blot analysis. Because infection with HIV may be asymptomatic, screening at-risk persons is critical in preventing the spread of this epidemic. HIV testing should be offered to all women diagnosed with or at risk for an STD (e.g., multiple sexual partners, history of STD). Screening is particularly important for women of reproductive age because antiretroviral treatment during pregnancy has significantly reduced the vertical transmission of HIV.

537

Although the natural history of the disease is variable, the median time from infection to the development of AIDS is about 10 years. This interval can be significantly altered by the use of antiretroviral therapy. Therapy for HIV/AIDS is guided by following the viral load and CD4 T-cell count. The goals of therapy include the suppression of viral load, restoration of the immune system, and improved quality of life. Multidrug therapy is best at accomplishing these goals. Specific treatment regimens are beyond the scope of this text, and HIV-positive women should be referred to an infectious disease specialist with experience treating HIV.

Viral Hepatitis

Hepatitis was initially described as *type A* or *infectious* hepatitis and *type B* or *serum hepatitis.* With the improvement in diagnostic testing, five different hepatitis viruses have been isolated: hepatitis A virus, hepatitis B virus, hepatitis C virus, hepatitis D virus, and hepatitis E virus. Although these viruses do not manifest their symptoms in the female genital tract, they are mentioned here because transmission of some types of hepatitis is associated with sexual exposure. Vaccination for hepatitis A and B should be recommended for any persons at risk for exposure to the virus.

URINARY TRACT INFECTIONS

UTIs are one of most common reasons for physician visits made by women in the United States and are a significant source of morbidity. A thorough understanding of the pathophysiology of UTIs, including common pathogenic organisms, is necessary to identify patients at risk and to prevent serious morbidity and mortality. Advances in therapy have shortened treatment courses and decreased morbidity for the majority of patients with UTI, but complicated infections of the urinary tract remain a significant challenge.

Urethritis

Women with urethritis typically complain of dysuria, frequency, and urgency. The urethra may be tender on examination, and pus may occasionally be expressed from the urethra, particularly if the periurethral glands are infected. Symptoms usually develop over a longer period of time than cystitis. Although urethritis commonly occurs with cystitis, the infections can be distinct. The "urethral syndrome" has similar symptoms to urethritis except that no organisms can be identified and symptoms are long lasting. In patients in whom no causative organism can be identified, interstitial cystitis and suburethral diverticulum should also be ruled out.

Organisms commonly isolated in patients with urethritis include gonococcus, *C. trachomatis*, trichomonas, and yeast. Urinary cultures usually have low counts of bacteria or no growth on culture, although white blood cells can be seen on urinalysis. Urethral and vaginal cultures should be performed for sexually transmitted infections. Therapy should be directed at the specific organism identified on the culture specimen. If no specific organism is identified, a full course of doxycycline or azithromycin should be prescribed to treat possible fastidious organisms.

Cystitis

Symptomatic lower UTIs are among the most common bacterial infections, responsible for as many as 8 million physician office visits and more than 100,000 hospital admissions annually. Even more infections are treated solely by phone consultation. The majority of these infections occur in young, healthy women and can be viewed as uncomplicated UTIs. These require minimal evaluation and therapy, provided that the patient has experience with the symptoms.

Women appear to be at higher risk for developing a UTI in part due to the short length of the female urethra (4 cm), as well as the short distance between the urethra and the rectum. Fecal flora can thus easily migrate to the urethra and ascend into the urinary tract, causing symptoms. Sexual activity increases this risk, as well as diaphragm or spermicide use.

Symptoms of a UTI include dysuria, frequent urination, small-volume voids, and urinary urgency, which have a high rate of sensitivity for diagnosis. Some patients might also report hematuria, suprapubic pain, or rarely, urinary retention.

Diagnosis can usually be made by means of a careful history in young, nonpregnant women, although urine culture is required for definitive diagnosis. In-office diagnosis can be made using a standard urine dipstick on a clean-catch urine specimen. Nitrite or leukocyte esterase can be used as indicators of bacteriuria. If equipment is available, a Gram stain of the urine for bacteria or microscopy for leukocytes (pyuria) and bacteria is also reliable.

Patients who have recently had a UTI treated with antibiotics require a formal urinalysis and urine culture with antibiotic sensitivities before the initiation of therapy. Classically, a UTI was defined as greater than 100,000 (10^5) colony-forming units of bacteria, but more recent studies have recommended that the threshold be lowered to 10^2 to 10^3 colony-forming units in symptomatic patients. Women with symptoms but negative in-office test results should be treated presumptively while culture results are pending because dipstick tests can miss low-count infections.

More than 75% of acute, uncomplicated UTIs are caused by *Escherichia coli*, which in some cases may be a distinctly virulent strain known to have factors associated with uropathogens. These include the type 1 pilus and the adhesin molecule FimH. *Staphylococcus saprophyticus* is the second most common pathogen, causing up to 15% of uncomplicated infections. Other UTIs are caused by enterococci, Gram-negative rods other than *E. coli* such as *Klebsiella* species, and more rare pathogens. Infections due to urea-splitting bacteria such as *Proteus* species require closer attention because of the risk of struvite kidney stone formation with persistent bacteruria.

Risk factors for complicated UTIs in women include pregnancy, advanced age, hospitalization, recent or current catheterization/instrumentation, anatomic abnormality, immunosuppression from chemotherapy or drugs, sickle cell disease, diabetes mellitus, recent antibiotic use, and recent UTI. All of these patients require urine cultures and close clinical attention. Very young females with UTIs should be evaluated for anatomic abnormalities or sexual abuse.

In otherwise healthy nonpregnant women with acute uncomplicated cystitis, 3-day therapy has been found to be effective at resolving symptoms and preventing recurrence without increasing bacterial resistance. Trimethoprim-sulfamethoxazole (TMP-SMX, Bactrim DS) is the standard therapy in this patient population (Box 22-10). Therapy with trimethoprim (TMP) alone or a fluoroquinolone for 3 days is also effective. Fluoroquinolones, however, are significantly more expensive than the TMP-containing regimens and are not recommended as initial therapy for this reason, as well as to prevent resistance to these valuable drugs.

However, resistance is growing to TMP-SMX, and in communities where resistance rates are known to be greater than 10% to 20%, fluoroquinolones

---

Box 22-10 Antibiotic Regimens for Urinary Tract Infection

Three-day regimen
Trimethoprim-sulfamethoxazole
  Double strength
Trimethoprim
Norfloxacin
Ciprofloxacin
Ofloxacin

Seven-day regimen
Amoxicillin
Nitrofurantoin
Cefixime
Amoxicillin-clavulanate
Trimethoprim-sulfamethoxazole
  Double strength

can be used as initial therapy. Any antibiotic use within the past 3 months has been linked to resistance and should prompt fluoroquinolone use. Fluoroquinolones are contraindicated in pregnancy.

Therapy involving nitrofurantoin (Macrodantin) for 7 days is growing in use in areas of high resistance to TMP-SMX. However, it is less effective against gram-negative bacilli other than *E. coli*. For 3-day therapy, β-lactam medications such as ampicillin and amoxicillin are less effective.

In women with severe irritative symptoms, phenazopyridine (Pyridium or Uristat) is available over the counter for analgesia. However, most patients with UTI get symptomatic relief after 72 hours of antibiotic therapy, and this is not usually necessary.

Radiographic imaging is rarely needed in simple UTIs but may be required for pyelonephritis or after multiple infections. For uncomplicated infections, no follow-up care or testing is needed. More than 90% of these patients will have eradication of bacteriuria.

Recurrent UTIs may involve the same bacteria as the initial infection, separated by an asymptomatic period. Of all women who are diagnosed with UTI, 10% to 20% will have another within a few months. These may be related to persistence of pathogenic fecal flora in the periurethral area. These women may also have genetic factors that predispose them to increased bacterial adhesion to the uroepithelium.

Prophylactic antibiotic therapy can be considered in specific situations but should not be overused to prevent antibiotic resistance. Patients with three or more UTIs in the past year or two within 6 months are candidates for continuous antibiotic prophylaxis, which involves TMP-SMX, TMP alone, or nitrofurantoin given daily at a low dose. In patients with fewer infections, patient-initiated self-treatment may be more appropriate. These patients have a prescription on hand that they can fill when they become symptomatic. A smaller number of patients can relate symptoms to sexual intercourse and are candidates for postcoital prophylaxis, using either single-dose fluoroquinolone or double-dose TMP-SMX.

Multiple nonpharmacologic therapies have been tried throughout the years. There is some evidence that cranberry juice will help treat or prevent UTI, possibly by decreasing adhesion of pathogenic bacteria to the uroepithelium. However, studies do not support sole therapy with cranberry juice, and it should only be used as an adjuvant therapy to appropriate antibiotics. Evidence does not link UTI with mode of wiping after voiding, type of undergarments, postcoital voiding, douching, or use of hot tubs. Topical estrogen cream has been shown to decrease the incidence of UTIs in postmenopausal women.

Some patients are found to have bacteriuria in the absence of symptoms of UTI. Asymptomatic bacteriuria is particularly common in elderly persons and patients with other medical problems, such as diabetes or an indwelling urinary catheter. Treatment can be frustrating for the patient and physician because the colonizing bacteria are difficult to permanently eradicate and frequently recur without serious long-term sequelae. Thus, most cases of asymptomatic bacteriuria do not need to be treated.

Pyelonephritis

Pyelonephritis is defined as infection and inflammation of the kidney and renal pelvis. Its diagnosis is clinical, and symptoms include back or flank pain with costovertebral angle tenderness on examination, fever (temperature higher than 38°C), bacteriuria, and possibly nausea and vomiting. Dysuria is a less common presenting symptom for pyelonephritis. *E. coli* accounts for up to 80% of cases. Other causative organisms include species of *Klebsiella, Proteus, Enterobacter, Pseudomonas, Serratia,* and *Citrobacter* species.

All patients with suspected pyelonephritis require a urinalysis and culture with sensitivity tests. Pyuria is almost universal in pyelonephritis, and white cell casts on urinalysis indicate upper urinary tract involvement. Infected patients can have an elevated white blood cell count, erythrocyte sedimentation rate, and C-reactive protein. Imaging is not usually required to make the diagnosis of pyelonephritis.

In patients with a mild infection without fever or other systemic complications, outpatient therapy is appropriate. All other patients should be hospitalized, particularly any patient who fits criteria for a complicated infection (e.g., immunocompromised patients, patients with urinary tract anomalies or infection associated with urologic surgery) or who may not be compliant. All pregnant patients with pyelonephritis should be hospitalized due to the risk of escalating infection, preterm labor, and possible sepsis with acute respiratory distress syndrome.

Recommended outpatient therapy includes a fluoroquinolone for 7 days or TMP-SMX for 14 days if the organism is known to be susceptible. For a gram-positive infection, amoxicillin or amoxicillin/clavulanic acid (Augmentin) can be used alone. Treatment can be refined once antibiotic sensitivities are available.

For inpatient therapy, parenteral therapy is recommended. This may consist of a fluoroquinolone, an aminoglycoside such as gentamicin with or without ampicillin, or an extended-spectrum cephalosporin with or without an aminoglycoside. After improvement and resolution of fever, the patient can be discharged to home with orders to complete 2 weeks of therapy. Ideally, culture-proven sensitivities can be used to design this regimen. For all treatment regimens, CT imaging or renal ultrasonography should be considered to rule out perinephric or intrarenal abscesses if no improvement of symptoms is seen within 72 hours.

CONCLUSIONS

A thorough knowledge of common causative organisms, appropriate diagnostic modalities, and treatment recommendations based on local antibiotic sensitivities is essential for the adequate care of patients presenting with genitourinary tract infections. In persons with sexually transmitted infections, care should be taken to test for concurrent infections including viral hepatitis and HIV. Counseling regarding risky behavior and evaluation and treatment of sexual partners is necessary to limit the spread of many of the sexually transmitted infections.

KEY POINTS

1. Patients diagnosed with a sexually transmitted infection should be offered testing for human immunodeficiency virus and viral hepatitis.
2. Vaginal discharge and pruritus should be evaluated with an examination, wet mount, vaginal pH, and cultures as indicated.
3. Attention should be paid to treating the sexual partners of any patient with a sexually transmitted disease.
4. Treatment of sexually transmitted infections should follow the current recommendations of the Centers for Disease Control and Prevention, with local antibiotic-resistance patterns taken into account.
5. Physicians should maintain a low threshold for the treatment of suspected pelvic inflammatory disease.
6. Young, healthy women with uncomplicated urinary tract infections can be treated with 3-day therapy using TMP-SMX as an outpatient without need for laboratory testing.
7. Risk factors for complicated urinary tract infections in women include pregnancy, advanced age, hospitalization, recent or current catheterization/instrumentation, anatomic abnormality, diabetes mellitus, or any recent antibiotic use, including medication for a recent urinary tract infection. All of these patients require urine cultures and closer clinical attention.
8. Uncomplicated pyelonephritis can be treated with outpatient antibiotic therapy.
9. Failure of symptoms to resolve within 72 hours of the start of antibiotic therapy for pyelonephritis should prompt radiologic evaluation for perinephric or infrarenal abscesses.

SUGGESTED READING

Beigi RH, Weisenfeld HC: Pelvic inflammatory disease: New diagnostic criteria and treatment. Obstet Gynecol Clin North Am 30:777–793, 2003.

Centers for Disease Control and Prevention; Workowski KA, Berman SM: Sexually transmitted diseases treatment guidelines, 2006. MMWR 55:1–94, 2006.

Eschenbach DA, Wolner-Hanssen P, Hawes SE, et al: Acute pelvic inflammatory disease: Associations of clinical and laboratory findings with laparoscopic findings. Obstet Gynecol 89:184–192, 1997.

Faro S: New considerations in treatment of urinary tract infections in adults. Urology 39:1–11, 1992.

Fihn SD: Clinical practice: Acute uncomplicated urinary tract infection in women. N Engl J Med 349:259–266, 2003.

McLaughlin SP, Carson CC: Urinary tract infections in women. Med Clin North Am 88:417–429, 2004.

Ness RB, Soper DE, Holley RL, et al: Effectiveness of inpatient and outpatient treatment strategies for women with pelvic inflammatory disease: Results from the Pelvic Inflammatory Disease Evaluation and Clinical Health (PEACH) Randomized Trial. Am J Obstet Gynecol 186:929–937, 2002.

Peipert JF: Clinical practice: Genital chlamydial infections. N Engl J Med 349:2424–2430, 2003.

Rubenstein JN, Schaeffer AJ: Managing complicated urinary tract infections: The urologic view. Infect Dis Clin North Am 17:333–351, 2003.

Stamm WE, Hooton TM: Management of urinary tract infections in adults. N Engl J Med 329:1328–1334, 1993.

Warren JW, Abrutyn E, Hebel JR, et al: Guidelines for antimicrobial treatment of uncomplicated acute bacterial cystitis and acute pyelonephritis in women: Infectious Diseases Society of America (IDSA). Clin Infect Dis 29:745–758, 1999.

Wise GJ, Marella VK: Genitourinary manifestations of tuberculosis. Urol Clin North Am 30:111–121, 2003.

23

PELVIC ORGAN PROLAPSE AND PELVIC FLOOR DYSFUNCTION

Andrew I. Sokol and Mark D. Walters

INTRODUCTION

Pelvic organ prolapse (POP) is a poorly understood condition affecting millions of women and is currently one of the most common indications for hysterectomy in the United States. Studies have shown that the prevalence of POP and pelvic floor dysfunction increases with advancing age. According to the U.S. Census Bureau, the number of women aged 60 years and older will almost double between 2000 and 2030. As this population ages, the impact of these disorders on quality of life and health care delivery will be profound. Additionally, increased attention to disorders of the pelvic floor and improved diagnostic and therapeutic modalities continue to increase the demand for health care services related to the pelvic floor.

Epidemiology of Prolapse

POP results in more than 300,000 surgeries per year. Studies suggest that up to 11% of all women will undergo a surgical procedure for POP or urinary incontinence by the age of 80 years, with a reoperation rate approaching 30%. Among ambulatory women, the prevalence of POP varies between 30% to 93%, depending on the population studied and the definitions used. Some studies suggest that the rate of mild to moderate prolapse approaches 50% in gynecologic populations not seeking care for POP, whereas the rate of severe prolapse (beyond the hymen) is only 2%. Because the symptoms of prolapse are nonspecific and its diagnosis requires examination, the true incidence and prevalence of POP are difficult to study. Adding to the difficulty in estimating its prevalence, prolapse is probably significantly underreported. Reasons for this are many, including patient embarrassment, fear of social stigmatization, and physician failure to inquire about the symptoms of prolapse.

Cost of Prolapse

The annual cost of POP is difficult to approximate, but the direct cost of surgical therapy for POP has been estimated to exceed $1 billion annually in the United States; this number can be expected to increase as the population ages and the number of older adults continues to grow. Costs associated with POP include the cost of protective undergarments, costs from loss of productivity, and direct and indirect medical expenses relating to prolapse. The true cost of prolapse, however, may be much higher than has been previously estimated because prolapse is underreported. Additionally, the costs of urinary and fecal incontinence, which often coexist with POP, are difficult to separate from those relating to POP.

Natural History of Prolapse

The natural history of POP is poorly understood. Most prolapse is mild, with fewer than 5% protruding outside of the introitus. Longitudinal studies of POP suggest that mild forms of prolapse may progress or recede, with the likelihood of regression being higher in milder cases. Regression is less likely with more advanced stages of POP.

TERMINOLOGY

The terminology and staging schemes used to describe POP have evolved over recent years. Although various staging systems exist, the following scheme has been recommended by the International Continence Society as a standardized way of assessing and reporting prolapse severity. The nomenclature for describing prolapse is described below. The staging of prolapse will be described later in the chapter.

Anterior Vaginal Wall Prolapse

Anterior vaginal prolapse is pathologic descent (beyond stage 0) of the anterior vaginal. The term *anterior vaginal prolapse* is preferred over *cystocele* because information obtained at the physical examination does not allow the exact identification of structures behind the prolapsing vaginal wall. If the bladder is identified behind the prolapsing anterior vaginal wall (by ancillary tests), the term *cystocele* may be used.

Posterior Vaginal Wall Prolapse

Posterior vaginal prolapse is pathologic descent (beyond stage 0) of the posterior vaginal wall. The term *posterior vaginal prolapse* is preferred over *rectocele* because information obtained at the physical examination does not allow the exact identification of structures behind the vaginal wall. If the anterior wall of the rectum is identified behind the prolapsing posterior vaginal wall (by ancillary tests), the term *rectocele* may be used.

Uterovaginal or Apical Prolapse

Uterine or apical prolapse is pathologic decent (beyond stage 0) of the uterus or vaginal apex (in women who have previously undergone hysterectomy).

Enterocele

An enterocele is a cul-de-sac abnormality containing peritoneum and intra-abdominal contents and involving the apical, anterior, or posterior compartments of the vagina. Enterocele may be a separate entity from apical prolapse.

ANATOMY AND MECHANISMS OF NORMAL SUPPORT

Pelvic Floor

An understanding of normal pelvic anatomy and support is needed before attempting to understand the pathophysiology and treatment of POP. This section briefly describes the anatomy and mechanisms of pelvic support, which maintain organs in their correct abdominopelvic positions. Reproductive anatomy is more thoroughly discussed in Chapter 4, Gynecologic Anatomy.

With the progression to an erect posture, the pelvis and vertebral column of humans underwent evolutionary changes to create a balance between intra-abdominal pressure and visceral support. The lumbosacral curve, a specific human characteristic, directs abdominal pressure forward onto the abdominal wall and pubic bones. Downward pressure is directed backward onto the sacrum and levator ani muscles, which fill in the pelvic cavity.

The pelvic floor is made up of muscular and fascial structures that enclose the abdominal-pelvic cavity, external vaginal opening, urethra, and rectum. The muscular components are described in more detail below. The fascial components consist of parietal and visceral (endopelvic) fascia. Parietal fascia covers the pelvic skeletal muscles and provides attachment of muscles to the bony pelvis; it is characterized histologically by regular arrangements of collagen. Visceral fascia is less discrete and exists throughout the pelvis as a meshwork of loosely arranged collagen, elastin, and adipose tissue through which the blood vessels, lymphatics, and nerves travel to reach the pelvic organs. By surgical convention, condensations of visceral endopelvic fascia have been described as discrete "ligaments" (such as the cardinal or uterosacral ligaments).

Pelvic Diaphragm

The broad name for the supportive striated muscles of the pelvic floor is the *levator ani muscle*. The levator ani muscle is, in fact, made up of a group of muscles that form part of the musculofascial diaphragm (i.e., pelvic diaphragm) that makes up the pelvic floor. The pelvic diaphragm collectively consists of the levator ani muscle and associated connective tissue attachments to the pelvis. The diaphragm is stretched like a hammock between the pubis and coccyx and is attached along the lateral pelvic walls to a thickened band in the obturator fascia, the arcus tendineus levator ani (Fig. 23-1). The levator ani functions as a unit but is described in two main parts: the diaphragmatic part (coccygeus and iliococcygeus muscles) and the pubovisceral part (pubococcygeus and puborectalis muscles).

The coccygeus muscles are paired and run from the lateral borders of the coccyx and sacrum to the ischial spines on each side, with the sacrospinous ligaments forming the tendinous components. The sacrospinous

545

Figure 23-1

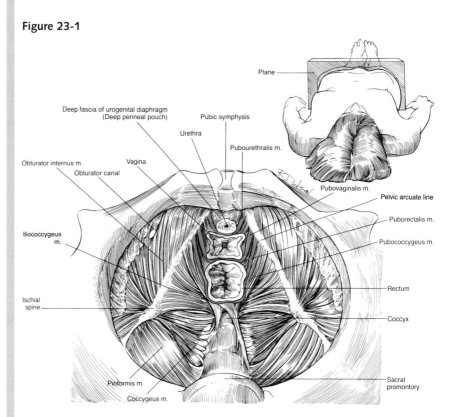

ligaments extend from the ischial spines on each side to the lower portion of the sacrum and coccyx. The fibromuscular coccygeus muscle and sacrospinous ligament are basically the same structure and thus are called the coccygeus-sacrospinous ligament (C-SSL). The fibromuscular coccygeus is attached directly to the underlying sacrotuberous ligament. Posterior to the C-SSL and sacrotuberous ligament are the gluteus maximus muscle and the fat of the ischiorectal fossa. The pudendal nerves and vessels lie directly posterior to the ischial spine. The sciatic nerve lies superior and lateral to the C-SSL. Also, an abundant vascular supply that includes the superior gluteal vessels and a hypogastric venous plexus lies superior to the C-SSL. The iliococcygeus muscles arise from the lateral pubic symphysis, travel over the pelvic sidewall (i.e., obturator internus muscle) attached to the arcus tendineus levator ani laterally, and meet in the midline at the anococcygeal raphe and the coccyx to form the levator plate (see Fig. 23-1).

The pubovisceral portion of the levator ani arises from the inner surface of the pubic bones and passes backward to insert into the anococcygeal raphe and the superior surface of the coccyx. The levator crura are formed by the pubococcygeus and puborectalis muscles, which have attachments to the lateral aspects of the vagina and rectum. The puborectalis forms a sling behind the rectum and contributes to anal continence. The genital hiatus is the space between the levator crura through which the rectum, vagina, and urethra pass.

The levator ani exhibits constant baseline tone and can also be voluntarily contracted. The muscle contains both type I (slow-twitch) fibers to maintain constant tone, and type II (fast-twitch) fibers to provide reflex and voluntary contractions. Innervation is provided primarily through the anterior sacral nerve roots of S2, S3, and S4 through the nerve of the levator ani.

Perineal Membrane

The perineal membrane is a triangular sheet of dense fibromuscular tissue that spans the anterior half of the pelvic outlet. It had previously been called the *urogenital diaphragm;* this change in name reflects the appreciation that it is not a two-layered structure with muscle in between (it is not a true diaphragm), as had been thought. The vagina and urethra pass through the perineal membrane and are supported by it. Cephalad to the perineal membrane is the striated urogenital sphincter muscle, which compresses the distal urethra.

547

Mechanisms of Normal Support

Normal support of the pelvic organs as well as urinary and fecal continence are maintained by a complex interplay between the striated muscles of the pelvic floor (i.e., levator ani muscle group) and their ligamentous attachments to the bony pelvis. Under most conditions, the pelvic muscles are the primary support for the pelvic organs, providing a firm yet elastic base on which they rest. The connective tissue attachments stabilize the pelvic organs in the correct position to receive optimal support from the pelvic muscles. When the pelvic muscles are relaxed during micturition or defecation, the connective tissue attachments help maintain support of the pelvic organs.

When the vagina is normally supported, it provides support to the bladder and urethra, cervix, and rectum. Other than the cervix, the uterus does not have fixed supports, as indicated by its ability to enlarge without restriction during pregnancy. The upper two thirds of the vagina are in a nearly horizontal orientation in a standing woman. Connective tissue attachments stabilize the vagina at different levels, as described by DeLancey and others (Fig. 23-2). The superior and lateral connective tissue attachments (cardinal-uterosacral ligament complex, or level I) support the cervix and upper vagina over the levator plate and away from the genital hiatus. The mid vagina is supported by lateral attachments to the arcus tendineus fasciae pelvis (also called the "white line"; level II). The lower vagina is supported predominantly by connections to the perineal membrane anteriorly and the perineal body posteriorly (level III).

PATHOPHYSIOLOGY OF POP AND PELVIC FLOOR DYSFUNCTION

POP can result when normal pelvic organ supports are chronically subjected to increases in intra-abdominal pressure or when defective genital support responds to normal intra-abdominal pressure. Individual organs that pass

Figure 23-2

Levels of support of the vagina. In level I (suspension), the endopelvic fascia suspends the vagina from the lateral pelvic walls. Fibers of level I extend both vertically and posteriorly toward the sacrum. In level II (attachment), the vagina is attached to the arcus tendineus fasciae pelvis and the superior fascia of the levator ani muscles. In level III, the vagina fuses with the perineal membrane, levator ani muscles, and perineal body. (From DeLancey JOL: Anatomic aspects of vaginal eversion after hysterectomy. Am J Obstet Gynecol 166:1717–1728, 1992.)

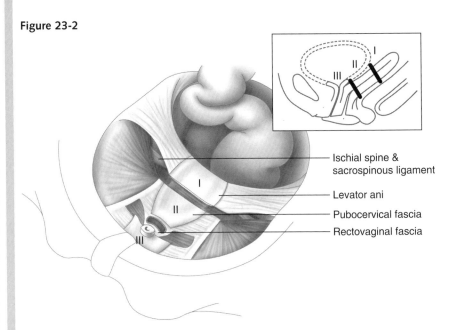

Ischial spine & sacrospinous ligament

Levator ani

Pubocervical fascia

Rectovaginal fascia

through the pelvic floor can lose support singly or in combination, resulting in various degrees and combinations of POP. This loss of support occurs as a result of damage to any of the pelvic supportive systems. These systems include the following structures: (1) the bony pelvis, to which the soft tissues ultimately attach; (2) the pelvic diaphragm, with the levator ani muscles and their fibromuscular attachments to the pelvic organs; (3) the subperitoneal retinaculum and smooth muscle component of the endopelvic fascia (the cardinal and uterosacral ligament complex); and (4) the perineal membrane. The perineal body and the walls of the vagina can lose tone and weaken from pathologic stretching from childbirth and the attenuating changes of aging and menopause. The vaginal epithelium covering the connective tissue is not important in maintaining normal support.

The pathophysiology of POP is poorly understood, and multiple theories explaining its etiology have been proposed. Some studies suggest that connective tissue abnormalities significantly contribute to prolapse, with the excessive synthesis of the weaker type III collagen in women with prolapse. Others have suggested that chronic increases in abdominopelvic pressure result in stretching and weakening of the pelvic floor musculature, with resultant pelvic floor relaxation and POP.

Richardson believed that the connective tissue around the vaginal tube (i.e., endopelvic fascia) does not stretch or attenuate but rather breaks at specific definable points (site-specific defects). By integrating the concepts of the suspension of level I with breaks in the pelvic connective tissue, one can conclude that vaginal apex or uterine prolapse, for instance, results from specific defects of the presacral endopelvic fascia (cardinal-uterosacral ligaments) where they connect to the apex of the vagina. Loss of support or integrity of the anterior and posterior vaginal walls results in anterior and posterior vaginal wall prolapse, respectively. Furthermore, when the muscles of the pelvic diaphragm weaken as a result of congenital factors, childbirth injury, pelvic neuropathy, or aging, the levator ani muscles lose resting tone and fail to contract quickly and strongly with increases in intra-abdominal pressure. Muscular atrophy and a wider levator hiatus result; weak and less rapid muscle contractions with rises in intra-abdominal pressure contribute to related symptoms of urinary and fecal incontinence.

Apical enterocele is a common defect seen in women with prior hysterectomy. In this case, the anterior vaginal wall muscularis (i.e., pubocervical muscularis), the rectovaginal muscularis posteriorly, or the rectovaginal fascia (also called *Denonvilliers' fascia*) have separated from the supportive endopelvic fascia (uterosacral ligaments) at the apex of the vagina. With apical and posterior enterocele, a defect occurs at the superior or transverse portion of rectovaginal muscularis allowing a peritoneal sac with intra-abdominal contents to herniate between the rectum and vaginal apex. A poorly supported vaginal apex or posterior vaginal wall often prolapses with the enterocele, leading to concurrent apical and posterior vaginal wall prolapse.

The pathophysiology of POP is probably multifactorial, resulting from a variety of factors that vary among individuals. As the mechanisms of support and prolapse become further elucidated, more effective therapies can be developed. Additionally, as understanding about the mechanisms of support and the pathophysiology improves, focus can be shift from treatment to prevention.

RISK FACTORS FOR PROLAPSE AND PELVIC FLOOR DYSFUNCTION

Multiple risk factors have been identified that increase the risk of POP, with certain demographic groups being more prone than others (Box 23-1). Although data are limited, most studies show that the prevalence of POP increases with age, with studies demonstrating a 16% to 20% increased odds of having prolapse per decade of life. Studies on racial differences in prolapse rates are controversial, with some showing a higher prolapse rate in white versus non-white women, whereas others show

Box 23-1 Possible Risk Factors for Prolapse
Nonmodifiable
Increasing age
White race
Menopause
Modifiable
Increasing parity
Operative vaginal delivery
Chronic increases in intra-abdominal pressure
Obesity

higher prolapse rates in African American or Hispanic women compared with white women. Most epidemiologic studies, however, have limited minority representation; reasons for possible racial differences in prolapse rates might include genetic, anatomic, or cultural factors as well as differences in the reporting and diagnosis of prolapse in certain ethnic groups. Data on the effects of menopause and estrogen on prolapse are limited. Although most prolapse occurs in postmenopausal women, few studies have evaluated the effects of menopause after controlling for age. Furthermore, data on exogenous estrogen replacement for prolapse prevention or treatment are very limited.

In addition to the above-mentioned nonmodifiable risk factors, several potentially modifiable risk factors for prolapse have been identified. Several studies show that increasing parity is linked to an increased prevalence of prolapse, with the prolapse risk doubling after the first birth and increasing approximately 10% to 20% for each subsequent pregnancy. Other studies suggest that the largest risk increase comes with the first pregnancy, with more modest increases for subsequent pregnancies. The role of mode of delivery (vaginal, operative, or abdominal) on POP is not completely understood. Some studies have identified operative vaginal delivery (with vacuum or forceps) as a risk factor for the future surgical treatment of prolapse or urinary incontinence.

Some evidence suggests that conditions and life situations that chronically increase intra-abdominal pressure can predispose to uterine or vaginal prolapse. These factors include heavy lifting at work, chronic coughing, and bowel dysfunction. Data on the relationship between smoking and POP are controversial, with some studies showing up to a doubled risk for POP and others showing a paradoxical protective effect. Most studies show higher rates of prolapse in overweight or obese women. Some studies show increasing prolapse rates with increasing body mass index (with more than 30 kg/m^2 defining obesity), whereas other studies show higher rates of prolapse in those with greater hip circumference measurements (i.e., truncal obesity). The magnitude of the effect seems to vary by anatomic site, with the strongest effect on posterior vaginal wall prolapse.

Distortions of the normal vaginal axis during reconstructive pelvic surgery are known to predispose women to the development of prolapse at an anatomic site opposite to where the repair was performed. Examples of this are the development of posterior vaginal wall prolapse after colposuspension procedures for stress incontinence and the development of anterior vaginal wall prolapse after suspension of the vaginal apex to the sacrospinous ligament.

DIAGNOSIS OF PROLAPSE

Symptoms

Mild forms of POP are often asymptomatic and may not require treatment. In these cases, the patient should be informed of the possibility that the prolapse may or may not require future intervention. Symptoms related to prolapse may include the sensation of a vaginal mass or bulge, pelvic pressure, low back pain, and sexual difficulty. Oftentimes, symptoms are worse after long periods of standing or straining and may be somewhat relieved by lying down.

Patients with anterior vaginal prolapse may complain of symptoms directly related to vaginal protrusion or associated symptoms such as urinary incontinence or voiding difficulty. Stress urinary incontinence commonly occurs in association with anterior vaginal prolapse. Voiding difficulty may result from advanced prolapse. Women may require vaginal pressure or manual replacement of the prolapse to accomplish voiding. Women may relate a history of urinary incontinence that has since resolved with worsening of their prolapse. This can occur with urethral kinking and obstruction to urinary flow; women in this situation are at risk for incomplete bladder emptying, recurrent or persistent urinary tract infections, and possible upper urinary tract injury.

Women with enterocele often have concomitant vaginal support defects. Symptoms are complex and cannot be attributed solely to the enterocele. Nonetheless, women with large enteroceles often experience pelvic pressure, fullness, vaginal protrusion, and low backache. Women with uterovaginal or apical prolapse may report similar symptoms. Additionally, women may experience irritation, spotting, and ulceration from exposure of the vaginal epithelium overlying the exposed enterocele or apical prolapse. Although extremely rare, evisceration of bowel through the vagina and small bowel incarceration in enterocele sacs has been described in patients with severe enterocele. Large enteroceles may also be associated with outlet type constipation.

In addition to pelvic pressure or protrusion, women with rectocele may experience difficulty when evacuating bowel contents (often described by the patient as constipation). In severe cases, the patient may have to splint the posterior vaginal wall by placing her fingers into the vagina to achieve evacuation, effectively decreasing the amount of stool trapped in the prolapsed "pocket."

Physical Examination

When evaluating women with POP, attention should be paid to all aspects of pelvic support, including a focused neurologic examination and test of pelvic muscle strength. The physician must determine the specific sites of damage for each patient, with the ultimate goal of restoring both anatomy and function. A more complete description of the physical examination can be found in Chapter 6, Preventive Health Care for Women.

The physical examination begins with a thorough inspection of the external genitalia, noting any masses protruding through the introitus, evidence of vulvovaginal atrophy, or ulcerations. After the external genitalia are inspected, a focused neurologic examination should be conducted to test the integrity of perineal sensation, pudendal reflex arcs (clitoral and anal wink responses), and pelvic floor muscle strength.

After the external examination, the labia are gently spread to expose the vestibule and hymen. The integrity of the perineal body is evaluated, and

551

the approximate size of all prolapsed parts is assessed (see further discussion). A retractor, half of a speculum, or a Sims' speculum can be used to depress the anterior and posterior vaginal walls sequentially to aid in visualization of the opposite vaginal wall. After the resting examination, the patient is instructed to strain down forcefully or to cough vigorously. During this maneuver, the order of descent of the pelvic organs is noted, as is the relationship of the pelvic organs at the peak of straining. Anterior vaginal wall descent usually represents bladder descent with or without concomitant urethral hypermobility. Rarely, an anterior enterocele can mimic a cystocele on physical examination. Posterior vaginal wall descent usually represents rectocele but may also include enterocele. Cervical or apical descent may occur with or without concomitant enterocele. After the supine straining examination is completed, the patient can be reexamined in the standing position while resting and straining to ensure that maximal prolapse has been observed.

STAGING OF PROLAPSE

The Pelvic Organ Prolapse Quantification System

Pelvic organ anatomy is described during a physical examination of the external genitalia and vaginal canal. Segments of the lower reproductive tract (i.e., anterior, posterior, or apical vaginal wall) replace the terms *cystocele, rectocele, enterocele,* and *urethrovesical junction* because these terms imply an unrealistic certainty as to the structures on the other side of the vaginal bulge, particularly in women who have had previous prolapse surgery. The examiner sees and describes the maximum protrusion noted by the patient during her daily activities. The details of the examination, including criteria for the end point of the examination and full development of the prolapse, should be specified. Suggested criteria for demonstration of maximum prolapse include one or all of the following: (1) any protrusion of the vaginal wall has become tight during straining by the patient; (2) traction on the prolapse causes no further descent; (3) the patient confirms that the size of the prolapse and the extent of the protrusion seen by the examiner are as extensive as the most severe protrusion she has had (a small handheld mirror to visualize the protrusion may be helpful); and (4) a standing/straining examination confirms that the full extent of the prolapse was observed in the other positions used. Details about the patient position, types of vaginal specula or retractors, the type and intensity of straining used to develop the prolapse maximally, and the fullness of the bladder should be stated.

This descriptive system contains a series of site-specific measurements of the woman's pelvic organ support. Prolapse in each segment is evaluated and measured relative to the hymen (not introitus), which is a fixed anatomic landmark that can be identified consistently and precisely. The anatomic position of the six defined points for measurement should be centimeters above (proximal) to the hymen (negative number) or centimeters below (distal) to the hymen (positive number), with the plane of the hymen being defined as zero. For example, a cervix that protrudes 3 cm distal to the hymen should be described as "+3 cm."

The Pelvic Organ Prolapse Quantification (POPQ) system begins with the patient in the dorsal supine lithotomy position. All measurements (except the total vaginal length) are done with the patient performing a Valsalva maneuver. Six points (two on the anterior vaginal wall, two in the superior vagina, and two on the posterior vaginal wall) are located with reference to the plane of the hymen (Fig. 23-3). The reference point for measurements along the anterior vaginal wall is the external urethral meatus. The reference point for measurements along the posterior vaginal wall is the hymen. On both the anterior and posterior vaginal walls, two points are determined in the midline—points A and B (see Fig. 23-3). Point A is always 3 cm from either the urethra (Aa; "a" is for anterior) or the hymen (Ap; "p" is for posterior). By definition, the range of position of points Aa and Ap relative to the hymen are −3 (proximal to the hymen) to +3 cm (distal to the hymen). Point B is more complicated to understand and refers to any prolapse that extends beyond any measured by point A; if there is no prolapse beyond A, then B is equal to A. If the vagina is prolapsed between point A and the apex, then B will render a value equal to the centimeters proximal (−) or distal (+) to the reference point (the urethra or hymen). If small bowel appears to be present in the rectovaginal space, the examiner should comment on this fact and describe the basis for this clinical impression. Point C is the distance from the cervix—or vaginal apex if the cervix is absent—to the hymen. Point D is only measured if a cervix is present and represents the distance from the

553

Figure 23-3

Six sites (points Aa, Ba, C, D, Bp, and Ap), genital hiatus (gh), perineal body (pb), and total vaginal length (tvl) used for pelvic organ support quantification in the Pelvic Organ Prolapse Quantification system. (From Bump RC, Mattiasson A, Bo K, et al: The standardization of terminology of female pelvic organ prolapse and pelvic floor dysfunction. Am J Obstet Gynecol 175:10–17, 1996.)

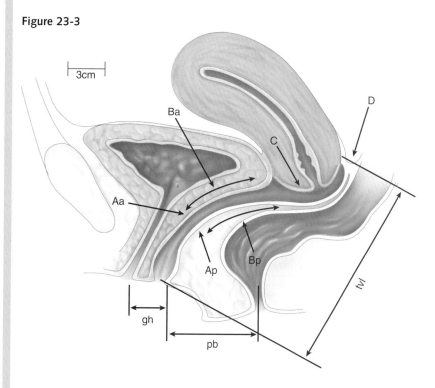

posterior fornix to the hymen. The total vaginal length is measured with the prolapse completely reduced and without the patient bearing down; it is the greatest depth of the vagina. Two perineal measures remain: the perineal body (pb) and genital hiatus (gh). The distance from the center of the anus to the posterior fourchette of the vagina is Pb. The distance from the middle of the urethral meatus to the posterior midline hymen is gh.

The positions of points Aa, Ba, Ap, Bp, C, and (if applicable) D with reference to the hymen are measured and recorded. Positions are expressed as centimeters above or proximal to the hymen (negative number) or centimeters below or distal to the hymen (positive number), with the plane of the hymen defined as zero. Measurements can be recorded as a simple line of numbers (e.g., $-3, -3, -7, -9, -3, -3, 9, 2, 2$ for points Aa, Ba, C, D, Bp, Ap, total vaginal length, genital hiatus, and perineal body, respectively). Alternatively, a 3×3 cm grid can be used to concisely organize the measurements, as shown in Figure 23-4, or a line diagram of a configuration can be drawn, as shown in Figures 23-5 and 23-6. Figure 23-5 is a grid and line diagram contrasting measurements indicating normal support to those of posthysterectomy vaginal eversion. Figure 23-6 is a grid and line diagram representing predominant anterior and posterior vaginal wall prolapse with partial vault descent.

Stages are assigned according to the most severe portion of the prolapse when the full extent of the protrusion has been demonstrated. For a stage to be assigned to an individual subject, it is essential that her quantitative description be completed first. The five stages of pelvic organ support (0 through IV) are described in Box 23-2.

Ancillary techniques for describing POP include performance of a digital rectal examination while the patient is straining; digital assessment of the contents of the rectovaginal septum during examination to differentiate between a "traction" enterocele (the posterior cul-de-sac is pulled down by the prolapsing cervix or vaginal cuff but is not distended by intestines) and a "pulsion" enterocele (the intestinal contents of the enterocele distend the rectal-vaginal septum and produce a protruding mass); cotton swab testing for the measurement of urethral axis mobility (Q-tip test);

Figure 23-4

Three-by-three centimeter grid for recording quantitative description of pelvic organ support. (From Bump RC, Mattiasson A, Bo K, et al: The standardization of terminology of female pelvic organ prolapse and pelvic floor dysfunction. Am J Obstet Gynecol 175:10–17, 1996.)

Anterior wall **Aa**	Anterior wall **Ba**	Cervix or cuff **C**
Genital hiatus **gh**	Perineal body **ph**	Total vaginal length **tvl**
Posterior wall **Ap**	Posterior wall **Bp**	Posterior fornix **D**

Figure 23-5

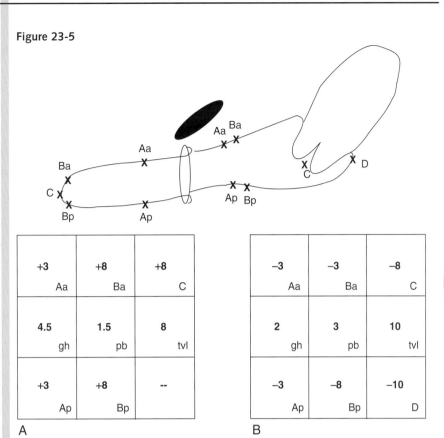

A, Grid and line diagram of complete eversion of vagina. Most distal point of anterior wall (point Ba), vaginal cuff scar (point C), and most distal point of the posterior wall (point Bp) are all at same position (+8) and points Aa and Ap are maximally distal (both at +3). Because total vaginal length equals maximum protrusion, this is stage IV prolapse. **B,** Normal support. Points Aa and Ba and points Ap and Bp are all −3 because there is no anterior or posterior wall descent. Lowest point of the cervix is 8 cm above hymen (−8) (point C) and posterior fornix is 2 cm above this (−10) (point D). Total vaginal length (tvl) is 10 cm, and genital hiatus (gh) and perineal body (pb) measure 2 and 3 cm, respectively. This represents stage 0 support. (From Bump RC, Mattiasson A, Bo K, et al: The standardization of terminology of female pelvic organ prolapse and pelvic floor dysfunction. Am J Obstet Gynecol 175:10–17, 1996.)

A

+3	+8	+8
Aa	Ba	C
4.5	1.5	8
gh	pb	tvl
+3	+8	--
Ap	Bp	

B

−3	−3	−8
Aa	Ba	C
2	3	10
gh	pb	tvl
−3	−8	−10
Ap	Bp	D

measurement of perineal descent; measurement of the transverse diameter of the genital hiatus or of the protruding prolapse; measurement of vaginal volume; description and measurement of rectal prolapse; and examination techniques differentiating between various types of defects (e.g., central versus lateral defects of the anterior vaginal wall). Cystoscopy and photography can be useful in describing POP. Imaging procedures include ultrasonography, contrast radiography, computed tomography, and magnetic resonance imaging. Intraoperative evaluation of pelvic support defects is of unproven value because the effects of anesthesia, diminished muscle tone, and loss of consciousness are of unknown magnitude and direction. It is important to note that, although a standardized staging system for prolapse has been accepted by the International Continence Society, there is no consensus as to what level of physical findings (i.e., what stage) defines clinically significant prolapse; the POPQ system does not incorporate patient symptoms into its staging categories.

As stated previously, evaluation and measurement of the pelvic floor muscle function also include an assessment of the patient's ability to selectively contract and relax the pelvic muscles without abdominal straining and a measurement of the strength of contraction. These measurements are subjective and usually based on a scale of I (weak) to V (strong). Assessment of pelvic floor muscle strength should be documented along with the findings of the focused neurologic examination.

Figure 23-6

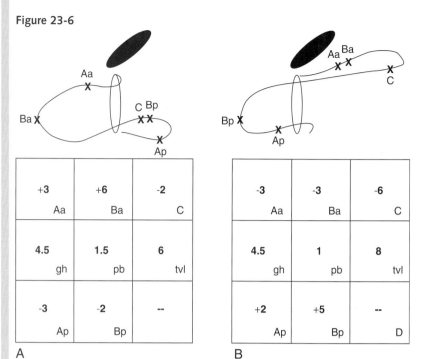

A, Grid and line diagram of predominant anterior support defect. Leading point of prolapse is upper anterior vaginal wall, point Ba (+6). There is significant elongation of bulging anterior wall. Point Aa is maximally distal (+3) and vaginal cuff scar is 2 cm above hymen (C = −2). Cuff scar has undergone 4 cm of descent because it would be at −6 (total vaginal length [tvl]) if it were perfectly supported. In this example, total vaginal length is not the maximum depth of the vagina with the elongated anterior vaginal wall maximally reduced, but rather depth of the vagina at the cuff with point C reduced to its normal full extent, as specified in text. This represents stage III Ba prolapse. **B,** Predominant posterior support defect. Leading point of prolapse is the upper posterior vaginal wall, point Bp (+5). Point Ap is 2 cm distal to hymen (+2) and the vaginal cuff scar is 6 cm above the hymen (−6). The cuff has undergone only 2 cm of descent because it would be at −8 (total vaginal length) if it were perfectly supported. This represents stage III Bp prolapse. (From Bump RC, Mattiasson A, Bo K, et al: The standardization of terminology of female pelvic organ prolapse and pelvic floor dysfunction. Am J Obstet Gynecol 175:10–17, 1996.)

	Box 23-2	Stages of Pelvic Organ Prolapse

Stage 0	No prolapse is demonstrated. Points Aa, Ap, Ba, and Bp are all at −3 cm, and either point C or D is between −TVL (total vaginal length) cm and −(TVL-2) cm (i.e., the quantitation value for point C or D is ≤[TVL-2] cm). Fig. 23-5B, represents stage 0.
Stage I	The criteria for stage 0 are not met, but the most distal portion of the prolapse is >1 cm above the level of the hymen (i.e., its quantitation value is less than −1 cm).
Stage II	The most distal portion of the prolapse is ≤1 cm proximal or distal to the plane of the hymen (i.e., its quantitation value is greater than or equal to −1 cm but less than or equal to +1 cm).
Stage III	The most distal portion of the prolapse is >1 cm below the plane of the hymen but protrudes no further than 2 cm less than the total vaginal length in centimeters (i.e., its quantitation value is greater than +1 cm but less than +[TVL-2] cm). Fig. 23-6A represents stage III Ba and Fig. 23-6B represents stage III Bp prolapse.
Stage IV	Essentially, complete eversion of the total length of the lower genital tract is demonstrated. The distal portion of the prolapse protrudes to at least (TVL-2) cm (i.e., its quantitation value is greater than or equal to +[TVL-2] cm). In most instances, the leading edge of stage IV prolapse is the cervix or vaginal cuff scar. Fig. 23-5A represents stage IV C prolapse.

From Bump RC, Mattiasson A, Bo K, et al: The standardization of terminology of female pelvic organ prolapse and pelvic floor dysfunction. Am J Obstet Gynecol 175:10–17, 1996.

Diagnostic Tests

After a careful history and physical examination, few diagnostic tests are needed to evaluate patients with POP. A urinalysis should be performed to evaluate for urinary tract infection if the patient complains of any lower urinary tract dysfunction. Hydronephrosis occurs in a small proportion of women with prolapse; however, even if identified, it does not change management in women for whom surgical repair is planned. Therefore, routine imaging of the kidneys and ureters is not necessary.

If urinary incontinence is present, further diagnostic testing is indicated to determine the cause of the incontinence. Urodynamic (simple or complex), endoscopic, or radiologic assessments of filling and voiding function are generally indicated only when symptoms of incontinence or voiding dysfunction are present. Even if no urologic symptoms are noted, voiding function should be assessed to evaluate for completeness of bladder emptying. This procedure usually involves a timed, measured void followed by urethral catheterization to measure residual urine volume.

In women with severe prolapse, it is important to check for urinary continence after the prolapse is repositioned. Some women with severe prolapse may be continent because of urethral kinking; when the prolapse is reduced, urethral dysfunction may be unmasked with occurrence of incontinence (called *potential* or *occult incontinence*). A pessary or vaginal packing can be used to reduce the prolapse before office bladder filling or electronic urodynamic testing. If urinary leakage occurs with coughing or Valsalva maneuvers after reduction of the prolapse, the surgeon can choose an anti-incontinence procedure in conjunction with the vaginal prolapse repair. If urinary incontinence is not demonstrated after prolapse reduction, an anti-incontinence procedure is usually not indicated. It should be noted that the accuracy of testing for potential incontinence is unknown and that methods for unmasking potential incontinence have not been standardized.

Enterocele may occur in association with rectocele, and these may be difficult to differentiate on physical examination. Rectovaginal examination may demonstrate the rectocele as distinct from the bulging sac that arises from a point higher in the vagina, often near the apex. Visual inspection of the posterior vaginal wall may reveal a transverse furrow between the two hernias, and oftentimes, loops of small bowel can be palpated through the vaginal wall overlying the enterocele. Occasionally, peristalsis of small bowel loops filling the enterocele sac may be seen during the examination. Further imaging studies may be helpful to differentiate between enterocele and rectocele, but these are rarely indicated because imaging studies rarely affect the treatment approach.

NONSURGICAL MANAGEMENT OF PROLAPSE

Expectant Management

Prolapse is rarely life threatening and usually does not need to be treated if symptoms are not bothersome to the patient. In these cases, expectant management is a reasonable option. Women with prolapse who opt for expectant management should be reexamined at their annual visits and evaluated for progression or regression of the prolapse.

Behavior Modification

Behavior modification for POP usually involves the identification of modifiable risk factors for prolapse and the treatment or alteration of habits that increase the risk of prolapse. Examples of behavioral modifications that may improve the symptoms of prolapse include weight loss, treatment for chronic constipation or cough, and refraining from chronic heavy lifting. The literature on these behavior modifications is sparse.

Data regarding the effects of vaginal delivery on future prolapse are also limited. Although the literature suggests that women who undergo cesarean section have a comparatively lower risk of future urinary incontinence than those who undergo vaginal delivery, few data exist evaluating the effect of delivery mode on prolapse risk. Elective cesarean section is controversial but may be acceptable if the patient is fully informed about its risks and benefits.

Other treatments that have been shown to be beneficial for the treatment of urinary incontinence, such as behavioral therapy, biofeedback, and electrical stimulation, have not been shown to be of benefit for the treatment of prolapse.

Pessary

The nonsurgical management of POP usually consists of pessary placement. A pessary is a prosthetic device inserted into the vagina to manually reduce the prolapse. Most pessaries are constructed of latex rubber, silicone, or acrylic. With its low morbidity, pessary placement is usually attempted before surgical repair is undertaken. Unexplained vaginal bleeding and vaginal, urinary, or pelvic infection are contraindications to pessary use. Pessaries are often successful in decreasing symptoms and improving the quality of life for women with POP. Many women choose pessaries as their final treatment option, thus avoiding the need for surgical repair with its attendant risks; others use pessaries as a temporizing measure before undergoing surgical repair. Pessaries may also be used to unmask coexisting urinary incontinence ("potential incontinence") after the prolapsed organs are reduced. Pessaries are available in a number of shapes and sizes (Fig. 23-7), and pessary fitting should be individualized to the patient. A general rule of pessary fitting is to start with one of the more inexpensive, user-friendly varieties and then move to the more expensive, less user-friendly types.

Before pessary placement, women with vaginal atrophy should be treated with vaginal estrogen or oral hormone replacement therapy; this makes wearing the pessary more comfortable for the patient and improves compliance. A prescription for vaginal estrogen cream can be given with the pessary and used twice weekly when inserting the pessary (if the woman changes her own pessary). Otherwise, the patient can be instructed to apply vaginal estrogen cream twice per week. If vaginal estrogen cream is contraindicated, Trimo-San vaginal gel (Milex Products, Inc., Chicago, IL) can be used to help maintain normal vaginal pH and to prevent bacterial

Figure 23-7

Varieties of pessaries. **A** to **C,** Smith-Hodge (with and without support). **D,** Gehrung. **E,** Risser. **F** to **H,** Incontinence ring (with and without support). **I** and **K,** Ring (with and without) support). **J,** Incontinence dish. **L** and **M,** Cube. **N,** Inflato-ball. **O,** Donut. **P** to **R,** Gellhorn. (From Harvey MA, Versi E: Urogynecology and pelvic floor dysfunction. In Ryan KJ, Berkowitz RS, Barbieri RL [eds]: Kistner's Gynecology, 7th ed. St. Louis, Mosby, 1999, pp 570–609.)

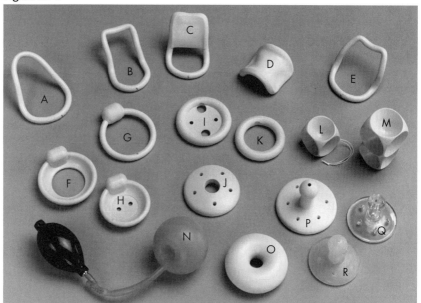

overgrowth. An appropriately sized pessary should be comfortable for the patient, should not become displaced with straining, and should leave enough space to pass a finger between the pessary edge and the vaginal wall when in place. A typical fitting sequence is demonstrated in Box 23-3.

Box 23-3   Suggested Sequence for Fitting Pessaries for Prolapse

Apical prolapse: vaginal vault, uterus
1. Ring with support
2. Incontinence dish with support
3. Shaatz
4. Donut
5. Gelhorn (for uterine prolapse)
6. Inflato-ball
7. Cube (rarely used; see text)

Anterior vaginal wall prolapse
1. Ring with support
2. Incontinence dish or dish with support
3. Contraceptive diaphragm (Ortho Pharmaceuticals, Raritan, NJ)
4. Gehrung
5. Donut

Posterior vaginal wall prolapse
1. Ring with support
2. Gehrung

Devices made by Milex Products, Chicago, IL, except as noted. Adapted from Nygaard I, Dougherty MC: Genuine stress incontinence and pelvic organ prolapse: Nonsurgical treatment. In Walters MD, Karram MM (eds): Urogynecology and Reconstructive Pelvic Surgery, 2nd ed. St. Louis, Mosby, 1999, pp 145–158.

Once the pessary is placed, the patient should be instructed to strain forcefully and then to mimic physical exertion with walking or heel-bouncing. Women must demonstrate their ability to void before leaving the office. Women who are physically able should be taught how to remove, clean, and replace the pessary. Women who are unable to do so should be seen by a visiting nurse or instructed to return to the office at regular intervals for pessary cleaning and vaginal inspection. Return visit intervals vary by pessary type. Guidelines for pessary care and follow-up are demonstrated in Box 23-4.

Despite its low morbidity, pessary use can be associated with complications. This most often results from poor pessary care rather than the pessary itself (except in the cased of a poorly sized pessary). Women who report vaginal bleeding or a foul-smelling discharge should be instructed to arrange for an evaluation so the pessary can be removed, the vagina inspected, and any infection or ulceration treated. More serious complications of pessary use are rare but include vaginal abrasions or erosions, urinary retention, and incarceration with or without fistula formation to adjacent organs (usually resulting from a "forgotten" pessary). Complication rates vary by pessary type and maintenance regimen, but complications are rare when diligent pessary maintenance is observed.

Box 23-4 Pessary Care Instructions

Initial pessary use
Estrogen cream, if needed
Pessary fitting
Vigorous activity in office
Void in office
Home with pessary

First follow-up visit (1 week; 1 to 3 days for cube)
Examine vagina
Adjust type and size as needed
Teach insertion and removal
Visiting nurse referral (possibly—see text)

Long-term follow-up
If woman can insert and remove:
    Return visits: 2 weeks, 3 months later, every 6 to 12 months
    Remove pessary each night or at least once per week
    Leave out overnight
    Use estrogen cream on pessary as lubricant
If woman cannot insert and remove:
    Return visits: 2 weeks, 4 weeks later, 6 weeks later, etc., up to 3 months
    Determine appropriate pessary removal interval
    Optimal: Remove and have nurse reinsert in morning (or vice versa)
    Estrogen: Systemic or cream three times per week
    Triple sulfa cream or buffered acid jelly may decrease discharge

Adapted from Nygaard I, Dougherty MC: Genuine stress incontinence and pelvic organ prolapse: Nonsurgical treatment. In Walters MD, Karram MM (eds): Urogynecology and Reconstructive Pelvic Surgery, 2nd ed. St. Louis, Mosby, 1999, pp 145–158.

SURGICAL REPAIR TECHNIQUES

Treatment of symptomatic prolapse usually involves surgical repair. The goal of surgical treatment of POP is to give the patient a durable repair that relieves her of prolapse (and associated incontinence) symptoms and improves her quality of life. A secondary goal is to restore anatomy and to provide the patient with a functional vagina (unless the patient is sexually inactive and does not desire future coital function). Most patients with POP have prolapse of multiple vaginal segments; surgical repair should be aimed at repairing all of the prolapsed segments.

Operations for Enterocele and Uterine or Vaginal Vault Prolapse

Hysterectomy

Uterine prolapse is generally treated with hysterectomy combined with a vault suspension procedure (see further discussion). Hysterectomy can be accomplished by the vaginal, abdominal, or laparoscopic route. The procedure is covered in more detail in Chapter 29, Hysterectomy. It should be noted that hysterectomy alone is not ample treatment for uterine prolapse; the vaginal vault should be resuspended to the uterosacral ligaments to treat the prolapse and prevent future enterocele formation or vault prolapse. A number of vault suspension techniques are available, some of which are described below.

561

Modified McCall Culdoplasty

McCall described the technique of surgical correction of enterocele and a deep cul-de-sac during vaginal hysterectomy. The McCall culdoplasty closes the redundant cul-de-sac and associated enterocele, provides apical support, and lengthens the vagina. In a randomized study, Cruikshank and Kovac demonstrated the superiority of McCall culdoplasty to uterosacral plication and simple peritoneal closure in the prevention of posthysterectomy enterocele. For this reason, most pelvic surgeons advocate McCall culdoplasty after vaginal hysterectomy even in the absence of prolapse. With posthysterectomy prolapse and enterocele, a high McCall-type culdoplasty or uterosacral ligament vaginal vault suspension can be performed.

To perform a high McCall culdoplasty, the uterosacral ligament remnants are identified and placed on tension after the enterocele has been entered. The remnants of uterosacral ligaments are found posterior and medial to the ischial spines and can be identified by placing Allis or Kocher clamps on the vaginal epithelium at approximately 4 and 8 o'clock (at the old hysterectomy scar) and placing tension on structures of the pelvic sidewall. A permanent No. 0 suture is passed through the uterosacral ligament as high as possible. The needle is passed from lateral to medial to reduce the risk of ureteral entrapment. Successive bites are then taken at 1- to 2-cm intervals across the anterior serosa of the sigmoid colon until the opposite uterosacral ligament is reached and incorporated. This suture is left untied. Occasionally, one to three more identical sutures are placed caudally, progressing toward the posterior vaginal cuff. The goal is obliteration of the entire dependent portion of the cul-de-sac. After the internal permanent sutures have been placed, their ends are held laterally without tying. A No. 0 delayed absorbable suture is then placed from the vaginal lumen just below the middle of the cut edge of the posterior vaginal cuff, through the peritoneum, and through the left uterosacral ligament. Successive bites are taken across the cul-de-sac, as before, and into the right uterosacral ligament. This suture is passed back through the peritoneum and vaginal epithelium, adjacent to the point of entry (Fig. 23-8). The permanent sutures are tied sequentially, and an additional suture of No. 0 delayed absorbable suture can be placed through the plicated uterosacral ligaments and positioned in the anterior vaginal epithelium at the point of the new vault. Cystocele repair is performed as needed, the excess vaginal epithelium is trimmed, and the delayed absorbable vault suspension stitches are positioned at the new apex. The vaginal epithelium is closed and the vault suspension stitches are tied, elevating the vault toward the uterosacral ligaments and obliterating the cul-de-sac. Cystoscopy is performed after intravenous indigo carmine is given to inspect for ureteral patency after all sutures have been tied. Rectocele and perineal repair are then completed as necessary. Enterocele recurrence rates of 4% to 5% have been reported after McCall culdoplasty.

Figure 23-8

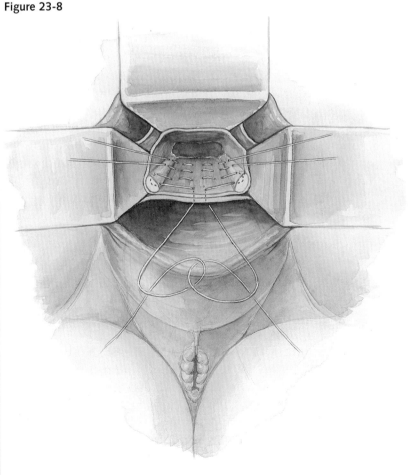

McCall culdoplasty technique. Note that the lowest suture incorporates the posterior vaginal wall, thus providing additional support. (From Shull BL, Bachofen CB: Enterocele and rectocele. In Walters MD, Karram MM [eds]: Urogynecology and Reconstructive Pelvic Surgery, 2nd ed. St. Louis, Mosby, 1999, pp 221–234.)

Uterosacral Ligament Vaginal Vault Suspension

Uterosacral ligament vaginal vault suspension can be performed either transvaginally, transabdominally, or laparoscopically. According to Shull and Bachofen, this operation follows the principles of hernia surgery: the identification of a fascial defect, reduction of intra-abdominal contents, and closure and reinforcement of the defect. The enterocele must be closed and the vagina—both anterior and posterior walls—must be reliably suspended at the apex.

In this procedure, the enterocele is identified and the edges of the vaginal epithelium are dissected sharply away from the enterocele sac. The enterocele sac is opened and bowel is packed out of the operative field. Occasionally, an enterocele is not present and entry into the peritoneal cavity is not possible. In these cases, an extraperitoneal suspension to the uterosacral ligaments, iliococcygeus fascia suspension, or sacrospinous ligament suspension is done (see further discussion). After the enterocele sac is entered, the ischial spines and uterosacral ligaments are identified, and a series of interrupted nonabsorbable (or delayed absorbable) sutures are placed in each uterosacral ligament beginning at the level of, but posterior and medial to, the ischial spine. The needle is driven from lateral to medial to decrease the risk of ureteral injury. After the first suture is placed, the second is placed in a more cephalad and medial position (toward the sacrum), and the third is placed cephalad and medial to the second.

After the suspensory sutures have been placed, the surgeon should perform any required cystocele repair and/or bladder neck suspension or sling, as needed. The suspensory sutures in the uterosacral ligaments are then systematically placed into the most apical portions of the pubocervical and rectovaginal muscularis. The most cephalad suspensory sutures (closest to the sacrum) are sewn to the most medial portions of the pubocervical and rectovaginal muscularis. The sutures caudal to that one are placed more laterally into the pubocervical and rectovaginal muscularis. The most caudal (delayed absorbable) sutures are placed most laterally into the pubocervical and rectovaginal muscularis and passed out the vaginal epithelium laterally at the 3 and 9 o'clock positions (Fig. 23-9).

The patient is given intravenous indigo carmine, and the suspensory sutures are tied sequentially. Once the suspensory sutures have been tied, the apex of the vagina should be in the hollow of the sacrum and the connective tissue tube closed at the vaginal apex. Cystoscopy is performed to ensure ureteral patency; if no flow of urine is seen from one of the ureters, the sutures are removed on that side one at a time from lateral to medial. This usually restores ureteral patency. If not, then cul-de-sac exploration and ureteral stent placement might be necessary. The vaginal epithelium is tailored to the contour of the vagina by excising excess tissue, and the epithelial incision is closed vertically or horizontally with an absorbable suture.

Several studies have described outcomes of series of patients with vaginal prolapse after uterosacral ligament vaginal suspension. Shull and colleagues described the results of 302 consecutive women who underwent

Figure 23-9

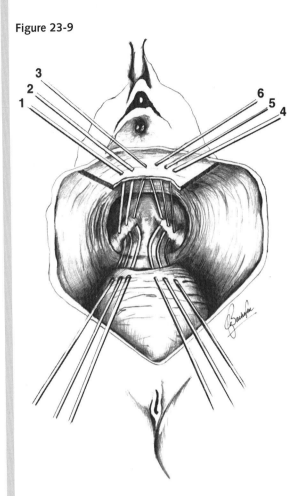

Suspension of the vaginal apex to the cardinal-uterosacral ligament complex using endopelvic fascia. Note the correct placement of each numbered suture posterior and medial to the ischial spines. (From Shull BL, Bachofen CB: Enterocele and rectocele. In Walters MD, Karram MM [eds]: Urogynecology and Reconstructive Pelvic Surgery, 2nd ed. St. Louis, Mosby, 1999, pp 221–234.)

uterosacral ligament vaginal suspension. Eighty-seven percent of the women had optimal anatomic outcomes with no prolapse at any site in the vagina at follow-up examination. Only 5% of patients had development of stage II or greater prolapse at any site, and most recurrences were in the anterior wall. Intraoperative ureteral obstruction has been described in 1% to 11% of cases, necessitating cystoscopy to check for ureteral patency after the procedure is performed.

Vaginal Enterocele Repair

Enterocele usually exists with other support defects, and concurrent vaginal vault suspension, cystocele, and rectocele repair are often necessary. Vaginal enterocele repair is performed by opening the vaginal epithelium over the enterocele and identifying and entering the enterocele sac. Multiple purse-string sutures are placed to obliterate the enterocele sac, making sure to incorporate the uterosacral remnants. When the enterocele sac is difficult to distinguish from the rectum, differentiation is aided by a rectal examination with simultaneous dissection of the enterocele sac from the rectal wall. At times, distinguishing the enterocele sac from a large cystocele may prove difficult. When this occurs, placement of a curved uterine sound into the bladder or transillumination with a cystoscope may be helpful. Anterior colporrhaphy, posterior colporrhaphy, and vaginal vault suspension are then performed, as indicated. Cystoscopy is performed to ensure ureteral patency after intravenous indigo carmine is given.

Sacrospinous Ligament Suspension

To safely perform a sacrospinous ligament suspension, the surgeon must be familiar with the anatomy of the C-SSL and its surrounding structures. The anatomy has been previously described and is covered in depth in Chapter 4, Gynecologic Anatomy. Before the procedure is started, the ischial spine and C-SSL should be identified with pelvic examination. In unilateral sacrospinous ligament suspension, the apex of the vagina is grasped with two Allis clamps, and downward traction is used to determine the extent of the vaginal prolapse and associated pelvic support defects. The vaginal apex is reduced to the sacrospinous ligament, usually on the right, and then tagged with two sutures for its later identification. Anterior colporrhaphy should be completed as necessary. The posterior vaginal wall is then incised and opened just short of the apex, leaving a small vaginal bridge 3 to 4 cm wide. If an enterocele sac is present, it should be dissected off the posterior vaginal wall and closed with a high purse-string suture. Next, the perirectal space is opened by bluntly breaking through the rectal pillar with an index finger or tonsil clamp. Once the perirectal space is entered, the ischial spine is identified and, with dorsal and medial movement of the fingers, the C-SSL is palpated and bluntly cleared while retracting the rectum medially. Usually, two sutures are passed through the C-SSL two fingerbreadths medial to the ischial spine and then passed through the muscularis of the apex (if permanent suture is used) or through the full thickness of the apex (if delayed absorbable suture is used). The suture may be passed through the C-SSL ligament with a Deschamps ligature carrier, Miya hook, or a Capio disposable ligature carrier (Microinvasive/Boston Scientific, Inc., Natick, MA). These sutures are then tied, directly opposing the vaginal vault to the C-SSL (Fig. 23-10). Posterior colpoperineorrhaphy is then completed as needed, and rectal examination is performed to ensure integrity of the rectum.

Although infrequent, serious intraoperative complications can occur with sacrospinous ligament fixation. Potential complications of the procedure include hemorrhage from the veins around the C-SSL complex, buttock pain, pudendal nerve injury, rectal injury, stress urinary incontinence, and vaginal stenosis. Objective cure rates between 70% and 94% have been reported, with the highest risk of failure occurring in the anterior compartment.

Iliococcygeus Fascia Suspension

Iliococcygeus fascial suspension is often performed when vaginal vault eversion is present but no enterocele is present and the peritoneal cavity cannot be entered. In this procedure, the everted vaginal apex is bilaterally fixed to the iliococcygeus fascia just below the ischial spines.

Figure 23-10

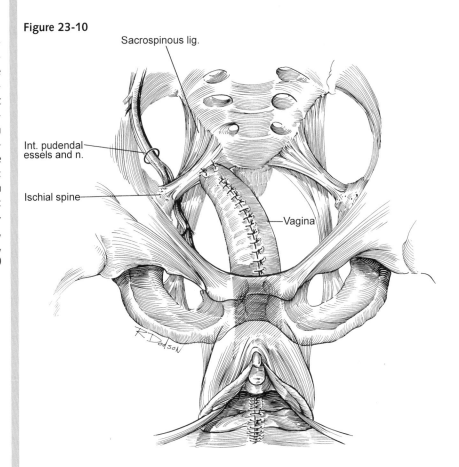

Diagrammatic representation of a sacrospinous fixation of the vaginal vault to correct vaginal vault prolapse. Int., Internal; n., nerve. (From Beck PR: Abnormalities of support in the female genital tract: Genital prolapse. In Copeland LJ [ed]: Textbook of Gynecology. Philadelphia, W.B. Saunders, 1993, p 733.)

To perform this procedure, the posterior vaginal wall is opened in the midline as for a posterior colporrhaphy, and the rectovaginal spaces are bilaterally dissected widely to the levator ani muscles. The dissection is extended bluntly toward the ischial spines. With the surgeon's nondominant hand pressing the rectum downward and medial, an area 1 to 2 cm caudal and posterior to the ischial spine in the iliococcygeus muscle and fascia is exposed, and a single No. 0 delayed absorbable suture is placed deeply into the levator muscle and fascia. Both ends of the suture are passed through the ipsilateral posterior section of vaginal apex and held with a hemostat. This is repeated on the opposite side. The posterior colporrhaphy is completed and the vagina closed. Both sutures are tied, elevating the posterior vaginal apices.

From 1981 to 1993, Shull and Meeks used the iliococcygeus fascial suspension to treat 152 patients with posthysterectomy vault prolapse or total uterine procidentia. Intraoperative complications were rare but included one rectal and one bladder laceration and two cases of hemorrhage requiring transfusion. Thirteen (8%) patients developed recurrent pelvic support defects at various sites 6 weeks to 5 years after the initial procedure; two had vault prolapse, eight had anterior vaginal wall relaxation, and three had posterior wall defects.

In a more recent retrospective study, Maher et al. compared the results of iliococcygeus fascia suspension to sacrospinous ligament suspension in 128 patients. Objective cure (defined as no vaginal prolapse beyond the halfway point of the vagina) was found in 53% of patients after iliococcygeus fascia suspension and in 67% after sacrospinous ligament suspension; most recurrences of prolapse were in the anterior vaginal wall.

Abdominal Sacral Colpopexy

Abdominal sacral colpopexy involves suspension of the vagina to the sacral promontory with a graft via an abdominal approach. In women who have other indications for abdominal surgery, it is the procedure of choice. Retropubic procedures, such as Burch colposuspension and paravaginal defect repair, can be performed as needed through the same laparotomy incision. This procedure may also be performed laparoscopically.

Many different graft materials have been used for abdominal sacral colpopexy. Autologous materials that have been used include rectus fascia, fascia lata, and dura mater. Synthetic materials include polypropylene mesh, polyester fiber mesh, polytetrafluoroethylene mesh, Dacron mesh, and Silastic silicone rubber. Few studies have compared the efficacy of the various graft materials, and individual reports of long-term rates of cure are generally good. Decreased success rates have been reported with the use of cadaver fascia. Most surgeons prefer either polypropylene or polyester fiber mesh because of their high success and relatively low erosion rates.

To perform abdominal sacral colpopexy, the patient should be placed in Allen stirrups so that the surgeon can place a sponge stick or EEA sizer, (US Surgical Corp., Norwalk, CT) in the vagina for manipulation of the apex. Laparotomy is performed through a low transverse or midline incision, and the bowels are packed out of the surgical field. If the uterus is present, a hysterectomy should be performed and the vaginal cuff closed. The depth of the cul-de-sac and the length of the vagina when completely elevated are estimated. While the vagina is elevated cephalad using a sponge stick or EEA sizer, the bladder and rectum are dissected from the anterior and posterior vaginal walls. Three to five pairs of nonabsorbable No. 0 sutures are placed in the posterior vaginal wall, transversely, 1 to 2 cm apart. Sutures are placed through the full fibromuscular thickness of the vagina but not into the vaginal epithelium. Sutures are then fed through the graft in pairs and tied. The graft should extend down the length of the posterior vaginal wall. Another piece of mesh is affixed to the anterior vaginal wall. This piece of mesh is then sewn to the posterior piece of mesh, which will be attached to the sacrum. Alternatively, a full length piece of mesh can also be attached anteriorly to be sutured to the sacrum.

A longitudinal incision is made in the peritoneum over the sacral promontory and extended into the cul-de-sac. Care must be taken to identify the aortic bifurcation, common and internal iliac vessels, middle sacral vessels, and right ureter so that these structures can be avoided. The left common iliac vein is medial to the left common iliac artery and is partic-

567

ularly vulnerable to damage during this procedure. Blunt and sharp dissection caudally can be used to create a subperitoneal tunnel into the full depth of the cul-de-sac so that the graft can be extraperitonized. A 3- to 4-cm segment of the anterior longitudinal ligament is carefully cleared over the sacral promontory with sharp dissection, blunt dissection, and electrocautery. Special care should be taken to avoid the delicate plexus of presacral veins that is often present, especially as one dissects more caudally.

Although some authors have advocated connecting the graft material at S3 and S4 level (the normal vaginal axis in a nulliparous woman), life-threatening hemorrhage from presacral vessels at this low level on the sacrum has been described. Thus, the graft is usually fixed to the upper third of the sacrum, near the sacral promontory, thus improving safety without sacrificing outcome or future vaginal function (Fig. 23-11). Using a stiff but small half-curved tapered needle with permanent No. 0 suture, two to four sutures are placed through the anterior sacral longitudinal ligament, over the sacral promontory. The graft is trimmed to the appropriate length and the sutures are fed through the graft in pairs and tied. The appropriate amount of vaginal elevation should provide gentle tension without undue traction on the vagina. The peritoneum over

Figure 23-11

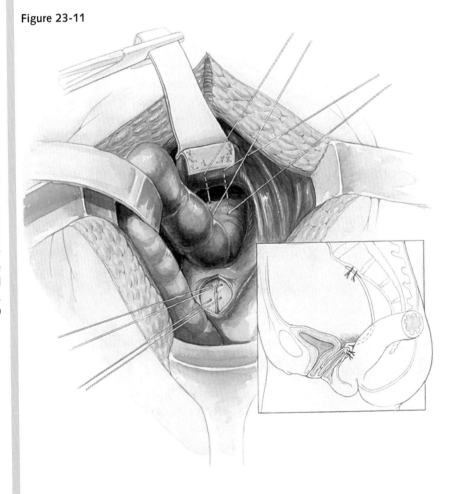

Abdominal sacral colpopexy. Note that Halban technique is used to obliterate cul-de-sac below graft. Inset, Graft connects vagina to sacrum and lies without tension in the deep pelvis. (From Karram MM, Sze EHM, Walters MD: Surgical treatment of vaginal vault prolapse. In Walters MD, Karram MM [eds]: Urogynecology and Reconstructive Pelvic Surgery, 2nd ed. St. Louis, Mosby, 1999, pp 235–256.)

the presacral space is closed with a running absorbable suture. The deep cul-de-sac can be obliterated as needed with multiple horizontal (Halban) or semicircular (Moschcowitz) sutures. When appropriate, retropubic urethropexy or paravaginal repair should be accomplished at this time. Posterior colporrhaphy and perineoplasty are generally performed to treat the remaining rectocele and perineal defect.

Recurrences of vaginal vault prolapse are uncommon if attention has been paid to repairing all the support defects of the vagina at the time of sacral colpopexy. The durability of abdominal sacral colpopexy has been demonstrated in multiple studies with good long-term follow-up; success rates between 93% and 99% have been reported. Failures of this procedure are usually attributable to avulsion of the mesh off of the vaginal apex, reinforcing the need to suture the suspensory mesh to the posterior and anterior vaginal apex over an extended area.

Intraoperative complications are uncommon but can be life threatening. When bleeding from presacral vessels is encountered, hemostasis can be difficult to achieve because these veins may retract beneath the bony surface of the anterior sacrum and recede into the underlying channels of cancellous bone. Packing of the presacral space may control bleeding temporarily, but it often recurs when the pack is removed, and packing may further lacerate delicate veins. Sutures, metallic clips, cautery, and bone wax should be used initially. If these measures are not successful, sterilized stainless steel thumbtacks can be placed on the retracted bleeding presacral vein to treat life-threatening hemorrhage that has not responded to other measures.

Other complications of abdominal sacral colpopexy include enterotomy, ureteral damage, cystotomy, proctotomy, extrafascial wound infections, and persistent granulation tissue in the vaginal vault. Graft rejections are exceedingly rare. Small bowel obstructions caused by incarceration of bowel loops under the mesh have been reported. This problem underscores the importance of reperitonization of the mesh to prevent small bowel from getting trapped in the cul-de-sac or behind the graft.

Uteropexy

Occasionally, uterine prolapse develops in a younger patient who desires future fertility. If pessary use fails to improve the patient's symptoms, abdominal or laparoscopic sacral uteropexy can be performed. In this procedure, a piece of mesh is sutured to the posterior aspect of the cervix and distal uterosacral ligaments and retroperitoneally to the anterior longitudinal ligament overlying the sacrum, as in abdominal sacral colpopexy. Data regarding the success of this procedure are few.

Obliterative Operations

LeFort Colpocleisis

The LeFort colpocleisis is an obliterative procedure that can be performed yielding minimal blood loss with the patient under general, regional, or local anesthesia. It is used as a last resort to treat severe prolapse in medically fragile patients who are no longer interested in sexual function. This procedure, performed in a patient with a uterus, reduces the uterovaginal prolapse and opposes the anterior and posterior vaginal walls, thus eliminating a functional vagina. In this procedure, panels of vaginal epithelium are removed from the prolapsed anterior and posterior vaginal walls. The cut edge of the anterior vaginal wall is sutured to the cut edge of the posterior vaginal wall with delayed absorbable suture, creating epithelial-lined channels bilaterally. The uterus and prolapsed vagina are gradually reduced by the sutures and are completely inverted (Fig. 23-12). This procedure is often performed with a concurrent incontinence procedure because it results in postoperative urinary stress incontinence in up to 30% of cases. Additionally, perineorrhaphy is commonly performed after this procedure to narrow the introitus.

Figure 23-12

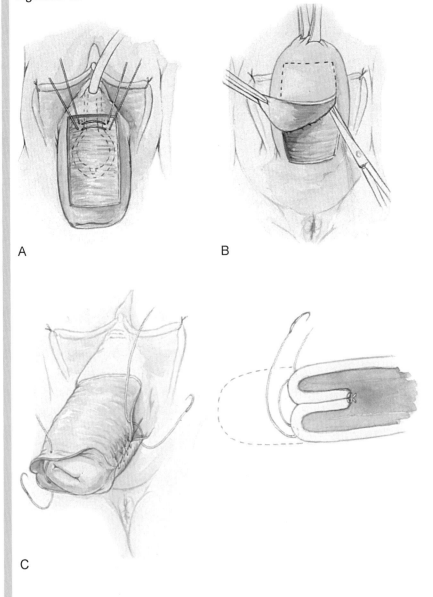

A

B

C

Technique of LeFort partial colpocleisis. **A,** Anterior vaginal wall has been removed and plication stitch is placed at the bladder neck. **B,** Posterior vaginal wall is removed. **C,** Cut edge of anterior vaginal wall is sewn to cut edge of posterior vaginal wall in such a way that the uterus and vagina are inverted. (From Karram MM, Sze EHM, Walters MD: Surgical treatment of vaginal vault prolapse. In Walters MD, Karram MM [eds]: Urogynecology and Reconstructive Pelvic Surgery, 2nd ed. St. Louis, Mosby, 1999, pp 235–256.)

Colpectomy and Colpocleisis

Colpectomy with colpocleisis is another obliterative procedure commonly used in elderly, medically fragile patients with severe posthysterectomy vaginal prolapse when surgical time is best kept to a minimum and future sexual activity is not anticipated. In this procedure, the vaginal epithelium is completely excised and the underlying vaginal muscularis and endopelvic fascia is reduced with a series of delayed absorbable purse-string sutures. Bladder neck plication, posterior colporrhaphy with high levator plication, and perineorrhaphy are often performed with colpectomy. Good anatomic results and symptomatic relief have been reported at rates between 86% and 91% with both LeFort colpocleisis and colpectomy with colpocleisis. Other studies demonstrate prolapse recurrence rates as low as 2.5%.

Operations for Anterior Vaginal Wall Prolapse

Anterior Colporrhaphy

The objective of anterior colporrhaphy is to plicate the pubocervical muscularis in the midline and to reduce the protrusion of the bladder and vagina.

To perform this procedure, a transverse or diamond-shaped incision is made in the vaginal epithelium near the apex. If a vaginal hysterectomy has been performed, the incised apex of the anterior vaginal wall is grasped transversely with two Allis clamps and elevated. A third Allis clamp is placed about 1 cm below the posterior margin of the urethral meatus and pulled up. Hemostatic solutions (such as 0.5% lidocaine with 1:200,000 epinephrine) or saline may be injected submucosally, along the midline of the anterior vaginal wall, to aid in dissection. The points of a pair of curved Mayo scissors are inserted between the vaginal epithelium and the vaginal muscularis and gently forced upward while being partially opened and closed, undermining the vaginal epithelium. The vaginal epithelium is then incised in the midline, and the incision is continued to the level of the mid urethra. As the vagina is incised, the edges are grasped with Allis clamps and drawn laterally for further mobilization. Vaginal flaps are then developed bilaterally until the entire extent of the anterior vaginal prolapse has been dissected (Fig. 23-13).

Once the vaginal flaps have been developed, the urethrovesical junction is identified by pulling the Foley catheter downward until the bulb obstructs the vesical neck. Repair should begin at the urethrovesical junction, using No. 2-0 or 0 delayed absorbable suture. The first plicating stitch is placed into the periurethral pubocervical muscularis and tied. One or two additional stitches are placed to support the urethrovesical junction. After the stitches for vesical neck plication have been placed and tied, No. 2-0 or 0 delayed absorbable sutures are placed in the pubocervical muscularis medial to the vaginal flaps and multiple imbricating sutures are placed to reduce the prolapse. The vaginal epithelium is then trimmed from the flaps bilaterally, and the remaining anterior vaginal wall is closed with a running No. 2-0 or 3-0 locking suture (Fig. 23-14).

Anti-incontinence operations are often performed concurrently with anterior colporrhaphy. Urethral suspension procedures (e.g., sling procedures

Figure 23-13

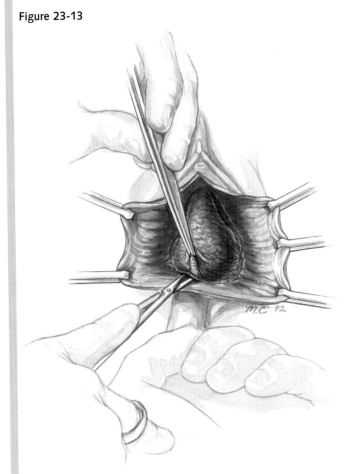

Sharp dissection is used to mobilize the bladder base from the vaginal apex during anterior colporrhaphy. (From Weber AM: Surgical correction of anterior vaginal wall prolapse. In Walters MD, Karram MM [eds]: Urogynecology and Reconstructive Pelvic Surgery, 2nd ed. St. Louis, Mosby, 1999, pp 211–219.)

572

or retropubic urethropexies) may effectively treat mild anterior vaginal prolapse associated with urethral hypermobility. More advanced anterior vaginal prolapse will not be treated adequately, and in these cases, anterior colporrhaphy should be performed as well. If anterior colporrhaphy is combined with a sling procedure, the cystocele should be repaired first.

Paravaginal Defect Repair

This procedure is performed when anterior vaginal wall prolapse results from a lateral detachment of pubocervical muscularis from the arcus tendineus fasciae pelvis rather than from a central defect in the pubocervical muscularis. The objective of paravaginal defect repair is to reattach the lateral vagina to its normal place of attachment at the level of the arcus tendineus fasciae pelvis. This can be accomplished using a retropubic or vaginal approach.

To perform the procedure vaginally, vaginal flaps are developed bilaterally as in anterior colporrhaphy. The retropubic space is entered bluntly and the obturator internus muscle and arcus tendineus fasciae pelvis are identified by palpation and visualization. Using No. 0 or 2-0 nonabsorbable suture, a series of four to six stitches are placed into the arcus tendineus

Figure 23-14

Technique of anterior colporrhaphy. **A,** After dissection of vaginal wall from the bladder and urethra, one to three plication sutures are placed into the periurethral endopelvic fascia at the urethrovesical junction. **B,** The plication sutures at the vesical neck are tied.

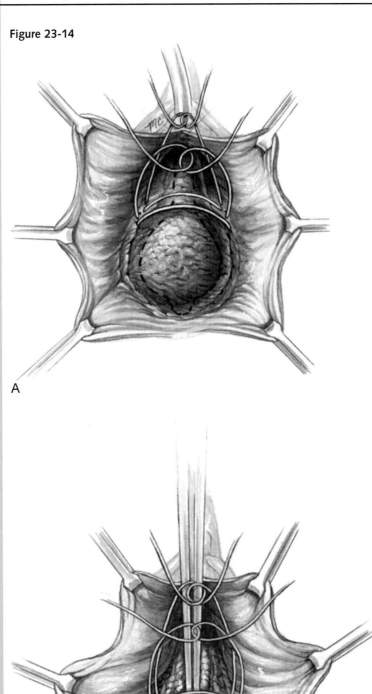

A

B

573

continued

Figure 23-14 Cont'd

C, A purse-string suture can be placed in the vaginal muscularis to reduce large cystoceles. **D,** The entire cystocele has been repaired with plication sutures, and the vaginal epithelium is trimmed before closure. (From Weber AM: Surgical correction of anterior vaginal wall prolapse. In Walters MD, Karram MM [eds]: Urogynecology and Reconstructive Pelvic Surgery, 2nd ed. St. Louis, Mosby, 1999, pp 211–219.)

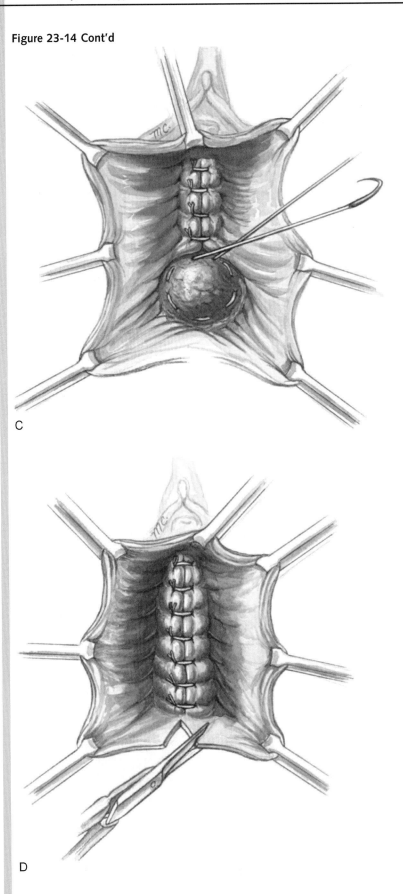

fasciae pelvis, starting at the level of the ischial spine and moving toward the urethrovesical junction. Sutures are then placed through the pubocervical muscularis and the underside of the vaginal epithelium using a three-point closure technique. The stitches are then tied in order from the urethra to the apex, alternating from one side to the other. If it has not already been performed, vaginal muscularis can then be plicated in the midline with several interrupted stitches using No. 0 delayed absorbable suture. The vaginal flaps are trimmed and closed with a running interlocking delayed absorbable suture.

Abdominal (or laparoscopic) paravaginal defect repair is performed by entering the retropubic space, as in Burch urethropexy. After the retropubic space has been entered, blunt dissection is carried out inferolaterally on both sides to identify the arcus tendineus fasciae pelvis. The obturator neurovascular bundle should also be visualized as dissection is carried toward the ischial spines. Once the dissection is complete, the lateral vaginal attachments to the arcus tendineus fasciae pelvic are visualized (level II support) and defects are noted. The defects are then repaired with No. 0 or 2-0 permanent or delayed absorbable suture, starting with the sutures closest to the ischial spines. Burch urethropexy is then performed as needed. It should be noted that paravaginal defect repairs are used for anterior vaginal wall prolapse, not stress urinary incontinence, because failure rates for incontinence are higher for paravaginal defect repair than for Burch urethropexy.

Operations for Posterior Vaginal Wall Prolapse

Posterior Colporrhaphy and Perineorrhaphy

Although the repairs of a relaxed perineum and posterior vaginal wall prolapse are usually performed together, they are two distinct operative procedures. Traditional posterior colporrhaphy involves plication of the rectovaginal muscularis in the midline; the technique is similar to anterior colporrhaphy. Special care must be taken during posterior colporrhaphy and perineorrhaphy not to narrow the introitus and vaginal canal excessively because this can lead to dyspareunia and difficulties with sexual intercourse. The ultimate size of the vaginal orifice is determined by placing Allis clamps on the inner aspect of the labia minora bilaterally and approximating them in the midline; the final vaginal opening should comfortably admit three fingers.

To begin the posterior colporrhaphy, Allis clamps are placed bilaterally on the posterior perineum. A triangular incision is made in the perineal body, and the overlying perineal skin is removed. The vaginal epithelium is undermined and divided in the midline with Mayo scissors, as in anterior colporrhaphy. The dissection is extended to the apex of the vagina and bilaterally in the rectovaginal space using blunt and sharp dissection, separating the vaginal epithelium from the rectovaginal muscularis laterally to mobilize the perirectal fascia and expose the medial margins of the puborectalis muscles.

Vertical mattress sutures are used to plicate the rectovaginal muscularis and perirectal fascia over the rectal wall. If the rectocele and levator hiatus are large, additional No. 0 delayed absorbable sutures are placed deeply into the medial portions of the puborectalis muscles, and the muscles are brought together in the rectovaginal space. Although levator plication effectively treats rectocele, it also tends to decrease the caliber of the vaginal lumen and to create a transverse ridge in the posterior vaginal wall, both of which may lead to dyspareunia. After the rectovaginal muscularis and levator muscles are plicated as appropriate, redundant vaginal epithelium is trimmed bilaterally, and the posterior vaginal epithelium is closed with No. 2-0 or 3-0 delayed absorbable running suture.

During perineorrhaphy, the components of the perineal body, including the anal sphincter, superficial and deep transverse perinei muscles, bulbocavernosus muscles, and the junction of the rectovaginal muscularis to the anal sphincter, are reconstructed. This can be performed after posterior colporrhaphy by placing deep sutures into the perineal muscles and fascia to build up the perineal body. The overlying vulvar skin is closed with No. 2-0 or 3-0 running subcuticular suture. A vaginal pack is placed after anterior and posterior colporrhaphy to compress the surgical beds; this is removed the first postoperative day.

The complications of posterior colporrhaphy and perineorrhaphy include blood loss requiring a transfusion, unintended proctotomy, and dyspareunia. Proctotomy should be repaired in layers at the time of the injury. After repair, management of the patient's diet is individualized. Use of a stool softener for 10 to 14 days may be beneficial but is not mandatory.

Discrete Rectovaginal Fascia Defect Repair

An alternative for the treatment of posterior vaginal wall prolapse is the site-specific repair of defects in the rectovaginal fascia (Denonvilliers' fascia). Isolated defects can be seen most readily when the vaginal epithelium is dissected sharply from the underlying rectovaginal fascia. Identification of rectovaginal defects is aided by rectal examination with the surgeon's finger elevated toward the vagina. Transverse defects may occur most superiorly along the posterior wall of the cervix or at the vaginal apex. In these patients with a "high rectocele," an enterocele is sometimes present as well. Transverse defects may also occur at mid vagina or, more commonly, where the rectovaginal fascia should be connected to the perineal body. The transverse defects may extend laterally and be associated with a tear or separation of the rectovaginal fascia from its normal attachment to the fascia over the levator muscles. Midline defects may occur in association with or separately from the other defects. The repairs of various defects are shown in Figure 23-15. This type of repair preserves vaginal caliber and may decrease the risk of postoperative dyspareunia.

Overall success rates of 80% to 90% have been reported for both types of repairs, but few studies have compared the long-term success of the different posterior colporrhaphy techniques. Some studies show discrete rectovaginal fascia defect repair to be as effective as posterior colporrhaphy for the treatment of posterior vaginal prolapse, whereas others show posterior colporrhaphy to have higher success rates. Most studies

Figure 23-15

A, Midline defect of the rectovaginal septum. Inset demonstrates reapproximation after repair. B, Transverse defect of the rectovaginal fascia in the mid to upper vagina. Inset depicts reapproximation after repair.

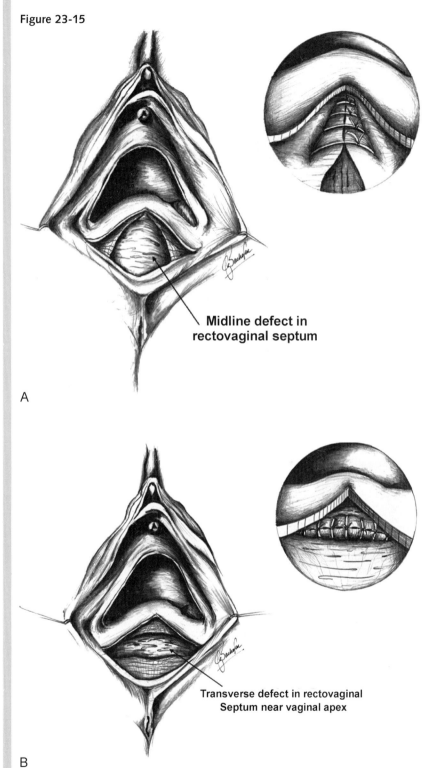

Midline defect in rectovaginal septum

A

Transverse defect in rectovaginal Septum near vaginal apex

B

577

continued

Figure 23-15 Cont'd

C, Transverse defect near the junction of the rectovaginal fascia to the perineal body. Inset depicts reapproximation after repair. **D,** Lateral defect in rectovaginal fascia. Inset demonstrates repair with interrupted sutures. (From Shull BL, Bachofen CB: Enterocele and rectocele. In Walters MD, Karram MM [eds]: Urogynecology and Reconstructive Pelvic Surgery, 2nd ed. St. Louis, Mosby, 1999, pp 211–219.)

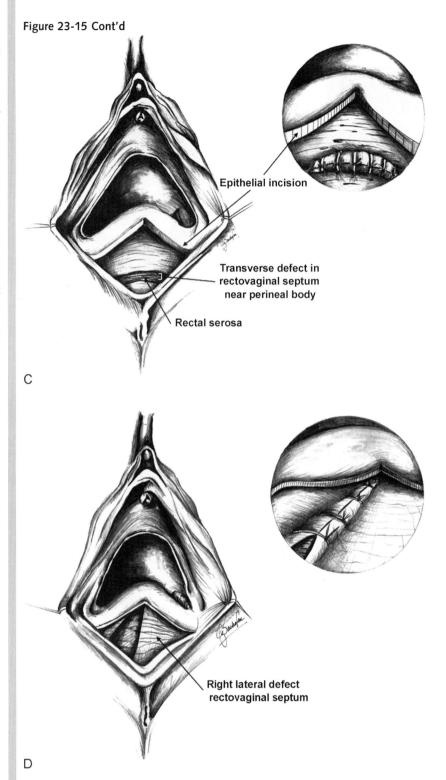

Epithelial incision

Transverse defect in
rectovaginal septum
near perineal body

Rectal serosa

C

Right lateral defect
rectovaginal septum

D

demonstrate higher rates of dyspareunia after posterior colporrhaphy compared with discrete rectovaginal fascia repair. More studies comparing the techniques are needed. Early recurrence after rectovaginal fascia defect repair is probably caused by failure to identify and individually repair all support defects. Late recurrence may be caused by the subsequent weakening of the patient's support tissue occurring with advancing age, chronic straining, estrogen deficiency, and other factors. The intraoperative complications of discrete rectovaginal fascia defect repair are similar to those of posterior colporrhaphy.

Grafts in Pelvic Reconstructive Surgery

Increasing attention is being paid to the addition of either autologous, xenographic, or synthetic grafts to reconstructive pelvic procedures to bolster surgical success rates and to decrease the risk of prolapse recurrence. However, data on the repairs with various graft materials are limited and restricted to mainly case series. Few randomized trials comparing repairs with grafts to those without have been conducted. No current evidence clearly demonstrates the superiority of repairs with grafts versus those without. However, many series have demonstrated significant complications with various graft materials. More evidence is needed before recommendations can be made regarding the use of graft materials in reconstructive pelvic surgery.

CONCLUSIONS

POP is relatively common, and its prevalence will continue to increase as the population ages. Although the pathophysiology of POP is probably multifactorial, a thorough understanding of pelvic anatomy, normal supportive mechanisms, and risk factors for prolapse is required to adequately treat patients suffering from the disorders. Current treatment options for patients with POP mainly include pessary use and surgery. As the predisposing factors and pathophysiology of prolapse become further understood, a shift from treatment to prevention may be seen in the future.

KEY POINTS

1. Normal pelvic organ support is maintained by a complex interplay between the striated muscles of the pelvic floor (i.e., levator ani muscle group) and their ligamentous attachments to the bony pelvis (i.e., endopelvic fascia).
2. The pathophysiology of pelvic organ prolapse (POP) is probably multifactorial and may be related to connective tissue disorders, pelvic neuropathy, chronic increases in abdominal pressure, or specific breaks in the endopelvic fascia.

Continued

KEY POINTS—CONT'D

3. Risk factors for POP include increasing age, pelvic floor injury during childbirth, chronic increases in intra-abdominal pressure, obesity, and distortions of the normal vaginal axis during pelvic reconstructive surgery.

4. POP is diagnosed with a careful history and physical examination assessing all aspects of pelvic support. During the examination, the patient should confirm that the maximum extent of the prolapse has been visualized. Ancillary testing is rarely required to diagnose POP.

5. When describing POP, segments of the lower reproductive tract (i.e., anterior, posterior, or apical vaginal wall) replace the terms *cystocele, rectocele, enterocele,* and *urethrovesical junction* because these terms imply an unrealistic certainty as to the structures on the other side of the vaginal bulge.

6. POP is staged in relation to the hymen and should be described in accordance with the Pelvic Organ Prolapse Quantification system.

7. Prolapse usually does not need to be treated if symptoms are not bothersome to the patient.

8. Pessaries are often successful in treating prolapse symptoms and may obviate the need for surgery.

9. The goal of surgical treatment of POP is to give the patient a durable repair that relieves her prolapse symptoms and improves her quality of life. A secondary goal is to restore anatomy and provide the patient with a functional vagina (unless the patient does not desire future coital function).

10. Most patients with POP have prolapse of multiple vaginal segments; surgical repair should be aimed at repairing all of the prolapsed segments.

SUGGESTED READING

American College of Obstetricians and Gynecologists: Surgery and patient choice: The ethics of decision making. ACOG Committee Opinion No. 289. Obstet Gynecol 102:1101–1106, 2003.

Bump RC, Mattiasson A, Bo K, et al: The standardization of terminology of female pelvic floor dysfunction. Am J Obstet Gynecol 175:10–17, 1996.

Colombo M, Milani R: Sacrospinous ligament fixation and modified McCall culdoplasty during vaginal hysterectomy for advanced uterovaginal prolapse. Am J Obstet Gynecol 179:13–20, 1998.

Cruikshank SH, Kovac SR: Randomized comparison of three surgical methods used at the time of vaginal hysterectomy to prevent posterior enterocele. Am J Obstet Gynecol 180:859–865, 1999.

DeLancey JOL: Anatomic aspects of vaginal eversion after hysterectomy. Am J Obstet Gynecol 166:1717–1728, 1992.

Given FT: "Posterior culdoplasty." Revisited. Am J Obstet Gynecol 153:135–139, 1985.

Handa VL, Garrett E, Hendrix S, et al: Progression and remission of pelvic organ prolapse: A longitudinal study of menopausal women. Am J Obstet Gynecol 190:27–32, 2004.

Hendrix SL, Clark A, Nygaard I, et al: Pelvic organ prolapse in the Women's Health Initiative: gravity and gravidity. Am J Obstet Gynecol 186:1160–1166, 2002.

Maher CF, Murray CJ, Carey MP, et al: Iliococcygeus or sacrospinous fixation for vaginal vault prolapse. Obstet Gynecol 98:40–44, 2001.

McCall ML: Posterior culdoplasty. Obstet Gynecol 10:595–602, 1957.

Nichols DH, Randall CL: Vaginal Surgery. Baltimore, MD, Williams & Wilkins, 1989.

Norton P, Boyd C, Deak S: Abnormal collagen ratios in women with genitourinary prolapse. Neurourol Urodyn 11:2–4, 1992.

Olsen AL, Smith VJ, Bergstrom JO, et al: Epidemiology of surgically managed pelvic organ prolapse and urinary incontinence. Obstet Gynecol 89:501–506, 1997.

Richardson AC: The anatomic defects in rectocele and enterocele. J Pelvic Surg 1:214–221, 1995.

Shull BL, Bachofen C, Coates KW, Kuehl TJ: A transvaginal approach to repair of apical and other associated sites of pelvic organ prolapse with uterosacral ligaments. Am J Obstet Gynecol 183:1365–1374, 2000.

Snyder TE, Krantz KE: Abdominal-retroperitoneal sacral colpopexy for the correction of vaginal prolapse. Obstet Gynecol 77:944–949, 1991.

Swift S, Pound T, Dias J: Case-control study of the etiology of severe pelvic organ prolapse. Int Urogynecol J 12:187–190, 2001.

Tulikangas PK, Walters MD, Brainard JA, Weber AM: Enterocele: Is there a histologic defect? Obstet Gynecol 98:634–637, 2001.

Walters MD and Karram MM (eds): Urogynecology and reconstructive pelvic surgery, 2nd ed. St. Louis Mosby, 1999.

Weber AM, Abrams P, Brubaker L, et al: The standardization of terminology for researchers in female pelvic floor disorders. Int Urogynecol J 12:178–186, 2001.

24

URINARY INCONTINENCE

Eric R. Sokol

INTRODUCTION

Urinary incontinence (UI) is the involuntary loss of urine from the urethra sufficient to be a problem. Even though 10% to 70% of women living in a community setting are affected by UI at an estimated annual cost in excess of $20 billion, only one in four women consults a health care professional to obtain treatment for this condition. Epidemiologic studies show that approximately 10% to 30% of women younger than 64 years of age have UI, and 15% to 30% of persons older than 65 years are incontinent. UI is even more prevalent in long-term care facilities, where more than 50% of patients experience it. In fact, UI is a major cause of institutionalization among elderly persons.

UI adversely affects the physical and psychological well-being of persons who experience it. Adverse events associated with UI are sleep deprivation from nocturia, urinary tract infections, urosepsis associated with urinary retention and indwelling catheters, and perineal irritation and breakdown from constant moisture. Among elderly patients, UI is also a major cause of hip fractures sustained during falls that occur while patients rush to the toilet. Adverse psychological impacts from UI include depression, sexual dysfunction, and social isolation. Moreover, the cost of incontinence pads, laundry, and medications for UI can be a hardship for patients on a fixed income.

UI may go unreported because of a number of factors. Patients may not report symptoms of incontinence because of the perceived social stigma, because of the belief that UI is an inevitable part of aging, or because of a lack of knowledge about available treatment options. In addition, when UI is reported, many health care providers are ill prepared to manage it. As a result, UI is vastly underdiagnosed and undertreated. With a growing elderly population, it is reasonable to expect a growing population of patients with UI. Such a common and treatable medical condition as UI deserves an increased amount of attention from all health care providers. In this chapter, we address the different types and causes of UI, prevention strategies, diagnostic techniques, and medical and surgical management techniques for UI.

A detailed discussion of female pelvic anatomy can be found in Chapter 4, Gynecologic Anatomy. This section will review only anatomic topics related to female UI. Female continence is maintained by the interaction of muscle, connective tissue, and nerves in the pelvic floor. The three layers of the pelvic floor function as a sheet of musculofascial tissue that spans the bony pelvis and provides critical support to the pelvic viscera. The first and innermost layer of the pelvic floor is the endopelvic fascia, which connects the vagina, urethra, and rectum to the sidewalls of the pelvis. The fascia is associated intimately with the pelvic viscera and the second layer of the pelvic floor, the levator ani muscle.

The second layer consists of the levator ani, a muscle complex consisting of three smaller muscles functioning as a group: the iliococcygeus, puborectalis, and pubococcygeus muscles. It attaches anteriorly to the bony pelvis at the pubic bones, laterally to the ischial spines and arcus tendineus levator ani, and posteriorly to the sacrum and coccyx. The levator ani muscle extends in a U shape around the rectum, attaching to the vagina and urethra as it passes by them. On contraction, the muscles of the levator ani complex lift the rectum, vagina, and urethra anteriorly, compressing the lumens of each structure.

The third and most superficial layer of the pelvic floor consists of the anal sphincter, the perineal membrane, and the external and internal urethral sphincters. The perineal membrane is a triangular fibrous layer that attaches the perineal body and vaginal side walls to the pubis. The perineal membrane does not provide primary support to the pelvic viscera, but instead functions to prevent excessive downward movement of the perineal body and pelvic organs when the levator ani muscles are relaxed, as during urination, defecation, and childbirth.

The external urethral sphincter is located cranial to the perineal membrane and is made up of the bilateral compressor urethrae, the urethrovaginal sphincter, and the sphincter urethrae muscles. These muscles surround the central portion of the urethra and play a minor role in maintaining resting urethral pressures and a major role in increasing urethral pressures in response to a sudden increase in intra-abdominal pressures.

The internal urethral sphincter is located at the vesical neck, where the urethra transverses the bladder wall. It is made up of the trigonal ring and detrusor loop muscles, which are smooth involuntary muscle extensions of the detrusor muscle of the bladder. The internal urethral sphincter is the primary contributor to resting pressures in the urethra. The urethral mucosa, which is rich in estrogen receptors and mucosal and submucosal vessels, provides additional resting pressure and aids in coaptation of the urethra at rest.

When abdominal pressure increases, such as with a cough, the urethra stays closed by maintaining a pressure higher than intravesical pressure. Connective tissues attaching the suburethral fascia to the levator ani muscles as well as to the fascia of the arcus tendineus create a firm platform that remains relatively stable in the face of the downward force generated by a cough. As the downward force is halted, the urethra is compressed and continence is maintained. However, if damage occurs to the endopelvic fascia or the levator ani muscles, downward force will displace the urethra caudally, and there will be insufficient urethral pressures to counterbalance the intravesical pressures, allowing leakage of urine. In addition, if the internal urethral sphincter is damaged and resting pressures are low, leakage can occur with sudden increases in intra-abdominal pressure, even if the external urethral sphincter and levator ani muscles are functioning properly.

NEUROPHYSIOLOGY

Bladder function cannot be fully understood without basic knowledge of neurophysiology. The bladder is unique because it is an "involuntary" organ that is under voluntary control. As the bladder fills during the urine storage phase, the detrusor muscle remains quiescent, with little change in intravesical pressure. There is a gradual increase in urethral resistance, known as the *guarding reflex,* to prevent urine loss during the filling phase. When the bladder is filled to a specific volume, tension receptors in the bladder sense fullness, and when appropriate, the external urethral sphincter is relaxed and a voluntary micturition reflex is initiated.

The lower urinary tract receives innervation from three sources: the sympathetic division of the autonomic nervous system, which controls urine storage; the parasympathetic division of the autonomic nervous system, which controls bladder emptying; and somatic innervation, which controls voluntary function of the pelvic floor musculature and the striated external urethral sphincter. Efferent sympathetic nerves arise from spinal cord segments T11 through L2, run through the hypogastric nerve plexus, and innervate the pelvic organs including the lower urinary tract, the rectum, and internal genital organs. Parasympathetic neurons arise from spinal levels S2 through S4 and run through the pelvic nerve and the hypogastric nerve plexus, meet with the sympathetic nerve fibers in Frankenhauser's plexus, and then continue to the bladder and other pelvic organs. Spinal levels S2 through S4 also give rise to the pudendal nerve, which is responsible for somatic and sensory innervation to the pelvic floor and urethral and anal sphincters. Figure 24-1 summarizes the neural pathways responsible for urine storage and micturition.

In the autonomic nervous system, the preganglionic neurotransmitter is acetylcholine. Likewise, in the parasympathetic division, the postganglionic neurotransmitter is acetylcholine. The detrusor muscle is filled with muscarinic cholinergic receptors that, when stimulated, respond with detrusor contraction and bladder emptying. This explains why anticholinergic medications are the mainstay of treatment for patients with detrusor overactivity. The postganglionic neurotransmitter for the sympathetic autonomic system is norepinephrine, which stimulates adrenergic receptors. α-Adrenergic receptors, found in the urethra and bladder neck, regulate vasoconstriction and smooth muscle contraction. When stimulated, the tone of the urethra will increase, helping to maintain continence.

Figure 24-1

Peripheral innervation of the female lower urinary tract. (From Walters MD, Karram MM [eds]: Urogynecology and Reconstructive Pelvic Surgery, 2nd ed. St. Louis, Mosby, 1999.)

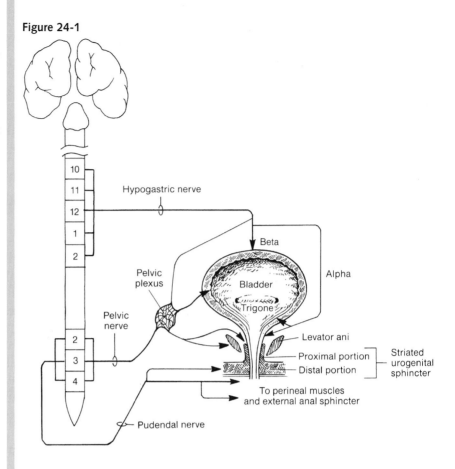

β-Adrenergic receptors are found in the bladder wall and function to relax the smooth muscle of the bladder and allow storage of urine.

Intact innervation of the urethra and periurethral muscles is paramount to maintaining continence. When the bladder fills, reflex stimulation of the α-adrenergic receptors within the smooth muscle of the bladder neck and urethra occurs, increasing outlet resistance. Voluntary and reflex stimulation of the muscles of the pelvic diaphragm also occurs, resulting from increased efferent pudendal nerve activity.

There are multiple complex facilitative and inhibitory pathways that function under the control of higher centers. Above the level of the spinal cord, the most important facilitative motor center for micturition is the pontine micturition center located in the brain stem. The cerebellum is the major center for controlling pelvic floor relaxation and the rate and force of detrusor contractions. The basal ganglia are involved in inhibition of detrusor contractions. The cerebral cortex (primarily the frontal lobes) is important in inhibiting the pontine micturition reflex.

A promising area for developing new stress urinary incontinence (SUI) treatments involves the role of the external urethral sphincter. The origin of somatic nerves to the external urethral sphincter is Onuf's nucleus in the sacral spinal cord. This nucleus has a high density of serotonin 2 (5-HT$_2$) receptors that, when stimulated, increase sphincter tone.

Researchers hope to develop medications by targeting the neurons of Onuf's nucleus to increase external urethral sphincter tone, thus decreasing incontinence.

CLASSIFICATION

Current classifications of UI are based on the recommendations from the International Continence Society.

Stress Urinary Incontinence

SUI is the involuntary leakage of urine on effort or exertion, such as during sneezing or coughing. It is the most common cause of UI in young women and the second most common cause of UI in older women. The diagnosis of *urodynamic stress incontinence* (previously referred to as *genuine stress incontinence*) is made by urodynamic testing to confirm leakage of urine with increased intra-abdominal pressure in the absence of a detrusor contraction. Urodynamic stress incontinence is the most common cause of UI among ambulatory women, accounting for 29% to 75% of cases. *Intrinsic sphincter deficiency* (ISD) is a subtype of stress incontinence in which there is a failure of the internal urethral sphincter to maintain mucosal coaptation at rest or during minimal physical stress, leading to the involuntary leakage of urine. The diagnosis of ISD is made by urodynamic testing and is discussed later in this chapter. It is important to identify patients with ISD before therapeutic intervention because they may have higher failure rates with certain surgical procedures, such as retropubic suspensions.

Urge Urinary Incontinence

Urge UI is involuntary leakage accompanied by or immediately preceded by the feeling of urgency. Women with urge incontinence characteristically complain of a strong, irrepressible urge to void accompanied by leakage of moderate to large volumes of urine. Symptoms of urge incontinence also include increased daytime frequency (defined as more than eight voids in a 24-hour period) and nocturia (defined as waking more than once at night to void). Patients often report triggers for urge incontinence such as running water, cold weather, or putting a key in the door. *Detrusor overactivity incontinence* is a urodynamic diagnosis of leakage accompanied by involuntary detrusor muscle contractions. When the detrusor contractions are the result of a neurologic insult such as a spinal cord injury, the label *neurogenic detrusor overactivity* is used. *Overactive bladder, detrusor instability,* and *sensory urgency* are all terms previously used to describe urge UI. Detrusor overactivity accounts for 7% to 33% of incontinence cases.

Mixed Incontinence

Mixed incontinence is an involuntary leakage of urine associated with urgency and exertion, such as effort, coughing, sneezing, or laughing. Overall, this is the most common form of UI in women. Although the exact mechanism of mixed incontinence is still under investigation, the condition is widely believed to be caused by a combination of detrusor overactivity and impaired urethral sphincter function. Clinically, it helps to determine which symptoms bother the patient more and to address them accordingly. Because patients with mixed incontinence can present with variable symptoms, multichannel urodynamic testing can help to guide clinical therapy.

Overflow Incontinence

Overflow incontinence is a condition of urinary dribbling or continuous leakage associated with incomplete bladder emptying caused by outlet obstruction or impaired detrusor contractility. The International Continence Society deems the term *overflow incontinence* to be confusing and therefore recommends using terms that describe the symptoms and pathophysiology (such as *bladder outlet obstruction*). Other appropriate descriptive terms include *chronic retention of urine* and *acute retention of urine.* Although acute retention of urine is common in older men, this form of obstruction is relatively rare in women and is usually caused by prior corrective surgery for UI. In women, chronic or acute retention is also associated with severe genital prolapse, postsurgical obstruction, diabetes, or neurologic disease. Patients with chronic retention may present with symptoms of stress incontinence, urge incontinence, or mixed incontinence, but the symptoms will not improve unless the underlying cause is diagnosed and treated. The sensation of incomplete bladder emptying and consistently elevated postvoid residuals are suggestive of chronic retention of urine.

Extra-Urethral Incontinence

Extra-urethral incontinence encompasses less common causes of UI such as ectopic ureters and fistulas. Women with extra-urethral incontinence often describe constant urinary leakage, even during the night and without exertion. If constant urinary leakage has been present since the patient was born, an ectopic ureter should be suspected. A fistula is usually associated with a history of obstructed labor, previous pelvic surgery, or pelvic radiation. Fistulas are discussed in more detail in Chapter 26, Urinary Tract Injury and Genital Tract Fistulas.

Uncategorized Incontinence

Some patients with a normally functioning bladder and urethra are unable to make it to the toilet because of physical impairments such as limited mobility or mental impairments due to dementia or oversedation from medications. Sometimes a simple intervention, such as a walker or a bedside commode, can have a profound impact on a patient's quality of life by reducing episodes of UI.

PREDISPOSING FACTORS

Increasing awareness of the detrimental effects UI has on quality of life has lead to a growing body of research aimed at identifying risk factors. Modifiable risk factors include bladder irritants such as caffeine, urinary tract infections, and bladder stones. Chronically increased intra-abdominal pressure associated with UI can be caused by such conditions as morbid obesity, chronic obstructive pulmonary disease, chronic cough, and chronic constipation. Neurologic factors such as strokes or dementia are risk factors, whereas a familial predisposition to UI has been suggested in some studies. Developing a prevention program to address modifiable risk factors in women alone could reduce new cases of incontinence by approximately 50,000 cases annually.

Two important risk factors for UI are age and female sex. Data from the Norwegian Epidemiology of Incontinence in the County of Nord-Trøndelag (EPINCONT) group demonstrate a clear pattern of increasing prevalence of stress incontinence with advancing age. The association between aging and urge incontinence may be partially explained by ultrastructural changes in the bladder and accumulated interruptions in the central nervous system inhibitory pathways such as those that occur with cervical spinal stenosis or stroke. Elderly persons are especially at risk for transient causes of incontinence, including delirium, infection, severe depression, restricted mobility, and stool impaction. Medications often used by the elderly, such as α-blockers and sedative-hypnotics, can also adversely affect bladder function or may be so sedating that patients are unaware of the need to void. Table 24-1 summarizes the effects of common medications on bladder function. Older persons may experience a number of comorbid conditions that either directly or indirectly affect function of the lower genitourinary tract, and at least one third of elderly patients have multiple predisposing conditions.

Gender is also a significant risk factor, since the risk of developing UI has been associated with increasing parity as well as vaginal delivery. Trauma occurring during vaginal delivery can weaken the collagen fibers that provide fascial support to the pelvic organs, contributing to UI and pelvic organ prolapse. Passage of the baby through the birth canal has been postulated to damage and stretch the pudendal nerve, thereby weakening the levator ani muscles that are crucial to continence. Several large trials have demonstrated a moderate to large attributable risk for vaginal delivery in the development of UI and pelvic floor dysfunction. However, a study by Buchsbaum and colleagues also showed the incidence of UI to be almost 50% in a group of 149 nulliparous nuns. These conflicting studies highlight the fact that vaginal delivery is only one of a number of factors that can lead to the development of incontinence, and that all women, regardless of pregnancy or childbirth history, should be asked about symptoms of UI.

PATIENT HISTORY

A carefully taken history can result in a working diagnosis for and guide the diagnostic workup of UI. It is important to ask all women specifically about symptoms of UI during a gynecologic visit because at least half of incontinent persons will not report the problem to their health care

Table 24-1

Medications	Effect on the Bladder Function
Diuretics	Polyuria, frequency, and urgency
Caffeine	Aggravation or precipitation of urge symptoms
Anticholinergic agents	Urinary retention, overflow incontinence, fecal impaction
Psychotropic agents:	
Antidepressants	Anticholinergic actions, sedation
Antipsychotics	Anticholinergic actions, sedation, rigidity, and immobility
Sedatives/hypnotics/CNS depressants	Sedation, delirium, immobility, muscle relaxation
Narcotic analgesics	Urinary retention, sedation, delirium (and fecal impaction)
α-adrenergic blockers	Urethral relaxation
α-adrenergic agonists (present in many cold and diet over-the-counter preparations)	Urinary retention
β-adrenergic agonists	Urinary retention
Calcium channel blockers	Urinary retention

CNS, Central nervous system.

providers. A thorough urogynecologic workup can be time-consuming, so it may help to have the patient fill out a questionnaire at home, giving her the opportunity to fully consider her symptoms, thus providing more accurate information. The questionnaire should be reviewed with the patient at a subsequent visit. Although patient histories can be helpful for diagnosis, studies of the use of history alone to predict stress or urge UI have shown sensitivities of 70% to 90% and specificities of 50% to 55%. Further diagnostic testing is therefore indicated before treatment is initiated.

When taking a patient's history, lower urinary tract symptoms can be divided into three groups: storage, voiding, and postmicturition symptoms. Symptoms occurring during the storage phase of the bladder include urinary frequency, urgency, nocturia, urge incontinence, stress incontinence, and nocturnal enuresis. Symptoms experienced during the voiding phase include slow stream, splitting or spraying of the urine stream, straining, hesitancy, or terminal dribble. Symptoms occurring immediately after micturition include the feeling of incomplete bladder emptying and postmicturition dribbling. Questions should be phrased to clearly distinguish these three different phases.

To determine the best course of treatment, it is important to distinguish whether the patient has SUI, urinary frequency, urinary urgency, urge incontinence, or mixed incontinence. If she has mixed incontinence, are the stress or urge symptoms more prominent? Questions about dysuria and irritative bladder symptoms (e.g., urgency, frequency, and nocturia) can screen for common conditions such as urinary tract infections. Any complaints of incomplete bladder emptying should also be elicited because obstructive conditions such as pelvic organ prolapse or previous incontinence surgery are relatively common in this group of patients. Also, direct questioning about the severity of the problem, such as the need for pad use and the degree to which symptoms are troublesome to the patient, help to determine a course of treatment.

A useful tool for the physician and the patient is a bladder diary. Diaries help to record signs that suggest lower urinary tract dysfunction. The patient keeps such a diary for 24 to 48 hours, and the results can be used to quantify the amount and type of daily fluid intake, urine output, frequency, and number of incontinent episodes. This information helps the physician to assess whether excessive fluid or caffeine intake is part of the problem and can help gauge the severity of the incontinence. Studies have shown that the simple act of keeping a bladder diary has therapeutic effects for patients. The diary can also chart the progress of treatments as they are tried.

The physician should also screen for conditions frequently associated with UI, such as pelvic organ prolapse, defecatory dysfunction, and urinary tract infections. Does the patient note a vaginal bulge, and is it necessary for her to manually replace the bulge in order to void or defecate? Does she have trouble with fecal incontinence or constipation? Is she sexually active, and if not, is the abstinence due to incontinence? Patients with hematuria, especially smokers or women with a history of exposure to aniline dyes, should be screened for renal and bladder cancer.

The physician must obtain a full medical, neurologic, surgical, obstetric, gynecologic, and pharmacologic history. The medical and neurologic history should include any history of asthma, renal disease, diabetes mellitus, poliomyelitis, stroke, arthritis, radiculopathies, sciatica, multiple sclerosis, syphilis, and vitamin B_{12} deficiency. The surgical history should screen for hysterectomy, previous prolapse surgery, previous incontinence surgery, and urethral dilation. Obstetric history should include any history of prolonged labor or complicated delivery, as well as the weight of the largest baby. Carefully examining the medication list can help the physician to determine whether there might be an iatrogenic component to the incontinence.

PHYSICAL EXAMINATION

The physician should perform a complete general examination, including examinations of the cardiovascular system (to look for evidence of volume overload), abdomen (to evaluate for masses and tenderness), extremities (to assess for mobility), and pelvis. In addition, a neurologic examination should include sensory and motor strength testing of the lower extremities. During the pelvic examination, further neurologic evaluation should include testing the bulbocavernosus reflex and the "anal wink." This testing should be done at the beginning of the pelvic examination because these reflexes accommodate to touch and are less likely to be elicited later in the examination. The bulbocavernosus reflex confirms proper function of the sacral reflex arcs and can be elicited by gently touching a cotton-tipped applicator lateral to the clitoris and observing contraction of the external anal sphincter. The anal wink can be elicited by gently touching a cotton-tipped applicator lateral to the external anal sphincter and observing its contraction. These reflexes are absent in about 15% of healthy patients. In addition, the voluntary contraction of the external anal sphincter suggests intact innervation of the pelvic floor muscles through the pudendal nerve.

The pelvic examination continues with inspection of the external genitalia, noting evidence of genital atrophy or excoriation and irritation, possibly due to contact with wet pads or undergarments. If the vulva is irritated, petroleum-based barrier products (such as those used for diaper rash) and frequent pad changes should be encouraged. Vaginal examination should include an assessment for pelvic organ prolapse, hypoestrogenic vaginal epithelium, and anatomic abnormalities. The physician should examine the base of the bladder, and the urethra should be evaluated for evidence of a diverticulum and for any discharge from the urethral meatus. Furthermore, pelvic muscle tone can be assessed both at rest and with a voluntary contraction. Support defects of the anterior, apical, and posterior segments of the vagina should be independently staged using the Pelvic Organ Prolapse Quantification system (see Chapter 23, Pelvic Organ Prolapse and Pelvic Floor Dysfuction). A Q-tip test can evaluate for mobility of the urethral-vesical junction. In patients with SUI, upward deflection of the tip of the cotton swab greater than 30 degrees with straining suggests that the patient's symptoms will respond to surgical correction.

A rectovaginal examination should be performed to rule out fecal impaction or rectal masses, as well as to assess for external anal sphincter tone and squeeze pressure. It can also screen for any palpable defects in the rectovaginal septum suggestive of a rectocele. Occult blood testing should be performed if it has not been done recently. A full bimanual examination should be performed to assess for uterine or adnexal abnormalities and pelvic masses. For an adequate bimanual examination to be performed, the patient's bladder must be empty because a full bladder can interfere with the evaluation of the pelvic organs. If the patient's bladder is full before the pelvic examination, the patient should be asked to cough and perform the Valsalva maneuver to see whether transurethral leakage of urine occurs. Observing involuntary urine leakage that occurs with coughing or the Valsalva maneuver confirms the presence of SUI. Leakage of urine from channels other than the urethra is highly suggestive of a fistula.

If the patient reports a sensation of incomplete bladder emptying or has risk factors for urinary retention, the physician should measure a postvoid residual volume using a sterile bladder catheter or bladder ultrasound. Finally, a urine specimen should be sent for urinalysis and culture to rule out infection and hematuria, and urine cytology can be sent to screen for urothelial cancer in patients with risk factors such as a history of hematuria, smoking, or exposure to aniline dyes.

URODYNAMIC TESTING

Routine urodynamic testing is not recommended for all patients reporting symptoms of UI. However, many urogynecologists will proceed with urodynamic testing if the clinical picture is unclear, if the patient's condition has failed to respond to previous medical or surgical therapy, or if surgical intervention is planned. Urodynamic testing is the gold standard for the assessment of lower urinary tract function. The data from urodynamic testing can be used to inform clinical decisions and can provide objective outcome measures for research studies. Urodynamic testing protocols often include uroflowmetry, simple or multichannel cystometry, abdominal leak point pressure measurement and/or urethral pressure profilometry, and a pressure-voiding study.

Uroflowmetry is a screening tool for voiding dysfunction in which the patient voids into a special commode that measures flow in milliliters per second versus time, thereby assessing urine flow patterns. Intermittent, interrupted, or prolonged uroflow patterns suggest a voiding disorder such as an underactive detrusor muscle or outlet obstruction that should be further evaluated by pressure-flow studies. Various uroflow patterns are illustrated in Figure 24-2. A postvoid residual urine check can be made with a urethral catheter or bladder ultrasound measurement. Although normal values for postvoid residual urine volumes have not been established, volumes less than 50 mL indicate adequate bladder emptying. Repetitive postvoid residuals ranging from 100 to 200 mL or higher may indicate urinary retention, which can cause overflow incontinence.

Cystometry is a test of detrusor muscle function that can be used to assess bladder sensation, capacity, and compliance. Cystometry is also used to determine the presence and magnitude of both voluntary and involuntary detrusor contractions. A simple cystometry can be performed

593

Figure 24-2

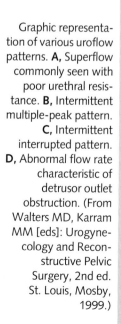

Graphic representation of various uroflow patterns. **A,** Superflow commonly seen with poor urethral resistance. **B,** Intermittent multiple-peak pattern. **C,** Intermittent interrupted pattern. **D,** Abnormal flow rate characteristic of detrusor outlet obstruction. (From Walters MD, Karram MM [eds]: Urogynecology and Reconstructive Pelvic Surgery, 2nd ed. St. Louis, Mosby, 1999.)

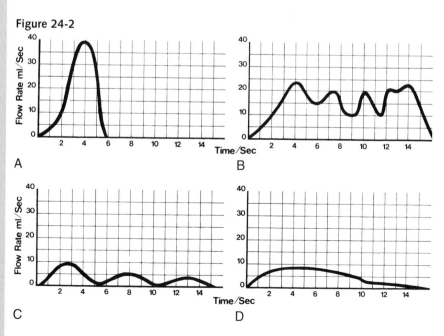

by filling the bladder in a retrograde fashion with a 60-mL syringe (without its plunger) connected to a catheter. Water is poured into the syringe in 60-mL aliquots, and the patient's first bladder sensation and bladder capacity are noted. If the water level in the syringe begins to rise or overflow during filling, an uninhibited bladder contraction may be occurring. A standing cough stress test and supine empty bladder cough stress test can be performed at this time. The complex cystometrogram is performed by placing a pressure catheter into the vagina or rectum to measure abdominal pressure and a double-sensor catheter in the urethra and bladder. By subtracting the abdominal pressure from the vesical pressure, the detrusor pressure can be measured while the bladder is filled with sterile saline or water. The cystometrogram is performed with the catheters in place, with the goal of differentiating urodynamic stress incontinence from detrusor overactivity. The patient is asked to cough or perform Valsalva maneuvers at different times during bladder filling, and any resulting leakage is noted. If the patient leaks at the exact moment of increased abdominal pressure without a concomitant rise in detrusor pressure, then she has urodynamic stress incontinence. If, on the other hand, any significant rise occurs in the true detrusor pressure during filling or provocation, detrusor overactivity is demonstrated.

Two tests can be used to assess intrinsic urethral sphincter function. Abdominal leak point pressures are performed by recording pressures with a Valsalva maneuver at the time of urinary leakage. Urinary leakage that occurs at less than 60 cm of water pressure suggests a diagnosis of ISD. The second test is the urethral pressure profile, which is performed by pulling the urethral catheter along the length of the urethra while measuring closure pressures. A maximum urethral closure pressure of less than 20 cm H_2O is another parameter that suggests the diagnosis of ISD. This test can also measure the functional urethral length; that is, the length of the urethra that maintains a pressure above that of the bladder.

Finally, a pressure-flow voiding study can be performed by having the patient void with the catheters in place, which allows for assessment of the voiding mechanism. A normal voiding mechanism involves urethral relaxation with detrusor pressure elevation. Especially in elderly persons, a prolonged uroflow pattern can sometimes be found in the absence of a functional outlet obstruction. Usually these patients are found to have poor detrusor contractions, which can be documented during this examination.

BEHAVIORAL APPROACHES

Simple behavior modifications can have a large impact on a patient's incontinence. For example, patients who admit to using excessive caffeine should be instructed to decrease intake or switch to noncaffeinated beverages because caffeine is both a diuretic and bladder irritant. Also, overweight patients may benefit from an exercise and diet regimen because weight loss can reduce episodes of UI.

Bladder training aimed at increasing the interval between voiding has been shown to be beneficial for urge, stress, and mixed UI. The patient is instructed to determine the longest interval she can wait between voids without risking an urge incontinence episode. She is then instructed to void on this initial schedule, increasing the interval by 15 to 30 minutes every week or two. For example, if a patient voids every hour during the day, then this is the interval that is initiated. She then progressively increases this interval, with a goal interval being every 3 to 4 hours. If the patient feels the urge to void sooner, she is instructed to suppress the urge by performing three quick Kegel squeezes. By flexing the levator ani muscles, it is theorized that a reflex arc is interrupted, allowing the bladder to relax.

Pelvic muscle exercises, also called *Kegel exercises,* have been shown to reduce the frequency of urine loss in patients with SUI and can also improve the symptoms of urge incontinence. To teach a patient to perform Kegel exercises, she should be instructed to squeeze her pelvic muscles around the physician's fingers during a pelvic examination as if she were trying to stop the flow of urine or hold back gas. Once the patient has learned the proper muscles to flex, she should be instructed to perform 10 repetitions of these exercises from three to eight times a day (between 30 and 80 repetitions). These exercises should be performed daily for 3 months for the best results.

Other treatments include pessaries such as the incontinence dish and the incontinence ring. These devices can create a physical obstruction to the urethra and can stabilize the proximal urethra and bladder neck, reducing episodes of leakage caused by urethral hypermobility. Some patients with mild symptoms may find that a diaphragm or a tampon used during exercise can prevent leakage.

PHYSIOTHERAPY OF THE PELVIC FLOOR

In the treatment of UI, pelvic muscle exercises can be used alone or augmented with biofeedback therapy or vaginal weight training. Pelvic floor electrical stimulation is another modality that can be used for pelvic muscle rehabilitation. Biofeedback can help patients identify and strengthen their pelvic floor muscles, thereby maintaining the bladder neck in a favorable position during stress maneuvers. Biofeedback is performed by placing a sensor in the vagina and having the patient isolate her levator ani muscle from visual cues on a computer screen. In one study, biofeedback led to symptom improvement in 66% of patients with SUI and in 33% of patients with detrusor overactivity. Specially designed vaginal weights can also be used to augment pelvic muscle exercise programs.

Pelvic floor electrical stimulation uses vaginal or anal sensors or surface electrodes to produce contractions of the levator ani muscles and the external urethral and anal sphincters. This treatment modality is theorized to work by promoting growth of motor axons to the pelvic floor muscles.

Adverse reactions are minimal and include discomfort. Some studies have shown a modest improvement in the symptoms of stress incontinence and detrusor overactivity.

MEDICAL MANAGEMENT

Stress Urinary Incontinence

The rationale for using pharmacologic therapy in SUI caused by urethral sphincter insufficiency is based on selecting agents targeted toward the high concentration of α-adrenergic receptors in the bladder neck, bladder base, and proximal urethra. Sympathomimetic drugs with α-adrenergic agonist activity presumably cause muscle contraction in these areas, thereby increasing bladder outlet resistance. However, adverse effects such as hypertension have limited the use of these medications. Duloxetine is a selective serotonin reuptake inhibitor that has some α-adrenergic properties and holds particular promise as a medical treatment for SUI.

Because the bladder and urethra are rich in estrogen receptors, oral and vaginal estrogen supplementation has been used to try to improve symptoms of incontinence. However, recent studies have suggested an increase in UI with estrogen therapy.

Detrusor Overactivity

A number of pharmacologic agents appear to be effective in the treatment of urinary frequency, urgency, and urge incontinence. These agents can be broadly classified into anticholinergic agents, tricyclic antidepressants, musculotropic drugs, and a variety of less commonly used medications.

Anticholinergic agents are effective treatments for UI because they block contractile activity of the bladder. Oxybutynin has both anticholinergic and direct smooth muscle relaxant properties and is available in immediate release (IR), extended release (ER), and transdermal formulations. The generic IR formulation is less expensive than the ER formulation. The initial dosage for the IR formulation is 5 mg to 10 mg daily, followed by titration as needed up to 30 mg/day in divided doses. The ER formulation is started at 5 mg once daily and is titrated as needed up to 30 mg once daily. The rapid onset of action of the IR preparation makes it useful when protection is wanted at specific times, and it can decrease urinary frequency even if incontinence is not abolished. The efficacy of oxybutynin may continue to increase beyond 2 weeks, suggesting that physicians should avoid escalating the dose too quickly or abandoning therapy too soon.

Several randomized controlled studies have shown oxybutynin to be effective in the treatment of UI. In six studies of middle-aged outpatients, oxybutynin reduced urge incontinence frequency by 15% to 58% compared with placebo. In two of these studies, 43% and 67% of subjects became subjectively continent, a much better result than occurred with placebo. Oxybutynin has also been effective and well tolerated when instilled into the bladder of study patients, primarily those with neuropathic bladder.

Adverse effects from oxybutynin have been noted in all studies and include dry skin, blurred vision, change in mental status, nausea, constipation, and marked xerostomia (dry mouth). Severity of the adverse effects increased with dosage, with severe xerostomia occurring in 84% of subjects receiving 5 mg of oxybutynin four times per day. Dry mouth may be less frequent with the ER and transdermal preparations.

Tolterodine is another anticholinergic agent that is similar in effectiveness. The IR formulation is taken as a 1- or 2-mg tablet twice a day. The ER formulation can be taken as a 2- or 4-mg tablet once daily and is well tolerated by most patients. Tolterodine causes dry mouth less frequently than IR oxybutynin 5 mg three times daily but has similar adverse effects to ER oxybutynin 10 mg/day. A meta-analysis found that oxybutynin and tolterodine have similar clinical efficacy, but tolterodine is better tolerated (dry mouth relative risk [RR], 0.54; 95% confidence interval [CI], 0.48 to 0.61; study withdrawal because of side effects RR, 0.63; 95% CI, 0.46 to 0.88). A subsequent randomized trial confirmed these findings. However, there have been case reports of cognitive adverse effects mimicking dementia with tolterodine, and tolterodine is more expensive than generic oxybutynin IR. All anticholinergic drugs are contraindicated in patients with documented narrow-angle glaucoma.

Trospium (20 mg twice daily) was recently approved by the U.S. Food and Drug Administration (FDA) for the treatment of overactive bladder with symptoms of urge incontinence, urgency, and urinary frequency. In a randomized trial of 523 patients with overactive bladder and urge incontinence, patients who received trospium had a larger decrease in the number of daily episodes of incontinence compared with placebo (from 3.9 to 1.6 episodes with trospium versus decrease from 4.3 to 2.4 episodes with placebo). Constipation occurred in 10% of patients, and dry mouth occurred in 22% of patients treated with trospium.

Darifenacin (7.5 to 15 mg daily) and solifenacin (5 to 10 mg daily) were also recently approved by the FDA for the treatment of overactive bladder with symptoms of urge incontinence, urgency, and urinary frequency. Darifenacin and solifenacin are more selective for M3 muscarinic receptors in the bladder, though it is unclear whether this increased selectivity improves clinical outcomes. One randomized trial of solifenacin showed a decrease in the number of incontinence episodes in 24 hours compared with placebo, but not significantly more than with tolterodine 2 mg twice daily. Rates of dry mouth with solifenacin 5 mg, solifenacin 10 mg, tolterodine, and placebo were 14%, 21%, 19%, and 5%, respectively; rates of constipation were 7%, 8%, 3%, and 2%.

Tricyclic antidepressants such as imipramine can be tried as a second-line therapy for detrusor overactivity in patients whose conditions fail to improve with oxybutynin or tolterodine. Imipramine acts to decrease bladder overactivity through its anticholinergic effects and can increase closing pressures in the proximal urethra through its α-adrenergic effects. Although a subset of patients respond favorably to imipramine, this drug carries a higher rate of adverse effects. The most common adverse effects are nausea and insomnia. Imipramine should be used with caution in elderly persons because anticholinergic side effects and orthostatic hypotension may be increased in these patients.

Other medications such as propantheline, dicyclomine, and hyoscyamine have been used for the treatment of urge incontinence with varying degrees of success, but data regarding the efficacy of these medications have been inconsistent in randomized, controlled trials.

SURGICAL MANAGEMENT

Although detrusor overactivity is primarily treated medically, surgery is the mainstay of treatment for SUI. The purpose of surgical repair often depends on the perceived cause of the incontinence. Surgeries for UI are performed to reestablish the normal anatomic relationships thought to be important to the continence mechanism; to stabilize the anterior vaginal wall, bladder neck, and urethra in a retropubic position; to increase urethral outlet resistance; or to create a "backboard" that allows for urethral compression during instances of increased intra-abdominal pressure. The following sections discuss the most commonly performed surgical procedures for UI.

Retropubic Procedures

Retropubic urethrovesical suspension for the treatment of SUI was first described by Marshall and colleagues in 1949. The purpose of the procedure was to stabilize the bladder neck and proximal urethra in a retropubic position, preventing descent of the bladder neck and creating a firm shelf of suburethral tissue to compress the urethra. There have been various modifications of the procedure since then, but the basic concept has remained unchanged. Retropubic urethropexies remain popular today because of their consistently high cure and improvement rates for SUI with urethral hypermobility.

Patient Selection for Retropubic Procedures
Patients with a diagnosis of SUI with urethral hypermobility are the best candidates for retropubic urethrovesical suspension procedures. Although patients diagnosed with ISD may derive some benefit from these procedures, studies show that more obstructive operations, such as suburethral slings, may provide better long-term results.

Patients are diagnosed with urodynamic stress incontinence using clinical and urodynamic parameters. They exhibit loss of urine at the urethral meatus under direct observation with increases in intra-abdominal pressure, such as during coughing. During urodynamic testing (simple or complex), urine loss is observed during episodes of increased abdominal pressure in the absence of detrusor muscle contractions. A positive upward deflection of the handle of a long cotton swab more than 30 degrees from the neutral position while straining is suggestive of urethral hypermobility. The presence of urinary leakage during an empty supine cough stress test, a maximum urethral closure pressure less than 20 cm of H_2O and/or a Valsalva leak point pressure less than 60 cm H_2O is suggestive of ISD, and these patients may have higher failure rates after retropubic urethrovesical suspension procedures.

Burch Colposuspension

Burch colposuspension is performed with the patient in the supine position, with legs slightly abducted, to allow the surgeon to operate with his or her nondominant hand in the vagina and the other hand in the retropubic space. Access to the retropubic space is achieved through a Pfannenstiel or Cherney incision, and the surgeon dissects close to the pubic bones to expose the Retzius space. Once the retropubic space is entered, the bladder and urethra are depressed, and care is taken to avoid dissection in the midline to protect the urethra from surgical trauma. Blunt dissection is then used to expose the periurethral fascia and vaginal wall on either side of the urethra, facilitated by elevating the lateral anterior vaginal wall with the surgeon's nondominant hand in the vagina. The urethra and lower edge of the bladder are identified by palpating the Foley catheter balloon medial to the area of elevation and dissection. Once the glistening white layer of periurethral fascia and vaginal wall are seen, two sutures of 0 or 1 delayed absorbable or permanent suture are placed laterally in the anterior vaginal wall, with care taken to include the full thickness of the vaginal wall, but excluding the vaginal epithelium. The most distal suture is placed approximately 2 cm lateral to the proximal third of the urethra, and the proximal suture is placed approximately 2 cm lateral to the bladder wall at the level of the urethrovesical junction. These two sutures are placed in the same location on each side of the urethra and then attached to the ipsilateral Cooper's ligament on each side, creating two suspension sutures on each side of the urethra and urethrovesical junction. With a vaginal finger elevating the urethrovesical junction and proximal urethra to a neutral position, the distal suspension sutures are tied first, followed by the proximal suspension stitches. Absorbable gelatin sponge (Gelfoam) can be placed behind the suture bridges before tying them to facilitate hemostasis and scarring. Scarring of the periurethral and vaginal tissues to the fascia over the obturator internus muscle ultimately leads to vaginal and urethral support. When tying the suspension sutures, it is not necessary to have the vaginal wall apposed to the Cooper's ligaments, which may create too much tension across the vaginal wall and compress the urethra against the pubic symphysis, leading to voiding dysfunction. The Burch colposuspension procedure can be also be performed laparoscopically. Figure 24-3 illustrates the technique of an open Burch colposuspension.

Marshall-Marchetti-Krantz Procedure

Similar to the Burch urethropexy procedure, in the Marshall-Marchetti-Krantz (MMK) procedure the retropubic space is exposed and entered either through an abdominal incision or laparoscopically. With the surgeon's nondominant hand elevating the urethrovesical junction on either side of the urethra vaginally, double bites of delayed absorbable sutures

599

Figure 24-3

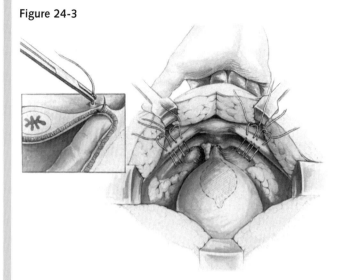

Technique of Burch colposuspension. (From Walters MD, Karram MM [eds]: Urogynecology and Reconstructive Pelvic Surgery, 2nd ed. St. Louis, Mosby, 1999.)

are placed at right angles to the urethra, lateral to the bladder neck, including the full thickness of the anterior vaginal wall but excluding the vaginal epithelium. After placement of one such suture lateral to the bladder neck on each side, the sutures are driven through the periosteum of the pubic symphysis and tied while elevating the urethrovesical junction with a vaginal finger. Use of the MMK procedure has decreased in recent years because of reports in the literature of postsurgical osteitis pubis in 0.74% to 2.5% of cases.

Paravaginal Defect Repair

Most surgeons do not use the paravaginal defect repair as a primary treatment for SUI because long-term results have been disappointing. The paravaginal defect repair aims to reattach the endopelvic fascia overlying the anterolateral vaginal sulcus to the fascia overlying the obturator internus and pubococcygeus muscles at the level of the arcus tendineus fascia pelvis. Avulsion of the lateral vaginal walls bilaterally can lead to rotational descent of the proximal urethra and bladder base with increases in intra-abdominal pressure, leading to SUI. The approach to paravaginal defect repair is similar to the Burch retropubic urethropexy procedure, and the retropubic space is entered in the same fashion. With the surgeon's nondominant hand in the vagina, the lateral vaginal wall is pulled medially, exposing the obturator internus muscle and obturator neurovascular bundle. The arcus tendineus fascia pelvis can then be identified in the lateral retropubic space as a thin band of white tissue running from the ischial spine, over the pubococcygeus and obturator internus muscles, to the back of the inferior edge of the pubic symphysis. With the surgeon's nondominant hand elevating the anterolateral vaginal sulcus, a permanent suture is then placed through the full thickness of the vaginal mucosa, excluding vaginal epithelium, and through the fascia over the obturator internus muscles or arcus tendineus fascia pelvis starting anterior to its origin at the ischial spine. The suture is then tied and additional sutures are placed at approximately 1-cm intervals out toward the pubic ramus. This procedure is performed bilaterally when paravaginal defects are identified on both sides. The paravaginal defect repair prevents rotational descent of the bladder base and urethra with increases in intra-abdominal pressure without causing overcorrection of the urethrovesical angle. The procedure can be performed via an abdominal, vaginal, or laparoscopic approach.

Complications of Retropubic Procedures

Immediate complications of retropubic procedures include sutures in the bladder, ureteral obstruction, and cystotomy, although direct injury to the urinary tract occurs in less than 2% of cases. Cystoscopy is often performed before completion of the surgical procedure to document ureteral patency and to rule out the presence of any intravesical sutures. Compromise of the lower urinary tract is usually easy to correct if identified intraoperatively. Postoperatively, the bladder is routinely drained for 1 to 2 days via a transurethral or suprapubic catheter, after which the patient undergoes a voiding trial to document adequate bladder emptying before the catheter is removed.

Prolonged voiding dysfunction rates are low and depend on the type of retropubic procedure performed, any concurrent reconstructive procedures, and preoperative voiding parameters as determined by urodynamic testing. A complication of retropubic procedures is detrusor overactivity, which can be demonstrated on cystometrogram in 7% to 27% of patients after Burch colposuspension. One study showed that this problem persisted for 3 to 5 years after surgery in 7% of cases. Although many of these patients remain asymptomatic, patients should be appropriately counseled about these potential complications before undergoing retropubic surgery.

Outcomes of Retropubic Procedures

Despite high reported success rates, the MMK has fallen out of favor as a primary treatment for SUI due to the complication of osteitis pubis. The paravaginal defect repair has also had inconsistent results as a primary treatment for SUI, and is now primarily used for repair of the anterior vaginal wall. However, studies continue to show consistently high cure and improvement rates for Burch colposuspension in the treatment of SUI in the absence of ISD, and many surgeons consider the Burch colposuspension to be the gold standard of treatment. A Cochrane review concluded that open retropubic colposuspension was the most effective treatment for SUI, with 85% to 90% of patients being continent after 1 year and 70% after 5 years. Other surgeons prefer suburethral slings for treating SUI, and there has been a recent trend toward performing less invasive mid-urethral slings, which will be discussed in the following sections.

Suburethral Sling Procedures

Traditionally, suburethral sling procedures have been used for the treatment of SUI caused by ISD. Slings likely work by restoring the normal urethrovesical junction support at rest, by creating a backboard upon which the urethra can compress when increases in intra-abdominal pressure occur, and by increasing outflow resistance via upward displacement with flexion of the rectus abdominis muscles.

Patient Selection for Suburethral Sling Procedures

These procedures have been traditionally used for the treatment of SUI with ISD, which can be demonstrated on urodynamic studies by low resting urethral closure pressures and low Valsalva leak point pressures. Patients with recurrent incontinence and with comorbidities that could increase the likelihood for surgical failure such as chronic obstructive pulmonary disease, obesity, athleticism, and congenital tissue weakness, are also appropriate candidates for suburethral slings. Indications for sling procedures are controversial, however, with many surgeons now performing these operations as the primary treatment of SUI. Numerous studies have demonstrated the efficacy and durability of sling procedures for the treatment of SUI, and many now consider mid-urethral slings to be the new gold standard of treatment for SUI.

Techniques for the Suburethral Sling Procedure

Two types of sling procedures are most commonly performed: traditional slings, which are placed underneath the urethrovesical junction, and mid-urethral slings, which rest under the middle of the urethra in a tension-free manner. Many variations for placing these slings exist, and there are few randomized controlled studies comparing the different approaches. The options for sling material include organic (such as autologous or cadaveric fascia) or synthetic (such as Mersilene polyester fiber mesh or polypropylene mesh). Although the risk of infection and erosion may be higher with synthetic slings, some studies suggest that these slings have slightly higher long-term success rates.

Most surgeons perform the sling procedure using a combined abdominal and vaginal approach, with the majority of the dissection being performed vaginally. Patients are placed in the dorsal lithotomy position and prepared and draped in the usual sterile fashion. A dilute epinephrine solution or saline is injected into the anterior vaginal wall, and a midline or U-shaped incision is made. Using sharp and blunt dissection, the vaginal mucosa is carefully separated from the periurethral and paravesical fascia to the level of the inferolateral aspect of the pubic rami bilaterally. The retropubic space is then entered, and the bladder neck is identified by placing gentle traction on the Foley catheter. If an anterior colporrhaphy is required, it should be performed at this time.

For the full-length sling, two small abdominal incisions are made lateral to the midline above the pubic symphysis and the rectus fascia is then incised. A long clamp or Pereyra needle carrier is then passed through the retropubic space, behind the pubis symphysis, and out through the vaginal incision just lateral to the bladder neck. One arm of the sling is then grasped and pulled back out through the abdominal incision. The same procedure is repeated on the opposite side, and the sling arms are then sewn to the rectus fascia with permanent sutures after proper tensioning. Cystourethroscopy is performed to rule out inadvertent injury to the ureters or bladder, and the abdominal and vaginal incisions are then closed. Transurethral or suprapubic bladder drainage is then used until a patient passes a voiding trial. Variations of the full-length sling, such as the patch sling, are placed in a similar fashion, except that permanent sutures are attached to the edges of the sling and are transfixed to the rectus fascia on each side.

Techniques for Midurethral Slings

Tension-free midurethral slings placed through the retropubic space or through the transobturator space are increasing in popularity because they are relatively easy to place, can be placed in an outpatient setting, and have high success rates. These surgeries can be performed with the patient under regional or local anesthesia in 30 minutes or less, are less invasive than traditional slings, and have good short- and long-term outcomes.

603

The tension-free vaginal tape (TVT) procedure (Gynecare, Ethicon, Inc., Somerville, NJ) is performed using specially designed needles attached to a synthetic sling material. The surgery may be done with the patient under local, regional, or general anesthesia. With the patient in the dorsal lithotomy position, the bladder is drained with an 18-French Foley catheter. A 22-gauge spinal needle is used to inject 25 mL of 0.25% bupivacaine (or other dilute anesthetic solution) with epinephrine along the posterior aspect of the pubic symphysis on each side of the urethra. These injections reduce postoperative analgesia, decrease bleeding, and help open the retropubic space. Two small stab incisions are made at the superior margin of the pubic symphysis approximately two finger-breadths lateral to the midline. Next, the anterior vaginal wall beneath and lateral to the midurethra is infiltrated with 10 mL of the dilute anesthetic solution, and a small midline anterior vaginal wall incision is made starting 0.5 cm proximal to the urethral meatus and continuing proximally to the bladder neck. Metzenbaum scissors are then used to create tunnels between the vaginal mucosa and pubocervical fascia to the inferior margin of the pubic rami on each side. With the bladder base and proximal urethra being deviated to the opposite side using a rigid catheter guide, the TVT needle tip is inserted into the vaginal incision, and the endopelvic fascia is perforated under the inferior ramus of the pubic bone. The needle is then guided behind the pubic bone, through the anterior rectus fascia, and out through the abdominal stab incision. This procedure is repeated on the opposite side, leaving the Prolene tape with its plastic sheath in a tension-free position below the mid urethra. The plastic sheaths are then sequentially removed and the excess tape cut on each side at the level of the skin. Cystoscopy is performed after passage of the needles to rule out trocar injury to the bladder. The vaginal and skin incisions are then closed.

The SPARC self-fixating sling system (American Medical Systems, Minnetonka, Minnesota) is essentially a TVT procedure in reverse; the needles are passed "top down" from the abdominal incisions, through the rectus fascia, behind the pubic bone, and out through the vaginal submucosal incision. The tape is then connected to the needle and pulled back out through the abdominal skin incisions, and the procedure is repeated on the opposite side.

A recent modification of midurethral sling placement involves passing the needle with its attached tape through the obturator membrane instead of the anterior rectus fascia, using helical needles. Transobturator slings probably work in a manner similar to the other midurethral slings by restoring the suburethral vaginal hammock. Transobturator slings take even less time to place than retropubic midurethral slings, and studies have shown lower rates of complications such as urinary retention. Long-term outcome studies of the effectiveness and durability of transobturator slings are ongoing.

Complications of Sling Procedures

Complications occurring after suburethral sling procedures include lower urinary tract injury, prolonged voiding dysfunction and urinary retention, worsened or *de novo* detrusor overactivity and irritative bladder symptoms, infection or erosion of mesh material, recurrent or persistent UI, the development of prolapse, hemorrhage into the retropubic space, and nerve damage.

Outcomes of Sling Procedures

Studies show cure rates of slings for SUI from 70% to 95%, but the studies are difficult to compare because different outcome parameters were measured, patients were followed up for variable lengths of time, and surgical techniques were not standardized. A study by Young and colleagues showed that a Mersilene mesh suburethral sling procedure performed on 200 women with SUI (complicated by recurrence, ISD, or chronically increased intra-abdominal pressure) resulted in a 93% objective cure rate after a mean follow-up of 30 months. Randomized controlled trials comparing different sling procedures, and different procedures for the treatment of SUI in general, are lacking.

A large, multicenter, prospective randomized trial comparing the outcome of 170 TVT procedures and 146 Burch colposuspensions for SUI showed similar objective cure rates at 6 months postoperatively. When followed up 2 years later, objective cure rates remained equivalent and durable. Also, a study evaluating long-term outcomes for the TVT procedure for SUI showed an 81% cure rate and 16% significant improvement rate at a mean follow-up of 7 years, illustrating the long-term benefits from these minimally invasive approaches. Long-term outcomes studies for the transobturator sling procedures are lacking, but initial reports have shown promise for these new technologies.

Transvaginal Needle Suspension Procedures

Used for similar indications as the Burch colposuspension procedure, transvaginal needle suspension procedures support the bladder neck and proximal urethra by using permanent sutures to attach the endopelvic fascia to the rectus fascia or pubic bone via a transvaginal approach. Various modifications of the original procedure described by Pereyra include the

Raz, Stamey, and Gittes procedures. The basic technique involves placing ligatures transvaginally into the endopelvic fascia on either side of the urethra. These sutures are then passed through the retropubic space with a long needle inserted above the pubic bone. A small abdominal incision is used to tie the sutures above the rectus fascia. A long discussion of needle suspension procedures is beyond the scope of this chapter because studies have shown considerably lower subjective and objective cure rates for needle suspension procedures than for retropubic operations or suburethral slings.

Injection of Bulk-Enhancing Agents

Periurethral bulking agents are used to treat isolated ISD without urethral hypermobility or to treat SUI in medically frail patients who are poor candidates for more invasive surgical procedures. Bulking agents work by increasing outflow resistance at the bladder neck by coapting the urethral lumen. The ideal bulk-enhancing agent would be biocompatible, be easy to inject, have a low complication rate, and have a low rate of degradation, and would not migrate to distant sites. The most commonly used bulking agents currently in use are glutaraldehyde-cross-linked bovine collagen (Contigen) and pyrolytic carbon-coated zirconium oxide beads (Durasphere), though other substances are being studied.

Technique for Periurethral Injection of Bulking Agents
Periurethral bulking agents are placed with the patient in the dorsal lithotomy position. Two percent lidocaine jelly is used to numb the urethra. With a 0- or 30-degree cystoscope in the mid urethra, a 22-gauge spinal needle is positioned periurethrally at the 4 or 8 o'clock position and advanced to the level of the bladder neck in the suburothelial plane. A dilute lidocaine solution can be injected through the spinal needle to enhance anesthesia and to confirm proper placement of the needle tip. When the needle tip is in the proper position, the bulking agent is injected until a wheel is raised that visually occludes the urethral lumen. The needle is then removed and the procedure is repeated on the opposite side. A cough stress test is performed, and bulking agent is added until continence is demonstrated.

Technique for Transurethral Injection of Bulking Agents
Bulking agents are injected transurethrally by advancing a specially designed injection needle through the operative port of a 0-degree cytoscope into the mucosa of the urethra just below the internal urethral sphincter. The bulking agent is then injected at the 4 or 8 o'clock position until the urethral lumen is visibly occluded, and the procedure is repeated on the opposite side. Because this technique can be performed in the office or with the patient under local anesthesia, the patient can then be asked to cough to ensure continence before ending the procedure.

Complications of Injection of Bulk-Enhancing Agents
Complications after the injection of bulk-enhancing agents for the treatment of SUI are rare. Short-term complications can include transient urinary

605

retention requiring intermittent self-catheterization, sterile abscess formation, irritative voiding symptoms, and urinary tract infections. Transient urinary retention can occur in up to 25% of patients but almost always resolves within 48 hours. Rates of urinary tract infection can be reduced by prescribing a 3-day course of oral antibiotics after injection. Long-term obstructive symptoms are exceedingly rare.

Outcomes of Injection of Bulk-Enhancing Agents

Available data suggest that the injection of periurethral or transurethral bulking agents results in short-term symptomatic improvement, but few prospective randomized studies have been performed. The widely divergent improvement and cure rates reported in the literature are probably a result of differences in study inclusion criteria, operative technique, injection materials, and outcome measures. In one prospective randomized study, Lightner and colleagues demonstrated that both Durasphere and Contigen achieved dryness and improvement rates of 70% to 80% at 1-year follow-up.

SUMMARY

Due to an ever-aging population, UI is increasingly becoming a major public health problem. Although the consequences of incontinence are not generally life-threatening, they can be socially isolating, economically draining, and emotionally devastating to patients. Gynecologists and urogynecologists are in a unique position, through proper diagnosis and treatment, to positively affect the quality of life of women experiencing UI.

KEY POINTS

1. Stress urinary incontinence is the involuntary leakage of urine on effort or exertion or when sneezing or coughing.
2. Urge urinary incontinence is involuntary urine leakage accompanied by or immediately preceded by the feeling of urgency.
3. Mixed incontinence is an involuntary leakage of urine associated with urgency and exertion, such as effort, coughing, sneezing, or laughing.
4. Overflow incontinence is a condition of urinary dribbling or continuous leakage associated with incomplete bladder emptying caused by outlet obstruction or impaired detrusor contractility.
5. Increasing age, female sex, and increasing parity are risk factors for urinary incontinence.
6. The basic evaluation of patients with urinary incontinence should include a history, physical examination, measurement of a postvoid residual, and a urinalysis.

Continued

KEY POINTS—CONT'D

7. Routine urodynamic testing is not necessary for all patients being evaluated for symptoms of urinary incontinence. However, many urogynecologists will proceed with urodynamic testing if the clinical picture is unclear, if the patient's condition has failed to respond to previous medical or surgical therapy, or if surgical intervention is planned.

8. Pelvic floor training is an effective treatment for stress and mixed incontinence, and behavioral therapy improves symptoms of urge and mixed incontinence. These conservative modalities can be recommended as a noninvasive treatment in many women.

9. Detrusor overactivity is usually treated with anticholinergic medications.

10. When conservative treatment approaches fail, stress urinary incontinence is usually treated surgically with retropubic colposuspension procedures, pubovaginal slings, mid-urethral slings, or injection of periurethral bulking agents.

SUGGESTED READING

Abrams P, Cardozo L, Fall M, et al: The standardization of terminology of lower urinary tract function: Report from the standardization sub-committee of the International Continence Society. Neurourol Urodyn 21:167–178, 2002.

American College of Obstetricians and Gynecologists Practice Bulletin No. 63: Urinary incontinence in women. Obstet Gynecol 105:1533–1544, 2005.

Association of Professors of Gynecology and Obstetrics: Clinical Management of Urinary Incontinence. Crofton, MD, APGO, 2004.

Buchsbaum GM, Chin M, Glantz C, et al: Prevalence of urinary incontinence and associated risk factors in a cohort of nuns. Obstet Gynecol 100:226–229, 2002.

DeLancey JOL: Structural aspects of the extrinsic continence mechanism. Obstet Gynecol 72:296–301, 1988.

Fantl JA, Newman DK, Colling J, et al: Acute and Chronic Management. Clinical Practice Guidelines No. 2, 1996 Update. Public Health Service, Agency for Health Care Policy and Research. *AHCPR* Publication No. 96–0682. Urinary Incontinence in Adults: Rockville, MD, U.S. Department of Health and Human Services, March 1996.

Hendrix SL, Cochrane BB, Nygaard IE, et al: Effects of estrogen with and without progestin on urinary incontinence. JAMA 293:935–948, 2005.

Lapitan M, Cody DJ, Grant A: Open retropubic colposuspension for urinary incontinence in women. Cochrane Database Syst Rev Jul 20:CD002912, 2005.

Lightner D, Calvosa C, Andersen R, et al: A new injectable bulking agent for treatment of stress urinary incontinence: Results of a multicenter, randomized, double-blind study of Durasphere. Urology 58:12–15, 2001.

Petros PE, Ulmsten UI: An integral theory of female urinary incontinence, experimental and clinical considerations. Acta Obstet Gynecol Scand Suppl 153:7–31, 1990.

Pickard R, Reaper J, Wyness L, et al: Periurethral injection therapy for urinary incontinence in women. Cochrane Database Syst Rev 2:CD003881, 2003.

Rortveit G, Daltveit AK, Hannestad YS, Hunskaar S: Norwegian EPINCONT Study: Urinary incontinence after vaginal delivery or cesarean section. N Engl J Med 348:900–907, 2003.

Ward K, Hilton P: Prospective multicentre randomised trial of tension-free vaginal tape and colposuspension as primary treatment for stress urinary incontinence. United Kingdom and Ireland Tension-free Vaginal Tape Trial Group. BMJ 325:67–70, 2002.

Young SB, Howard AE, Baker SP: Mersilene mesh sling: Short- and long-term clinical and urodynamic outcomes. Am J Obstet Gynecol 185:32–40, 2001.

25

BOWEL DISORDERS

Jorge A. Lagares-Garcia, Adam A. Klipfel, and Steven Schechter

INTRODUCTION

Disorders of the colon and rectum commonly affect pelvic organs, so it is imperative for a well-versed gynecologist to have knowledge of the more common diseases that may affect the pelvis or anorectal area. Simple benign diseases amenable to successful surgical or medical treatments will be treated in the outpatient clinic. Furthermore, it is important for a gynecologist to be able to recognize signs and symptoms of more severe diseases of the colon and rectum, such as inflammatory bowel disease and colon cancer, because women often seek care from their gynecologist first.

ANATOMY OF THE ANORECTAL RING

The sigmoid colon is the most distal part of the large intestine. As the sigmoid colon enters the pelvic inlet, the three taenia coli become a single longitudinal layer of smooth muscle during the transition to the upper rectum. In females, the rectum is covered by a serosal layer anteriorly to the level of the rectovaginal septum. Posteriorly, the rectum is invested by the *mesorectum*, which is not a major area of vascular supply but is an area of lymphovascular drainage.

Caudally, the rectum is divided into the mid and distal rectum before it becomes the anus. At the perineal portion of the rectum, the inner circular layer of smooth muscle thickens to become the internal anal sphincter, which is responsible for 85% of the resting tone of the anal canal. The outer longitudinal layers of smooth muscle thicken anteriorly and posteriorly and connect to the perineal body and coccyx. Externally, striated muscle is differentiated into three different fascicles that collectively make up the external anal sphincter. This muscle works in concert with the puborectalis muscle and can be voluntarily contracted to help maintain continence.

The anal canal extends the full length of the internal anal sphincter, which is demarcated at its top by the puborectalis muscle and at its distal end by the intersphincteric groove between the internal and external sphincter muscles. Within the anal canal is the *anal transition zone*, which extends from the dentate line (which is in the mid portion of the anal canal) to the top of the anal canal. The other important landmark is the *anal margin,* which extends from the intersphincteric groove, or the bottom of the anal canal, to the perianal skin. This distinction is important because cancers of the anal area are treated differently depending on whether they are in the anal canal or in the anal margin; this will be discussed later in this chapter.

HISTORY AND PHYSICAL EXAMINATION

An accurate patient history is necessary for proper diagnosis and therapy of bowel disorders. Symptoms can present in a variety of ways, so reports of the type and quality of pain (if present), timing of the onset of symptoms, symptom radiation, any aggravating or alleviating factors, changes in bowel habits, weight and appetite changes, and hematochezia or melena should be elicited. It is also important to ask about the quality of stools and any problems with evacuation of the bowels or bowel incontinence.

Anorectal pathology often causes rectal bleeding, which may be accompanied by pain indicating pathology past the dentate line. The characteristics of the pain recorded in the history will provide the interviewer with an idea of the pathology: "knife-like" pain may indicate an anal fissure, dull and deep continuous pain may indicate an anal abscess, or the sudden onset of throbbing pain may indicate a thrombosed hemorrhoid (Fig. 25-1). Furthermore, mucous discharge is often found in inflammatory bowel disease, full thickness rectal prolapse, or a large rectal polyp (Fig. 25-2).

The patient's screening history for colorectal cancer by colonoscopy or flexible sigmoidoscopy should be investigated for every individual. Special situations such as a family history of malignancy, familial adenomatous polyposis, or inflammatory bowel disease elevate the patient's risk for developing a primary colorectal carcinoma. Also, routine screening should

Figure 25-1

Grade IV prolapsing hemorrhoids.

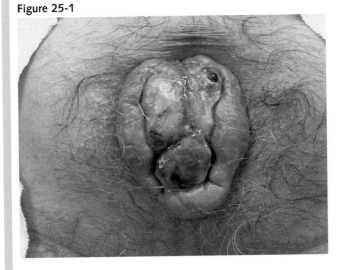

Figure 25-2

Large carpet-like polypoid lesion of the anorectal area.

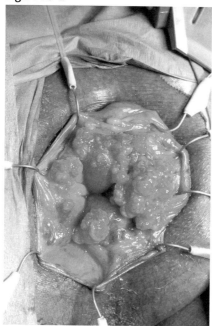

be recommended for any patient older than 50 years of age. Current screening guidelines from the American Society of Colon and Rectal Surgeons are shown in Box 25-1.

Physical examination should start with a gentle inspection retracting the buttocks close to the anal verge. Visualization of pathology such as a fissure or excoriation from a fistula or furuncle may truncate the rest of the examination because these clinical entities can be very painful. An important part of the examination is to position the patient on a toilet seat and recreate the normal action of evacuation to visualize prolapsing tissue that otherwise would not be seen in the prone position.

Digital rectal examination is performed to assess for masses such as hemorrhoids or cancer, to test the resting and squeeze tone, and to look for pain or bleeding. Also, the cervix and the uterus can be felt via trans-rectal examination. Fecal occult blood testing should be performed to rule out subclinical bleeding.

DIAGNOSTIC TESTS

Anoscopy or rigid or flexible sigmoidoscopy should complement the examination because these well-tolerated diagnostic tests can be performed in the clinic without anesthesia. Computed tomography (CT) is helpful in the staging and follow-up of cancer of the colon, rectum, and anus. Retrorectal tumors are also best visualized with this modality. Magnetic resonance imaging (MRI) and dynamic MRI with an endorectal coil have been more

---

Box 25-1 Current Screening Guidelines from the American Society of Colon and Rectal Surgeons

Screening persons at average risk

Fecal occult blood testing (FOBT) yearly: two samples each from three consecutive stools

Flexible sigmoidoscopy every 5 years

FOBT + flexible sigmoidoscopy every 5 years

Colonoscopy every 10 years

Double-contrast barium enema every 5 years

Screening persons at increased risk

If patient has a first-degree relative with colon cancer or adenomatous polyps diagnosed at an age younger than 60 years or two first-degree relatives diagnosed at any age, he or she should have colonoscopy at the age of 40 years or 10 years younger that the earliest diagnosis in the family.

If patient has a first-degree relative with colon cancer or adenomatous polyp diagnosed at an age younger than 60 years or two second-degree relatives with colorectal cancer, then colonoscopy is indicated at the age of 40 or 10 years earlier, whichever comes first, and every 5 years thereafter.

If patient has one second- or third-degree relative with colon cancer, screening should be initiated at the age of 50 years.

If familial adenomatous polyposis is present, start flexible sigmoidoscopy at the age of 10 to 12 years.

If hereditary nonpolyposis colorectal cancer is present, colonoscopy should be undertaken every 1 to 2 years starting at the age of 20 to 25 years or 10 years younger than the earliest cancer. Genetic testing should be offered to first-degree relatives of persons with inherited mismatch repair gene mutation.

Adapted from Winawer S, Fletcher R, Rex D, et al: Colorectal cancer screening and surveillance: Clinical guidelines and rationale—update based on new evidence. Gastroenterology 124:544–560, 2003.

---

recently used with excellent results in the evaluation of defecatory disorders and rectal cancer staging. MRI is also extremely sensitive for the detection of unsuspected fistulas or abscesses. More familiar to gynecologists, endorectal ultrasonography (ERUS) has gained an increasing importance in the evaluation and treatment of anorectal diseases. Two different probes can be used for this test: the 7.0-MHz transducer or a 12-MHz transducer for higher-resolution images. ERUS is the primary imaging modality used to identify sphincter defects in patients with fecal incontinence (Fig. 25-3) and can be used for staging rectal cancers with accuracy rates ranging from 84% to 93%.

BENIGN DISEASES

Colonic Diseases

Diverticular Disease

Approximately 60% of the population by the sixth decade of life will develop diverticular disease. It is only after microperforations form that diverticular disease will become symptomatic. Clinical presentation may range from microabscesses to full fecal peritonitis. The typical clinical picture includes

Figure 25-3

Combined anterior internal and external anal sphincter defect.

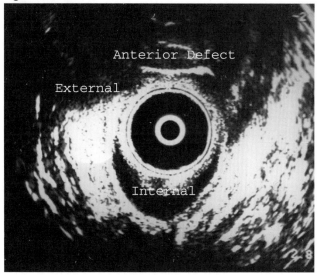

pelvic and left lower quadrant pain along with changes in bowel habits with constipation, mucous discharge or hematochezia, fever, and leukocytosis. The differential diagnosis of acute diverticulitis includes inflammatory bowel disease, irritable bowel syndrome, ischemic colitis, colon cancer, and gynecologic and urologic diseases. CT scan shows inflammation and fat streaking in early stages. Localized pelvic abscesses are also found in late stages (Fig. 25-4). An advanced clinical picture with frank free air and fluid in the abdomen can be also seen, though this presentation is rarer.

Figure 25-4

Large diverticular pelvic abscess.

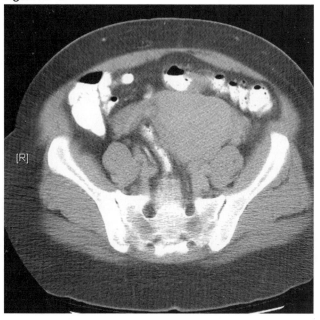

In patients without obvious peritoneal signs who have uncomplicated diverticulitis, initial intravenous hydration and broad-spectrum antibiotics as well as bowel rest is recommended. It is our practice to start ciprofloxacin at 400 mg/day given intravenously and metronidazole 500 mg given intravenously three times per day. When abdominal pain has nearly disappeared, a clear liquid diet is started, and if no worsening of symptoms occurs, the patient is advanced to a low-residue diet and the antibiotics are switched to oral dosage. Patients with localized abscesses should undergo percutaneous drainage along with intravenous broad-spectrum antibiotics. Elective colonic resection should be recommended for patients younger than 50 years of age who have had one episode of complicated disease (e.g., abscess, fistula) or two documented attacks. It is our practice to perform laparoscopic resections with or without ureteral stent placement depending on the original attack and amount of inflammation on subsequent CT scans. Before elective surgical resection, patients must undergo a full colonoscopy to rule out other causes of colonic perforation such as colon cancer.

Primary sigmoid resection with anastomosis is performed in patients who meet criteria for a safe anastomosis, including adequate mechanical bowel preparation, healthy bowel, good blood supply, and no tension on the anastomosis. A two-stage operation, generally Hartmann's procedure, is commonly performed for patients with fecal or purulent peritonitis.

Inflammatory Bowel Disease

Mucosal Ulcerative Colitis

Mucosal ulcerative colitis (MUC) is a chronic inflammatory disorder affecting the mucosal lining of the colon. The etiology of the disease is uncertain. High sugar consumption, decreased dietary fiber intake, and certain infectious agents may contribute to the pathogenesis of this disease. There is certainly a genetic component because patients with a family history of the disease have an increased risk of experiencing MUC themselves.

Clinical remissions and exacerbations are the hallmarks of MUC. The rectum is almost invariably affected with a retrograde involvement ranging from proctitis or proctosigmoiditis to a full proctocolitis. In certain instances, the terminal ileum may be affected by "backwash ileitis," representing retrograde inflammation of the small intestine by reflux of diarrhea.

Patients will typically present to the clinician with diarrhea and bleeding of varying intensity. Multiple frequent bowel movements with mucous components and hematochezia are common. Weight loss, malaise, and anemia are also long-standing disease findings. Abdominal distension, tachycardia, and toxic signs with or without peritoneal signs may represent a surgical emergency in the form of toxic megacolon. Extracolonic manifestations include mild hepatic dysfunction or primary sclerosing cholangitis (7.5%), with 7% of those transforming to bile duct carcinoma in some reported series. Other manifestations are indicated in Box 25-2. Clinically quiescent disease in pregnancy is likely to remain quiescent. However, initial onset or active disease will likely worsen during the course of the pregnancy, especially during the first trimester.

Endoscopy is the standard for diagnosis since the disease invariably starts in the rectum. Ulcerations and edema, friable mucosa, and atypical

Box 25-2	Extracolonic Manifestations of Mucosal Ulcerative Colitis

Hepatic dysfunction
Primary sclerosing cholangitis
Bile duct carcinoma
Arthritis
Ankylosing spondylitis
Erythema nodosum
Pyoderma gangrenosum
Episcleritis, uveitis, iritis, and conjunctivitis

lesions in long-standing disease may be seen. The presence of skip areas is more indicative of Crohn's disease than MUC.

Additional testing such as barium enema may show the characteristic "lead pipe" of the colon or "collar button" deep ulcers. Pathology invariably reveals the presence of leukocytes in the lamina propria, crypts, and surface of the epithelium. Differential diagnoses include Crohn's disease, infectious colitis (*Clostridium difficile, Campylobacter* species, *Salmonella* species, cytomegalovirus, etc.), and collagenous colitis.

MUC increases the risk of developing colorectal carcinoma in affected persons; approximately 20% of patients will develop colorectal cancer after 10 years of disease, and 50% to 75% of patients will develop colorectal cancer after 30 to 40 years of disease. Multiple endoscopic biopsies every 10 cm are therefore recommended to rule out dysplasia.

MUC is initially controlled medically. Multiple compounds are used alone or in combination to induce remission and to keep the disease quiescent. Mesalamine is a compound of unknown exact mechanism of action that is metabolized by the liver and intestine and primarily excreted in the feces. In lactation the safety is unknown, and it is a class B drug in pregnant patients. In the acute setting, it is taken by mouth at 800 mg three times per day for 3 to 6 weeks and reduced to 800 mg by mouth twice daily for maintenance. Also, rectal suppositories (1000 mg per rectum daily) can be given for 3 to 6 weeks if the disease is limited to the distal portion of the rectum.

Due to the large number of pills required when using mesalamine, better patient tolerance is achieved with olsalazine 500 mg twice a day. It is classified as a pregnancy class C drug and is possibly unsafe during lactation. Minimal proctitis or proctosigmoiditis can be treated with hydrocortisone by enema administration (100 mg/60 mL) or 10% rectal foam. It is metabolized by the liver and excreted in the urine. There is inadequate literature to assess the risk during lactation, and it is a class C drug during pregnancy. Adult administration is a 100-mg enema per rectum before bedtime for 21 days.

In patients for whom continued dosage of steroids is needed, azathioprine induces and maintains remission of MUC. The initial dosage is 50 mg taken by mouth daily with a maximum dosage of 2.5 mg/kg/day. This compound is metabolized in the liver and excreted in urine. Azathioprine is a pregnancy class D drug, and animal and human data demonstrate potential or actual effects transmitted to infants and breast milk. Another immunosuppressant is the antimetabolite mercaptopurine. It is metabolized in the liver to an active form. Initial dosage starts at 50 mg daily by mouth to a maximum of 1.5 mg/kg/day. Both of the previous medications require monitoring of the complete blood count as well as liver functions tests. For acute induction, intravenous methylprednisolone can be used in dosages ranging from 10 to 250 mg every 4 to 8 hours, to be tapered in an oral dosage of prednisone.

Emergent surgical indications include toxic colitis despite maximized medical management, hemorrhage, or perforation. The most common surgical option is total abdominal colectomy with end Brooke ileostomy and Hartman's closure of the rectal stump or mucous fistula. A second staged procedure will be required to perform an ileal pouch anal anastomosis to reestablish intestinal continuity with or without ileostomy (Fig. 25-5).

Elective surgical options are mandated by medical resistance to therapy, presence of carcinoma, or dysplasia on biopsy. Choices of treatment include open or laparoscopic total proctocolectomy with ileal pouch anal anastomosis with or without diverting loop ileostomy, total proctocolectomy with end Brooke ileostomy, or continent ileostomy. Before permanent surgical options are undertaken, patient counseling is important due to the significant morbidity of the surgery. Infertility, pelvic adhesions, pouch-vaginal fistulae, perineal wound complications, ileostomy complications, and pelvic sepsis may occur. However, quality of life is clearly improved when these operations are successful, and most patients live active healthy lives after surgery, with the ability to become pregnant. Controversy exists regarding the method of delivery (i.e., vaginal or cesarean) in such patients, and close discussion between the obstetrician and colorectal surgeon should be established before term.

Crohn's Disease

Originally described in 1932 by Crohn, Ginzberg, and Oppenheimer at Mount Sinai Hospital in New York City, Crohn's disease was originally thought to be a terminal ileitis. Now, Crohn's disease is known to manifest

Figure 25-5

Stapled ileal J-pouch before anal anastomosis.

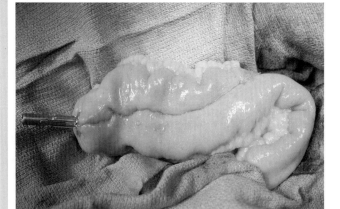

itself anywhere from the mouth to the anus. The main treatment is medical, though many adverse effects and complications can occur, and surgical therapy is mainly reserved to treat complications of the disease.

Crohn's disease is a transmural inflammatory disease of the bowel. Because of its transmural nature, Crohn's disease can result in fistulas to almost any surrounding organs, with or without abscesses. The other consequence of this inflammation can be stenosis or hemorrhage. The stenosis or stricturing can manifest as obstruction, and the hemorrhage can be either small or massive. Crohn's is a segmental disease, often sparing the rectum, whereas ulcerative colitis has more continuous involvement and often will start in the rectum. However, there are similarities to ulcerative colitis, and patients often present with a similar clinical picture. In fact, there are patients who have manifestations consistent with both, a phenomenon that is termed *indeterminate colitis* and creates a difficult problem in the decision of how to manage these patients.

The cause of Crohn's disease is unclear. There are many theories ranging from genetic to infectious, and the truth may be somewhere in between. The fact that the condition responds to steroids and anti-inflammatory agents makes an autoimmune mechanism likely, but what begins the inflammatory process and keeps it recurring is still uncertain. Crohn's disease occurs in about 60 to 70 per 100,000 persons and is far more prevalent in industrialized nations. The age at presentation is most often between 15 and 30 years old, but there is a second peak around 55 to 60 years old.

There are various types of Crohn's disease that are categorized based on their presentation, and the treatment is based on the presentation and manifestation of the disease. The main types are stenosing, fistulizing, and hemorrhagic. The presentation of these patients can range anywhere from crampy abdominal pain with diarrhea to frank perforation with abscess and sepsis. More often, the initial signs and symptoms are subtle and often can be confused with other diagnoses. The extraintestinal manifestations of the disease can be a clue (Box 25-3).

Many of these symptoms will improve with treatment. The liver and joint symptoms generally do not improve despite treatment of the disease. Other symptoms that are related to the disease, especially if significant

---

Box 25-3 Extraintestinal Manifestations of Crohn's Disease

Skin	Liver
Pyoderma gangrenosum	Sclerosing cholangitis
Erythema nodosum multiforme	Pericholangitis
Vasculitis	Granulomatous hepatitis
Aphthous stomatitis	

Eyes	Joints
Conjunctivitis	Arthritis
Iritis	Ankylosing spondylitis
Uveitis	Osteoarthropathy
Episcleritis/iridocyclitis	

small bowel disease is present, include malabsorption and nutritional deficiencies. Also, patients can present with gallstones and kidney stones related to the small bowel disease.

The fistulas associated with Crohn's disease are usually of two types. One type is the perianal fistula, which can range from mild to severe "watering can perineum," including perianal abscesses. The second type is from the bowel to other loops of bowel or to adjacent structures such as bladder, vagina, and even skin. The treatment often involves antibiotics and drainage of the infection. In perianal disease, the avoidance of deep incisions and fistulotomies is advised in favor of placing draining setons and allowing the infection to settle and medical treatment to take effect. Intra-abdominal fistulas are treated by resection of the inflamed bowel segment on one side and simple closure of the target organ on the other side.

The mainstay of treatment for Crohn's disease is medical. The initial treatment for most exacerbations is steroids, taken orally or intravenously, depending on the functional status of the bowel. Once the acute inflammation had resolved, medical treatment usually includes 6-mercaptopurine or infliximab. Infliximab was initially used for perianal-fistulizing disease, but its indications are being expanded, and it is now being used on a more regular basis for maintenance therapy.

Surgical therapy is reserved for those patients who are very sick and cannot undergo a trial of medical therapy, or those who are not responding to the usual medical therapies. The goal is for preservation of bowel length to prevent malabsorption and its sequelae.

The surgical options are different from ulcerative colitis, where a total proctocolectomy is curative. Surgical options for Crohn's disease are related to the complication being treated. Resection of the inflamed, stenotic, or bleeding segment of bowel and reanastomosis should be performed if possible. Drainage of any intra-abdominal or perianal abscesses is also warranted. Treatment for perianal disease should be conservative, and large resections should be avoided because healing is poor in this area and it may take time for the infection to pass. Surgical therapy for Crohn's disease can be frustrating and problematic because relapses can occur despite meticulous application of technique.

Defecatory Disorders

Constipation

Constipation is the most common colorectal disorder. It can be challenging to treat because of its varied causes, which can include poor fiber intake, inadequate fluid intake, or slow colonic transit time due to decreased intrinsic bowel motility. Other causes of constipation include occult malignancy and obstructive defecation, which can result from rectoceles, internal intussusception, or hypertonic puborectalis with anorectal dysfunction.

A thorough history and determination of the time frame and sequence of development of the constipation can provide important information. For example, a 32-year-old woman who says she has been constipated her whole life may require a different workup than a woman who is 80 years old, lives in a nursing home, and is taking several psychiatric medications. Workup often includes a barium study or colonoscopy to evaluate for any intracolonic lesions. Once a mass is ruled out, the diagnosis can often be made through dietary and medication history. The other tests often used are the Sitz Marker study or colonic transit study, in which radiopaque markers are ingested and serial abdominal films are taken. The presence and distribution of the markers will help to give the diagnosis. If the markers are absent at day 4 to 5, severe constipation is ruled out. If the majority of the markers are still present on day 4 to 5 but they are grouped in the rectosigmoid area, the diagnosis of outlet obstruction is made. If the majority of the markers are present and distributed throughout the colon, slow transit constipation is diagnosed.

Treatment is dictated mainly by the source of the constipation. Dietary adjustment, increase in fluid intake, and addition of stool softeners and fiber constitute the mainstay of therapy. One of the more common errors in using stool softeners and fiber is not using enough. Additionally, patients often do not realize that caffeinated beverages such as tea and soda actually cause diuresis and loss of fluids, leading to dehydration and hard stools. Cathartics can be classified as stimulant (e.g., cascara sagrada, senna), saline (e.g., magnesium sulfate, milk of magnesia), osmotic (e.g., GoLYTELY), bulk-forming (e.g., psyllium, methylcellulose), or lubricant (e.g., mineral oil).

The surgical treatment of slow-transit constipation is with a subtotal colectomy with ileorectal anastomosis. This surgery works well in selected patients; however, patients often experience the development of frequent bowel movements. The treatment of outlet obstruction caused by a failure of the puborectalis muscle to relax during defecation is with biofeedback and retraining of the pelvic floor muscles to have more coordinated function. Rectoceles, discussed below, are common causes of outlet obstruction and are amenable to surgical repair by a gynecologist.

Rectocele

A rectocele is an outpouching of rectum into the vagina caused by a weakness in the rectovaginal septum. Rectoceles are often not recognized as causes of bowel dysfunction because the symptoms do not always correlate with the amount of defect seen on physical examination or radiologic studies. One commonly used radiologic study is called a *defecogram,* which is a functional study observing the process of defecation during fluoroscopy. Barium paste can be seen getting caught in the rectocele, thus identifying the likely source of the obstructed defecation. A thorough history and physical examination are often all that are needed to identify a symptomatic rectocele.

Obstetric injury caused by vaginal delivery has been implicated in the development of rectoceles, which occur almost entirely in women. Weakness in the septum between the rectum and the vagina allows a pouch to form from the pressure of the stool passing through the rectum. The pouch will usually form just above the top of the anal sphincter. There are patients who also have concurrent damage to the anal sphincter, requiring repair of both.

Surgical repair has many variations and approaches. Colorectal surgeons tend to repair the defect transanally, and gynecologists tend to repair rectoceles vaginally. However, the basic principles of surgical repair are the same—to plicate the intact and strong tissue of the rectovaginal septum and to close the defect of the rectocele. This will often require resection of redundant tissue, namely rectal or vaginal mucosa, after plication of the rectovaginal septum. The end result is straightening and strengthening of the rectovaginal septum, which causes the stool to be redirected to pass out of the anal canal rather than becoming stuck in the pouch of the rectocele, thus improving bowel function. A thorough discussion of rectoceles and their treatment can be found in Chapter 23, Pelvic Organ Prolapse and Pelvic Floor Dysfunction.

Benign Anorectal Disease

Fecal Incontinence

Fecal incontinence occurs when a person cannot control the act of defecation. Patients can be either partially or completely incontinent to gas, liquid, or solid stool. Patients with fecal incontinence may experience social embarrassment, which can lead to social isolation. In a recent study, the incidence of fecal incontinence was shown to be almost 25% among patients older than 65 years of age.

Many disease states can mimic fecal incontinence. Hemorrhoidal, rectal mucosal, and full rectal prolapse can all lead to soiling and varying degrees of fecal incontinence. Patients with intractable diarrhea, irritable bowel syndrome, or inflammatory bowel disease may also present with poor fecal continence. The rectum serves as a reservoir and can increase its volume to minimize the pressure or sensation of urgency, giving the person time to defecate appropriately. If the rectum has a diseased state such as cancer, inflammatory bowel disease, pelvic infections, or reconstructive colorectal surgery, the patient can present with elements of fecal incontinence. A careful history is paramount in understanding whether the patient is truly experiencing fecal incontinence. The most common causes of fecal incontinence include obstetric trauma and anorectal surgery (Box 25-4).

When the history is taken, the patient needs to be asked about his or her stool consistency (i.e., liquid, formed, hard). The frequency and degree of incontinence is best recorded using a fecal incontinence score (FIS). The Cleveland Clinic Florida FIS has been very useful in this respect and has

---

Box 25-4 Etiologies of Fecal Incontinence

Obstetric trauma
Hemorrhoidectomy
Fistulotomy
Anal dilation
Internal anal sphincterotomy
Radiation
Congenital abnormalities (e.g., spina bifida)
Imperforate anus
Myelomeningocele
Pelvic trauma

been modified. The FIS score ranges from 0 to 20, with higher numeric scores being associated with more severe fecal incontinence (Table 25-1). The patient needs be asked about medications, prior obstetric history, prior anorectal or pelvic surgery, and the presence of inflammatory bowel disease or irritable bowel syndrome. If the patient reports excessive diarrhea, other etiologies need to be considered, such as lactose intolerance, laxative abuse, celiac disease, short gut syndrome, and intestinal parasitic or bacterial infections.

Beyond the routine physical examination, attention should be paid to the anal sphincter mechanism. The perianal area should be examined for any scarring caused by trauma, surgery, or prior infections. The presence of stool soiling the perianal area is an important finding. The anal opening may show a gap (Fig. 25-6) that is consistent with a sphincter

Table 25-1

Fecal Incontinence Grading Scale

	0 Never	1 Less than once a month	2 More than once a month	3 More than once a week	4 Daily
1. Do you have difficulty controlling solid stool?	A	B	C	D	E
2. Do you have trouble holding liquid stool?	A	B	C	D	E
3. Do you have trouble controlling gas?	A	B	C	D	E
4. Do you wear pads?	A	B	C	D	E
5. Does this condition affect your lifestyle?	A	B	C	D	E

Figure 25-6

Fully incontinent anal sphincter before repair.

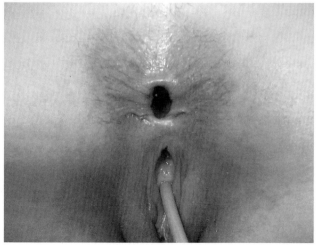

injury. The perineal body needs to be examined for thickness as well as evidence of obstetric trauma. Of course, one must be aware of the presence of hemorrhoidal prolapse or the presence of fistula. Gentle touching of the perianal skin should elicit a wink response. Gentle digital examination reveals the resting tone and, on command, the squeeze tone. The length of the anal canal should also be noted. The anal canal is composed of anoderm as well as distal rectal mucosa, which should be smooth and not fibrotic. The presence of a rectocele or palpable sphincter defects, along with palpation of the puborectalis muscle, can be noted. Anoscopy as well as sigmoidoscopic examination (rigid and/or flexible) are important to rule out any underlying mucosal disease that can mimic fecal incontinence. Endoanal ultrasound is highly sensitive and specific for the diagnosis of both internal and external anal sphincter defects, and it is the diagnostic test of choice before any surgical repair with sphincteroplasty is attempted. Other diagnostic tests that may lend useful information before therapy for fecal incontinence include anal manometry and pudendal nerve terminal motor latency testing, though studies evaluating the role of nerve conduction velocities have been mixed and these tests are falling out of favor.

Nonsurgical treatment of fecal incontinence includes a bowel management program with bulking agents, adequate fluid intake, and stool softeners or constipating medications. Additionally, perineal exercises (i.e., Kegel exercises) and biofeedback may improve symptoms. Less invasive techniques include signaling devices such as the Procon system (Anatech Inc. LLC, Houston, TX), sacral nerve stimulation, anal plugs or radiofrequency energy delivery (SECCA, Curon Medical Inc., Freemont, CA).

The mainstay of surgical therapy is sphincteroplasty. Multiple techniques have been described including apposition, overlapping, and reefing or plication. Sphincteroplasty leads to improvement of the symptoms of fecal incontinence in up to 85% of patients in some studies, with 52% of patients experiencing excellent results. However, results of sphincteroplasty may deteriorate over time. More complex operations including postanal repair, gracilis muscle transposition with or without stimulation, or artificial bowel sphincters are also practiced in selected cases. Normally, patients view a colostomy as a final resort; however, when performed, functional results and quality of life may be as good as surgical choices of sphincter repair.

Rectal Prolapse

Rectal prolapse or rectal procidentia occurs when the rectum protrudes through the anal canal and sphincter mechanism. The prolapsed rectum appears as a large thick tube containing full thickness mucosa/submucosa and muscle propria and its associated blood supply. The rectum is inverted in that the dentate line maintains its position while the more proximal portion of the rectum serves as the lead point of the prolapse. The most common pelvic floor abnormalities found in patients with rectal prolapse include loss of anal sphincter tone, a deep cul-de-sac, poor posterior rectal fixation, diastasis of the levator ani muscles, and a redundant sigmoid colon.

Patients who present with the report of rectal prolapse are often distressed with the amount of tissue that prolapses along with the attendant incontinence. Besides stool, patients report drainage of mucus and bleeding. Although the rectal prolapse occurs during straining at defecation, patients often report spontaneous prolapse, difficulty pushing the prolapse back into place, or both. This disorder can present in childhood and may be associated with cystic fibrosis and neurologic disorders of the spinal canal. Patients with advanced rectal prolapse may develop severe bleeding, incarceration, and gangrene of the rectal wall.

On physical examination, the prolapse appears to harbor full-thickness rectal wall along with classic circumferential mucosal folds. Prolapsed hemorrhoids have a radial distribution. In mild cases, only mucosal prolapse will be evident. A complete digital examination should be performed to evaluate the resting and squeeze pressures, allowing evaluation of the internal and external anal sphincters respectively. Office sigmoidoscopy or colonoscopy is appropriate to evaluate for the presence of colorectal neoplasia. Anal manometry will allow a standardized clinical assessment of the sphincter complex. When the internal anal sphincter pressure is below 10 mm Hg, it is unlikely that patient will recover fecal continence, and the patient may require a permanent colostomy.

Rectal prolapse can be treated surgically using an abdominal or transperineal approach (Box 25-5). Our preferred approach is the laparoscopic. However, laparotomy and sigmoid colon resection with rectal suspension is performed. The rectum is then mobilized and fixated posteriorly, pulling it up and tethering it to the sacral hollow just below the promontory. The reanastomosis is carried out so that the rectum is also held by the splenic flexure attachment to the colon. Recurrence rates after this procedure have been reported to be less than 5%.

Unfortunately, many patients with rectal prolapse are elderly women with comorbidities that make abdominal surgery risky. Perineal repairs for rectal prolapse can be performed with the patient under general or intravenous sedation and may be better tolerated by elderly persons. The most popular perineal procedure in the United States is the rectosigmoidectomy. In this procedure, the rectal prolapse is pulled into view and the bowel wall is divided with subsequent division, clamping, and tying of the blood supply. A new anastomosis is then created.

Some authors have supplemented this operation with an anterior or posterior levator ani repair. The Delorme procedure, or perineal rectal sleeve resection, is a simpler operation in that after the rectum is completely prolapsed, the patient has the mucosal and submucosal portion of the prolapse

---

Box 25-5 Abdominal Correction of Rectal Prolapse

Abdominal Approach
Ripstein repair
Wells procedure
Frykman-Goldberg procedure

Perineal Approach
Thiersch wire method
Delorme procedure
Altemeier procedure
    (rectosigmoidectomy)

excised in sleeve-like fashion, leaving the muscular propria of the rectum and distal internal sphincter complex intact (Fig. 25-7). A reefing up of the smooth muscle coat and internal sphincter creates a new anal canal/internal sphincter. An anastomosis is then carried out between the rectosigmoid mucosa and anoderm. This procedure can be carried out in lithotomy or prone position with intravenous sedation, regional block, or general anesthesia. Although these procedures are better tolerated and therefore suited for elderly patients, the recurrence rates can vary between 15% and 20%.

Overall, patients are satisfied with the anatomic correction of the rectal prolapse, though restoration of fecal continence occurs in only two thirds of patients. Patients with rectal prolapse who experience constipation may require some form of sigmoid resection. Careful evaluation of these patients is needed to identify underlying disorders, such as colonic inertia, which will require a total abdominal colectomy.

Hemorrhoidal Disease

Hemorrhoidal disease has an estimated prevalence of 4.4%, affecting approximately 10 million persons in the United States. Most patients do not seek medical advice and instead self medicate with over-the-counter products. An accurate diagnosis will allow appropriate treatment and a speedy recovery.

Hemorrhoids can be divided into two anatomic types that influence their presentation and treatment. Internal hemorrhoids are proximal to the dentate line and are covered by columnar epithelium, whereas external hemorrhoids are distal and covered by squamous epithelium (i.e., anoderm). In general, hemorrhoids are naturally very vascular cushions of the anal canal and serve to protect the sphincter mechanism from the trauma of defecation. It is only when the hemorrhoids become diseased that symptoms arise. The etiology of hemorrhoidal disease is multifactorial. Clearly, family

Figure 25-7

Mucosal dissection of Delorme repair of rectal prolapse.

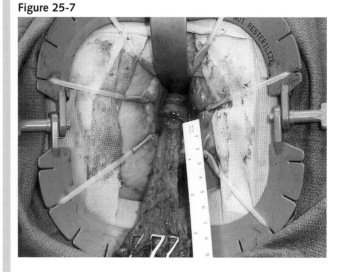

history plays a major role. Chronic alteration of the defecatory mechanism by diarrhea or constipation plays a major role.

External hemorrhoids present with symptoms of perianal pain associated with a localized swelling. The diagnostic term often used in this setting is a *thrombosed hemorrhoid* because trauma causes thrombus formation, inflammation, and pain. Bleeding is rare but may occur if the overlying anoderm develops ulceration or cracking. Most thrombosed hemorrhoids develop spontaneously within hours and peak in terms of symptoms over the next 3 to 5 days. By 1 week's time, the pathologic process has retreated. Conservative management such as with warm sitz baths, psyllium seed, a high-fiber diet, and stool softeners can reduce the time of experiencing symptoms. Treatment centers on eliminating underlying constipation, which can cause trauma and worsening of the hemorrhoid. If the pain is debilitating, the healing process prolonged, or bleeding develops, excision of the thrombosed hemorrhoid is recommended. This is often accomplished with the patient under local anesthesia in the office setting with minimum morbidity and a rapid return to normal function.

Internal hemorrhoids are classified into four grades based on their degree of prolapse and persistence, as outlined in Table 25-2. Patients report bleeding, but no pain is present. The more the hemorrhoid is diseased, the more it will prolapse externally from the anal canal. The diagnosis and evaluation of internal hemorrhoidal disease begins with a thorough history and physical examination. The patients need to explain their dietary and bowel habits, along with other underlying systemic disease, if present. Physical examination centers on careful visual examination of the perianal area as well as digital examination and anoscopy. Other disease processes such as proctitis, Crohn's disease or ulcerative colitis, rectal cancer, squamous cell cancer of the anal canal, fissures, fistulas, and sexually transmitted diseases need to be excluded from consideration. Flexible or rigid proctosigmoidoscopy can aid with the differential diagnosis. Anoscopy will reveal inflamed and enlarged hemorrhoidal cushions.

Treatment is usually dependent on the degree of internal hemorrhoidal prolapse. Grade 1 internal hemorrhoids often respond to dietary fiber, psyllium seed or stool softeners, and hydrocortisone (25 mg) suppositories nightly over 7 to 10 days. Internal hemorrhoids that are grade 2 or worse need more aggressive intervention. Persistent grade 1, 2, and/or 3 internal hemorrhoids respond to rubber band ligation and infrared

Table 25-2

Internal Hemorrhoid Staging and Symptoms

Grade	Degree of Prolapse	Symptoms
1	Absent	Painless bleeding
2	Present with spontaneous reduction	Bleeding, discharge
3	Requires manual reduction	Bleeding, itch, soiling of underwear
4	Tissue is incarcerated	Bleeding, discomfort, pain, soiling of underwear, poor hygiene

coagulation. Sclera therapy has been successfully used but has fallen out of favor in the United States. Some grade 3 and most grade 4 internal hemorrhoids require a hemorrhoidectomy performed in the operating room (Table 25-3).

Anal Fissure

An anal fissure is a common disorder that can cause significant morbidity. Patients report severe pain and bleeding upon defecation. The typical anal fissure is a split in the anoderm at the anal verge, usually directly in the posterior midline (90%). Anterior midline fissures are noted 10% of the time and usually occur in women. Careful examination allows this diagnosis to be made without a digital examination, which can elicit much discomfort. At the base of the fissure, fibers in the internal sphincter are often visualized. The exposed internal sphincter often goes into spasm, which generates much of the pain the patient experiences. Often, the patient reports severe constipation or passing a particularly large and hard stool, causing the initial breach in the anoderm.

The differential diagnosis of an anal fissure usually depends on the location in the perianal area. When the fissure is identified either posteriorly or anteriorly in the midline, it is most often benign. When a fissure is identified to be lateral, the possibility of inflammatory bowel syndrome, anal cancer, tuberculosis, syphilis, or ulcer associated with human immunodeficiency virus (HIV) must be raised. Anal fissures usually start at the dentate line; if they are found to be proximal and affect the rectal mucosa, these other entities must be considered and the appropriate biopsy and culture specimens taken.

The majority of patients who experience a fissure will respond to conservative medical therapy. Conservative therapy centers on gaining control of any underlying constipation. Of course, patients with severe diarrhea can also develop problems with anal fissures. To control constipation, patients are often instructed to take psyllium seed as a bulking agent, along with a stool softener. The usage of topical anesthetic agents is discouraged because the attendant additives can lead to pruritus ani and do not treat the underlying problem. Topical steroids have not been proved to be effective. After 3 to 4 weeks of medical treatment, if the patient's condition does not improve, topical nitroglycerin (diluted to

Table 25-3

Treatment of Internal Hemorrhoids

Grade	Treatment
1	Conservative/medical, infrared coagulation, hemorrhoidal banding, sclera therapy
2	Conservative/medical, infrared coagulation, hemorrhoidal banding, sclera therapy
3	Conservative/medical, infrared coagulation, hemorrhoidal banding, sclera therapy, operative hemorrhoidectomy
4	Excisional hemorrhoidectomy, possible rubber band ligation
Acute	Urgent hemorrhoidectomy within 24 hours

0.2%) given on a schedule of two or three times daily is recommended for 6 weeks. Nitroglycerin has been shown to decrease anal resting pressure and internal sphincter spasm, resulting in less traumatic bowel movements and decreased pain with defecation. Fifty to seventy-five percent of patients have excellent relief and healing with this treatment. A common adverse effect is a low-grade headache, which often responds to acetaminophen or ibuprofen.

When a patient's anal fissure fails to respond to medical treatment, surgery is recommended. Originally, a standard fissurectomy was used, but these often lead to a "keyhole" deformity in which chronic drainage from the posterior wound occurs. Eisenhammer reported a technique called a *lateral internal sphincterotomy* to avoid this problem; today, this is the standard procedure and can be carried out with the patient under intravenous, regional, and/or local anesthesia. The open technique involves a small lateral incision over the intersphincteric groove (between the internal and external sphincter muscles) and identification of the white fibers of the distal internal sphincter. The internal sphincter is cut up to the dentate line or up to the most proximal portion of the fissure, slightly distal to the dentate line. The wound is closed with an absorbable suture, and the patient has immediate relief. A closed sphincterotomy is performed by placing a thin small scalpel into the intersphincteric groove laterally and then rotating the scalpel 90 degrees toward the anal canal. The muscle is then cut gently via pressure exerted from the scalpel toward the anal canal, where the surgeon's finger is resting over the anoderm. Both methods are highly successful and can be performed either in an ambulatory surgical center or in the surgeon's office procedure room. Occasionally fissures can recur, and if medical treatment fails again, a lateral internal sphincterotomy can be carried out on the opposite side.

Anal Stenosis
Anal stenosis is a condition in which the anal opening becomes narrowed to the point of obstructive defecation. The most common etiology is excessive excision of the anoderm during hemorrhoidectomy or excision of lesions such as condyloma. Other causes include chronic diarrhea or excessive laxative use in elderly persons and chronic anal disorders such as perianal Crohn's disease. Patients report pain with defecation as well as the inability to fully evacuate stool. Bleeding may occur as fissures can develop in this setting. Medical therapy for anal stenosis entails the usage of stool softeners as well as bulking agents such as psyllium seed. Fleet or warm tap enemas may assist in changing the firm stool to a liquid consistency that can be evacuated. Self-dilation is inappropriate and can lead to painful trauma.

Multiple surgical procedures have been developed to treat anal stenosis. The simplest approach is controlled dilation in the operating theater with the patient under anesthesia. Progressively larger-caliber dilators are passed transanally until the surgeon's index finger can pass without difficulty, with care taken not to overdilate the anus, which could lead to fecal incontinence. Often, the surgeon will find a tight distal internal sphincter

627

band that will require a lateral sphincterotomy. Occasionally, the anal stenosis is severe, and an advancement flap is required (Fig. 25-8). Complications from this surgery such as infection, wound breakdown, and tissue necrosis have been documented. The overall success and satisfaction rates are high.

Anal Fistula

An anal fistula is a relatively common disorder in which the rectum or anal canal is connected to the perianal skin via a tract. A fistula develops as a consequence of a perianal abscess. Glandular tissue at the level of the dentate line can become infected and is often benign (e.g., cryptitis). These infections can spread along lymphatics, allowing bacteria to break through the anal wall and infect the surrounding ischiorectal plane. An abscess thus develops. After the abscess is surgically drained or spontaneously ruptures, persistent drainage may develop from this site. This is a hallmark of a fistula.

A patient with an anal fistula will report perianal drainage, bleeding, and local irritation. A history of having a recent painful lump that spontaneously or was incised by a physician is commonly reported. On physical examination, an external opening in the perianal area can be identified. Digital examination reveals induration in the region of the fistula due to an inflammatory process. Anoscopy allows direct visualization at the level of the dentate line, where an internal opening can often be seen (Fig. 25-9). Often, pus can be identified coming from both the internal and external fistula openings. A probe can be placed gently through the external opening toward the anal canal to confirm the diagnosis, though this may be difficult because of the pain elicited. Patients with underlying inflammatory bowel disease, such as Crohn's disease, often have complicated fistula tracts descending deep into the rectum.

Fistulas have been classified by the path they take and their relationship to the internal and external sphincter complex (Box 25-6). Most fistulas

Figure 25-8

House flap anoplasty for anal stricture.

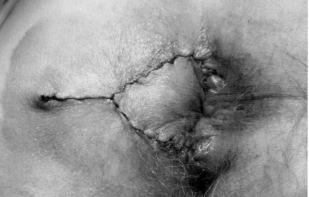

Figure 25-9

Complex transsphincteric fistula placed to drain with a seton.

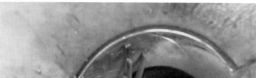

629

Box 25-6
Classification of Anal Fistula

I. Intersphincteric
II. Transsphincteric
III. Suprasphincteric
IV. Extrasphincteric

(70%) are the intersphincteric type. Since the diagnosis is clinical, radiologic studies are often unnecessary. When the fistula tract appears to be complicated and no clear internal opening is identified, a fistulogram can be obtained by injecting contrast media through a small angiocatheter via the external opening. Flat-plate radiography of the area is then carried out. A pelvic CT scan or an MRI, or both, may be required to identify a complex fistula. Also, transanal ultrasonography in conjunction with peroxide injection of the tract is a highly sensitive test.

Surgical treatment of fistula disease is required to prevent extension of the fistula or repeated perianal abscesses that will lead to chronic pain, poor hygiene, and injury to the sphincter mechanism over time. Examination in the operating room allows clear identification of the external and internal openings, the tract, and its relationship to the sphincter complex. Fibrin glue has recently been used to fill the tract with subsequent migration of fibroblasts, creating a cellular matrix that obliterates the tract; unfortunately, results have been less than satisfactory.

The standard surgical repair of a fistula is called the "lay open" technique. The overlying anoderm is incised over a probe, opening the entire tract, which is then curetted free of debris. The wound edges can be marsupialized with absorbable suture (3-0 Vicryl or 3-0 chromic). Often a small portion of the internal sphincter is involved distally, and this can be safely transected as well. Problems arise when a portion of the external sphincter is involved. Care must be taken not to transect more than 30% to 50% of the external sphincter because fecal incontinence can result. These techniques are summarized in Box 25-7.

Another treatment option is placement of a seton, which is often made of rubber, silk, or another soft braided material. The seton is placed through the tract and tied to prevent the tract from closing off. The seton method can be used to slowly cut through the muscle involved in the tract and can be carried out on an outpatient basis. The slow cutting through

Box 25-7 Surgical Treatment of Anal Fistula
Lay open technique
Fibrin glue
Seton technique (cutting)
Seton technique (drainage)
Fistulectomy
Fistulectomy with rectal mucosal advancement flap

the sphincter complex often leads to fibrosis and limits the amount of fecal incontinence that can develop. Sometimes the seton is placed loosely through the tract (especially when a large portion of the external sphincter is involved) and left in place. This method is often used in patients with underlying Crohn's disease. When in doubt, it is best not to transect the internal sphincter or injure it.

A fistulectomy allows the surgeon to excise the entire tract down to the muscle complex from the outside and then to core out the fistula tract from the inside. This technique is often combined with a rectal mucosal advancement flap to improve outcomes. In the operating room, the surgeon mobilizes the rectal mucosa and excises the internal opening at the dentate line. The external tract is excised with a fistulectomy up to the sphincter complex. The mucosal flap is then brought up and sutured to the dentate line while the external opening is left open for drainage. More recently, the rectal mucosal advancement flap has been combined with fibrin glue to minimize the dissection with promising results.

The most common complications after fistula surgery include urinary retention, hemorrhage, and fecal impaction. Recurrence rates have been reported to be in the range of 10% to 25%. Treatment failures may be due to complex fistulas where the true internal opening was missed during surgical repair or to the presence of underlying inflammatory bowel disease.

MALIGNANT DISEASES

Colorectal Cancer

Colorectal cancer is the third leading cause of cancer-related death in the United States. Approximately 106,000 and 40,000 new cases of colon and rectal cancer, respectively, were estimated for the year 2004. Ten percent of all cancer-related deaths are attributed to colorectal cancer.

Increased dietary fat intake, carcinogenic potential of bile acids, and low fiber intake have been epidemiologically linked to the development of colorectal cancer. The progression from adenoma to carcinoma is well documented and is caused by progressive mutations in the genetic material of the colonic cell. Oncogenes such as *K-ras* (chromosome 12) and tumor suppressor genes such as *APC* (chromosome 5), *DCC* (chromosome 18), and *p53* (chromosome 17) are involved in the development of colorectal carcinoma. The genetic pathways recently described include the loss of heterozygosity or replication error pathways. A complete description of current theories is beyond the scope of this text, and interested readers are referred to the Suggested Reading list.

Loss of heterozygosity includes sporadic colorectal cancer, familial colorectal cancer, and inherited polyposis syndromes (e.g., familial adenomatous polyposis [Fig. 25-10], Gardner's syndrome, Turcot's syndrome, and hereditary flat adenoma syndrome/attenuated adenomatous polyposis). Replication error also includes sporadic and familial forms and the inherited nonpolyposis colorectal carcinoma syndromes (e.g., Lynch I and Lynch II syndromes, Muir-Torre syndrome, and Turcot's syndrome). Of special interest to gynecologists, Lynch II syndrome is related to carcinomas of the endometrium, ovaries, pancreas, stomach, larynx, urinary system, small bowel, and bile duct.

The age of onset for colorectal cancer is between 40 and 45 years, and clinical presentation may be subtle with occult blood in the stool or frank hematochezia with mucous components. Anemia resulting from long-standing subclinical bleeding may be mistakenly attributed to menstrual or fibroid hypermenorrhea. Changes in bowel habits may occur and can include constipation or diarrhea, pencil-thin stools, urgency, tenesmus, or even dyspareunia in low-lying rectal tumors. Differential diagnoses include diverticular disease, inflammatory bowel disease, or benign anorectal conditions.

The diagnosis is readily made with colonoscopy or office flexible sigmoidoscopy (for low-lying lesions). Approximately 20% of patients will have a

Figure 25-10

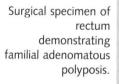

Surgical specimen of rectum demonstrating familial adenomatous polyposis.

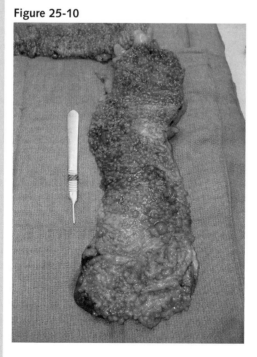

synchronous lesion in the colon, so upon diagnosis of a colonic malignancy, a full evaluation on the entire colon must be undertaken.

The clinical staging and metastatic workup depends on the location of the tumor. Endoscopic ultrasonic staging of the tumor in the colon tends to under-stage the depth of penetration; however, for rectal cancers, ERUS has become the main imaging modality. Comparative studies determining the depth of invasion between ERUS, CT, or MRI with endorectal coil clearly favor ERUS, with accuracy ranging from 77% to 95% compared with 60% to 94% for CT and 58% to 82% for MRI. Recent improvements in the three-dimensional representation of ultrasound as well as the software and quality of the magnets of the MRI have increased the accuracy to 90% for either modality. However, due to cost, not all institutions can provide MRI with endorectal coil, and ERUS is a simple, safe, and relatively inexpensive tool of assessment. In our practice, ERUS is the preferred technique for assessment of rectal cancers for tumor staging as well as lymph node involvement. CT along with liver function testing should be performed on patients with invasive carcinomas of the colon and rectum to evaluate for metastases.

Current staging of colon and rectal cancer is shown in Box 25-8. Since the publication of the American Clinical Outcomes of Surgical Therapy (COST) Study Group trial in 2004 by Nelson and colleagues, there has been a shift in the surgical approach for colon cancer. Laparoscopic resections for colon cancer have been demonstrated to be oncologically equal to open resections in experienced hands. Right, transverse, left, or sigmoid colectomies can be performed totally laparoscopically or by hand-assisted techniques. The advantages of the laparoscopic approach include a shorter length of hospital stay, faster return of gastrointestinal function, and sooner return to daily activities. The COST trial, however, was not designed to evaluate outcomes for the surgical treatment of rectal cancers.

The use of neoadjuvant therapy (e.g., 5-fluorouracil [FU] and leukovorin) as well as radiotherapy (4500 to 5000 cGy) as a combined treatment modality for advanced rectal cancer has been shown to down-stage approximately 60% of lesions, with a 20% complete response rate in final pathologic specimens. The timing between last radiotherapy treatment and surgical resection with colonic reconstruction and anastomosis is approximately 6 to 8 weeks.

Abdominoperineal resection or Miles procedure once considered the standard of care for rectal cancer, is rarely used in our practice. Very low lying lesions with sphincter involvement or an inability to obtain proper 2-cm distal margins are indications for abdominoperineal resection. Most of the time, sphincter-preserving techniques with low coloanal anastomosis are used (Fig. 25-11). Construction of a rectal reservoir is performed using a colonic J-pouch or a coloplasty. For any lesions less than 5 cm from the anal verge or with previous chemotherapy or radiation therapy, a temporary diverting loop ileostomy is recommended to allow healing of the coloanal anastomosis.

Increasing literature favors the use of the transanal microscopic surgery technique (better field view and complete resections achieved). Local

Box 25-8   Colon Cancer Staging

Tumor, node, and metastasis (TNM) definitions
Primary tumor (T)
TX: Primary tumor cannot be assessed
T0: No evidence of primary tumor
Tis: Carcinoma *in situ*: intraepithelial or invasion of the lamina propria*
T1: Tumor invades submucosa
T2: Tumor invades muscularis propria
T3: Tumor invades through the muscularis propria into the subserosa, or into nonperitonealized pericolic or perirectal tissues
T4: Tumor directly invades other organs or structures, and/or perforates visceral peritoneum[†,‡]

*Note: Tis includes cancer cells confined within the glandular basement membrane (i.e., intraepithelial) or lamina propria (i.e., intramucosal) with no extension through the muscularis mucosae into the submucosa.
[†]Note: Direct invasion in T4 includes invasion of other segments of the colorectum by way of the serosa, for example, invasion of the sigmoid colon by a carcinoma of the cecum.
[‡]Note: Tumor that is adherent macroscopically to other organs or structures is classified T4. If no tumor is present in the adhesion microscopically, however, the classification should be pT3. V and L substaging should be used to identify the presence or absence of vascular or lymphatic invasion.

Regional lymph nodes (N)
NX: Regional nodes cannot be assessed
N0: No regional lymph node metastasis
N1: Metastasis in 1 to 3 regional lymph nodes
N2: Metastasis in 4 or more regional lymph nodes

Note: A tumor nodule in the pericolorectal adipose tissue of a primary carcinoma without histologic evidence of residual lymph node in the nodule is classified in the pN category as a regional lymph node metastasis if the nodule has the form and smooth contour of a lymph node. If the nodule has an irregular contour, it should be classified in the T category and also coded as V1 (microscopic venous invasion) or V2 (if it was grossly evident), because there is a strong likelihood that is represents venous invasion.

Distant metastasis (M)
MX: Distant metastasis cannot be assessed
M0: No distant metastasis
M1: Distant metastasis

AJCC stage groupings
Stage 0
  Tis, N0, M0
Stage I
  T1, N0, M0
  T2, N0, M0
Stage IIA
  T3, N0, M0
Stage IIB
  T4, N0, M0
Stage IIIA
  T1, N1, M0
  T2, N1, M0

continued

633

Box 25-8   Colon Cancer Staging–Cont'd

Stage IIIB
  T3, N1, M0
  T4, N1, M0
Stage IIIC
  Any T, N2, M0
Stage IV
  Any T, Any N, M1

Figure 25-11

Rectal cancer specimen with a 2-cm distal margin.

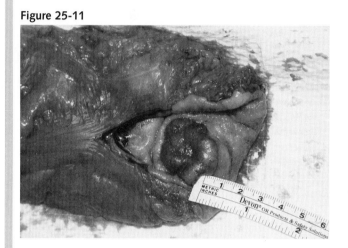

excision for rectal cancers should be limited to well-differentiated lesions that are less that 3 cm in diameter, are mobile, and are T1 well-differentiated staged lesions. Stage 3 and 4 colorectal cancers are treated with additional chemotherapy. Current treatments include 5-FU and leukovorin, FOLFOX 4, oxiliplatin and irinotecan, or anti–vascular endothelial growth factor (VEGF) (for advanced tumors). The reader is referred to the Suggested Reading list for dosages and protocols.

Anal Neoplasia

Anal neoplasia is similar to cervical neoplasia in that human papilloma virus (HPV) plays a causative role. Current research focuses on the relationship between HPV, condyloma, anal dysplasia, and the progression to invasive anal cancer. Patients infected with HIV are at particularly high risk for the development of condyloma and anal cancers.

The rate of infection with HPV is known to be very high in the general population, and HPV is said to be the most widely spread sexually transmitted disease on college campuses. HPV can be silent in women and often does not manifest as a clinical lesion in the vagina or cervix. Rates of HPV infection are thought to be even higher in HIV-positive patients and anal-receptive men. The presence of anal condyloma is often the first sign that an HPV infection is present, although the infection can be present for years without any signs of condyloma or other lesions.

The treatment of anal condyloma is removal, whether by topical application of dichloroacetic acid or podophyllin, which burn the warts, or imiquimod (Aldara), which is an immunomodulator. These techniques are feasible for small numbers of warts and external condyloma. If the warts are numerous, or if they are located in the internal canal, excision and fulguration of the warts is recommended. The warts can also be sent for typing because "high-risk" strains including HPV 16 and HPV 18 are associated with an increased risk for transformation into anal cancer.

Anal Intraepithelial Neoplasia

The term *anal intraepithelial neoplasia* (AIN) is used to describe various forms of dysplasia—AIN I, II, III, represent mild, moderate, and severe dysplasia, respectively. Other terms that are used include high- and low-grade squamous intraepithelial lesion (HSIL and LSIL, respectively). These terms describe similar pathology, with LSIL being equivalent to AIN I and II, and HSIL being equivalent to AIN III. Bowen's disease (described below) is similar to AIN III, but with a palpable or visible lesion, whereas *AIN* describes cells that have a dysplastic appearance under microscopy.

Bowen's Disease

Bowen's disease is a squamous cell carcinoma *in situ*, which is thought to be the next step in the progression of AIN. It will often present as a scaly erythematous rash; however, it is often subtle and the margins of the lesion are not discrete. Traditionally, Bowen's disease was treated by a full-thickness excision to remove all evidence of abnormal-appearing cells, with large flaps and extensive anorectal reconstruction (Fig. 25-12). However, it is increasingly thought that these lesions are very slow growing,

Figure 25-12

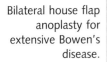
Bilateral house flap anoplasty for extensive Bowen's disease.

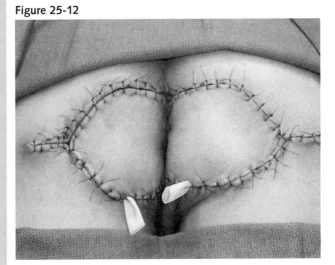

with only 5% of lesions progressing to cancer. The utility of extensive surgery is therefore coming into question. Many clinicians are treating these patients conservatively with observation and biopsies of any palpable lesions. Others are trying less invasive treatments such as infrared coagulation and topical 5-FU in an effort to eradicate the lesions, though these treatments are not well tolerated by patients. The best treatment for Bowen's disease has yet to be determined.

Paget's Disease

Paget's disease is much less common than Bowen's disease but has a similar appearance in the perianal area, with a scaly erythematous rash that is often described as eczematous. Paget's disease is an *in situ* adenocarcinoma that should be treated with wide local incision. Patients with this condition can also have a synchronous lesion in the colon, and a colonoscopy is warranted. Patients with Paget's disease should be followed up closely for recurrence, which can again be excised locally. The overall prognosis is good unless the lesion progresses to invasive cancer.

Invasive Anal Carcinoma

Squamous cell cancer (SCCA) of the anal area has two forms: SCCA with lesions inside the anal canal and SCCA with lesions on the anal margin (i.e., perianal skin). SCCA with lesions inside the anal canal were traditionally treated with wide excision, often requiring abdominal perineal resection. These lesions are now treated with radiation and chemotherapy, which has better results than surgery. Surgery can still be used for early lesions and is still required if there is failure of chemoradiation. The stage of the lesion can be evaluated with endoanal ultrasonography, examining the depth of invasion and the presence of any enlarged lymph nodes. Endoanal ultrasonography can also be used to follow up with these patients post-treatment to look for recurrences. SCCA with lesions on the anal margin are treated with wide local excision.

Another lesion that is very uncommon is anal melanoma. These lesions often are discovered at a late stage and are uniformly fatal, no matter which treatment modality is used. Radical excisions have similar mortality rates to those of wide local excisions because most treatment failures are caused by distant metastases. Patients with anal melanoma usually report perianal pain and itching, and there is often a palpable mass with or without ulceration.

KEY POINTS

1. A thorough history and physical examination will often provide a clinical diagnosis in patients who report anorectal problems. Flexible sigmoidoscopy or colonoscopy, when indicated, will aid to confirm the diagnosis.

2. The mainstay of treatment for diverticular disease is antibiotic therapy for uncomplicated diseases. Recurrent or complex disease is an indication for surgical treatment.

Continued

636

KEY POINTS—CONT'D

3. Medical treatment for ulcerative colitis is indicated to maintain remission. Total proctocolectomy with ileal pouch anal anastomosis is the appropriate surgical treatment in patients who are resistant to medical therapy, in the presence of carcinoma, or when dysplasia is present on biopsy.

4. Control of sepsis with sphincter-sparing techniques in anorectal Crohn's disease is mandatory. Medical therapy to induce remission is indicated after active infections have been adequately treated.

5. Fecal incontinence due to a sphincter defect is an indication for surgical sphincteroplasty.

6. Perineal techniques for rectal prolapse offer a low-morbidity surgical choice for high-risk patients. Abdominal rectopexy with or without sigmoid resection provides for a lower recurrence rate in appropriately selected patients.

7. Dietary bulking agents and local skin care lead to resolution of symptoms in most hemorrhoidal grades.

8. The cornerstone of fistula treatment is sphincter preservation and eradication of perianal infections.

9. Surgical treatment for colorectal cancer is the standard of care. Sphincter-preserving surgery for rectal cancers can be accomplished if patients are given preoperative chemoradiation.

10. Anal cancer will respond to chemoradiation, allowing for the avoidance of a permanent colostomy. For recurrences, an abdominoperineal resection is indicated.

SUGGESTED READING

Allen JI: Molecular biology of colorectal cancer: A clinician's view. Perspect Colon Rectal Surg 8:181–202, 1995.

Beck DE, Wexner SD: Fundamentals of Anorectal Surgery. Philadelphia, W.B. Saunders, 1998.

Gordon PH, Nivatvongs S: Principles and Practice of Surgery for the Colon, Rectum and Anus, 2nd ed. St. Louis, Quality Medical Publishing, Inc, 1999.

Green F, Page D, Flemming I, et al: Colon and rectum. In American Joint Committee on Cancer: AJCC Cancer Staging Manual, 6th ed. New York, Springer, 2002, pp 113–124.

Wexner SD, Rosen L, Lowry A, et al: Practice parameters for treatment of mucosal ulcerative colitis. Dis Colon Rectum 40:1277–1285, 1997.

Wexner SD, Vernava AM: Clinical Decision Making in Colorectal Surgery. New York, Igaku-Shoin Medical Publishers, Inc, 1995.

Wong DW, Wexner SD, Lowry A, et al: Practice parameters for the treatment of sigmoid diverticulitis. Dis Colon Rectum 43:289–297, 2000.

URINARY TRACT INJURY AND GENITAL TRACT FISTULAS

Vivian W. Sung and Kyle J. Wohlrab

INTRODUCTION

The female urinary tract is vulnerable to injury during many of the abdominal and vaginal surgeries performed by obstetrician-gynecologists. In fact, between 50% and 80% of all surgical complications involving the lower urinary tract are associated with gynecologic surgery. The following chapter will review the most common types of urologic injuries encountered by surgical gynecologists, as well as their prevention, intraoperative, and postoperative management. Genitourinary fistulas, which can be caused by complications after gynecologic surgery or can arise from other pelvic conditions, will also be reviewed.

URINARY TRACT INJURIES

Epidemiology

Approximately 600,000 women undergo hysterectomies annually, and approximately 75% of the lower urinary tract injuries that occur during major gynecologic surgery occur during this procedure. The majority of lower urinary tract injuries occur during "routine" benign pelvic surgery. In a retrospective review of published cases, Gilmour and colleagues noted an overall rate of urinary tract injury of 1.6 per 1000 major gynecology cases. Ureteral injury has been reported to occur in 0.4% to 2.5% of benign pelvic procedures, and bladder injury rates range from 0.4% to 1.8%. Actual rates are suspected to be higher because many injuries may be unreported. Furthermore, numerous reviews have found that up to 30% of injuries are unsuspected and not diagnosed until postoperative cystoscopy. The intraoperative recognition of an injury and correction of the defect leads to significantly reduced postoperative morbidity.

Most urinary tract injuries occur in patients without identifiable risk factors. However, the potential for injury is multiplied when there is a distortion of the normal anatomy or when substantial dissection is necessary for adequate surgical exposure. Conditions that predispose women to lower urinary tract injury include pelvic malignancy, large ovarian masses, pelvic inflammatory disease, endometriosis, and intraoperative complications such as hemorrhage. Other risk factors include previous pelvic surgery, broad ligament fibroids, and history of pelvic radiation. Other less common risk factors include congenital abnormalities such as ectopic ureter, ureteral duplication, and ectopic kidney (Box 26-1). An intimate knowledge and understanding of the normal anatomy and its most common variations are of paramount importance for the prevention of complications and injuries.

Special Considerations: Type of Procedure

The route of hysterectomy and the type of procedure may also play a role in the risk of urinary tract injury. A case-control study by Carley and colleagues found the incidence of bladder and ureter injury to be 0.58% and 0.35%, respectively, for abdominal hysterectomy, and 1.86% and 0%, respectively, for vaginal hysterectomy. As expected, women with a fibroid uterus were more likely to have an abdominal procedure whereas women with pelvic organ prolapse were more likely to undergo a vaginal procedure. The higher rate of bladder injury during vaginal hysterectomy may be related to a decreased area of exposure.

Laparoscopic hysterectomies have gained popularity as surgeons and hospitals have noted decreased postoperative recovery time and perioperative analgesia requirements. However, a Finnish study performed in 1998 found that laparoscopic hysterectomies had a high rate of ureteral injury (13.9 per 1000 cases) compared with abdominal procedures (0.4 per 1000 cases). Theorized factors contributing to this discrepancy include the learning curve of a new procedure, the alteration in surgical visualization, and the use of thermocoagulation for dissection. Indeed, Altgassen and colleagues demonstrated that surgeons who had completed 30 or more laparoscopic hysterectomies had decreased complications compared to their less experienced counterparts.

However, the rate of laparoscopic urinary tract injury has not been comprehensively documented in the literature. A review by Ostrzenski et al. found the overall incidence of ureteral injury during laparoscopic

---

Box 26-1 Patient Risk Factors for Urinary Tract Injury During Gynecologic Surgery

Malignancy
Previous pelvic surgery
Endometriosis
History of pelvic inflammatory disease
Fibroid uterus
Ovarian neoplasms
Renal anomalies; ectopic or double ureter
History of pelvic radiation
Pelvic organ prolapse

surgery to be 1% to 2%, which is likely an underestimation because the study included only reported cases. The authors found that 20% of injuries occurred during laparoscopic-assisted vaginal hysterectomy (LAVH) and that only 8.6% of cases were recognized intraoperatively. When location of the injury was specified, most injuries occurred at the pelvic brim.

The urinary tract can also be injured during urogynecologic and pelvic reconstructive procedures. A retrospective review of 526 women who underwent routine cystoscopy at the time of urogynecologic and major vaginal reconstructive procedures found a total of 26 (4.9%) unsuspected significant findings; fifteen (2.9%) of these findings required intervention, with ureteral compromise occurring in 1.7% of cases (Kwon et al., 2002). Anterior colporrhaphy accounted for almost half of the cases for which intervention was required. Other studies have shown that for uterosacral ligament plication or suspension, ureteral injury rates may vary from 1% to as high as 11%. Box 26-2 lists the incidence of various urinary tract injuries during different gynecologic procedures.

Obstetric procedures are associated with bladder injury, and less commonly, iatrogenic ureteral injury. Urologic consultation for suspected injury during cesarean section occurs in 0.3% of cases, with more than 90% of urinary tract injuries occurring during emergent cesarean sections. Most commonly, the dome of the bladder is involved. Intraperitoneal exploration during a repeat cesarean section may reveal dense scarring of surrounding structures to the lower uterine segment and bladder. A study of women who underwent repeat cesarean sections demonstrated a fourfold increase in bladder injury compared with women who underwent primary cesarean sections. Another obstetric event that can lead to lower urinary tract injuries is uterine rupture during attempted vaginal birth after cesarean. Uterine rupture of the lower segment has the potential for concurrent bladder rupture. Controversy remains concerning subclinical uterine rupture and the potential for vesicovaginal fistulas.

Prevention

A complete history and physical examination before surgery should focus on eliciting potential sources of pelvic scarring such as a history or symptoms of endometriosis or a family history of renal anomalies. These clues

---

Box 26-2   Incidence of Various Urinary Tract Injuries per 1000 Operations

Laparoscopic hysterectomy, 1.9 to 13.5
Major laparoscopic surgery, 4.2
Total abdominal hysterectomy, 0.4 to 8.5
Subtotal abdominal hysterectomy, 0.3 to 2.4
Major abdominal surgery, 0.7 to 14.6
Vaginal hysterectomy, 0 to 4.7
Major vaginal surgery, 6.3
Adnexal surgery, 1.8
Reconstructive pelvic floor surgery, 26.8
Laparoscopic Burch colposuspension, 0 to 16.9
Open Burch colposuspension, 0 to 4.3

may allow the surgeon to anticipate a more complicated procedure and dissection. The prevention of urinary tract injuries is dependent on knowledge of the anatomy and the potential aberrant course of the ureter that may be encountered during surgery.

Preoperative imaging studies are most useful in identifying anatomic variations that may increase the risk for urinary tract injury during gynecologic surgery. Intravenous pyelography may be useful in illustrating the course of an ectopic ureter, especially in those patients with a history of pelvic malignancy, pelvic radiation, or leiomyomatous uteri greater than 12 weeks' gestational size. Despite its ability to depict the proximity of the ureter to the surgical site, intravenous pyelography has not been shown to decrease the rate of ureteral injuries. The added cost and the lack of prevention of injuries have deferred its routine preoperative use. Similarly, contrast-enhanced computed tomography (CT) scans of the pelvis have been described as tools in identifying areas of possible injury even before the first surgical incision, but they have failed to demonstrate a decrease in the rate of urinary tract injuries when used preoperatively.

The preoperative placement of ureteral stents cystoscopically was originally described in colorectal surgery as a method to reduce ureteral injury by allowing for easier intraoperative identification of the ureters. Some gynecologists argue that placement of ureteral stents may increase the difficulty of ureterolysis and mobilization, possibly increasing the risk of injury to the ureter. Also, studies have not shown a decrease in rates of ureteral injury with the preoperative placement of ureteral stents. Proponents for preoperative stent placement counter that stents allow for the identification of intraoperative injuries, making immediate surgical management more likely. Kadar and Lemmerling recommend the use of prophylactic stents as aids to diagnose unrecognized ureteral ligations, especially in laparoscopic-assisted vaginal hysterectomies.

Anatomy

Identification of the ureter and its course should be considered routine during hysterectomy. As the ureters descend into the pelvis, they are 1.5 to 2.0 cm lateral to the lateral margin of the sacral promontory. They enter the pelvis by coursing medial to the bifurcation of the iliac vessels and form the boundaries of the avascular pararectal space along with the cardinal ligament. The ureter then passes under the uterine artery, approximately 1.5 cm lateral to the cervix at the level of the internal cervical os. Finally, the ureter passes medially over the anterolateral vaginal fornix to enter the bladder trigone. A study by Buller et al. on cadavers found the mean distance between the ureter and the uterosacral ligament to be 0.9 ± 0.4 cm, 2.3 ± 0.9 cm, and 4.1 ± 0.6 cm in the cervical, intermediate, and sacral portions of the uterosacral ligament, respectively. The distance from the ischial spine to the ureter was 4.9 ± 2.0 cm.

Techniques for identification of the ureter are best used near areas in which injury is most likely to occur. The 22- to 30-cm tubule is most commonly injured as it enters the pelvis near the pelvic brim during ligation of the gonadal vessels (Fig. 26-1). Another site of injury that occurs during

Figure 26-1

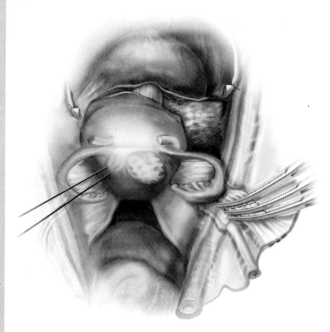

Transection of the infundibulopelvic ligament. The proximity of the ureter is noted coursing over the common iliac vessels. (From Baggish MS, Karram MM [eds]: Atlas of Pelvic Anatomy and Gynecologic Surgery. Philadelphia, Saunders, 2001.)

Figure 26-2

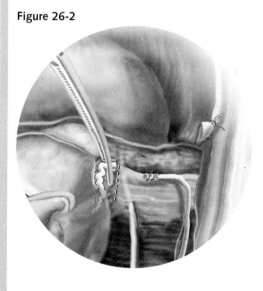

Transection of the uterine artery. The proximity of the ureter is noted approximately 1.5 cm lateral to the cervix and inferior to the uterine artery. Its medial course makes it susceptible to injury at the time of uterine artery ligation during hysterectomy. (From Baggish MS, Karram MM [eds]: Atlas of Pelvic Anatomy and Gynecologic Surgery. Philadelphia, Saunders, 2001.)

pelvic lymph node dissection is the location at which the ureter passes immediately medial to the bifurcation of the iliac vessels. During hysterectomy, ligation of the uterine vessels may place the ureter at risk (Fig. 26-2). Finally, care at the time of dissection of the bladder from the vagina will help to prevent injury at the anterolateral fornix of the vagina.

Abdominal Surgery

The abdominal incision should provide adequate exposure to identify vital structures during abdominal surgery. After the round ligament is divided during abdominal hysterectomy, the lateral peritoneum is dissected in a cephalad direction. Division of the anterior and posterior leafs of the broad ligament to enter the retroperitoneal space affords the surgeon the best possible view of the ureter. Gentle blunt dissection with the suction catheter displaces the loose areolar tissue laterally. The ureter should then be easily identifiable on the medial aspect of the dissected plane. Distinguishing the ureter from vascular structures is best accomplished by the visualization of ureteral peristalsis. If the ureter is not immediately identifiable, gentle stroking of the suspected tubule with a blunt tool usually provokes peristalsis. Palpation alone of the ureter is not recommended as the sole technique to identify the structure because vascular bundles may be deceivingly band-like. The location of the ureter by observation of peristalsis remains the most accurate method of detecting its course and avoiding iatrogenic injury.

Vaginal Surgery

During vaginal hysterectomy or pelvic reconstructive surgery, in addition to the previously mentioned precautions, an adequate vesicouterine space should be developed to protect the ureters from injury. Downward traction on the cervix with upward traction beneath the bladder during vaginal hysterectomy will help keep the ureters out of the immediate operative field (Fig. 26-3).

During anterior colporrhaphy, care should be taken to avoid placing sutures too far lateral, which may cause injury or kinking of the ureter, and placing them too deeply should be avoided to prevent needle injury to the bladder or ureter. Uterosacral plication and vaginal vault suspension can also cause kinking or ureteral obstruction (Fig. 26-4), which should be ruled out by cystoscopy after performance of these procedures.

Laparoscopic Surgery

During laparoscopy, the ureter should again be identified before ligation of the gonadal vessels. Visualization can be accomplished by direct visualization behind the peritoneum covering the pelvic side wall or by retroperitoneal exploration. By noting its course, the surgeon is able to place a stapling device, cautery, or ligation sutures across the infundibulopelvic ligaments away from the site of the ureter. If pelvic scarring or broad ligament fibroids are present, it may be prudent to further dissect the retroperitoneal structures cephalad. Because the ureter crosses medially over the iliac vessels as it enters the pelvis at the level of the sacral promontory, this provides a useful landmark for identification of the ureters.

A case series by Koh found that when ureters were identified through a peritoneal window during LAVH, no ureteral injuries were sustained. Kadar and colleagues noted that the bladder and ureters are exposed to injury most frequently during LAVH when the bladder is dissected caudally under laparoscopy and the vaginal cuff is closed distally via a vaginal approach. The authors recommend laparoscopic closure of the cuff if dissection was initially performed laparoscopically. If the bladder was dissected vaginally, the authors advise closing the cuff vaginally distal to the site of bladder dissection.

Figure 26-3

Dissection of the pubocervical fascia during vaginal hysterectomy. Dense adhesions may complicate the surgery with risk of iatrogenic cystotomy. **A,** Sharp dissection along the uterine surface will avoid iatrogenic cystotomy. **B,** Blunt dissection with a surgeon's finger in cases of dense adhesions may cause bladder trauma. (From Baggish MS, Karram MM [eds]: Atlas of Pelvic Anatomy and Gynecologic Surgery. Philadelphia, Saunders, 2001.)

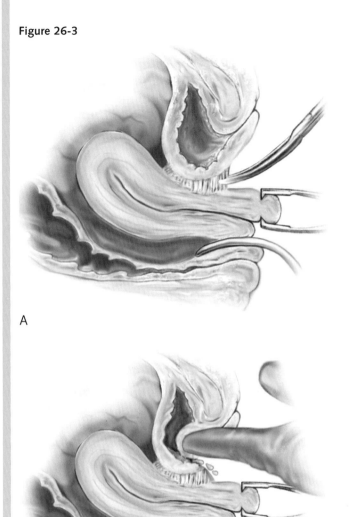

A

B

There are other considerations during laparoscopic surgery. Ostrzenski noted electrocoagulation to be the most common laparoscopic tool involved in ureteral injury, accounting for 24% of injuries reviewed. Thermal spread from bipolar cautery ranges from 0.4 to 1.3 cm depending on the type of tissue cauterized and the duration of thermocoagulation. Monopolar cautery causes thermal spread ranging from 0.6 to 2.1 cm. Laparoscopic oophorectomy is the most common procedure in which thermal spread causes ureteral injury. Because the infundibulopelvic ligament and the gonadal vessels are closest in proximity to the ureter as it passes over the bifurcation of the iliac vessels, risks of transection, crush injury, or thermal spread are greatest at this location.

Figure 26-4

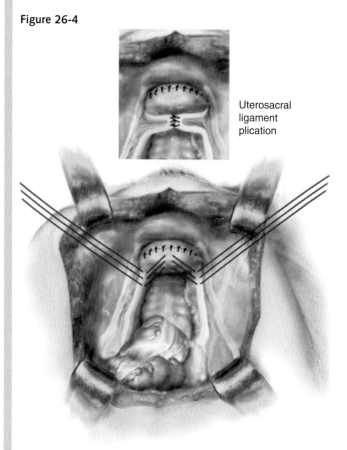

Uterosacral ligament plication

646

Other Considerations

Devascularization of the ureter is a rare complication of routine hysterectomies and is more often encountered after extensive retroperitoneal dissection. Lymph node sampling and radical hysterectomy are the two most common offending surgeries. The vasculature of the ureter is derived from branches of the renal, ovarian, internal iliac, and inferior vesical arteries. Devascularization of one segment of the ureter may result in partial or complete loss of function. In the pelvis, the blood supply for the ureter travels medially in the adventitial layer. During complex operative cases, especially in cases in which a malignancy is suspected and retroperitoneal dissection is necessary, the ureter may need to be mobilized and isolated. Chan recommends preservation of as much of the mesentery of the ureter as possible, especially along the medial aspect of the peritoneum where vascular collaterals lie. Dissection of the ureter from the lateral pelvic wall will aid in the preservation of the medial fibrofatty tissue containing the vascular collaterals.

Ureteral Injury

Intraoperative Recognition

Intraoperative recognition of an injury to the ureter or bladder gives the surgeon an opportunity to manage the complication immediately and avoid further postoperative morbidity. Gilmour and colleagues found that only 11.5% of injuries are detected intraoperatively. Undiagnosed injuries can potentially lead to renal damage, voiding dysfunction, detrusor instability, bladder stone formation with recurrent urinary tract infection, and urogenital fistula formation.

Intraoperative detection of ureteral or vesicular injury can be facilitated by the aid of intraoperative cystoscopy. Ferro and colleagues reviewed eight urinary tract injuries, four of which were not recognized intraoperatively and were later detected at the time of cystoscopy. Before the cystoscopy, 5 mm of intravenous indigo carmine can be given intravenously. Three to 5 minutes after the instillation, the surgeon should note bilateral ureteral jets. The absence of a ureteral jet should warn the surgeon that ureteral injury may have occurred. Absence of jets bilaterally may also be due to dehydration. An intravenous bolus with the intravenous administration of a diuretic such a furosemide may expedite the visualization of effusion. If effusion is still absent, ureteral stents can be placed to ensure ureteral patency. Complications of ureteral stent placement include urinary tract infection, pyelonephritis, reflex anuria, and ureteral perforation. It is recommended that the surgeon consult with a urologist or urogynecologist if the placement of ureteral stents is considered. Conversely, it should not be forgotten that the visualization of bilateral jets may falsely reassure the surgeon when, in fact, a stricture or proximal injury may have occurred. Dandolu et al. noted that of five patients diagnosed with ureteral injury postoperatively, three had undergone immediate postoperative cystoscopy that failed to diagnose the injury. These patients were further evaluated with ultrasound and intravenous pyelography, demonstrating partial obstruction of the ureters.

The role of routine postoperative cystoscopy remains controversial. The cost effectiveness of the procedure becomes justified as the rate of ureteral injury approaches 1.5% for abdominal hysterectomy and 2% for vaginal hysterectomy (Visco et al., 2001). Unfortunately, rates of urinary tract injury are likely underreported and, although rare, some injuries may remain unrecognized for many years. The use of postoperative cystoscopy is recommended for all procedures in which the integrity of a ureter or bladder is questionable.

Surgical Management

When an injury is detected, management is dependent on the nature and location of the injury. Ureteral stents can be placed to aid in the diagnosis of injury, and in cases of very small injuries, may be left in place for conservative management. Identification of ureteral obstruction caused by ligating sutures may be easily resolved with removal of the offending suture. Crush injuries to ureters are often more difficult to recognize intraoperatively. A misplaced surgical clamp may disrupt ureteral peristalsis proximally, but not distally. Intraoperative management of a crush injury should consist of immediate placement of ureteral stents to avoid possible stricture. If an intravenous pyelogram 10 days postoperatively ensures ureteral function and patency, the stents can be removed. If the injury is severe enough to compromise the muscularis and expose ureteral lumen, transection and debridement should be performed with the reanastomosis of noninjured ends or reimplantation into the bladder. There are reports of laparoscopic repair of ureteral injuries.

Iatrogenic transection of the ureter must be managed appropriately according to the location of the injury because this will determine how much viable ureter can be preserved. Key principles include a tension-free repair, preservation of vascular and neurologic supply of the ureter, and meticulous hemostasis. An injury involving the abdominal ureter or portion more than 2 cm from the ureterovesicular junction can be repaired with ureteroureterostomy because there may not be enough proximal ureter left to reach the bladder for reimplantation. This technique is best accomplished over ureteral stents. The ureteral orifices are spatulated and reapproximated with fine absorbable suture in an end-to-end fashion. An omental fat pad can be used to provide an additional blood supply. Utrie recommends leaving a 7-French ureteral drain to closed suction until urine extravasation is no longer present. This technique should prevent against the formation of a urinoma compromising the repair. Three weeks postoperatively, the stents can be removed after a normal pyelogram.

Transection below the mid pelvis should consist of an ureteroneocystostomy. These injuries most commonly occur within 4 to 6 cm of the trigone. This technique is best accomplished by the reimplantation of healthy ureter through an oblique incision in the bladder dome above the trigone. Splaying of the ends of the ureter allows the surgeon to first perform a mucosal-to-mucosal repair followed by a serosal-to-serosal reapproximation for further stabilization. A tension-free repair is paramount to its success. Mobilization of the bladder using a psoas hitch or Boari flap technique may be needed to ensure a tension-free closure.

When a substantial length of ureter has been injured, it may no longer be possible to reanastomose the ureter to itself. In this case, a transureteroureterostomy may be required. This is an end-to-side anastomosis of the proximal ureter to the contralateral ureter. Stenosis at the anastomotic site often makes this procedure a last resort.

Contraindications to immediate surgical management of a ureteral injury include intra-abdominal infections or urinary tract infection. Conservative management with ureteral stents or percutaneous nephrostomy tubes can be used until definitive surgical treatment is possible. Case reports have demonstrated resolution of severe crush injuries with conservative management alone. Diverting techniques including transureteroureterostomy, ileal conduits, and percutaneous nephrostomy tubes have been well described in the urology literature. These techniques provide useful tools to aid in the diversion of urine after ureteral repair, allowing the site of anastomosis to heal.

Bladder Injury

Intraoperative Recognition and Management

Retrograde instillation of 30 to 60 mL of sterile milk or methylene blue–stained fluid allows the surgeon to fully investigate the bladder dome and its relation to the peritoneal reflection. Filling the bladder also aids in the diagnosis of a bladder laceration or puncture. Extravasation of fluid into the abdominal cavity illustrates to the surgeon that a defect is present. An intentional cystotomy can be created for full exposure to the bladder mucosa. During laparoscopy or an abdominal procedure, an incision in the dome of the bladder is made and a watertight closure is ensured with a purse string of absorbable suture surrounding the cystotomy. A 5-mm laparoscope or cystoscope can then be advanced through the cystotomy for further evaluation of ureteral patency or bladder integrity. The cystotomy may also afford the surgeon the opportunity to place a suprapubic catheter, if desired, during this procedure. After repairs are made, the purse string is simply closed and a Foley catheter is left in place, allowing the cystotomy to heal for at least 48 hours. More commonly, traditional cystoscopy can be performed to evaluate the integrity of the ureters and bladder, without the need for an intentional cystotomy.

649

An injury to the dome of the bladder is best repaired with a small, absorbable, two-layer closure. Sokol et al. used animal models to demonstrate decreased rates of vesicovaginal fistulas with two-layer closures (Fig. 26-5). The investigators further speculated that cystotomy from thermocoagulation may benefit from the excision of 5 mm of surrounding tissue to ensure excision of the burned area as well as an omental flap to facilitate healing and vascularity of the affected area. Evans and colleagues describe a technique using 2 mm of fibrin sealant over the

Figure 26-5

Two-layer closure of bladder cystotomy. (From Baggish MS, Karram MM [eds]: Atlas of Pelvic Anatomy and Gynecologic Surgery. Philadelphia, Saunders, 2001.)

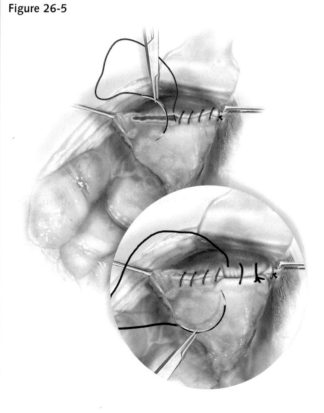

suture line to ensure a watertight closure and to help expedite recovery. Defects disrupting the trigone or bladder neck necessitate intraoperative consultation with a urologist or urogynecologist.

Postoperative Management

A postoperative Foley or suprapubic catheter allows the bladder to heal completely and prevents disruption of the suture line. A catheter left in place for 1 week provides ample time for healing. If a patient is discharged, close follow-up and a trial of void should be performed in the office 1 to 2 weeks postoperatively, following removal of the catheter. The patient should be instructed to return if she experiences fever, back pain, anuria, or vaginal leaking of fluid. If ureteral stents have been placed, they should be left in place for 30 to 45 days. A postoperative evaluation including an intravenous pyelogram before their removal will help to confirm the return to normal function. The postoperative testing of blood urea nitrogen and creatinine levels has not been demonstrated to be cost-effective in patients sustaining intraoperative ureteral injury but may aid in the diagnosis of an unsuspected injury. A comparison CT scan may be warranted in patients with urinoma or hydronephrosis to ensure a return to normal anatomy.

Postoperative Recognition of Injury

Early manifestations of urinary tract injury include hematuria, fever, flank pain, hyponatremia, and a rise of serum blood urea nitrogen or creatinine concentrations. The most common postoperative presenting symptoms include urinary leakage in 44%, pain and discomfort (especially in the flank region) in 33%, fever in 5%, and urosepsis in 12% of patients. Patients may present with symptoms from 3 days to 4 years postoperatively, with a median time to diagnosis of 10 days. Radiologic imaging modalities used to diagnose ureteral injuries include intravenous pyelogram, CT scan, voiding cystourethrogram (VCUG), and renal ultrasound. Renal ultrasound, which relies on the finding of ureteral dilatation, has a false-negative rate of 25% for the identification of ureteral obstruction. Intravenous dye is associated with nephrotoxic effects and should be used with caution in patients who have impaired renal function. CT proves most useful when evidence of an urinoma or retroperitoneal ascites is evident. A negative CT scan result does not rule out ureteral damage and may be especially confusing in postoperative patients, in whom a moderate amount of free fluid is expected. An intravenous pyelogram may also be considered but must be used cautiously in patients in whom a ureteral fistula is suspected.

Cystoscopy should be considered postoperatively in any case in which ureteral injury is suspected, even in cases in which a postoperative cystoscopy was performed. Several cases of repeat postoperative cystoscopy have diagnosed suture and erosions of the bladder mucosa from 3 days to 5 years postoperatively. Intravenous administration of indigo carmine is given to test for ureteral jets. Methylene blue may also be used, but this is slowly cleared and has been associated with transient disruptions of pulse oximeters due to the addition of the intravenous blue dye. No data exist supporting the subjective strength of the effusion as a marker for renal function. A sluggish jet in the setting of suspicion of ureteral damage should be further investigated, especially when a robust contralateral efflux is noted.

Urethral Injury

Urethral injury is most commonly encountered during specialized vaginal surgery, including anti-incontinence procedures. Laceration of the urethra during sling revision has also been described. Urethroscopy aids in the immediate recognition of the injury and allows for prompt surgical correction. The use of a small delayed absorbable suture closed in two layers is the preferred method of correction. A Foley catheter placed for 1 week postoperatively allows the repair to heal and may decrease the rate of postoperative fistula formation.

651

GENITAL TRACT FISTULAS

Introduction

Genital tract fistulas can be devastating and may have profound effects on the quality of life for women. Historically, successful repair of these defects was rare. Milestones leading to increased success include the discovery of antibiotics, the development of general and regional anesthesia, and the use of muscle and omental flaps.

Etiology/ Epidemiology

The etiology and epidemiology of genital tract fistulas vary by geography. In developing countries, fistulas are usually associated with obstructed childbirth. It is estimated that two million women throughout developing countries have genital tract fistulas. In parts of Nigeria, it is estimated that one to three deliveries per 1000 will be complicated by a urogenital fistula. The prevalence is likely considerably underestimated since reporting of vesicovaginal fistulas in developing countries is based on women receiving treatment. Women experiencing obstructed labor in developing countries may wait many days before the decision is made to seek further help. From there, many other obstacles must be overcome, including obtaining transportation to a health center that can adequately care for the woman and having the resources, such as money, to provide care to the woman. Many women do not even live within reach of a health care facility. Many women may remain in obstructed labor until they deliver a stillborn child or they die.

Contributing to the problem is the fact that many of these women are adolescents and the consequences are lifelong. Young women and adolescents may have smaller pelvises, not fully developed yet for childbirth, increasing the risk of obstructed labor. Prolonged pressure from the fetal head can then cause necrosis of the anterior vaginal wall and bladder as well as the posterior vaginal wall and rectum, leading to fistula development. Other factors possibly associated with fistula development include short stature and poor nutritional status. Recently, the International Federation of Gynecology and Obstetrics (FIGO) Initiative for the Prevention and Treatment of Vaginal Fistulas was formed. FIGO and other nongovernmental organizations have formed a strategy to both promote fistula prevention and improve access to fistula repair.

In contrast, genital fistulas in industrialized countries are primarily related to pelvic surgery. Using data from the National Patient Insurance Association in Finland from 1990 to 1995, Harkki-Siren and colleagues found the overall incidence of vesicovaginal fistula after hysterectomy to be 0.8 of 1000. The incidence of vesicovaginal fistula after laparoscopic hysterectomy was one in 455, after abdominal hysterectomy was one in 958, and after vaginal hysterectomy was one in 5636. In the United States, estimates of urogenital fistula formation range from less than 0.5% after simple hysterectomy to 10% after radical hysterectomy.

The pathogenesis of a vesicovaginal fistula after hysterectomy likely begins with an unrecognized bladder injury. Urinoma formation occurs, which ultimately drains through the suture line of the vaginal cuff. This leads to the development of a mucosa-lined tract between the bladder and the vagina. A second likely mechanism occurs when sutures are placed between the vaginal cuff and the base of the bladder. Tissue necrosis occurs, leading to fibrosis, induration, and eventual fistula tract formation. There are also reports of fistulas occurring after anti-incontinence procedures including needle suspension, sling, colporrhaphy, colposuspension, and periurethral collagen injection. Other causes of fistulas include malignancy, radiation, inflammatory bowel disease, and foreign bodies such as pessaries and diaphragms. Box 26-3 lists a summary of etiologic factors for genitourinary fistula formation.

Presentation

The most common complaint associated with a genitourinary fistula is continuous or intermittent urine leakage. Complaints of vulvar irritation and recurrent vaginal infections are common as a result of constant dampness and contact of the perineum to urine and sanitary pads. Most fistulas are painless; however, some postradiation fistulas may be associated with pain. When associated with hysterectomy, leakage of urine most commonly occurs 7 to 12 days postoperatively. Early diagnosis

---

Box 26-3   Etiologic Factors of Genitourinary Fistulae

Obstetric
Obstructed labor

Gynecologic
Hysterectomy
Malignancy
Anti-incontinence procedures

Other
Radiotherapy
Foreign body
Inflammatory bowel disease

may sometimes be delayed as a result of postoperative vaginal cuff edema, which may obscure the incision line and make a thorough examination difficult. In contrast, after pelvic irradiation, fistulas may occur at any time interval.

Diagnosis

An exact diagnosis is imperative for the successful treatment of a genitourinary fistula. A complete algorithm for the workup of a suspected urogenital fistula is shown in Figure 26-6. Externally, the vulva may appear reddened and excoriated. There may be a strong odor of urine. There may also be greenish-gray crystalloid deposits present on the vulva or along the fistula opening.

Figure 26-6

Workup of a suspected genitourinary fistula. IVU, Intravenous urography; VCUG, voiding cystourethrography; EUA, examination under anesthesia. (From Baggish MS, Karram MM [eds]: Atlas of Pelvic Anatomy and Gynecologic Surgery. Philadelphia, Saunders, 2001.)

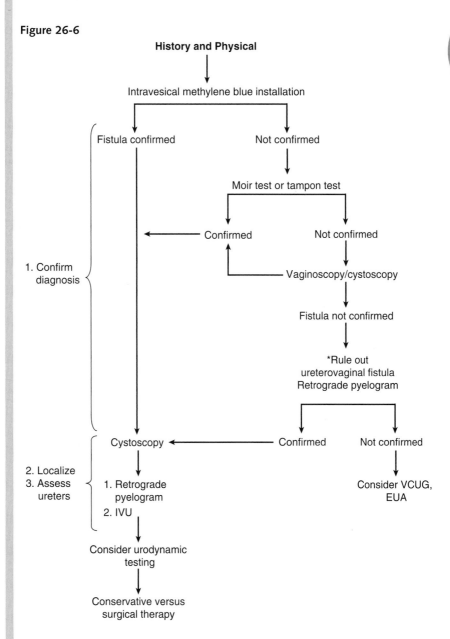

A careful speculum examination should be performed with the patient in the lithotomy position in a head-down tilt. The most common location of a vesicovaginal fistula after hysterectomy is at the level of the vaginal cuff. The anatomic location of the fistula should be clearly documented if seen on examination and should be identified, if possible, as a vesicouterine, vesicovaginal, or urethrovaginal fistula. There may be pooling of urine in the vaginal fornices and at the vaginal apex. The fistula may appear as a small, red area of granulation tissue. Sometimes, an actual hole or opening can be seen. The amount of urinary leakage that can be visualized may vary with the size of the fistula. Women with a very small fistula may only have a small amount of leakage that may also be dependent on patient positioning. If the fistula is visualized, assessment of any significant induration or fibrosis around the tract, vaginal mucosal integrity, and overall vaginal dimensions and visualization should be performed for surgical planning purposes. Finally, the entire vaginal caliber should be inspected because there may be more than one fistula tract.

If a fistula tract is not readily identified on speculum examination, the bladder should be filled retrograde with methylene blue–stained fluid. Asking the patient to cough or perform a Valsalva maneuver during a speculum examination may allow visualization and localization of the fistula tract. Attention should be given to the anterior vaginal wall and vaginal cuff. If this is unsuccessful, three cotton swabs or a tampon may be inserted into the vagina (the Moir test). The patient is then asked to ambulate, and the swabs or tampon are removed and inspected. Blue staining on the swabs or tampon confirm the diagnosis of a fistula; however, this test may not provide any information on the location of the fistula tract or whether multiple fistulous tracts are present. In theory, wetness with clear fluid on the swabs may indicate an ureterovaginal fistula, whereas blue staining would support the diagnosis of a vesicovaginal fistula. A similar test can also be performed using oral phenazopyridine (Pyridium), which produces orange staining of the urine.

Some authors support performing a combined vaginoscopy-cystoscopy for fistula identification. During this procedure, a cystoscopy is performed in the usual fashion with a 10-mm, 0-degree laparoscope used for vaginoscopy. Urinary leakage can be viewed simultaneously by passing a guidewire through the cystoscope and vaginal wall. The authors argue that this allows precise identification of the fistula position and allows better surgical planning. And because several tests are performed at the same time, it is also a time-saving procedure.

Further Investigation

After diagnosis of a fistula, further investigation is still warranted to allow for surgical planning. A cystoscopy should always be performed, even if the diagnosis of genitourinary fistula is clear on vaginal examination. Cystoscopy will provide further information about the location and size of the fistula. It will also provide critical information regarding the proximity of the fistula to one or both ureteral orifices as well as the urethra. Furthermore, it can also provide further information on the possibility of multiple tracts, tissue edema, necrosis, and cautery injury. In patients with cancer, it is recommended that a biopsy specimen be taken upon identification of the fistulous tract.

Ureteral involvement in vesicovaginal fistulas is reported to occur in 10% to 15% of patients. Therefore, it is important to further assess ureteral integrity with either intravenous urography (IVU) or retrograde pyelography. An IVU is useful for noting hydronephrosis, a duplicated ureter, or ureteral obstruction. However, it is less helpful for the direct visualization and diagnosis of an ureterovaginal fistula. For example, hydronephrosis may be absent if the ureter decompresses into the fistula. Furthermore, an IVU may miss a ureteral leakage immediately adjacent to the bladder trigone since dye filling the bladder may obscure visualization of a small leak in that area. Contraindications to IVU include a history of severe reaction to contrast media and moderate to severe renal failure.

In retrograde pyelography, contrast medium is injected into the upper urinary tract through a catheter during cystoscopy. The pressure applied while injecting the contrast medium will help to reveal any dye extravasation on fluoroscopy. Many authors consider retrograde pyelography to have the highest diagnostic accuracy for diagnosing a ureterovaginal fistula alone or in combination with a vesicovaginal fistula. Retrograde pyelography may be contraindicated in women with known allergic reactions to contrast media or very recent lower urinary tract trauma or surgery.

A voiding cystourethrogram (VCUG) is a dynamic study that can be used to evaluate the bladder and urethra. It may be helpful to further determine fistula presence and location, and may also be helpful for identifying lower urinary tract abnormalities. The test involves retrograde filling of the bladder with a water-soluble contrast medium. The patient is instructed to void under fluoroscopy, allowing evaluation of the bladder and urethra in conjunction with assessment of bladder function and capacity. More advanced imaging modalities, such as CT scan, can be useful in the identification of genitourinary fistulas, particularly if they are associated with malignancy.

Some authors support urodynamic testing in women with genitourinary fistulas. Hilton and colleagues performed urodynamic testing on 30 patients with urogenital fistulas and found that 47% had genuine stress incontinence, 40% had detrusor instability, and 17% had impaired bladder compliance. Thomas et al. support documentation of detrusor instability and impaired sphincter function before surgical repair of genitourinary fistulas to allow for appropriate counseling and discussion of patient expectations.

Treatment

This section will be restricted to a discussion of vesicovaginal fistulas.

Conservative Management

Most authors recommend a trial of conservative therapy consisting of continuous urethral catheter drainage, though outcomes are unpredictable and dependent on the length of time since fistula formation. In one series of 151 vesicovaginal fistulas, three (2%) were successfully managed by continuous catheter drainage. Other authors report success rates ranging from less than 1% to 7%. Conservative management is less likely to be successful in a mature fistulous tract. Vulvar dermatitis and irritation during this time can be treated with zinc oxide barrier ointment or sitz baths. Most authors agree that if spontaneous closure does not occur within 4 weeks of conservative management, surgical therapy should be considered.

Another possible option for conservative therapy is transvesical or transvaginal electrocautery or physically abrading the fistula tract. Both techniques seek to disrupt the tract leading to an inflammatory response and, possibly, ultimate fistula closure. In one series by Stovsky and colleagues, 17 women with small fistulas were treated with electro-fulguration followed by 2 weeks of catheter drainage. Seventy-three percent (11 of 17) had complete resolution of symptoms. This technique is not recommended for immature, inflammatory, or malignant fistulas.

Timing of Repair

Traditionally, surgical repair of fistulas was deferred for 3 to 6 months to allow resolution of any inflammation or edema. However, these recommendations were based largely on experience with obstetric fistulas. The important principle is that optimal results are obtained when surgery is performed on a mature tract without induration or inflammation. Therefore, the timing of surgical repair should be individualized. Many authors have reported excellent results with early repair. Factors to consider include infection, size of the fistula, tissue quality, and general health of the patient. Early repair may not be appropriate in cases associated with radiation, infection, or extensive tissue loss. In developing countries, nutrition should be optimized and any untreated chronic infection should be treated before repair. If necessary, patients should be reexamined at 2-week intervals to determine optimal timing of repair. Box 26-4 includes a summary of these principles regarding timing of fistula repair.

Surgical Management

Principles The most important principle in genitourinary fistula repair is that the first attempt at closure has the highest success rate and that subsequent attempts are less likely to achieve success. Therefore, care should be taken in surgical planning and preoperative workup. Important principles for the surgical management of fistulas are listed in Box 26-5. These include ensuring a watertight, tension-free, and uninfected repair. Overlapping suture lines should be avoided. If necessary, a well-vascularized interposition flap should be used.

Box 26-4 Principles of Proper Timing of Fistula Repair

No evidence of infection
Good tissue quality
No induration or inflammation
Mature fistula tract
Appropriate nutrition

> **Box 26-5** **Principles of Surgical Management of Fistula Repair**
>
> Perform thorough preoperative workup.
> Administer perioperative antibiotics.
> Ensure adequate visualization.
> Maintain hemostasis.
> Avoid devascularization of tissues.
> Perform tension-free, multilayer closure.
> Avoid overlapping suture lines.
> Use interposition flaps when repair is tenuous.
> Provide continuous postoperative urinary drainage for 10 to 14 days.

Preoperative Management

In women with poor-quality vaginal tissue, a course of topical estrogen can be prescribed. Prophylactic broad-spectrum antibiotics should be given preoperatively. Tomlinson and colleagues performed a randomized trial in West Africa evaluating prophylactic intraoperative antibiotics that did not show a difference in surgical success or urinary incontinence between the two groups. However, the antibiotic used in this study was ampicillin, which would not be considered a first choice for surgical prophylaxis in the United States. Most authors recommend continuing intravenous antibiotics for 24 to 48 hours postoperatively.

Surgical Approach

Fistulas can be successfully repaired with an abdominal, vaginal, or combined approach. The approach chosen is dependent on the location of the fistula, tissue quality, and surgeon preference. Proponents of the vaginal approach argue that there is less bladder dissection, less postoperative pain, and improved patient satisfaction. Cases involving significant vaginal fibrosis, limited visualization, or large tracts close to the ureteral orifices may be better suited to an abdominal approach.

Vaginal Approach A suprapubic catheter or urethral catheter is used for urinary drainage. If the fistula tract is in close proximity to the ureteral orifices, ureteral stents should be placed with cystoscopic guidance. Relaxing vaginal incisions can be made at a distance from the fistula to facilitate visualization, mobilization, and a tension-free closure. Vaginal retraction can be obtained using a self-retaining vaginal retractor.

A lacrimal probe can be used to identify the fistula and to dilate very small fistulas. Stay sutures can be placed close to the margins of the fistula, and a pediatric-sized Foley catheter can be threaded through the tract and inflated to aid in retraction and dissection. Some surgeons infiltrate the surrounding tissues with normal saline or a dilute solution of epinephrine (1:200,000). In a traditional vaginal approach, the fistula repair involves a split-flap dissection, mobilization of tissue planes, and a tension-free closure. After stay sutures are placed to help with mobilization, a vaginal incision is made circumscribing the fistula, and the fistulous tract is completely excised or the scarred edges are cut back until vascular tissue is identified. The vaginal epithelium is then sharply mobilized around the

657

fistula. Care is taken not to widely excise the fistula tract because over-excision may result in an excessively large defect that is difficult to close.

The bladder epithelium is then closed transversely in two layers of interrupted sutures. The first layer reapproximates the bladder submucosa whereas the second layer closes the bladder muscularis and reduces tension on the first layer. Sutures should be gently tied to avoid strangulation and compromise of blood supply. The vagina is then closed in one or two layers of interrupted sutures in a mattress fashion. The integrity of the closure is then tested using installation of methylene blue. A vaginal pack is placed overnight, and the bladder is drained continuously for 10 to 14 days. Figure 26-7 illustrates the traditional vaginal repair for vesicovaginal fistulas.

Simple vesicovaginal fistulas can also be repaired using the Latzko technique (Fig. 26-8). This technique involves less dissection than the traditional

Figure 26-7

Classic method of vaginal repair of vesicovaginal fistula. **A,** Stay sutures are placed for retraction, and a circumferential incision is made around the fistula. **B,** The fistula tract is completely excised or excised enough to expose healthy tissue. **C,** The bladder is closed in two to three layers. **D,** The vaginal mucosa is closed. (From Baggish MS, Karram MM [eds]: Atlas of Pelvic Anatomy and Gynecologic Surgery. Philadelphia, Saunders, 2001.)

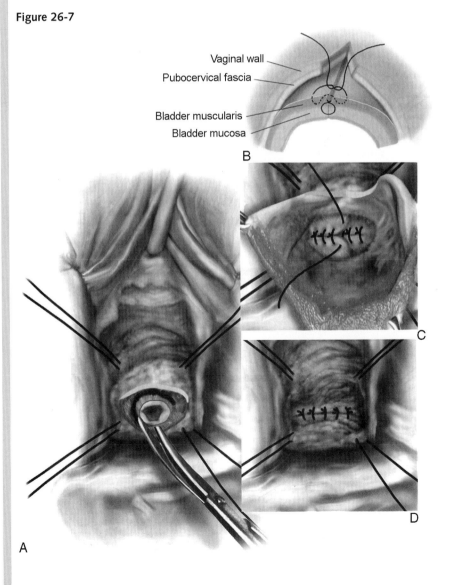

Vaginal wall
Pubocervical fascia
Bladder muscularis
Bladder mucosa

A

B

C

D

Figure 26-8

Latzko technique for vesicovaginal fistula repair. **A,** Stay sutures have been placed and a circumferential incision is made around the fistulous tract. Minimal dissection is performed, mobilizing the vaginal mucosa. **B,** The vaginal edges are approximated with delayed absorbable sutures. **C,** The vaginal mucosa is completely closed. (From Baggish MS, Karram MM [eds]: Atlas of Pelvic Anatomy and Gynecologic Surgery. Philadelphia, Saunders, 2001.)

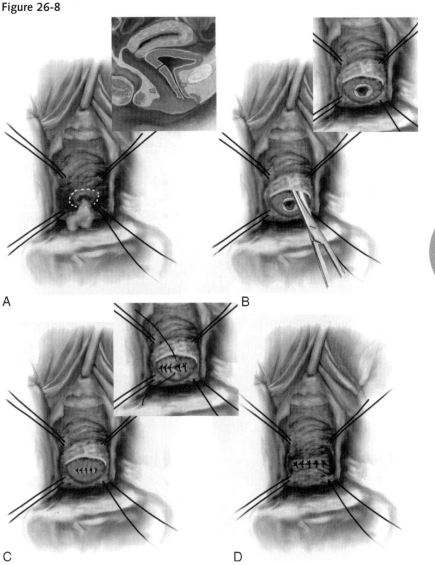

A

B

C

D

vaginal approach. After stay sutures are placed, the fistula is circumscribed and the vaginal mucosa mobilized approximately 2.5 cm in all directions. Interrupted delayed absorbable sutures are then used to close the fistula without any attempt at excision. If possible, a second layer of sutures are placed through the pubocervical fascia to reinforce the initial layer of sutures. Finally, the vaginal mucosa is reapproximated. Although vaginal depth may be compromised after large fistula repairs, most reports do not show a significant impact on sexual function.

Abdominal Approach

The abdominal approach is preferable in cases in which the fistula site cannot be adequately visualized, there are multiple tracts, or there is a need for ureteral reimplantation. Abdominal approaches can be either intraperitoneal or extraperitoneal. However, because one advantage to the abdominal approach is that the omentum can be mobilized as an interposition flap, many surgeons prefer an intraperitoneal technique. Ureteral stents can be placed to protect the ureters. The technique first reported by O'Connor and colleagues then involves bisection of the bladder to the level of the fistula. The bladder is then widely mobilized from the vaginal and the fistula tract is completely excised. The bladder and vagina are closed separately with absorbable sutures. Similar to the vaginal approach, the integrity of the repair should be tested. A suprapubic catheter or urethral catheter is then placed to allow for continuous drainage.

Interposition Flaps

When the viability of the tissues of the repair are questionable or the repair is tenuous, interposition flaps should be used. For vaginal repairs, the Martius flap is the most convenient source. This flap is a labial fat pad flap supplied by the pudendal artery. A vertical incision is made over one of the labia majora, exposing the deep labial fat pad. This is then mobilized from the bulbocavernosus muscle, taking care to preserve the pudendal vascular supply entering posteriorly. A tunnel is then created medial to the labium toward the vagina, which the fat pad is pulled through. The flap is sutured in place over the first two layers of the fistula repair, followed by closure of the vaginal layer over the flap. The labial incision is then closed in two layers. In large or very proximal fistulas, a gracilis flap can also be considered, although it may be associated with considerable scarring.

For abdominal repairs, the omentum is the preferred interposition flap. In one third of patients, the omentum will reach the pelvis without the need for any additional mobilization. However, if necessary, the omentum can be mobilized based on the right gastroepiploic artery from the transverse colon. If the omentum cannot be mobilized, a flap of the lateral pelvic peritoneum can also be used.

Postoperative Care

Continuous urinary drainage is necessary for 10 to 14 days. Drains and catheters should be carefully secured to prevent accidental removal or tension. Antibiotics for urinary tract infections can be used for prophylaxis. Most authors recommend a VCUG before catheter removal. If urinary extravasation is seen on VCUG, the catheter can be left in place for an additional 1 to 2 weeks.

Complications

The most common complications include fistula recurrence and ureteral injury. Approximately 85% of vesicovaginal fistulas are repaired successfully on the initial attempt. Occasionally, sutures in the bladder lumen may cause bladder stones or infections. Stress incontinence is most likely to occur in patients with obstetric fistula when the injury has involved the sphincter mechanism or in surgical fistulas involving the urethra or bladder neck.

SUGGESTED READING

Altgassen C, Michels W, Schneider A: Learning laparoscopic-assisted hysterectomy. Obstet Gynecol 104:308–313, 2004.

Aronson MP, Bose TM: Urinary tract injury in pelvic surgery. Clin Obstet Gynecol 45:428–438, 2002.

Barber MD, Visco AG, Weidner AC, et al: Bilateral uterosacral ligament vaginal vault suspension with site-specific endopelvic fascia defect repair for treatment of pelvic organ prolapse. Am J Obstet Gynecol 183:1402–1410, 2000.

Buller JL, Thompson JR, Cundiff GW, et al: Uterosacral ligament: Description of anatomic relationships to optimize surgical safety. Obstet Gynecol 97:873–879, 2001.

Carley ME, McIntire D, Carley JM, Schaffer J: Incidence, risk factors and morbidity of unintended bladder or ureter injury during hysterectomy. Int Urogynecol J Pelvic Floor Dysfunct 13:18–21, 2002.

Chan JK, Morrow J, Manetta A: Prevention of ureteral injuries in gynecologic surgery. Am J Obstet Gynecol 188:1273–1277, 2003.

Dandolu V, Mathai E, Chatwani A, et al: Accuracy of cystoscopy in the diagnosis of ureteral injury in benign gynecologic surgery. Int Urogynecol J 14:427–431, 2003.

Drake MJ, Noble JG: Ureteric trauma in gynecologic surgery. Int Urogynecol J 9:108–117, 1998.

Ferro A, Byck D, Gallup D: Intraoperative and postoperative morbidity associated with cystoscopy performed in patients undergoing gynecologic surgery. Am J Obstet Gynecol 189:354–357, 2003.

Fry DE, Milholen L, Harbrecht PJ: Iatrogenic ureteral injury: Options in management. Arch Surg 118:454–457, 1983.

Gilmour DT, Dwyer PL, Carey MP: Lower urinary tract injury during gynecologic surgery and its detection by intraoperative cystoscopy. Obstet Gynecol 94:883–889, 1999.

Gulmi FA, Felsen D, Vaughan ED: Pathophysiology of urinary tract obstruction. In Walsh PC (ed): Campbell's Urology, 8th ed. Philadelphia, Saunders, 2002, pp 426–428.

Handa VL, Maddox MD: Diagnosis of ureteral obstruction during complex urogynecologic surgery. Int Urogynecol J 12:345–348, 2001.

Harkki-Siren P, Sjoberg J, Tiitinen A: Urinary tract injuries after hysterectomy. Obstet Gynecol 92:113–118, 1998.

Hilton P: Urodynamic findings in patients with uro-genital fistulae. Br J Urol 81:539–542, 1998.

Kadar N, Lemmerling L: Urinary tract injuries during laparoscopically assisted hysterectomy: Causes and prevention. Am J Obstet Gynecol 170:47–48, 1994.

Koh LW, Koh PH, Lin LC, et al: A simple procedure for the prevention of ureteral injury in laparoscopic-assisted vaginal hysterectomy. J Am Gynecol Laparosc 11:167–169, 2004.

Kuno K, Menzin A, Kauder HH, et al: Prophylactic ureteral catheterization in gynecologic surgery. Urology 52:1004–1008, 1998.

Kwon CH, Goldberg RP, Koduri S, Sand PK: The use of intraoperative cystoscopy in major vaginal and urogynecologic surgeries. Am J Obstet Gynecol 187:1466–1471, 2002.

Liapis A, Bakas P, Giannopoulos V, Creatsas G: Ureteral injuries during gynecological surgery. Int Urogynecol J 12:391–394, 2001.

Meirow D, Moriel EZ, Zilberman M, Farkas A: Evaluation and treatment of iatrogenic ureteral injuries during obstetric and gynecologic operations for nonmalignant conditions. J Am Coll Surg 178:144–148, 1994.

Ostrzenski A, Radolinski B, Ostrzenska KM: A review of laparoscopic ureteral injury in pelvic surgery. Obstet Gynecol Surv 58:794–799, 2003.

Phipps M, Watabe B, Piscitelli JT, et al: Who should have intravenous pyelograms before hysterectomy for benign disease? Obstet Gynecol 69:541–545, 1987.

Sokol AI, Paraiso MF, Cogan SL, et al: Prevention of vesicovaginal fistulas after laparoscopic hysterectomy with electrosurgical cystotomy in female mongrel dogs. Am J Obstet Gynecol 190:628–633, 2004.

Tomlinson AJ, Thornton JG: A randomised controlled trial of antibiotic prophylaxis for vescio-vaginal fistula repair. Br J Gynaecol 105:397–399, 1998.

Tulikangas PK, Weber AM, Larive AB, Walters MD: Intraoperative cystoscopy in conjunction with anti-incontinence surgery. Obstet Gynecol 95:794–796, 2000.

Visco AG, Taber KH, Weidner AC, et al: Cost-effectiveness of universal cystoscopy to identify ureteral injury at hysterectomy. Obstet Gynecol 97:685–692, 2001.

Yossepowitch O, Baniel J, Livne PM: Urological injuries during cesarean section: Intraoperative diagnosis and management. J Urol 172:196–199, 2004.

661

27

INTERSTITIAL CYSTITIS AND CHRONIC PELVIC PAIN

Deborah L. Myers

INTERSTITIAL CYSTITIS

Background

Interstitial cystitis is a chronic condition of urinary urgency, frequency, and suprapubic pain in the absence of bacteruria. The condition was described in 1915 by Hunner, who evaluated patients with this constellation of symptoms cystoscopically. He described classic lesions in the bladder submucosa that became known as *Hunner's ulcers.* The word *ulcer* has proved to be a misnomer; the lesion is actually a coalescence of vessels.

Interstitial cystitis is one of the diagnoses in the differential diagnosis of painful bladder syndromes. Causes of painful bladder syndrome include tuberculosis, stones, malignancy, sarcoidosis, previous chemotherapy of the bladder or pelvic radiation, and interstitial cystitis. Interstitial cystitis is a diagnosis of exclusion when no other known cause of painful bladder can be identified. Interstitial cystitis is a chronic illness for which the etiology and optimum management have yet to be determined.

Epidemiology

The prevalence of urinary symptoms corresponding to probable interstitial cystitis is 450 in 100,000. Interstitial cystitis occurs in approximately 60 in 10,000 patients. Interstitial cystitis occurs predominantly in women with a female-to-male ratio of 9:1. It is therefore important for practitioners involved in women's health care to know about this condition. Using newer diagnostic techniques and a less stringent set of criteria for the diagnosis of interstitial cystitis, estimates of the number of women affected by interstitial cystitis in the United States range from 1.5 million to as high as 25 million women. Interstitial cystitis predominantly affects women between 40 to 60 years of age, but women younger than 30 years of age can be affected. Younger women are more often diagnosed with urethral syndrome or urgency/frequency syndrome, but they most likely have interstitial cystitis. Interstitial cystitis has also been diagnosed in children and adolescents. It is probable that male patients have been underdiagnosed. Recent studies have shown that men who have been diagnosed with chronic nonbacterial prostatitis, sterile prostatitis, and prostadynia may have interstitial cystitis, as treatment modalities used for interstitial cystitis improve their symptoms. Other risk factors for interstitial cystitis are white race and Jewish ancestry.

Etiology

The etiology of interstitial cystitis has long been debated. It is unclear whether it is an inherited condition or one that results from an insult to the bladder. In the mid 1980s, the theory of a causative infection, either bacterial or viral, was intensely investigated. The bacterial flora of the lower urinary tract in patients with interstitial cystitis are different from those of healthy women, but this difference may be due to increased bacterial colonization of an already damaged bladder mucosa. Ultimately, the theory of an infectious etiology for interstitial cystitis was disproved by electron microscopy studies.

An allergic cause has also been investigated as an etiologic factor because many patients with interstitial cystitis have various environmental, drug, and food allergies. An increased number of mast cells have been found on bladder biopsies in patients with interstitial cystitis, and mast cells are a known part of the allergic pathway. This increased number of mast cells has been a diagnostic marker for the disease; however, mast cells are also present in biopsies of normal bladders. It is likely that mast cells are activated by allergens penetrating an already damaged urothelium. Some of the cystoscopic findings seen in patients with interstitial cystitis, such as an injected appearance of the bladder wall, can be explained by the release of vasoactive substances by mast cells.

An autoimmune theory has also been proposed as an etiology for interstitial cystitis. In 1972, Jokinen and Oravisto studied a population of patients with interstitial cystitis and found that 85% of them had elevated antinuclear antibody titers. Silk has also found the presence of antibodies to bladder tissue in patients with interstitial cystitis. The chronic pattern of remissions and exacerbations of interstitial cystitis symptoms is similar to that of other autoimmune diseases; the increased number of mast cells seen in the bladder wall is also consistent with a potential autoimmune process.

Currently, the theorized cause of interstitial cystitis is a "leaky epithelium." Normally, the transitional epithelium of the bladder has an overlying protective mucous coat layer that consists of glycosaminoglycan (GAG) substances including hyaluronic acid, heparin, and dermatan sulfate. These substances are hydrophilic, thus forming a layer of micelles of water on the bladder epithelium. This micellar water layer acts as a barrier between the transitional cells and the urine. It has been theorized that a defect in or the lack of the protective GAG layer is the cause of interstitial cystitis. A "defect" in the GAG layer would allow the solutes (e.g., potassium) and toxins in the urine to penetrate into the bladder epithelium and muscle, thus causing irritation, inflammation, and pain. The cause of the leaky epithelium still remains unknown, but Keay and colleagues have identified proteins in the urine that affect the ability of the uroepithelium to regenerate and repair itself. Antiproliferative factor (APF), a small peptide of nine amino acids, is made by human bladder cells. APF inhibits the growth of the lining of the bladder. Patients with interstitial cystitis have increased levels of APF and demonstrate a lower rate of cell proliferation. Another protein, heparin-binding epidermal growth factor-like growth factor (HB-EGF), is required for epithelial growth and is decreased in patients with interstitial cystitis.

Whatever the etiology (e.g., allergic, infectious, autoimmune, or inherited deficient layer) that leads to increased permeability of the bladder epithelium, a complex cascade of interactions unfolds involving urinary cations, activated mast cells, sensory nerves, detrusor muscle overactivity, and spinal cord sensitization. The deficient GAG layer allows the diffusion of urinary cations such as potassium and other toxins to irritate the bladder musculature and produce the symptoms of interstitial cystitis.

Neurogenic inflammation also plays a role in the etiology of interstitial cystitis. Studies have shown increased nerve fiber density, including sympathetic nerves, in the bladders of patients with interstitial cystitis. Neurogenic inflammation is an important component of the cascade of interactions, whether or not it is a primary mechanism (Fig. 27-1). In response to a bladder insult, mast cells release substance P and other vasoactive substances such as histamines and prostaglandins. These vasoactive substances can cause pain. Inflammatory mediators also released by the sensory nerves stimulate visceral neural pathways and can cause pain. Substance P is a nociceptor transmitter and is integral in this part of the pathway as well. When released, substance P starts this inflammatory cascade, leading to further mast cell activation and degranulation. Increased levels of substance P have been found in the urine of patients with interstitial cystitis. It is theorized that the sensory C afferent nerve fibers of the bladder become up-regulated. Interstitial cystitis could be a type of reflex sympathetic dystrophy with abnormal spinal sympathetic activity.

Spectrum of Disease

A spectrum of disease for interstitial cystitis has been postulated. Young women may initially have symptoms of "urethral syndrome" (i.e., urgency

665

Figure 27-1

Neurophysiology of interstitial cystitis (IC). (Adapted from Parsons CL, Stanford EJ, Kahn BS, Sand PK: Tool for diagnosis and treatment. The Female Patient 27(Suppl):12–17, 2002.)

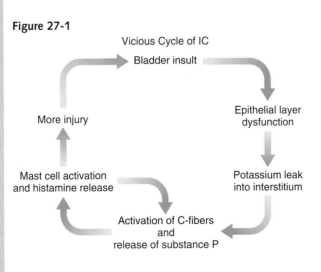

and frequency), although the patient may not complain of pain *per se*. Urethral syndrome symptoms usually do not interfere with the patient's quality of life to the extent that symptoms in the later stages of interstitial cystitis do. The spectrum of disease of interstitial cystitis is depicted in Figure 27-2.

Associated Conditions

Interstitial cystitis has also been associated with other diagnoses such as irritable bowel syndrome, migraine headaches, fibromyalgia, temporal-mandibular joint disorders, and collagen vascular diseases such as systemic lupus erythematosus. Patients with these disorders who develop voiding symptoms should have a workup to rule out interstitial cystitis. Many patients with interstitial cystitis have allergies to medications and environmental substances such as pollens, molds, dust, foods, dyes in foods, and perfumes.

There is also an association of interstitial cystitis with chronic pelvic pain, and 20% to 30% of patients with endometriosis have interstitial cystitis. Therefore, interstitial cystitis should be included in the differential diagnosis of women with chronic pelvic pain. Vestibulitis and vulvodynia are also associated with interstitial cystitis. Depression and anxiety are often seen in these women; however, this may be secondary to the chronic pain of interstitial cystitis. Women with interstitial cystitis score poorly on quality-of-life questionnaires; interstitial cystitis should not be considered a psychosomatic disorder.

Symptoms

Patients with interstitial cystitis will complain of urgency, frequency, and pain, which are also the classic symptoms for a urinary tract infection. Not surprisingly, many patients with interstitial cystitis have visited multiple physicians and have undergone chronic antibiotic therapy for supposed chronic urinary tract infections. Symptoms of interstitial cystitis also overlap with overactive bladder. During flare-ups, patients may complain of urinary frequency (e.g., voiding every 30 minutes), and nocturia is almost always present. Episodes of incontinence are rare, and patients can complain of difficulty voiding. Because these patients do not tolerate large volumes of urine in their bladders, they sense an urge to void at small bladder volumes. However, it is difficult for the bladder to empty efficiently at low urine volumes, so these women will often complain of a sensation of postvoid fullness.

Other conditions such as bladder tumors, stones, and carcinoma *in situ* can produce symptoms of bladder pain similar to those related to interstitial

Figure 27-2

Theoretical disease progression of interstitial cystitis (IC). UTI, Urinary tract infection; NIDDK, National Institute of Diabetes and Digestive and Kidney Diseases.

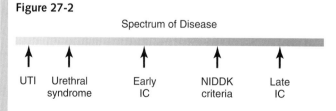

Spectrum of Disease

UTI   Urethral syndrome   Early IC   NIDDK criteria   Late IC

cystitis. Because of these similar symptoms, a urine cytology and cystoscopy are needed to evaluate painful bladder syndromes. A urinalysis that shows hematuria will also require a urologic evaluation.

Pain is a common symptom of interstitial cystitis, and patients with interstitial cystitis often complain of either cyclic or constant pelvic pain. Although some patients can localize their pain to the suprapubic region, patients will often describe diffuse pain in the pelvis. Other complaints include an inability to wear tight clothing or sleep on their stomachs, vaginal burning, and painful intercourse (Box 27-1). Symptoms are often increased with intercourse and near the menses. Consequently, symptoms of interstitial cystitis can mimic some gynecologic disorders including pelvic tumors, vaginal atrophy, vaginal infections, vulvodynia, vestibulitis, pelvic relaxation, endometriosis, endometritis, pelvic adhesive disease, levator ani myalgia, and undiagnosed chronic pelvic pain. Usually, patients with interstitial cystitis have had symptoms for approximately 7 years and have visited four to five physicians before diagnosis. Symptoms of interstitial cystitis can be debilitating and can fluctuate in severity over time.

667

Diagnosis

In 1988, the National Institute of Diabetes and Digestive and Kidney Diseases (NIDDK) developed inclusion and exclusion criteria for the diagnosis of interstitial cystitis for patient recruitment into clinical and drug trials (Box 27-2). Strict criteria were set up to ensure that the group of patients studied did, in fact, have interstitial cystitis and not any other condition. However, these criteria have limitations when applied to clinical practice because approximately 60% of patients judged by experienced clinicians to have interstitial cystitis fail to meet the NIDDK criteria.

Inclusion criteria for interstitial cystitis require that the patient complains of urinary urgency, frequency, or pain in the bladder and has the presence of either glomerulations or Hunner's ulcers in the bladder on cystoscopic examination. Exclusion criteria (see Box 27-2), however, may be too strict for general clinical use. There are patients who have interstitial cystitis but have an awake bladder capacity of more than 350 mL, have nocturia less than two times per night, have a "late" first sensation in their bladder greater than 100 mL, have diurnal frequency fewer than seven times per day, or have symptoms for less than 9 months. Also, the NIDDK criteria exclude women younger than 18 years of age; however, there are reports in the pediatric literature of children diagnosed with interstitial cystitis. Acute and chronic urinary tract infections need to be

---

Box 27-1   Symptoms of Interstitial Cystitis

Urgency
Frequency
Dysuria
Pelvic pain
Incomplete bladder emptying
Dyspareunia
Premenstrual flares

Box 27-2   NIH-NIDDK Diagnostic Criteria of Interstitial Cystitis

Category A—At least one of the following cystoscopic findings
Diffuse glomerulations (at least 10 per quadrant) in at least three quadrants
A classic Hunner's ulcer

Category B—At least one of the following symptoms
Pain associated with the bladder
Urinary urgency

Exclusion criteria
Age younger than 18 years
Daytime frequency of seven or fewer episodes
Nocturia, less than two episodes
Maximum bladder capacity >350 mL while awake
Absence of intense urge to void at 150 mL as measured by cystometry
Involuntary bladder contractions
Symptoms occurring for less than 9 months
Symptoms relieved by antimicrobial, anticholinergic, or anti-spasmodic agents
Urinary tract infection in the past 3 months
Active genital herpes
Vaginitis
Uterine, vaginal, cervical, or urethral cancer
Bladder or ureteral calculi
Urethral diverticulum
History of cyclophosphamide, chemical, tuberculous, or radiation cystitis
Benign or malignant bladder tumors

NIH, National Institutes of Health; NIDDK, National Institute of Diabetes and Digestive and Kidney Diseases.
Adapted from Gillenwater JY, Wein AJ: Summary of the National Institute of Arthritis, Diabetes, Digestive and Kidney Diseases Workshop on Interstitial Cystitis, National Institutes of Health, Bethesda, MD, August 28–29, 1987. J Urol 140:203–206, 1988.

ruled out, but patients with interstitial cystitis can have an occasional urinary tract infection. The exclusion criteria of active genital herpes, vaginitis, pelvic malignancy, bladder tumor, or urethral diverticulum are valid. The diagnosis of interstitial cystitis is made by exclusion (Box 27-3).

Evaluation

History taking should include a query for associated conditions and symptoms such as allergies, symptoms of irritable bowel, pain with intercourse, pelvic pain, and menstrual flares of bladder symptoms. Physical examination will most likely elicit only subtle findings. There may be only generalized

Box 27-3   Tools Used to Diagnose Interstitial Cystitis

Diagnosis of exclusion
Voiding diary
Screening questionnaire
Potassium sensitivity test result
Cystoscopy with hydrodistention under anesthesia

tenderness of the anterior vaginal wall, bladder, urethra, or bony structures such as the suprapubic tubercle or sacroiliac joints. These women also may have tender levator ani muscles as a result of muscle spasms caused by chronic pain. Palpating the levator ani muscles along the pelvic side walls during vaginal examination may detect trigger points. These women may have trouble performing a Kegel squeeze because the pelvic muscles are already maximally tight. Patients with interstitial cystitis can also have difficulty relaxing their pelvic muscles.

Pelvic examination will serve primarily to evaluate and rule out other causes of urinary urgency, frequency, and pelvic pain. One needs to rule out gynecologic causes such as pelvic infection, pelvic masses, endometriosis, vaginal infections, gastrointestinal causes, and other urinary causes such as urethral diverticulum, urinary tract infection, and known causes of painful bladder syndrome.

A urinalysis and urine culture and sensitivity are performed to rule out infection. A culture for acid-fast bacilli or yeast may be done depending on the physician's index of suspicion. These types of infectious agents would not show up on routine culture. Sexually transmitted diseases such as chlamydia should be screened for, if appropriate. Urine cytology is performed to screen for bladder cancer in at-risk patients (i.e., those with hematuria, older age, pain in the bladder, or a history of smoking or occupational exposure to organic dyes).

The patient is asked to complete a 24- to 48-hour voiding diary or "urolog." A voiding diary is a timed record of oral intake (i.e., amount and fluid type), spontaneous micturitions, and the volume voided. Patients with interstitial cystitis will usually have frequent voids and small voided volumes because they do not tolerate urine in the bladder. The average voided volume will be about 75 to 100 mL; the maximum volume may only be about 250 mL. Nocturia will usually be present. Upon reviewing the voiding diary, one can assess the type of fluid being consumed. Fluids that contain caffeine such as coffee, cola, and tea are bladder irritants. Citrus juices and carbonated beverages may also be bladder irritants in some patients.

Although full urodynamic studies may be helpful, they are not necessary because most women with this condition do not have problems of incontinence. However, patients with interstitial cystitis who do often complain of incomplete bladder emptying, so an assessment of postvoid residual urine volume by bladder ultrasound or catheterization is needed. There are about 5% of women with interstitial cystitis who have large bladder capacities (>1000 mL) as a result of a detrusor myopathy, and these women are prone to have large urine residuals. If urodynamics are performed, a cystometrogram often reveals early first sensation of bladder filling (50 mL), decreased maximum bladder capacity (<250 mL), and decreased bladder compliance as a result of a fibrotic detrusor muscle. Uroflowmetry tends to reveal prolonged flow times with normal residual urine volumes because these women are often "low-volume voiders."

Questionnaires have been developed to improve screening of patients with symptoms of urinary frequency, urgency, and pain. In 1997, O'Leary and colleagues developed two validated self-administered questionnaires to monitor symptoms (Table 27-1). Clemons et al. in 2002 found that a score of 5 or more on the symptom index was 94% sensitive in diagnosing interstitial cystitis. Parsons and colleagues developed the pelvic pain and urgency/frequency questionnaire as another tool to detect interstitial cystitis.

Table 27-1

The O'Leary-Sant Interstitial Cystitis Symptom and Problem Index

Interstitial Cystitis Symptom Index	Interstitial Cystitis Problem Index
	During the Past Month, How Much Has Each of the Following Been a Problem for You?
1. During the past month, how often have you felt the strong need to urinate with little or no warning? 0.___not at all 1.___less than 1 time in 5 2.___less than half the time 3.___about half the time 4.___more than half the time 5.___almost always	1. Frequent urination during the day? 0.___no problem 1.___very small problem 2.___small problem 3.___medium problem 4.___big problem
2. During the past month, have you had to urinate less than 2 hours after you finished urinating? 0.___not at all 1.___less than 1 time in 5 2.___less than half the time 3.___about half the time 4.___more than half the time 5.___almost always	2. Getting up at night? 0.___no problem 1.___very small problem 2.___small problem 3.___medium problem 4.___big problem
3. During the past month, how often did you most typically get up at night to urinate? 0.___none 1.___once 2.___2 times 3.___3 times 4.___4 times 5.___5 or more times	3. Need to urinate with little warning? 0.___no problem 1.___very small problem 2.___small problem 3.___medium problem 4.___big problem
4. During the past month, have you experienced pain or burning in your bladder? 0.___not at all 2.___a few times 3.___almost always 4.___fairly often 5.___usually	4. Burning pain, discomfort, or pressure in your bladder? 0.___no problem 1.___very small problem 2.___small problem 3.___medium problem 4.___big problem
Add the numerical values of the checked entries; total score: _____	Add the numerical values of the checked entries; total score: _____

From O'Leary MP, Sant GR, Fowler FJ, et al: The interstitial cystitis symptom and problem index. Urology 49:58–63, 1997.

An in-office test that screens for epithelial permeability and may help diagnose interstitial cystitis is the potassium sensitivity test. Parsons found that a mixture of 40 mEq of KCl per 100 mL H_2O instilled into the bladder will not be tolerated by 75% of women who have interstitial cystitis. This test is based on the theory that women with interstitial cystitis have a leaky epithelium. Without a protective GAG layer, the potassium chloride mixture penetrates through the transitional cell layer and stimulates sensory nerves, causing urgency and pain.

The potassium sensitivity test is performed by preparing two room-temperature solutions: the first solution is simply sterile water, and the second solution is 40 mEq of KCl in 100 mL of H_2O. Through a 14F catheter, 30 to 50 mL of the first solution (sterile H_2O) is instilled into the bladder. After 2 to 4 minutes, the patient is asked whether she has increased symptoms of urgency, frequency, or pain or if she feels the same. The patient then grades her symptoms on a severity scale ranging from 0 to 5. The bladder is then drained and the procedure repeated with the second (KCl) solution. A change in the baseline score of at least two points after instillation of the KCl solution is considered a positive test result and is indicative of interstitial cystitis. Importantly, a "rescue solution" composed of 10,000 units of heparin and 10 mL of 1% lidocaine can be instilled into the bladder if severe pain is provoked. Only 30- to 50-mL volumes are used when performing the potassium sensitivity test because larger volumes, in and of themselves, may trigger symptoms in women with interstitial cystitis. Although Parson demonstrated that 30% of women with interstitial cystitis will have a negative potassium sensitivity test result, it is still a simple and useful diagnostic tool.

The traditional method to diagnose interstitial cystitis is by cystoscopic hydrodistension of the bladder with the patient under anesthesia. First, a full cytoscopic evaluation of the bladder and urethra is performed to eliminate other causes of persistent symptoms. Hydrodistension is then performed by filling the bladder under gravity at 70 to 80 cm H_2O and holding at this capacity for 2 to 5 minutes. It may be necessary to manually compress the urethra around the cystoscope to maintain the distension media in the bladder. Upon draining the bladder, the capacity is recorded. Women with interstitial cystitis usually hold less than 1000 mL under anesthesia, and the average bladder capacity in patients with interstitial cystitis is reported to be 575 mL. Terminal hematuria is often found once the bladder is drained. Cystoscopy is then repeated and the bladder mucosa inspected for epithelial changes such as petechial hemorrhages, glomerulations (Fig. 27-3), Hunner's ulcers (Fig. 27-4), and linear cracking. Bladder biopsy specimens are taken in suspicious areas to rule carcinoma *in situ* and to quantitate the number of mast cells in the lamina propria and detrusor muscle. Although normal cystoscopic findings do not rule out the diagnosis of interstitial cystitis, findings such as reduced bladder capacity, terminal bloody effluent, and glomerulations are highly suggestive of the diagnosis. A bladder capacity less than 350 mL and Hunner's ulcers confirm the diagnosis of late interstitial cystitis.

Figure 27-3

Glomerulations.

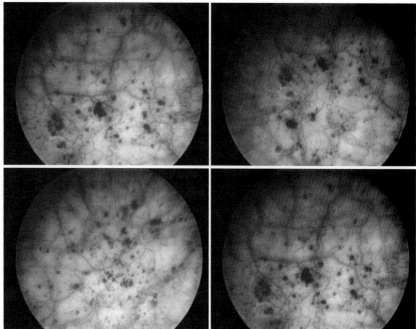

Figure 27-4

Hunner's ulcer.

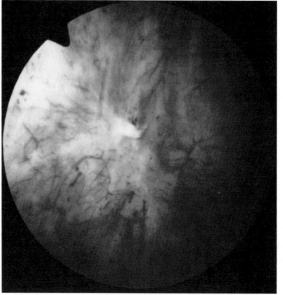

Pathology

Traditionally, random bladder biopsy specimens were taken to diagnose interstitial cystitis. Fibrosis, submucosal edema, and ulceration of the mucosa, a mononuclear infiltrate composed primarily of lymphocytes and plasma cells, and perivascular and perineural inflammation can be seen on biopsy. Histologic evaluation confirming the presence of a high number of degranulating mast cells in the lamina propria and detrusor muscle is highly suggestive of interstitial cystitis. Electron microscopy has demonstrated degranulating mast cells in close proximity to intrinsic nerves after hydro-distension of the bladder. Although these microscopic findings are not unique to interstitial cystitis, the changes support the theory that neurogenic inflammation is an important mechanism in the pathogenesis of the disease.

Treatment

Behavioral and Self Help

There are several initial treatment modalities that are simple and useful for patients with interstitial cystitis (Box 27-4). Patients can obtain information on the condition from the NIDDK (Bethesda, MD) or the Interstitial Cystitis Association (Rockville, MD). Patients can be referred to the website www.ichelp.org, which provides useful information to patients with interstitial cystitis. Just obtaining a diagnosis of interstitial cystitis can be psychologically therapeutic for patients who have been living with the debilitating symptoms without a diagnosis.

673

Treatment of patients with interstitial cystitis will vary according to the degree of symptoms and the patient's response to various interventions. Dietary modifications may be helpful. Clinicians have found that avoidance of certain beverages and foods will help relieve symptoms in some patients; these include carbonated, citrus, and caffeinated beverages; foods high in potassium content such as citrus fruits and tomatoes; foods with a high acid content, such as vinegar and vinegar-based products; and

---

Box 27-4 Treatment Modalities for Interstitial Cystitis

Behavioral
Bladder retraining
Dietary

Oral medications
Pentosan polysulfate
Tricyclic antidepressants
Hydroxyzine

Intravesical instillations
DMSO
BCG
Heparin
Hyaluronic acid (not FDA approved)
Anesthetic cocktails

Surgical
Hydrodistention
Cystoscopic destruction of lesions
Radical/extirpative procedures

Neurostimulation
TENS
Sacral neuromodulation (not FDA approved)

Physical therapy

DMSO, Dimethyl sulfoxide; BCG, bacillus Calmette-Guerin; FDA, U.S. Food and Drug Administration; TENS, transcutaneous electrical nerve stimulation.

alcoholic beverages and wines. Women often drink cranberry juice to prevent infections, but cranberry juice may worsen symptoms in women with this condition. Spicy foods and foods rich in tyrosine and tryptophan, such as aged cheese, may also increase symptoms. Women are asked to follow a diet eliminating these foods for 2 weeks. If symptoms improve, the patient will often want to maintain dietary restrictions. Once relief is obtained, the patient can begin to slowly add back one food at a time to see whether she is sensitive to that particular food. Dietary changes can be initiated even before diagnostic testing. If a patient's symptoms respond to dietary modification, the diagnosis of interstitial cystitis is suggested.

There are several over-the-counter products that may also be recommended to reduce the symptoms of interstitial cystitis. Calcium glycerophosphate (Prelief, AKPharma Inc., Pleasantville, NJ) can be used before meals to reduce the acidity in foods because alkalinization of the urine does reduce symptoms in some patients. One teaspoon of baking soda in an 8-ounce glass of water once or twice a day, or during flare-ups, can also be tried. Polycitra K can also be prescribed to basify the urine.

Other potentially useful over-the-counter products that may improve the symptoms of interstitial cystitis are chondroitin sulfate (taken 1000 mg daily) or the amino acid L-arginine (500 mg taken orally three times daily). Chondroitin sulfate has a molecular structure similar to the GAG layer and functions as a mast cell inhibitor. Chondroitin sulfate is often found in combination with glucosamine, which functions as a component of the GAG layer. The chondroitin/glucosamine preparation is said to reduce inflammation in arthritis and may do the same for patients with interstitial cystitis. L-arginine has been reported to relieve symptoms in some studies. Other herbal alternatives include Algonot Plus, CystoProtek, Algonot LLC, Sarasota FL and Cysta-Q, Farr Laboratories, Westwood, CA.

Bladder retraining can be initiated if symptoms are mild. Bladder retraining to increase the voiding interval can be done by either a patient repetitively resisting the urge to void or by practicing timed voids according to a predetermined schedule. Over a period of time, the patient is instructed to resist the urge to void for increasing durations or progressively increase their voiding interval by 15 minutes until their frequency decreases and bladder capacity increases.

Physical therapy is another treatment that can be beneficial for women with interstitial cystitis. Women with interstitial cystitis or chronic visceral pelvic pain syndromes can develop levator ani syndrome. Levator ani syndrome is an inflammation and spasm of the pelvic floor muscles; consequently, these muscles do not function properly. Levator spasm can cause further pelvic pain and can bring about symptoms of urinary frequency, urinary hesitancy, and incomplete bladder emptying. A physical therapist who specializes in treatment of pelvic floor dysfunction can help patients "re-educate" the levator ani muscles. Physical therapists will conduct a full assessment of the back, pelvis, and lower extremities. Trigger points locating musculofascial spasm can be identified. Biofeedback and electrical stimulation of the pelvic muscles are modalities that can be used by physical therapists for rehabilitation.

Oral Medications

Pentosan polysulfate (Elmiron, Ortho-McNeil, Raritan, NJ) is the only oral medication approved by the U.S. Food and Drug Administration (FDA) for the treatment of interstitial cystitis (see Box 27-4). In 1993, Parsons reported the use of oral Elmiron as a treatment for interstitial cystitis. Its chemical structure is similar to the GAG layer, and it has properties similar to heparin. Elmiron works to correct the permeability defect in the GAG layer. Bleeding problems have been reported with intravenous Elmiron therapy but are rare with the oral formulation. Elmiron is prescribed in a dose of 100 mg taken orally three times daily. The medication has occasional adverse effects of gastrointestinal distress, headache, and reversible hair loss. Approximately 60% of patients will experience relief of symptoms by 6 months. During this 4- to 6-month waiting period, other treatments can be instituted. Studies support the safety of the long-term use of Elmiron. Currently, investigators are evaluating the effectiveness of this medication for intravesical use.

675

Tricyclic antidepressants (TCAs) such as amitriptyline and nortriptyline have several properties that can be used to relieve the symptoms of interstitial cystitis: they have anticholinergic properties that reduce bladder spasm and urgency, they can increase the pain threshold by inhibiting the serotonin uptake in the presynaptic nerve endings, they are sedating (which can improve sleep), and as antidepressants, they act to elevate mood. Adverse effects include dry mouth, constipation, and sedation. TCAs need to be used with caution in elderly persons because these drugs can cause confusion and electrocardiogram changes. TCAs are prescribed at bedtime. When prescribing TCAs to a younger population, one can start at a dose of 25 mg and increase to 50 to 75 mg, but in elderly persons one should start at low doses of 10 to 20 mg. TCAs can give prompt relief of symptoms in patients with interstitial cystitis as shown in a recent randomized study by Van Ophoven et al. Other antidepressants such as doxepin (Sinequan, Pfizer, New York, NY), fluoxetine (Prozac, Eli Lilly and Co, Indianapolis, IN) and sertraline (Zoloft, Pfizer, New York, NY) have also been used.

Hydroxyzine (Atarax and Vistaril, Pfizer, New York, NY) is another medication used in the management of interstitial cystitis. Since degranulation of mast cells is involved in the pathophysiology of interstitial cystitis, control of this part of the cascade should be helpful therapy. Hydroxyzine blocks the release of histamines from the mast cells. The recommended dose is 25 to 50 mg taken orally at bedtime. Hydroxyzine also has a sedating effect and can thus improve sleep in this group of patients. Theoharides and Sant demonstrated a 40% reduction of interstitial cystitis symptoms with hydroxyzine and a 55% reduction of symptoms in patients with a history of allergies. Because of the association of interstitial cystitis with mast cells, hydroxyzine may be especially useful in patients who have allergies, spring and fall seasonal flares of their symptoms, or a high number of mast cells on bladder biopsy. However, a recent randomized trial failed to show significant statistical improvement of symptoms for either hydroxyzine or pentosan polysulfate

Medications that may relieve some symptoms of interstitial cystitis include anticholinergic medications such as oxybutynin, (Ditropan XL, Ortho McNeil, Raritan, NJ), hyoscyamine, and tolterodine (Detrol, Pfizer, New York, NY). This group of medications may improve urinary frequency and treat urge incontinence, if present. Phenazopyridine (Pyridium, Warner Chilcott, Rockaway, NJ) is a bladder analgesic that can relieve symptoms on an as-needed basis. Although these medications may control some of the symptoms of interstitial cystitis, they do not affect the physiologic pathways that lead to these symptoms.

Bladder Instillations

The long-standing treatment of interstitial cystitis is dimethyl sulfoxide (DMSO) (see Box 27-4). DMSO, a wood by-product, was introduced as a commercial solvent in 1953. It was popularized during the 1960s and 1970s as treatment for musculoskeletal problems because it has anti-inflammatory, analgesic, and antispasmodic properties. DMSO may also block peripheral C fiber nerves. In 1978, the FDA approved DMSO for the treatment of interstitial cystitis. DMSO (RIMSO-50) is prepared as a 50% solution and is instilled into the bladder through a catheter. DMSO works by causing degranulation of mast cells and their depletion in the bladder. Immediately after instillation there is an initial rise in symptoms due to increased mast cell degranulation, but then the symptoms resolve as the mast cells become depleted. Before instillation, a urine dipstick test is performed to rule out a bladder infection. Patients undergo bladder instillations every 7 to 14 days for six to eight treatments. The solution is held in the bladder for 15 to 20 minutes, and the bladder is emptied either by spontaneous voiding or by catheterization. About 50% of patients obtain relief with DMSO treatments. DMSO can be instilled along with a corticosteroid and sodium bicarbonate. Patients can also be taught how to self-administer DMSO at home if long-term maintenance treatments are needed.

DMSO is metabolized through the lungs and liver; patients will have characteristic garlic-like odor for 24 to 48 hours after treatment. There have been reports of high doses of DMSO in dogs causing cataracts. Because some patients may need to receive maintenance DMSO treatments every month for several years, chronic users should be monitored with periodic liver function tests and yearly eye examinations. DMSO bladder instillations can reduce symptoms for up to 6 months in 78% of patients receiving six weekly treatments, but resistance to the therapy can develop.

Various other medications have been instilled into the bladder to treat interstitial cystitis. Hypochlorous acid (Clorpactin), used to treat tuberculosis of the bladder during the 1940s, has been used to treat interstitial cystitis. Clorpactin acts like a detergent to strip the bladder lining and its nerve endings, theoretically promoting healing and rebuilding of a new lining. Clorpactin instillations are painful and are therefore performed with the patient under anesthesia.

Intravesical bacillus Calmette-Guérin (BCG) has also been used to treat interstitial cystitis. BCG works by stimulating the immune response in the bladder. In a prospective, double-blind, placebo-controlled study, treatment with BCG produced a 60% response rate, compared with a 27% placebo response rate at a mean follow-up of 8 months. Of those patients who received only 6 weekly treatments and responded favorably, 89% continued to have an excellent response with follow-up ranging from 24 to 33 months. Intravesical BCG appears to be effective and durable in the treatment of interstitial cystitis. A rare but reported complication after BCG instillation is disseminated infection.

Medications that have properties of replacing or simulating the GAG layer have also been instilled into the bladder. Heparin has a chemical structure similar to the components of the GAG layer and thus has been used for instillations. Heparin treatments provide good long-term relief, perhaps because of the similar molecular structure and their frequency and length of treatment. Women who have undergone heparin instillations are reported to be symptom free or have reduced symptoms for up to 2 years. Studies have shown that intravesical heparin can relieve bladder symptoms in a significant proportion of patients, and this may be associated with the restoration of mucosal integrity. The concentration of heparin solution used is 10,000 units in 50 mL of sterile saline. The solution is instilled into the bladder daily or at least three times per week for at least 4 months. Because of the frequency of instillations, patients are taught to self-administer the medication. Maintenance treatment is long term, often extending for 2 to 4 years.

677

Hyaluronic acid (Cystistat, Bioniche, Belleville, Ontario, Canada) has a similar chemical structure to the GAG layer and thus acts to replenish it. Again, the solution is instilled into the bladder and held for 20 to 30 minutes. These treatments are tolerated very well. It may take four to six treatments before women start to see relief. Currently, Cystostat is available only in Canada. There are currently trials ongoing in the United States to determine its effectiveness.

Anesthetic solutions have also been instilled into the bladder. One can use a combination of lidocaine (Xylocaine), a corticosteroid, heparin, and sodium bicarbonate to make a "cocktail" to be instilled into the bladder. There have been reports of systemic absorption of the anesthetic with toxic reactions, so no more than a total of 400 mg of Xylocaine should be used; 10 mL of Xylocaine in a 1% solution is recommended. Steroids are often used in cocktails because they have anti-inflammatory properties. Sodium bicarbonate is frequently also used in cocktails because it acts as a carrier and allows better penetration of medication into the bladder wall. Traditionally anesthetic cocktails have been used for treatment, but recently they have been advocated as an office diagnostic aid for interstitial cystitis. Unlike the potassium sensitivity test, which is used to diagnose interstitial cystitis by increasing symptoms, the instillation of an anesthetic agent would decrease symptoms.

Pain Management

If the pain associated with interstitial cystitis is severe or debilitating, it may be necessary to refer the patient to a pain clinic. Patients who live with chronic pain are often depressed and have low scores on standardized quality-of-life questionnaires. These patients may need the psychological support and resources that a pain clinic can provide. Neuroleptic pain medications such as gabapentin (Neurontin) and carbamazepine (Tegretol) are used for other types of neuropathies and chronic pain and have been used "off label" for treatment of the pain of interstitial cystitis. These medications serve to down-regulate the hyperesthesia seen in these patients.

Nerve Stimulation

Transcutaneous electrical nerve stimulation (TENS), which has long been used for the treatment of patients with chronic back pain, can be used for patients with interstitial cystitis. TENS units are used in an attempt to change the pain threshold. Sacral neuromodulation (InterStim, Medtronic Corp., Minneapolis, MN) is FDA approved for the treatment of urge incontinence, urinary retention, and urinary urgency/frequency, but not yet for interstitial cystitis. The electrode of the stimulator is placed surgically into the S3 nerve root foramen to reregulate the pelvic floor and "reset the thermostat" of the nerve impulses to the bladder. Case series have shown the effectiveness of sacral neuromodulation in managing the urinary frequency associated with interstitial cystitis. InterStim has also been shown to normalize the levels of APF and HB-EGF in patients with interstitial cystitis. The success of sacral stimulation and its management of pain in these patients remain preliminary. Additionally, patients may seek out alternative non-Western treatments such as acupuncture.

Surgical Treatment

Hydrodistension of the bladder was first described in 1930 by Bumpus. Hydrodistension is not only a diagnostic tool, but can also be a therapeutic one (see Box 27-4). It offers initial relief in approximately 60% of patients and its effects may last up to 6 months. Under anesthesia, the patient's bladder is distended with sterile water as previously described. The hydrodistension overstretches the epithelium, stimulating epithelial regeneration and repair. The sympathetic fiber density has been found to be decreased after bladder distension, explaining the relief of symptoms after the procedure. Hydrodistension has also been shown to decrease production of APF and increase levels of HB-EGF.

Other cystoscopic procedures performed for interstitial cystitis include cauterization or destruction of glomerulations and ulcerations with either yttrium aluminum garnet laser or electrocautery. Several case series have reported only minimal success with this method. Because interstitial cystitis involves the entire bladder, treatment of a specific site does not prove to be fruitful.

Other types of surgical therapy are more radical. Enterocystoplasty is a surgery that attaches a portion of small intestine to the bladder to increase capacity. Surgical procedures such as urinary diversion, denervating the bladder, and cystectomy are only used as a last resort. Unpredictably, despite more radical/extirpative surgical procedures that divert the urine or remove the entire bladder, patients can still have bladder or pelvic pain, or both. This phantom pain phenomenon happens in these patients with chronic pain due to the overexcitation of the nerve pathways in the pelvis or bladder that keeps the pain syndrome active.

CHRONIC PELVIC PAIN

Chronic pelvic pain is defined as pain in the pelvis of a duration longer than 6 months. This is a common disorder, and it is estimated that 24 to 147/100,000 women are afflicted. Porpora has shown that 36% of patients have normal findings when diagnostic laparoscopy is performed to evaluate the cause of chronic pelvis pain. The intimate juxtaposition of the urinary, reproductive, and gastrointestinal structures should remind the practitioner that any disease process of the gastrointestinal (e.g., colitis, diverticulitis, irritable bowel disease), genitourinary (e.g., cancer, stones, radiation therapy to the bladder), or reproductive systems can produce pelvic pain. In addition, conditions involving any of these organ systems can refer pain to other organ systems in the pelvis. This interaction occurs for several reasons. The pelvic floor and the bladder are both innervated by sacral nerve roots S2, S3, and S4. These nerve roots include motor/efferent pathways and the sensory/afferent pathways of both the somatic and visceral systems. Thus, neurogenic inflammation occurs between the visceral and the somatic pathways (i.e., viscerosomatic hyperalgesia), as well as between the viscera of one organ system and another (i.e., viscerovisceral hyperalgesia). Also, the urinary and reproductive systems are embryologically related. Both systems initially develop from the intermediate mesoderm of the embryo. The endoderm, which ultimately forms epithelium of the bladder trigone and urethra, also forms the epithelium of the lower third of the vagina and vestibule. Consequently, conditions that affect the bladder may also produce vaginal/vulvar symptoms and vice versa.

Hormonal links also exist between the urinary and reproductive tracts. Estrogen and progesterone receptors have been found in the bladder and urethra. In 1998, Tao confirmed the presence of luteinizing hormone and human chorionic gonadotropin receptors in the bladder trigone. Several investigators have studied the effects of estrogen and progesterone on the bladder. It is likely that such hormonal receptors are also present within the gastrointestinal tract. Women will report flares of their gastrointestinal symptoms premenstrually, and preliminary research has shown an improvement of symptoms in patients with irritable bowel syndrome who are treated with gonadotropin-releasing hormone agonists. The presence of these receptors throughout all of the pelvic organ systems would explain the fluctuation of disease symptoms in women in conjunction with their menstrual cycles.

Differential Diagnosis

Pain in the pelvis can be due to a variety of gynecologic disorders (Box 27-5). One must consider benign or malignant tumors, endometriosis, and acute or chronic pelvic inflammatory disease as possible causes of pelvic pain. The clinical presentations, diagnosis, and management of these gynecologic disorders are discussed in depth in other areas of this text.

Pelvic adhesive disease is a reported cause of chronic pelvic pain. Adhesions can result from pelvic inflammatory disease, endometriosis, ruptured appendicitis, and diverticulitis. However, it is difficult to determine whether adhesions cause pain, as pain mapping studies by Howard demonstrated that lysis of adhesions provided relief only 50% of the time. Also, treatment of adhesions by lysis is problematic because adhesions can simply reoccur. To prevent adhesion formation, minimally invasive surgical approaches and barrier methods such as oxidized regenerated cellulose (Interceed, Ethicon Inc., Somerville, NJ) and hyaluronic acid with carboxymethylcellulose (Seprafilm, Genzyme Biosurgery, Cambridge, MA) have been advocated. Various solutions such as high-molecular-weight complex sugar Dextran 70, heparin, and steroids have also been instilled into the pelvis in an attempt to prevent adhesion formation.

Vulvodynia can be a cause of chronic pelvic pain. The incidence of vulvodynia has been found to be as high as 15% in a private obstetrician-gynecologist practice. It predominates in white women (97%) as well as nulliparous women (62%), and the mean age of patients is 32 years with a range of 11 to 75 years. Surgical procedures should be limited in these

---

Box 27-5 Differential Diagnosis of Chronic Pelvic Pain

Gynecologic
Endometriosis
Pelvic inflammatory disease
Pelvic adhesions
Vulvodynia
Pudendal neuralgia

Musculoskeletal
Abdominal wall
Levator ani myalgia

Urologic
Interstitial cystitis
Bladder stones
Malignancy
Radiation therapy to bladder

Gastrointestinal
Diverticulitis
Irritable bowel syndrome
Malignancy
Adhesive disease

Psychological

---

patients. Patients with vulvodynia can usually localize their pain to the vulvar, urethral, or rectal areas; however, some patients may not be able to locate the precise site and simply describe pain in the pelvis. Symptoms consistent with neuralgia such as burning, pain with light touch (allodynia), paroxysmal stabbing pains, and hyperesthesia are described. Symptoms may not only be associated with intercourse; symptoms may be constant or intermittent. Physical findings are usually lacking, unlike findings in patients with vestibulitis. Vulvodynia may result from a pudendal neuralgia caused by prior pelvic surgery, back pain, cycling or horseback riding injuries, muscle spasm, or multiple sclerosis. Pudendal neuralgia can also develop if herpes virus has invaded the pudendal nerve; a course of antiviral suppression therapy may be indicated for patients in these circumstances. Sacral meningeal (Tarlov's) cysts demonstrated on magnetic resonance imaging studies can cause chronic vulvar/vaginal pain. These patients may benefit from topical anesthetic ointments and medications that are used for neuropathic pain such as amitriptyline, gabapentin, divalproex (Depakote), or carbamazepine.

681

Abnormalities of the abdominal wall can also cause chronic pelvic pain. Conditions such as nerve entrapment, inflammation of an intercostal nerve root or an anterior cutaneous nerve, rib tip syndrome, myofascial pain, trigger points, and hernias can cause pain. In 1926, Carnett developed the Carnett test to screen for abdominal wall causes of pelvic pain. The Carnett test involves palpating the abdomen while the patient goes from a supine to a sitting position. A positive test result (i.e., pain is elicited) indicates that the source of pain is most likely not from the viscera but from parietal structures. A negative test result indicates that the pain is from the viscera. Further evaluation of a positive test result may involve injecting the palpated area with a local anesthetic to confirm that the pain is from the abdominal wall. If the pain is abolished, then the patient most likely has neuralgia. Entrapment of the ilioinguinal or iliohypogastric nerves in a lower abdominal scar can occur in women who have had prior pelvic surgery. Entrapment of these nerves can also cause pain in the lower abdomen and the inner thighs. Hernias involving the inguinal and femoral canals, the umbilicus, prior incisions, ventral wall (i.e., spigelian hernia), sciatic foramen, obturator canal, or perineum need to be sought out and will need surgical correction.

Levator ani muscle myalgia is a condition that can either cause chronic pelvic pain or be a result of any condition of the pelvic organs (i.e., gastrointestinal, reproductive, or urinary system) that causes chronic pain. Patients can experience spasm of the levator ani and the related pelvic muscles. Spasm can develop in the sacroiliac region, external muscles of the pelvic girdle (piriformis muscle), and internal muscles of the pelvis (obturator internus muscle). Patients with levator ani myalgia will have a "tight" pelvic floor. They cannot contract their pelvic muscles any further (i.e., perform a Kegel squeeze), nor can they relax their pelvic muscles. Consequently, these patients will often have problems of dysfunctional voiding and urinary urgency and frequency. Treatment will often include medications to relieve skeletal muscle spasm and physical therapy. A series of exercises, myofascial release, and biofeedback/electric stimulation can be used to rehabilitate the pelvic floor muscles.

The clinician must also consider the possibility of benign and malignant colorectal tumors, colitis, irritable bowel syndrome, and diverticular disease when evaluating pelvic pain. Irritable bowel syndrome is a poorly understood condition of the gastrointestinal tract characterized by abdominal pain, bloating, and alternating constipation and diarrhea. It is a functional disorder that is more common in women than in men. The etiology is unknown. Irritable bowel syndrome affects 15% of Western and Chinese populations. Affected women often complain of a flare-up of symptoms premenstrually, which may be related to the abrupt decrease of progesterone. Women with irritable bowel syndrome also complain of painful intercourse, a sense of bloating, abdominal cramping, rectal urgency, and a sense of incomplete evacuation. Symptoms often begin in the late teen years. The common term *spastic colitis* is not accurate because irritable bowel syndrome is not characterized by inflammation. Patients with irritable bowel syndrome can be categorized into three groups based on their symptoms: (1) abdominal pain, gas, and bloating, (2) diarrhea dominant and (3) constipation dominant. Treatment is directed toward relieving the dominant symptoms. Often, a referral to a gastroenterologist or colorectal surgeon may be needed for evaluation and treatment.

As already discussed in detail, painful bladder syndrome and interstitial cystitis can be a source of chronic pelvic pain. In 2001, Parsons and colleagues studied 134 women with complaints of chronic pelvic pain in an office gynecology practice. A potassium sensitivity test was performed in these women. The researchers found that 114 of 134 women (85%) had a positive test result, indicating that interstitial cystitis should be considered as a diagnosis in this group of women. Similarly, Clemons et al. reported on 45 women undergoing diagnostic laparoscopy for chronic pelvic pain. Cystoscopy with hydrodistension was performed, and 17 of 45 women (38%) were diagnosed to have interstitial cystitis.

Many symptoms of interstitial cystitis (e.g., urinary frequency, dysuria, pelvic pain, dyspareunia, and the menstrual flare-up of symptoms) overlap with the symptomatology of the other conditions that cause pelvic pain. To complicate the picture even further, some gynecologic conditions, though not causes of chronic pelvic pain, can mimic flare-ups of interstitial cystitis (i.e., symptoms of increased urgency, frequency and dysuria). Chronic or recurrent vulvovaginitis, either due to herpes, trichomonas, bacterial vaginosis, or candidiasis, will mimic a flare-up of interstitial cystitis. Recurrent candidiasis will often present premenstrually and is associated with urinary urgency, frequency, and vulvar burning. Pruritus is often, but not always, a complaint. Herpes neuralgia in the pelvis can cause chronic bladder symptoms and urinary frequency. It is common to have recurrences just before menses, which can be associated with a flare-up of urinary symptoms. Urogenital atrophy can cause problems of urinary urgency, frequency, and dysuria. An increase in complaints of dyspareunia can result from the vulvar dermatoses such as lichen sclerosus, lichen planus, or vestibulitis.

Chronic pelvic pain can also be of psychological origin. Several studies have looked at the psychological profiles of patients with complaints of chronic pelvic pain and have demonstrated an increased incidence of psychiatric disorders and history of abuse or sexual assault. Conversely, chronic pelvic pain can lead to depression, anxiety, and domestic and marital discordance. Whether or not the patient has a psychological disorder, the clinician is obligated to rule out physical causes of chronic pelvic pain.

Diagnosis

Careful history taking and physical examination are critical to make an accurate diagnosis. A careful history will include a detailed review of the pertinent pelvic organ systems (i.e., reproductive, urinary, and gastrointestinal systems), as well as the musculoskeletal, neurologic, and psychosocial systems. Usually, these patients have visited several other health care providers and have already undergone diagnostic procedures and therapies. It is essential to obtain prior office records and operative reports to thoughtfully diagnose a patient. If possible, the clinician may have the patient stop all regimens to give the patient a "drug holiday." This will allow symptoms and physical examination findings to "return to baseline" so that the clinician can reevaluate the patient. Diagnostic tests can then be instituted in a sequential fashion.

Physical examination of the abdomen, pelvis, bladder, and rectum is characteristically done to rule out disease processes, but evaluation of the lower back, abdominal wall, and levator ani muscles is often overlooked. The clinician must be mindful of the musculoskeletal causes or sequelae of chronic pelvic pain. The muscles of the back can be assessed externally, and the pelvic muscles can be assessed by vaginal palpation. These muscles should be assessed bilaterally because unilateral abnormalities can be detected. The bulk of the muscle, defects or spasm in the muscle, and trigger points can be determined.

To evaluate a patient's associated symptoms of dysuria and dyspareunia, the clinician will need to evaluate for vaginal infections and urogenital atrophy. Atrophy of the urethra will manifest as distal urethral meatal stenosis or a "urethral caruncle." A Papanicolaou smear of the vagina can be performed to estimate the estrogen maturation index. Colposcopy with vaginal or vulvar biopsies, or both, may be needed to diagnose vulvar dermatoses. Evaluation of the vestibule using a moistened cotton swab will be needed to look for irritated vestibular glands. Frequent office visits to obtain urine samples, perform vaginal examinations, and obtain wet preparations and cultures may initially be needed to establish a patient's diagnosis.

All available diagnostic and imaging techniques such as ultrasonography, computed tomography, magnetic resonance imaging, pelviscopy, cystoscopy, colonoscopy, psychological assessment, and possible referral to other health care providers might be required to accurately diagnose a patient.

Treatment

Treatment will be directed at the cause or causes of the chronic pelvic pain. It would not be unusual for a patient to have more than one disease process or organ system involved due to the juxtaposition of the various structures and nervous system interactions that exist within the pelvis. Thus, treatment will often be multimodal. Collaboration with providers in other specialties such as urology, gastroenterology, psychiatry, and physicians who specialize in pain management, neurology, neurosurgery, orthopedic surgery, general surgery, colorectal surgery, and physical and massage therapy may be needed to comprehensively treat a patient. Pain clinics are valuable resources because they involve the expertise of pain management specialists, social workers, and psychologists/psychiatrists who specialize in chronic pain management. A multidisciplinary pelvic floor center where the clinicians have specialized training in women's pelvic floor disorders would be the ideal setting to provide a diagnosis and treatment for this challenging group of patients.

KEY POINTS

1. Interstitial cystitis is a chronic condition of urinary urgency, frequency, and suprapubic pain in the absence of bacteruria.
2. A "leaky uroepithelium" with a cascade of neurologic inflammation is involved in the pathophysiology of interstitial cystitis.
3. Interstitial cystitis is associated with irritable bowel syndrome, allergies, migraine headaches, fibromyalgia, temporal-mandibular joint disorders, and collagen vascular diseases.
4. Symptoms of interstitial cystitis can mimic some gynecologic disorders.
5. Interstitial cystitis should be included in the differential diagnosis of women with chronic pelvic pain.
6. The O'Leary-Sant and pelvic pain and urgency/frequency questionnaires have been developed to improve screening of patients with symptoms of urinary frequency, urgency, and pain.
7. Both cystoscopic hydrodistension performed with the patient under anesthesia and the potassium sensitivity test are used to diagnose interstitial cystitis.
8. Treatment of interstitial cystitis includes behavioral and dietary modifications, physical therapy, oral medications (e.g., pentosan polysulfate, amitriptyline, hydroxyzine), bladder instillations (e.g., dimethyl sulfoxide, heparin, and anesthetic solutions) pain control, and hydrodistension.
9. *Chronic pelvic pain* is a common disorder defined as pain in the pelvis of more than 6 months' duration.
10. Pain in the pelvis can be due to a variety of gynecologic, urologic, gastrointestinal, musculoskeletal, and psychological disorders.
11. Careful history taking and careful physical examination are critical to making an accurate diagnosis in patients with chronic pelvic pain.
12. Treatment of chronic pelvic pain will often be multimodal and interdisciplinary.

SUGGESTED READING

Baggish MS, Miklos JR: Vulvar pain syndrome: A review. Obstet Gynecol Surv 50:618–627, 1995.

Clemons JL, Arya LA, Myers DL: Diagnosing interstitial cystitis in women with chronic pelvic pain. Obstet Gynecol 100:337–341, 2002.

Costello K: Myofascial syndrome. In Steege JF, Metzger DA, and Levy BS (eds): Chronic Pelvic Pain: An Integrated Approach. Philadelphia, Saunders, 1998, pp 251–266.

Curhan GC, Speizer FE, Hunter DJ, et al: Epidemiology of interstitial cystitis: A population based study. J Urol 161:549–552, 1999.

Gillenwater JY, Wein AJ: Summary of the National Institute of Arthritis, Diabetes, Digestive and Kidney Diseases Workshop on Interstitial Cystitis, National Institutes of Health, Bethesda, MD, August 28–29, 1987. J Urol 140:203–206, 1988.

Hanno PM, Landis JR, Matthews-Cook Y, et al: The diagnosis of interstitial cystitis revisited: Lessons learned from the National Institutes of Health Interstitial Cystitis Database study. J Urol 161:553–557, 1999.

Keay SK, Zhang CO, Shoenfelt J, et al: Sensitivity and specificity of antiproliferative factor, heparin-binding epidermal growth factor–like growth factor, and epidermal growth factor as urine markers for interstitial cystitis. Urology 57(6 Suppl 1):9–14, 2001.

Moldwin R: The Interstitial Cystitis Survival Guide. Oakland, CA, New Harbinger Publications, Inc., 2002.

Mullholland SG, Hanno P, Parsons CL, et al: Pentosan polysulfate sodium for therapy of interstitial cystitis: A double-blind placebo-controlled clinical study. Urology 35:552–558, 1990.

O'Leary MP, Sant GR, Fowler FJ, et al: The interstitial cystitis symptom and problem index. Urology 49(5A Suppl):58–63, 1997.

Parsons CL: Interstitial cystitis: Clinical manifestations and diagnostic criteria in over 200 cases. Neurourol Urodyn 9:241–250, 1990.

Parsons CL, Bullen M, Kahn BS, et al: Gynecologic presentation of interstitial cystitis as detected by intravesical potassium sensitivity. Obstet Gynecol 98:127–132, 2001.

Parsons CL, Dell J, Stanford EJ, et al: Increased prevalence of interstitial cystitis: Previously unrecognized urologic and gynecologic cases identified using a new symptom questionnaire and intravesical potassium sensitivity. Urology 60:573–578, 2002.

Parsons L: Interstitial cystitis: Epidemiology and clinical presentation. Clin Obstet Gynecol 45:242–249, 2002.

Porpora MG, Gomel V: The role of laparoscopy in the management of pelvic pain in women of reproductive age. Fertil Steril 68:765–779, 1997.

Ringel Y, Sperber A, Drossman D: Irritable bowel syndrome. Ann Rev Med 52:319–338, 2001.

Sant GR: Intravesical 50% dimethylsulfoxide (DMSO-50) in treatment of interstitial cystitis. Urology 29:17–21, 1987.

Sant GR, Theoharides TC: The role of the mast cell in interstitial cystitis. Urol Clin North Am 21:41–53, 1994.

Theoharides TC, Sant GR: Hydroxyzine therapy for interstitial cystitis. Urology 49(5A Suppl):108–110, 1997.

Weiss JM: Pelvic floor myofascial trigger points: Manual therapy for interstitial cystitis and the urgency-frequency syndrome. J Urol 166:2226–2231, 2001.

685

EVALUATION AND MANAGEMENT OF THE GYNECOLOGIC SURGICAL PATIENT

Jeffrey L. Clemons

PREOPERATIVE EVALUATION AND PREPARATION FOR SURGERY

Preoperative evaluation of a female patient before gynecologic surgery is crucial in order to minimize intraoperative and postoperative complications. Important issues include the evaluation of her medical history and physical examination, a preoperative medical or anesthesia consultation to optimize her medical status, the identification of social or physical limitations that could impact her recovery, informed consent, the management of her expectations of what the surgical procedure will and will not accomplish, and an explanation of the limitations she can expect during her recovery.

Most postoperative problems can be anticipated preoperatively, and some can be eliminated or minimized. After thoughtful review of her condition, it may be found that medical or conservative surgical treatment is better than an aggressive surgical treatment. Careful preoperative assessment is perhaps the gynecologic surgeon's best method of risk management.

Preoperative Evaluation and Testing

Given that many intraoperative and postoperative complications can be anticipated, gynecologic surgeons need to be able to identify risk factors before scheduling surgery. A detailed history and physical examination will allow the physician to identify these risk factors and coordinate appropriate preoperative medical consultation. Important factors to assess include age, exercise tolerance, surgical risk, medical comorbidities, current medications (including herbal supplements and over-the-counter medicines), drug allergies, substance abuse, prior surgery, prior blood transfusion, and prior anesthetic complications. For complicated cases, proper communication between the surgeon, patient, medical consultant, primary care physician, and anesthesiologist is essential. Preoperative testing should be individualized, and routine panels of tests are no longer recommended.

Preoperative Consultation

Medical consultation should be obtained for women with medical disorders, especially if the medical conditions are not well controlled. Just because the patient has been "medically cleared" does not mean that she is free of risk from surgery. Commonly, a list of recommendations will be given, such as use of pneumatic compression boots or heparin for deep venous thrombosis (DVT) prophylaxis, β-blockers for myocardial infarction prophylaxis, or discontinuation of aspirin or nonsteroidal anti-inflammatory drugs 1 week before surgery. It is important to ensure that the consultant has addressed any specific medical issues, such as control of hypertension or diabetes. Additionally, an anesthesia consultation should be obtained in women with severe medical disorders or with a history of difficulty with previous anesthesia.

Age

Geriatric women often have many medical problems and are under the care of different physicians who prescribe multiple medications. Medical consultation is often necessary, and the patient's medical physicians should be aware of the upcoming surgery. In addition to obtaining a preoperative baseline electrocardiogram (ECG), the patient should be asked about her exercise tolerance because this is a good predictor of cardiac disease. Women who can climb one to two flights of stairs or walk two to four blocks usually have good cardiovascular health. Women with poor exercise tolerance due to fatigue, shortness of breath, or chest pain may have limited cardiac reserve and need further evaluation with a cardiac stress test. Some patients are difficult to assess due to limited mobility from degenerative joint disease, and these persons may benefit from medical consultation. The physician should inquire about the patient's living arrangements: does she live alone or with a partner? In her own home, with her family, or in assisted living? Do stairs exist in her home (she may need to move her bed to a lower floor temporarily if she has limited mobility)? Discharge planning is an important consideration preoperatively because arrangements may need to be made with her family, in-home nursing care, or a rehabilitation center for her postoperative care, especially if her partner is deceased, debilitated, or unable to assist her.

Although elderly women are at an increased risk of life-threatening events and may experience longer hospitalizations (typically due to delayed return of bowel function or difficulty with ambulation), they often seem to have less postoperative pain than younger women and usually recover well after surgery. Many elderly women are in excellent health; the decision to undergo surgery should be based on her overall health, not just her age.

Exercise Tolerance

A simple screening test for perioperative complications is self-reported exercise tolerance. Patients with low exercise tolerance, defined as the inability to walk four blocks or climb two flights of stairs without the symptom of shortness of breath, have twice the rate of serious perioperative complications compared with patients with good exercise tolerance (20%

versus 10%). Another simple screening assesses the number of metabolic equivalents (METs) that a patient can tolerate. The functional capacity measured by the Duke activity status index questionnaire correlates well with functional capacity measured in METs, as estimated during symptom-limited exercise treadmill testing. The ability to climb one flight of stairs or walk two blocks is equal to about 4 METs. Women who perform less than 4 METs have a poor functional capacity.

Surgical Risk

Intraoperative and postoperative complications are more often associated with high surgical risk procedures (e.g., emergency surgery, vascular surgery, and prolonged surgeries with large blood loss and/or fluid shifts). As noted below, many patients who undergo these high-risk procedures need an extensive preoperative evaluation. Most gynecologic procedures are of low (cone biopsy) to moderate (hysterectomy) surgical risk. High-surgical-risk gynecologic surgeries include radical hysterectomy or vulvectomy, laparotomy for ovarian cancer with severe ascites, abdominal hysterectomy of a large fibroid uterus suspicious for major bleeding, and pelvic exenteration. It may be prudent to reserve an intensive care unit bed to postoperatively monitor women who undergo high-risk procedures due to the possibility of fluid shifts resulting from large-volume blood loss, transfusion of multiple blood products, or removal of malignant ascites, especially when the patient has significant medical problems.

689

Medical Comorbidities

Cardiac and Cardiovascular Disease

Perioperative myocardial ischemia is the most important potentially reversible risk factor for mortality and cardiovascular complications after gynecologic surgery. However, according to the American College of Cardiology/ American Heart Association Guidelines, coronary revascularization before surgery is usually recommended only for a small subset of patients at very high risk. Therefore, coronary angiography is only recommended for the following patients: (1) patients with prior revascularization, now with recurrent symptoms, and (2) patients with a major clinical predictor of cardiac complications (e.g., recent myocardial infarction, unstable angina, decompensated heart failure, severe valvular disease, and significant severe arrhythmias). Noninvasive cardiac testing and possible coronary angiography is only recommended for patients with two of the three following risk factors: (1) an intermediate clinical predictor of cardiac complications (e.g., prior myocardial infarction, mild angina, compensated or prior heart failure, diabetes mellitus, or renal insufficiency); (2) poor functional capacity (less than 4 METs); or (3) high-surgical-risk procedure. Therefore, most women who undergo gynecologic surgeries are cleared to proceed to the operating room with various precautions and recommendations given.

β-Blockers are commonly recommended to protect the heart during surgery. They prevent tachycardia during and after surgery, which limits myocardial oxygen demand, thereby lowering the rate of perioperative myocardial infarction. β-Blockers also reduce mortality in patients who have or are at risk for coronary artery disease (e.g., persons with prior myocardial infarction, angina, or with two or more cardiac risk factors). A randomized, placebo-controlled study demonstrated that atenolol (given intravenously before and after surgery, then orally for the remainder of hospitalization) significantly lowered mortality compared with placebo over the next 6 months (0% versus 8%). The effect lasted for 2 years (10% versus 21% mortality), primarily due to a reduction in deaths from cardiac causes during the first 6 months.

Hypertension

Hypertension is a common condition that needs to be controlled preoperatively, reducing the patient's blood pressure to less than 170/110 mm Hg. β-Blockers are an excellent treatment option for the reasons noted above. A preoperative ECG and creatinine level should be obtained to assess cardiac and renal function. Elective surgery should be postponed if hypertension is not well-controlled. In emergent situations, intravenous medications can be used to control blood pressure.

Antihypertensive medications should be taken the morning of surgery and resumed postoperatively. If oral intake is limited postoperatively, it is important to remember that β-blockers and clonidine should not be stopped acutely. Intravenous labetalol or metoprolol should be given to patients taking β-blockers, and transdermal clonidine should be given to patients taking clonidine.

Prevention of Bacterial Endocarditis

If a hysterectomy or vaginal surgery is performed, women with a history of structural cardiac abnormalities will need antibiotic prophylaxis to prevent subacute bacterial endocarditis. If a murmur is discovered on physical examination, then an echocardiogram is needed to determine whether there is significant valvular heart disease that requires prophylactic antibiotics. A typical regimen includes ampicillin 2 g administered intravenously and gentamycin 1.5 mg/kg given intravenously (maximum dose of 120 mg), 30 minutes before surgery, with a repeat dose of ampicillin given 6 hours later. In penicillin-allergic women, a single dose of vancomycin 1 g (with gentamycin) given intravenously over 1 to 2 hours, 30 minutes before surgery, should be given. These regimens will also be sufficient for prevention of surgical site infection.

Asthma

Women with uncontrolled asthma or with chronic obstructive pulmonary disease will need consultation to determine what additional treatment is needed to improve their ability to ventilate. Women with an upper respiratory infection need to recover from their illness, and women who use tobacco should be encouraged to stop smoking at least 8 weeks before surgery (the nicotine patch is a helpful aid in smoking cessation). Obese women also have a restrictive breathing problem, which can compound obstructive pulmonary disease postoperatively. Surgery should be delayed until optimal management of the airway has been achieved. Regional anesthesia should be considered in these women. Preoperative pulmonary function testing may be needed in some women. All asthma medications including inhalers should be taken the morning of surgery and resumed postoperatively. Perioperative intravenous corticosteroids are recommended when the peak flow rate or forced expiratory volume in 1 second is less than 75% to 80%

of predicted, or for asthmatic women with wheezing, productive cough, chest tightness, or shortness of breath despite outpatient therapy. A standard dose is methylprednisolone (Solu-Medrol) 80 mg (range, 40 to 120 mg) every 8 hours. Postoperative incentive spirometry and nebulizers are especially important in the treatment of these women.

Diabetes   Women with diabetes mellitus are at risk of poor wound healing and post-operative infection. Good glucose control preoperatively is important to minimize these problems, but tight perioperative control is not necessary and may predispose patients to hypoglycemic episodes. Glucose will tend to be low preoperatively due to fasting, may rise during surgery due to the release of cortisol, and may decrease postoperatively due to poor appetite. Women with insulin-dependent diabetes will need to be managed with insulin and glucose to ensure uptake of glucose intracellularly. On the day of surgery, one third of the morning dose of long-acting insulin should be taken, but short-acting insulin and oral hypoglycemics should not be taken. Take advantage of an insulin pump if the patient has one, but only infuse the basal rate. Insulin drip protocols can also be used. Monitor glucose levels every 1 to 2 hours during and after surgery, until the patient has resumed eating. Metformin should be stopped the day before surgery to prevent lactic acidosis from anesthesia, although studies have shown that the risk of lactic acidosis is negligible. Diabetic women should be scheduled for surgery in the morning if possible.

Adrenal Suppression   Perioperative intravenous corticosteroids are recommended when there is potential adrenal suppression from chronic oral steroids, including women who have used 20 mg of prednisone per day for 3 weeks in the year before surgery. A standard dose is Solu-Medrol 80 mg (range, 40 to 120 mg) every 8 hours.

Total Joint Replacements   Bacteremia can cause hematogenous seeding of total joint implants for many years after implantation, especially in the first 2 years, and can cause late prosthetic implant infection. The American Urological Association and the American Academy of Orthopedic Surgeons do not recommend prophylaxis for healthy patients with total joint replacements, but they do recommend prophylaxis for patients with the following risk factors undergoing high-risk surgery (i.e., procedures associated with bacteremia): undergoing surgery within 2 years of the surgical implant; immunocompromised condition; prior prosthetic joint infection; diabetes, malignancy, human immunodeficiency virus infection; malnourished state. Although not specifically required for gynecologic surgery, prophylaxis should be considered in women with the above risk factors who undergo hysterectomy, vaginal surgery, or bowel surgery. The recommended regimen is a single preoperative intravenous dose of a quinolone (e.g., ciprofloxacin 500 mg) or ampicillin 2 g (or vancomycin 1 g, if allergic) and gentamycin 1.5 mg/kg.

Medications
Some medications need to be stopped before surgery, whereas some medications need to be taken the day of surgery (Box 28-1). It is reasonable to

---

Box 28-1 Medications That Must Be Stopped Before Surgery

Oral hypoglycemics and regular insulin: Stop the day of surgery
Metformin: Stop the day before surgery
Nonsteroidal anti-inflammatory drugs: Stop 2 days before surgery
Warfarin: Stop 4 days before surgery
Aspirin: Stop 7 days before surgery
Clopidogrel and ticlopidine: Stop 7 and 14 days before surgery, respectively
Monoamine oxidase inhibitors: Stop 3 weeks before surgery; obtain anesthesia
  consultation

---

recommend discontinuation of herbal supplements 1 to 2 weeks before surgery, due to unknown risks associated with their use. Gingko biloba may increase the risk of bleeding.

The following types of medication should be taken the day of surgery with a small amount (30 to 60 mL) of water: anti-hypertensives, including hydrochlorothiazide, cardiac medications, gastroesophageal reflux medications, psychiatric drugs (including antidepressants and anxiolytics), asthma medications and inhalers, and antiseizure medications. Only one third of the usual morning dose of long-acting insulin should be taken; women with an insulin pump should only continue the basal rate.

Allergies
Common drug allergies include antibiotics (especially penicillin and sulfa drugs) and intolerance to narcotics. Identification of these allergies is important because it will affect the choice of antibiotic prophylaxis or postoperative pain control. Cephalosporins should be avoided if the allergic reaction to penicillin was anaphylaxis or if the patient gives a history of "throat swelling." It is also important to note any allergies to latex, tapes, soaps, dyes, or foods (important for postoperative diet).

Substance Abuse
Persons who abuse alcohol are at risk of liver disease, and intravenous drug abusers are at risk of viral hepatitis and human immunodeficiency virus. Tobacco abusers are at risk of underlying pulmonary and cardiovascular disease, postoperative atelectasis and pneumonia, and potentially, impaired abdominal wall or vaginal wall wound healing due to chronic cough. Preoperative or postoperative identification of patient alcohol or drug abuse may require coordination with psychiatrists, behavioral medicine specialists, nutritionists, social workers, and discharge planners to address withdrawal symptoms and to get patients into appropriate treatment programs. The perioperative period may be a prime opportunity to address smoking, alcohol, or substance abuse problems.

Prior Surgery
A history of prior pelvic surgery may warrant review of prior operative notes, especially if the surgery was complicated. The risk of pelvic adhesions involving the small and large bowel, bladder, and pelvic sidewall

(i.e., ureter, pelvic vasculature) is increased in women with prior surgery, as it is for a history of endometriosis, diverticulitis, and pelvic inflammatory disease. It is helpful to anticipate adhesions of the bowel to the abdominal wall when entering the abdominal cavity and to use careful, sharp dissection. A mechanical bowel preparation should be considered in this situation, to minimize the risk of infection related to possible intestinal injury and repair (from enterotomy repair to resection of part of the bowel).

Laboratory Tests and Imaging Studies

Although routine panels of tests are no longer recommended, the following preoperative tests are generally recommended. Imaging studies should be used judiciously. Depending on the institution, normal blood tests are acceptable for 1 to 3 months, and normal ECG results for 1 to 6 months. These tests include the following:

- Pregnancy test (β–human chorionic gonadotropin): all premenopausal women (unless sterilized)
- Hematocrit: All cases with the potential for major blood loss
- Serum creatinine: All women older than 50 years of age, with renal or liver disease, or with cardiac risk factors (e.g., hypertension, diabetes, morbid obesity, vascular disease, and tobacco use of more than 40 pack-years)
- Prothrombin and partial thromboplastin times (PT, PTT): Only women with liver disease or using anticoagulants
- Liver function testing and/or hepatitis serology: Only women with liver disease, intravenous drug use, tattoos, sexually transmitted diseases, alcohol abuse, or medications associated with liver dysfunction
- Blood type and antibody screen: All women with prior transfusion or known antibody; otherwise, only if there is a high risk of hemorrhage, such as hysterectomy or malignancy. A crossmatch for blood (type and cross) should only be ordered in women who are likely to have major intraoperative bleeding requiring transfusion, in which case they should be offered autologous blood donation
- ECG: All women older than 50 years of age, or with cardiac risk factors (listed above), or with known cardiac or renal disease
- Chest x-ray: Only women with known cardiac or pulmonary disease, or in cases when metastatic disease must be ruled out; some recommend if patient is older than 65 years
- Pelvic ultrasound: Should be considered in women with a pelvic mass, especially to assess whether an ovarian mass is simple or complex
- Computed tomography (CT): Helpful in the evaluation of a pelvic mass and provides additional information regarding enlarged lymph nodes and the urinary tract
- Magnetic resonance imaging: Helpful in the evaluation of uterine disorders such as adenomyosis or leiomyomatosis
- Intravenous pyelogram: Should be considered in women with suspected ureteral injury from prior surgical procedures, severe endometriosis, malignancy, or pelvic inflammatory disease

Informed Consent

Informed consent is perhaps the most important patient encounter related to surgery. Although signing of the consent form and the discussion of her surgery will primarily occur at the preoperative visit, some of the issues discussed below need to be addressed as early as the initial consultation. Informed consent is better thought of as an educational process rather than a single preoperative visit. Managing the expectations of patients is paramount to the success of achieving patient satisfaction.

Essentially, a contract is negotiated between the woman and her physician regarding several issues related to the surgery, including the following: (1) the indication(s) for the surgery, expected benefits and outcomes of the procedure, and alternatives to the surgery (medical and surgical); (2) possible complications that may occur, including anticipated blood loss, likelihood of transfusion, and risks of transfusion; risks of infection; operative injuries that may occur; and potential life-threatening events (Reassure the patient by explaining the preventive steps that will be taken, such as prophylactic antibiotics to lower the risk of infection, pneumatic compression devices to prevent pulmonary embolism [PE], incentive spirometry to prevent pneumonia, or bowel preparation to prevent infection from intestinal surgery.); (3) the amount of expected postoperative pain, adverse effects from the procedure, and limitations during her recovery, including sexual function; 4) possible need for additional surgery due to unexpected findings. The patient should be encouraged to bring in a list of questions to ask about her surgery and recovery.

Although patients usually remember the discussion of the planned surgery, they often cannot recall talking about potential complications and alternatives to surgery. Having a family member present during this discussion can be very beneficial in helping the patient adhere to limitations during her recovery, and in the event that a medicolegal complication occurs. In addition to having the woman sign the consent form, the physician should enter a note into her records that "the risks, benefits, indications, and alternatives were discussed, and all questions were answered." Document the presence of any additional family members during the informed consent process.

Surgical Site Infection Prophylaxis

Antibiotic prophylaxis prevents surgical site infection by reducing the number of bacteria present in the injured tissue, not by destroying all bacteria. Essentially, it augments the immune system's response to infection and promotes wound healing to the extent that infection and inflammation are reduced. However, to be effective, the antibiotic should be present at the time of tissue injury. Ideally, the antibiotic used for prophylaxis should be effective against bacteria found in the vagina (or at the area of intended surgery) but not routinely used for treatment of postoperative infectious complications.

There is clear evidence that prophylactic antibiotics reduce infection in women undergoing vaginal hysterectomy because febrile morbidity is reduced from about 40% to 15% and pelvic infection from 25% to 5%. For abdominal hysterectomy, although the reduction in complications is smaller, there is less postoperative infectious morbidity and decreased length of hospitalization. For other gynecologic surgeries, there is no good evidence that antibiotic prophylaxis is beneficial. However, prophylactic antibiotics are commonly used for most gynecologic surgeries that involve the vagina, due to the volume and wide spectrum of organisms (both aerobic and anaerobic) found in the vagina.

Cephalosporins (e.g., cefazolin, cefoxitin, or cefotetan, 1 or 2 g) are the drug of choice for prophylaxis because of their low cost, relatively long half-life, broad antibacterial spectrum, and low incidence of allergic reaction. Ideally, prophylactic antibiotics should be given 30 to 60 minutes before surgery, but no more than 2 hours before or 1 hour after surgery, as the efficacy is markedly diminished. A second dose of the antibiotic should be given during prolonged surgeries (more than 3 to 4 hours) or when there is major blood loss (>1000 to 1500 mL). Additional postoperative doses are not beneficial. It is unknown whether additional doses of antibiotics are needed when using biologic or synthetic implants for pelvic reconstructive surgery, although they are commonly given.

Women with anaphylaxis or throat swelling from penicillin should not be given cephalosporins. In these women, or in cephalosporin-allergic patients, an alternative antibiotic should be used. Alternative antibiotics include doxycycline, metronidazole, clindamycin, and quinolones.

Additionally, perioperative shaving is no longer recommended because studies have demonstrated that shaving leads to a two- to three-fold increased risk of surgical site infection. Shaving causes small cuts in the skin that harbor bacteria and lead to infection. If the hair needs to be removed, it should be clipped in the operating room just before the antiseptic preparation is placed on the skin.

Bowel Preparation

Although evidence supporting mechanical bowel preparation is limited, mechanical bowel preparation is the standard of care before elective intestinal surgery because it limits fecal spillage into the peritoneal cavity, reduces the risk of infection, and limits the need for colostomy. However, it is important to note that if unprepared bowel is injured during surgery, simple repair and copious irrigation are generally sufficient.

For minor gynecologic surgery, no bowel preparation is needed. For routine cases of hysterectomy (abdominal or vaginal) and vaginal prolapse repairs, one to two enemas the night before surgery will reduce the bulk of stool in the rectum and sigmoid, allowing for improved exposure—and for vaginal surgery, contamination of the surgical field will be avoided (compared with the inevitable liquid stool contamination after mechanical bowel preparation). An enema may also allow women who experience constipation to have easier bowel movements after surgery and avoid straining, which can exert extra force and impair wound healing of the vagina or abdominal wall.

For complicated gynecologic surgeries in which there is a high risk of unintentional injury to the bowel, the gastrointestinal tract should be prepared before surgery (Box 28-2).

The two most popular methods of mechanical bowel preparation are polyethylene glycol (GoLYTELY) and sodium phosphate (Fleet Phospho-soda). With GoLYTELY, 4 L of polyethylene glycol must be consumed over 4 hours, and this can be difficult for some patients. Sodium phosphate is easier to ingest and is taken as two 45-mL doses several hours apart. However, polyethylene glycol is associated with less frequent electrolyte abnormalities than sodium phosphate. For either bowel preparation, hypovolemia, hypokalemia, and hyponatremia may occur, particularly in elderly persons, so it is important to anticipate dehydration, assess electrolytes, and replace depleted electrolytes intravenously as needed before the induction of anesthesia.

In addition to mechanical bowel preparation, oral and intravenous antibiotics are given to decrease bacteria within the bowel lumen, reduce contamination, and decrease the risk of wound infection or abscess. The postoperative infection rate can be decreased from 30% to 75% down to 10% with mechanical and antibiotic bowel preparation.

Typically, a clear liquid diet is started the day before surgery, and polyethylene glycol is started around 11 a.m. and consumed over 4 hours. Oral antibiotics with minimal absorption, such as neomycin and erythromycin (1 g each), are taken at 12 p.m., 2 p.m., and 11 p.m. (Metronidazole 500 mg can be substituted for erythromycin.) Intravenous fluids are begun at least 2 to 3 hours before surgery, and electrolyte levels are corrected as needed. An intravenous second-generation cephalosporin with good anaerobic and gram-negative coverage, such as cefoxitin or cefotetan, 1 to 2 g, is given 30 to 60 minutes before surgery.

Patient Positioning for Surgery

Careful positioning of the patient helps to prevent serious injury to the nerves, muscles, ligaments, and soft tissues. Neuropathy and pressure necrosis can occur with improper positioning. Given the medicolegal risk of these injuries, the gynecologic surgeon needs to ensure that the patient

---

Box 28-2 Surgical Risk Factors That Warrant Preoperative Bowel Preparation

Pelvic mass
Malignancy
Endometriosis
Severe pelvic inflammatory disease
Pelvic adhesions
Prior bowel surgery
Prior bowel obstruction
History of diverticulitis
Prior ruptured appendix
Prior pelvic radiation
Multiple prior pelvic or lower abdominal surgeries
"Frozen pelvis" on pelvic examination

is correctly positioned. The surgeon should note any preexisting neurologic abnormality (sensory and motor) or limitation to motion (arthritic or artificial joints) at the preoperative visit.

For abdominal procedures, the supine position (and occasionally the low lithotomy position) is an obvious choice. There should be appropriate padding and protection of the arms, without hyperextension, and the vagina should be prepared and a bladder catheter placed, when appropriate.

For vaginal, laparoscopic, or combined abdominal-vaginal procedures, the lithotomy position is used, and proper positioning of the hips and knees is essential. If the patient has limited range of motion of the back, hip, or knee (i.e., from arthritis, polio, joint replacement), consider positioning her while she is awake; symmetric positioning may not always be possible. Avoid hyperflexion of the hips because this may cause femoral neuropathy by compressing the femoral nerve against the inguinal ligament. Avoid hyperextension of the knee, and avoid pressure on the lateral aspect of the knee and lower leg because this may cause peroneal neuropathy. Padding is necessary to protect the soft tissues.

Universal Allen stirrups are advantageous because they can be used with the patient in the low or high lithotomy position. Make sure that the stirrup attachment to the table is at the level of the hip. For low lithotomy, the hips are only slightly flexed, and the boot surrounding the foot and lower leg will typically attach at the mid point of the stirrup arm. For high lithotomy, the hips will be hyperflexed if the boot remains at the mid point of the stirrup arm. Therefore, to minimize the risk of femoral nerve injury, slide the boot farther down the stirrup arm, a few centimeters from the end, such that when the stirrup arm is horizontal, the hips and knees are just slightly flexed, but when the stirrups are raised into the high lithotomy position, the hips and knees are normally flexed. This provides excellent exposure and minimizes the risk of hyperflexion during vaginal surgery.

697

POSTOPERATIVE CARE

Fever

Body temperature above 38.0°C (100.4°F) is common in the first few days after major surgery, occurring in 30% of women undergoing gynecologic surgery with a laparotomy. Fever-associated cytokines (interleukin [IL]-1, IL-6, tumor necrosis factor α, and interferon-γ) are released by tissue trauma, and the amount of tissue trauma correlates with the febrile response, as demonstrated by decreased tissue trauma and decreased temperatures associated with laparoscopic versus abdominal surgery. However, fever may also be caused by bacterial exotoxins and endotoxins, which stimulate cytokine release.

Early postoperative fever (within the first 24 to 48 hours) is most often caused by the inflammation and cytokine release associated with surgery and will resolve spontaneously. Allergic reactions to antibiotics, transfused blood products, or anesthetic agents (malignant hyperthermia) should also be considered. Atelectasis has often been claimed to be the cause of early postoperative fever, but studies suggest that this is more coincidence than causation. Urine and blood cultures are not usually necessary for early postoperative fever because they are low yield. However, high fever, prolonged fever, an elevated white blood cell count, an indwelling bladder catheter, malignancy, and bowel resection are risk factors for a postoperative infection. It is reasonable to suppress fever postoperatively for the first 48 hours with acetaminophen to minimize the physiologic stress and metabolic demands of fever because this is unlikely to mask a significant infection.

Febrile morbidity is fever that persists beyond the initial 48 hours after surgery. Common causes include urinary tract infection and surgical site infection. One study found the incidence of acquired bacteriuria to be about 5% per day with catheterization. Another study showed that, after 4 days with an indwelling bladder catheter draining to a closed system, 30% to 40% of patients will have bacteriuria. Surgical site infection includes superficial incisional (i.e., skin infection), deep incisional (i.e., dehiscence, necrotizing fasciitis, fascial abscess, vaginal cuff cellulitis), and organ/space infections (i.e., deep abscess or purulent drainage from the organ/space). Other causes of febrile morbidity include pneumonia, thrombophlebitis, ureteral obstruction, catheter site infection, and drug fever. Fever workup may include a wound or catheter site inspection (and culture), pelvic examination, chest x-ray, complete blood count, and urine and blood cultures. Administration of empiric broad-spectrum antibiotics can be started after 48 hours, and targeted antibiotic therapy can be given if a source is identified. Most patients respond in another 24 to 48 hours.

Persistent fever despite antibiotics may be a sign of a pelvic abscess, which requires drainage, or septic pelvic thrombophlebitis, which requires heparin therapy. Therefore, the workup at this point requires an imaging study such as a CT scan or ultrasound of the pelvis. If no fluid collection is found, the diagnosis is likely to be septic pelvic thrombophlebitis, and a course of intravenous heparin should be started. If a fluid collection is found on imaging, it may be a benign fluid collection, a hematoma, or an abscess. Needle aspiration, wound exploration, or laparotomy may be necessary to drain and treat the abscess. Less common causes of postoperative fever include gout, myocardial infarction, PE, and pancreatitis.

Respiratory Complications

Pulmonary complications occur commonly after surgery and are associated with significantly longer hospital stays. Anesthesia, analgesia, and postoperative pain combine to negatively affect pulmonary function by decreasing ciliary transport, increasing mucous production and bronchial hyper-reactivity, and decreasing respiratory volume.

Atelectasis, reactive airway disease, and pneumonia are the most common postoperative pulmonary complications. Risk factors for atelectasis include tobacco use (six times increased risk), asthma (four times increased risk), obesity, prolonged surgery, upper abdominal incision, and poor health status. Risk factors for aspiration pneumonia include depressed mental status or gag reflex, mechanical ventilation, and nasogastric tubes (which increase gastro-esophageal reflux). Regional anesthesia will reduce the risk of pulmonary complications.

Atelectasis is the most common pulmonary complication and typically resolves with incentive spirometry, adequate pain control, and early ambulation. Nebulizers with β-agonist medications and treatment from a respiratory therapist may be needed for more severe cases. Women with asthma commonly need to use more aggressive treatment postoperatively than they required preoperatively, including nebulizers and inhaled or systemic steroids. Optimal pulmonary toilet may require a respiratory therapist. For hospital-acquired pneumonia, second- or third-generation cephalosporins or quinolones are commonly used.

Thromboembolic Complications

Although not all are clinically symptomatic, approximately 25% of women undergoing surgery for benign conditions and 40% of women undergoing surgery for malignant conditions develop venous thrombophlebitis, as demonstrated on iodine-125 fibrinogen scanning, if no preventive measures are taken. Risks factors for perioperative thromboembolic disease include a prior thromboembolic event, malignancy, immobility, prolonged surgery, advanced age, pelvic infection, obesity, prior pelvic radiation, and thrombophilia.

It is now recognized that almost half of patients with thrombosis have an inherited identifiable thrombotic disorder. The most common of these causes are the factor V Leiden mutation (i.e., resistance to activated protein C) and the prothrombin gene mutation G20210A. Other inherited traits include protein C deficiency, protein S deficiency, antithrombin-III deficiency, and homocystinemia, as well as the acquired antiphospholipid antibody.

Studies have shown that unfractionated heparin can decrease DVT by 70% and PE by 40%. Studies have shown similar efficacy between unfractionated heparin and intermittent pneumatic leg compression. Studies also show similar efficacy for unfractionated heparin compared with low-molecular-weight heparin; however, low-molecular-weight heparin should not be used if the patient will undergo spinal or epidural anesthesia because of the risk of spinal or epidural hematoma. Therefore, the standard of care is to offer prophylaxis for DVT and PE.

There are four risk categories for thromboembolic disease when patients undergo surgery. Low-risk patients are younger than 40 years of age, have none of the above risk factors, and are undergoing minor surgery of less than 30 minutes. Without prophylaxis, the risk of DVT is less than 3% and the risk of PE is less than 0.01%. The recommendation for these women is early ambulation only.

Moderate-risk patients are between ages of 40 and 60 years with no risk factors, or younger than age 40 with one or more risk factors, and will undergo surgery for more than 30 minutes. Without prophylaxis, the risk of DVT is 5% to 20%, and the risk of PE is 0.1% to 0.7%. Effective measures to prevent DVT and PE include graduated compression stockings, low-dose unfractionated heparin twice daily, low-molecular-weight heparin, or intermittent pneumatic leg compression. The recommendation for these women is intermittent pneumatic leg compression.

High-risk patients include those older than the age of 60 years, or those with a malignancy, who are having surgery lasting more than 30 minutes. Without prophylaxis, the risk of DVT is 20% to 40%, and the risk of PE is 1% to 2%. Effective measures to prevent DVT and PE include low-dose unfractionated heparin three times daily, low-molecular-weight heparin, or prolonged (5 or more days) intermittent pneumatic leg compression. The recommendation for these women is prolonged intermittent pneumatic leg compression.

Very-high-risk patients include those with prior DVT or PE or with an inherited thrombophilia. There are not good data for recommendations in these women. Without prophylaxis, the risk of DVT is over 40%, and the risk of PE is 1% to 2%. Effective measures to prevent DVT and PE are combined low-dose unfractionated heparin three times daily and intermittent pneumatic leg compression, intravenous heparin continued through the surgical procedure to maintain the PTT at 1.5 times the control value, or preoperative placement of an inferior vena cava filter. The recommendation for these women is combined low-dose heparin and intermittent pneumatic leg compression.

Patients using oral contraceptives should consider stopping them for 4 to 6 weeks before surgery because the risk of thromboembolism doubles (although the absolute risk remains very low). However, an alternative method of contraception is essential to prevent pregnancy and its associated hypercoagulable state, and if a good alternative does not exist, it is reasonable to continue the oral contraceptive up until surgery. Hormone replacement therapy similarly increases the risk of venous thromboembolism and should also be discontinued. Low-dose vaginal estrogen cream, however, is recommended by some surgeons before pelvic reconstructive surgery, when there is significant vaginal atrophy, to improve healing.

The diagnosis of DVT is difficult to make. Compression ultrasonography combined with color Doppler ultrasonography is the primary diagnostic test used today. It is a noninvasive test, compared with the invasive historical gold standard of venography. Sensitivity and specificity are reported to be as high as 95% and 100%, respectively. Many protocols for the diagnosis of DVT exist, based on various clinical point scores that rank patients as at low, moderate, and high risk for DVT. Ultimately, the initial study is ultrasonography, and the final study is venography. In between are the possibilities of repeat ultrasonography, using D-dimer values (a value of 500 µg/L is 96% sensitive for DVT and 35% specific, useful to rule out a DVT if the D-dimer value is low).

Treatment is with unfractionated heparin to achieve an activated PTT value of 1.5 to 2.5 times the control value. The typical dose is 80 U/kg as an intravenous bolus and then 18 U/kg/hour. Heparin is continued for 5 days or more and therapeutically for at least 2 days. Warfarin is then used to continue treatment for a total of 3 to 6 months. Thrombolytic therapy is rarely needed for DVT. Inferior vena cava filters are rarely needed for DVT, unless there are recurrent PEs from the DVT despite adequate anticoagulation.

PE is characterized by dyspnea and tachypnea. Large PEs can cause syncope or cyanosis; smaller PEs can cause pleuritic chest pain and cough. Other findings include bulging neck veins, inverted T waves in leads V1 through V4 on an ECG, abnormal blood gasses, and abnormal chest radiographs.

The ventilation-perfusion scan is the primary diagnostic test for PE and is noninvasive. Its predictive value relies on the combination of a high-probability scan and a patient with a high pretest probability for PE. The gold standard is pulmonary angiography, but it is invasive. Recently, helical (spiral) CT scanning of the chest has been used to diagnose PE. Although it is very accurate for the central vessels and can evaluate other pulmonary sources of the symptoms, it is less accurate in detecting PE of the peripheral lung vasculature. In summary, there are a variety of protocols that can be used to make the diagnosis of PE. Again, D-dimer can be useful, with values less than 500 µg/L ruling out for PE. Due to the seriousness of the diagnosis, however, it is wise to start anticoagulation in a patient while awaiting the results of the testing.

Treatment of PE is similar to that of DVT, with an initial treatment with unfractionated heparin followed by treatment with warfarin for 6 months. Thrombolytic therapy may be necessary for a massive PE with associated cardiogenic shock or hemodynamic instability. Streptokinase (250,000 IU bolus, then 100,000 IU/hour for 24 hours) or urokinase (4400 IU/kg bolus, then 4400 IU/kg/hour for 12 hours) can be used. Tissue plasminogen activator can also be used, but is very expensive.

Wound Care and Infection

Remove the dressing the day after surgery. If there is serous or serosanguineous discharge, compress the wound edges to force more of the fluid out, so that the wound edges can approximate and heal. Staples should be removed between days 2 and 7 after surgery.

Hematomas and seromas are collections of blood and serum that can cause wound separation and wound infection. They can be minimized by attention to hemostasis before wound closure, avoidance of thermal injury from excessive use of electrocautery, and closure of subcutaneous tissue in obese women. Such fluid collections can be asymptomatic or cause pain, swelling, drainage, or infection. The diagnosis is usually made by inspecting and probing the wound. Ultrasound or CT scan may be needed to diagnose subfascial hematomas. Small hematomas and seromas can be managed expectantly, but larger fluid collections must be drained by opening all or part of the incision. If there is no infection and the wound is small, it can be closed. If the wound is large or is infected, pack the wound with gauze and perform dressing changes twice a day. The wound can then be closed secondarily when granulation tissue is present, usually within 4 to 7 days.

Wound infection occurs in 3% to 5% of clean wounds. Surgical site infection is reduced with the use of antibiotic prophylaxis at the time of surgery. Signs and symptoms of wound infection include fever and erythema, induration, pain, purulent drainage, and separation of the wound. If the wound appears intact, without drainage, but with surrounding erythema and warmth, then cellulitis is the likely diagnosis and treatment with antibiotics directed against gram-positive cocci is indicated. If there is drainage or separation, then the wound must be opened and explored to irrigate and clean the wound. Infected fluid must be drained. If there is devitalized tissue, the wound must be debrided. The wound is then packed with gauze and dressing changes are done twice a day. Antibiotics are not needed unless there are systemic symptoms or there is surrounding cellulitis.

Necrotizing fasciitis is a serious wound infection and is a surgical emergency. It often occurs in immunocompromised or diabetic patients and is characterized by dusky and friable subcutaneous tissue, and serous drainage from a small wound that may be separate from the incisional wound. The fascia is typically pale and devitalized. Treatment is surgical, and extensive debridement of devitalized fascia is necessary, sometimes requiring more than one return to the operating room. Necrotizing fasciitis must be treated promptly and aggressively because it is associated with a high mortality rate.

Urinary Retention

Urinary retention occurs in up to 50% of cases after urethropexy for stress incontinence or radical hysterectomy and occasionally occurs after hysterectomy, pelvic reconstructive surgery, or epidural or spinal anesthesia. The condition is usually transient and will resolve with a transurethral or suprapubic bladder catheter or intermittent self-catheterization for 2 to 7 days. When the patient returns for follow-up after a few days, her ability to void can be tested by instilling 300 mL of normal saline retrograde through the indwelling catheter into the bladder and measuring the amount voided; she should void at least 200 mL.

Prolonged need for a catheter may follow urethropexy procedures, and eventually consideration for urethrolysis will be needed. Prolonged retention may also follow radical hysterectomy, requiring bladder drainage for weeks or months, and bladder function often recovers over time. Prophylactic antibiotics may be given (i.e., nitrofurantoin 100 mg once a day), especially after a cystotomy in which a bladder catheter will be used for 7 to 14 days, but antibiotics will not always prevent urinary tract infections. Alternatively, the physician can simply treat those women that develop urinary tract infections. This may be the better strategy for women requiring long-term catheter use.

Although α-antagonists can cause severe stress incontinence from urethral relaxation and can treat voiding difficulty from prostatic hyperplasia, there is no evidence that they will improve voiding in women with urinary retention. Similarly, cholinergic agents such as bethanechol, thought to improve bladder contractility, are not effective in these women.

Ileus

Ileus, defined as bowel distension, decreased bowel sounds, and delay of defecation after surgery, occurs in approximately 5% of women who undergo abdominal gynecologic surgery. Studies have shown that intestinal motility is decreased after abdominal surgery, with small bowel function delayed for several hours and left colonic function delayed up to 3 days.

Traditionally, postoperative feeding after abdominal surgery was a gradual process that could take several days. Nasogastric tubes were used to prevent ileus and vomiting because it was thought that ileus would increase the risk of wound dehiscence and intestinal leaks, and vomiting would lead to aspiration pneumonia. Therefore, the nasogastric tube was not removed until bowel sounds, flatus, or both were present. If the patient tolerated removal of the nasogastric tube and bowel sounds were still present, then the administration of clear liquids would be started, and the diet would be advanced slowly to solids when flatus was passed.

However, a meta-analysis of 26 randomized trials that compared 3964 patients with and without nasogastric tube decompression after elective abdominal surgery showed no difference in the rate of postoperative vomiting (8% versus 10%) and fewer cases of aspiration pneumonia (6% with and 3% without). There was also no difference in postoperative wound dehiscence or intestinal leaks. These findings have been confirmed in gynecologic surgical studies. Therefore, routine postoperative nasogastric tube use is unnecessary.

Similarly, several randomized studies have shown that early postoperative feeding (clear liquids on the first postoperative day and, if tolerated, advancement to a solid diet) is safe after gynecologic abdominal surgery. Although in the early postoperative feeding group the rate of emesis is increased (40% to 50%), the hospital stay is decreased by a day, and there is no increase in the incidence of aspiration pneumonia, wound dehiscence, or intestinal leaks. General surgery studies have even shown that early postoperative feeding is safe after elective bowel resection. Therefore, early postoperative feeding should be the goal after major abdominal surgery.

When ileus does occur, the patient may complain of nausea or vomiting, and physical examination often shows a nontender, distended abdomen with decreased bowel sounds. Initial management is to eliminate all oral intake, continue intravenous hydration, and check serum electrolyte levels. Ingestion of oral fluids can be resumed once bowel function recovers, as demonstrated by bowel sounds, flatus, or both, and the diet can be advanced to solids as tolerated.

If vomiting persists, a nasogastric tube should be inserted, an antigastritis medication (i.e., ranitidine) should be prescribed, and a baseline abdominal x-ray series (i.e., radiographs of the abdomen, supine and upright, and the chest) should be performed. Maintenance intravenous hydration should be continued, and nasogastric fluid loss should be replaced with intravenous fluids containing potassium. It is prudent to check serum electrolyte levels and perform an abdominal series daily, and electrolytes should be replaced intravenously as needed. When bowel function recovers, as demonstrated by bowel sounds and/or flatus, the nasogastric tube can be clamped for 8 to 12 hours and, if tolerated, the tube can be removed and clear liquid administration begun. The diet can then be advanced to solids as tolerated.

Patients whose conditions do not improve after 48 hours of nasogastric decompression should have a CT scan of the abdomen and pelvis, with oral and intravenous contrast. Ileus can occur in the setting of an abscess or a urinary tract injury such as ureteral obstruction or urinary ascites from a cystotomy. Parenteral nutrition is recommended after 7 days without oral nutrition. Exploratory abdominal surgery is needed if the CT scan shows a bowel perforation, a urinary tract injury, or a bowel obstruction that does not respond to conservative management (nasogastric decompression), or if the woman's condition yields findings suggestive of a bowel perforation such as fever, peritoneal signs, or leukocytosis.

Neurologic Injury

Neuropathies after gynecologic surgery are relatively uncommon, with an incidence of approximately 1.5% to 2%. Neuropathies can be caused by nerve injury due to stretch, compression, transection, or ligation. Improper preoperative positioning in the lithotomy position can cause a stretch or compression injury. Prolonged time (>2 hours) in the lithotomy position is a risk factor for neuropathy. Patients in the lithotomy position can also sustain neuropathy from the surgeon causing excessive pressure by leaning against an extremity. Improper placement or positioning of self-retaining or fixed retractors can also cause a stretch or compression injury, particularly those with deep lateral retractor blades. Surgical dissection or extirpation can lead to transection or suture entrapment of the nerve.

The key to minimizing these injuries is to prevent them by carefully attending to the positioning of the patient and the retractors, and to avoid leaning against a vulnerable extremity. Patient positioning is described above. Lateral retractor blades should not compress the psoas muscle. Use the shortest retractor blade that effectively retracts the abdominal wall to minimize any injury to the femoral or genitofemoral nerves. In thin women, rolled towels or large packs may be placed between the retractor and the skin of the abdominal wall to elevate the blades. Retractor blades should be checked when placed, checked later during long cases, and released and repositioned to relieve pressure as needed.

Studies have found the most common nerves involved in nerve injuries are the femoral, genitofemoral, ilioinguinal/iliohypogastric, lateral femoral cutaneous, obturator, peroneal, and sciatic nerves. Most often there is weakness or sensory loss in the distribution of the affected nerve. With ligation or transection, there may also be pain. The majority of neuropathies (75%) are related to stretch and compression injuries, from lithotomy position or retractor blades. These injuries typically resolve over many weeks to months. Neuropathies that result from transection or suture ligation typically will not resolve without surgical intervention. Many patients will require physical therapy until their conditions improve.

KEY POINTS

1. Medical consultation should be obtained for preoperative patients with preexisting medical conditions to optimize the patient's health before surgery and provide recommendations for postoperative care.

2. The perioperative use of β-blockers has been shown to reduce mortality in patients at risk for coronary artery disease.

3. Women with structural cardiac abnormalities such as valvular heart disease who are undergoing gynecologic surgery require antibiotic prophylaxis to prevent bacterial endocarditis.

4. Perioperative intravenous corticosteroids are recommended for patients with poor results on pulmonary function testing and for persons with asthma who experience wheezing, productive cough, chest tightness, or shortness of breath despite outpatient therapy.

5. In patients with diabetes, good glucose control preoperatively is important to minimize problems of poor wound healing and postoperative infection, but tight perioperative glucose control is not necessary and may predispose patients to hypoglycemic episodes.

6. Women who have used chronic steroids in the year before surgery are candidates for perioperative intravenous corticosteroids for adrenal suppression.

7. Patients with total joint replacements should receive antibiotic prophylaxis to prevent bacterial seeding of joint implants if they have risk factors for infection or if they are undergoing high-risk surgeries associated with bacteremia.

8. Cephalosporins are commonly used in the treatment of surgical prophylaxis because of their low cost, relatively long half-life, broad antibacterial spectrum, and low incidence of allergic reactions.

9. Perioperative shaving is not recommended and leads to an increased risk of surgical site infection.

10. Pneumatic compression boots or heparin should be used perioperatively to decrease the risk of deep venous thrombosis and pulmonary embolism. Standard treatment of deep venous thrombosis and pulmonary embolism is heparin followed by warfarin for up to 6 months.

11. Early postoperative feeding should be the goal after major gynecologic or abdominal surgery because diet restriction has not been shown to be beneficial.

12. Neuropathies occur after approximately 1.5% to 2% of gynecologic surgeries. The risk for neuropathy can be minimized by proper patient positioning and avoidance of pressure from retractor blades.

SUGGESTED READING

American College of Obstetricians and Gynecologists: Antibiotics prophylaxis for gynecologic procedures. ACOG practice bulletin No 23. Washington, DC, American College of Obstetricians and Gynecologists, 2001.

American College of Obstetricians and Gynecologists: Prevention of deep venous thrombosis and pulmonary embolism. ACOG Practice Bulletin #21. Washington, DC, American College of Obstetricians and Gynecologists, 2000.

American Urological Association; American Academy of Orthopaedic Surgeons: Antibiotic prophylaxis for urological patients with total joint replacements. J Urol 169:1796–1797, 2003.

Bratzler DW, Houck PM, for the Surgical Infection Prevention Guideline Writers Workgroup: Antimicrobial prophylaxis for surgery: An advisory statement from the National Surgical Infection Prevention Project. Am J Surg 189:395–404, 2005.

Cardosi RJ, Cox CS, Hoffman MS: Postoperative neuropathies after major pelvic surgery. Obstet Gynecol 100:240–244, 2002.

Cheatham ML, Chapman WC, Key SP, Sawyers JL: A meta-analysis of selective versus routine nasogastric decompression after elective laparotomy. Ann Surg 221:469–476, 1995.

Dajani AS, Taubert KA, Wilson W, et al: Prevention of bacterial endocarditis: Recommendations by the American Heart Association. JAMA 277:1794–1801, 1997.

Davis JD: Prevention, diagnosis, and treatment of venous thromboembolic complications of gynecologic surgery. Am J Obstet Gynecol 184:759–775, 2001.

de la Torre SH, Mandel L, Goff BA: Evaluation of postoperative fever: usefulness and cost-effectiveness of routine workup. Am J Obstet Gynecol 188:1642–1647, 2003.

Eagle KA, Berger PB, Calkins H, et al: American College of Cardiology; American Heart Association: ACC/AHA guideline update for perioperative cardiovascular evaluation for noncardiac surgery: Executive summary: a report of the American College of Cardiology/American Heart Association Task Force on Practice Guidelines. J Am Coll Cardiol 39:542–553, 2002.

Emond SD, Camargo CA Jr, Nowak RM: 1997 National Asthma Education and Prevention Program guidelines: A practical summary for emergency physicians. Ann Emerg Med 31:579–589, 1998.

Fanning J, Andrews S: Early postoperative feeding after major gynecologic surgery: Evidence-based scientific medicine. Am J Obstet Gynecol 185:1–4, 2001.

Greer AE, Irwin MG: Implementation and evaluation of guidelines for preoperative testing in a tertiary hospital. Anaesth Intensive Care 30:326–330, 2002.

Guenaga KF, Matos D, Castro AA, et al: Mechanical bowel preparation for elective colorectal surgery. Cochrane Database Syst Rev CD001544, 2003.

Irvin W, Andersen W, Taylor P, Rice L: Minimizing the risk of neurologic injury in gynecologic surgery. Obstet Gynecol 103:374–382, 2004.

MacMillan SL, Kammerer-Doak D, Rogers RG, Parker KM: Early feeding and the incidence of gastrointestinal symptoms after major gynecologic surgery. Obstet Gynecol 96:604–608, 2000.

Mangano DT, Layug EL, Wallace A, Tateo I: Effect of atenolol on mortality and cardiovascular morbidity after noncardiac surgery: Multicenter Study of Perioperative Ischemia Research Group. N Engl J Med 335:1713–1720, 1996.

Maxwell GL, Synan I, Dodge R, et al: Pneumatic compression versus low molecular weight heparin in gynecologic oncology surgery: A randomized trial. Obstet Gynecol 98:989–994, 2001.

Naumann RW, Hauth JC, Owen J, et al: Subcutaneous tissue approximation in relation to wound disruption after cesarean delivery in obese women. Obstet Gynecol 85:412–416, 1995.

Nichols RL, Smith JW, Garcia RY, et al: Current practices of preoperative bowel prep among North American colorectal surgeons. Clin Infect Dis 24:619, 1997.

Reilly DF, McNeely MJ, Doerner D, et al: Self-reported exercise tolerance and the risk of serious perioperative complications. Arch Intern Med 159:2185–2192, 1999.

Stanley BM, Walters DJ, Maddern GJ: Informed consent: how much information is enough? Aust N Z J Surg 68:788–791, 1998.

Toglia MR, Nolan TE: Morbidity and mortality rates of elective gynecologic surgery in the elderly woman. Am J Obstet Gynecol 189:1584–1588, 2003.

Warner MA, Warner DO, Harper CM, et al: Lower extremity neuropathies associated with lithotomy positions. Anesthesiology 93:938–942, 2000.

Wessel TR, Arant CB, Olson MB, et al: Relationship of physical fitness vs. body mass index with coronary artery disease and cardiovascular events in women. JAMA 292:1179–1187, 2004.

29

HYSTERECTOMY
Matthew D. Barber

HISTORICAL PERSPECTIVE

Although surgical removal of uterus was described as early as the second century A.D. the first successful vaginal hysterectomy was performed by Conrad Johann Martin Langenbeck in 1813. In the United States, the first successful vaginal hysterectomy was performed for uterine cancer by Herman and Werneberg in 1832. Walter Burnham of Lowell, MA, performed the first successful abdominal hysterectomy in 1853, accidentally. Upon opening the patient to remove a large ovarian cyst, the patient vomited, expelling a large fibroid uterus. As Burnham was unable to put the enlarged uterus back into the peritoneal cavity, he removed it supracervically. In fact, many of the first attempts at abdominal hysterectomy involved uterine leiomyomas that had been misdiagnosed as ovarian cysts; laparotomy for ovarian cystotomy became increasingly common after Ephraim McDowell's initial success in 1809. The first planned elective abdominal hysterectomies were performed independently by Clay and Koeberle in 1863.

The early hysterectomies were fraught with hazard and the patients usually died of hemorrhage, peritonitis, and/or exhaustion. Early procedures were performed without anesthesia with a mortality of approximately 70%. In the latter half of the nineteenth century, with advances in medical science like the advent of anesthesia in 1846, Joseph Lister's treatise on asepsis in 1867, and his introduction of aseptic suture (silk soaked in carbolic) in 1869, surgery became considerably safer and more successful. In 1878, W. A. Freund refined total abdominal hysterectomy technique using anesthesia, antiseptic technique, the Trendelenburg position, and ligatures around major vessels and ligaments. His description included dissecting the bladder from the uterus and detaching the cardinal and uterosacral ligaments. In the late 1890s, Howard Kelly and his colleagues at Johns Hopkins Hospital further refined the technique of abdominal hysterectomy and reported a mortality rate of only 4% after 245 such operations, a remarkable achievement in the preantibiotic era.

At the turn of the century, the majority of hysterectomies were being performed for carcinoma of the cervix or uterine corpus. In 1890, Schauta performed the first radical vaginal hysterectomy for treatment of cervical cancer and had perfected it by 1909. In 1898, Ernst Wertheim, a student of Schauta, introduced and ultimately popularized radical abdominal hysterectomy, the foundation of the radical hysterectomy performed today. In the early 1900s, as the safety of both the vaginal and abdominal hysterectomy improved, hysterectomy came to be used more frequently for benign indications including leiomyomata, endometriosis, adenomyosis, menorrhagia, and pelvic inflammatory disease.

From the late 1890s to the early 1900s there was division regarding the preferred approach to hysterectomy. Vaginal and abdominal surgeons almost never used the alternative method, although eventually the wisdom of being able to use either route based on the circumstance became apparent. In 1929, E. H. Richardson standardized the technique for simple abdominal hysterectomy. Richardson's technique serves as the basis for the modern-day operation. In 1934, N. S. Heaney describes his technique for vaginal hysterectomy using a clamp, needle holder, and retractor of his own design. His method for closing the vaginal cuff that incorporates peritoneum, vessels, and ligaments is known as the "Heaney stitch." Like that of Richardson, Heaney's vaginal hysterectomy technique has endured the passage of time and is the basis of today's technique.

In the latter half of the twentieth century, improved anesthetic technique, the introduction of antibiotics and blood products, and refinements in instrumentation and suture material resulted in significant reductions in morbidity and mortality and the general acceptance of hysterectomy as an important tool for the treatment of gynecologic disease. The fundamental techniques have remained relatively static since Heaney and Richardson introduced them, but contributions by several authors have been significant. In 1941, Lash introduced his "coring" technique for debulking large myomatous uteri at the time of vaginal hysterectomy. In 1957, McCall introduced his posterior culdoplasty to prevent or treat enterocele at the time of vaginal hysterectomy. Operative laparoscopy was first used in gynecologic procedures by Raol Palmer in 1943. In 1988, Reich performed the first laparoscopic hysterectomy.

In the first half of the twentieth century, gynecologists had very few effective therapeutic options. As its safety improved, hysterectomy became the cornerstone of gynecologic practice and was performed liberally for a wide variety of maladies, many of which would not be considered appropriate indications for surgery today. With the development and widespread use of antibiotics, hormonal therapies including oral contraceptive pills, nonsteroidal anti-inflammatory drugs, and other medications in the latter half of the century, the options for gynecologists and their patients improved considerably. The use of hysterectomy became more restrictive and was often reserved for cases in which medical therapy was not effective. Over the last two decades we have seen the development of nonmedical alternatives to hysterectomy including endometrial ablation, hysteroscopic myomectomy, and uterine fibroid embolization, further improving options for patients. In spite of this, hysterectomy still remains an essential and important therapeutic option for many gynecologic conditions.

EPIDEMIOLOGY

Today, hysterectomy is second most frequent major operation performed on women in the United States, following only cesarean section. In 2002, more than 650,000 hysterectomies were performed with an estimated annual cost of over $5 billion. The hysterectomy rate of the United States is among the highest in the developed world. Approximately 42% of women will undergo a hysterectomy during the course of their life.

There has been a steady decline in the annual incidence of hysterectomy from a peak of 10.4 per 1000 women in 1975 to 5.5 per 1000 in 1999. In 2002, 64% of hysterectomies were performed abdominally, 21% were performed vaginally, 9% were performed with laparoscopic assistance, and 6% were supracervical (subtotal). According to estimates from the Centers for Disease Control and Prevention (CDC), uterine leiomyomas, uterine prolapse, and endometriosis are the most frequent indications, accounting for as many as 73% of all hysterectomies. Approximately 10% of hysterectomies in the United States are performed for malignancy.

Women aged 40 to 44 years have the highest incidence of hysterectomy (11.7 per 1000 woman-years) with 64% of all hysterectomies being performed in patients between the ages of 35 and 54 years. At the age of 35 years, a woman has a 12.9% probability of undergoing a hysterectomy in the next 10 years. At age 45, the probability is 11.7%. Although some studies have suggested racial differences in hysterectomy rates, the most recent CDC data demonstrate no overall difference in hysterectomy rates between black and white women. However, black women do have significantly higher rates than white women between the ages of 35 and 44 years, with lower rates at other ages. This is likely explained by the increased incidence of uterine leiomyoma seen in black women. Some studies suggest that Hispanic women have lower rates of hysterectomy compared with non-Hispanic white women. The reason for this is unclear.

Geographic region also appears to influence hysterectomy rates within the United States. Rates for women living in the south (6.5 per 1000) are significantly higher than for those in the west (4.8 per 1000) and northeast (4.3 per 1000). Similarly, the average age at the time of hysterectomy is significantly younger for women living in the south than those living in the northeast (44 versus 49 years old). The availability of gynecologists, the numbers of hospital beds per capita, the types of health care insurance available, and regional variations in patient and physician attitudes toward hysterectomy are thought to contribute to this geographic variation. Other known risk factors for hysterectomy include low education, high parity, and history of multiple miscarriages.

INDICATIONS FOR HYSTERECTOMY

Broadly speaking, the vast majority of hysterectomies are performed to relieve the symptoms of pain, bleeding, or both. A list of common disease processes for which hysterectomy is appropriate can be found in Table 29-1. Age has an important influence on the relative frequency of these indications. In women of reproductive age, uterine fibroids and menstrual irregularities are the most common indications. In postmenopausal women, uterine prolapse is the most frequent indication. Figure 29-1 demonstrates the cumulative risk of hysterectomy by indication over a woman's life span.

In general, the following criteria should be met before a hysterectomy for benign disease is considered: (1) the patient should have completed childbearing; (2) an adequate trial of medical or nonsurgical management has been attempted, if such therapy exists for the individual patient; (3) a workup has been performed to rule out nonuterine causes of the patient's symptoms or causes for which a hysterectomy would be inappropriate; and (4) an appropriate informed consent process has been undertaken that includes a detailed discussion of the risks and benefits of hysterectomy and a balanced discussion of hysterectomy alternatives. A detailed review of each of the indications listed in Table 29-1 is beyond the scope of this chapter, but many can be found elsewhere in this textbook. Certain indications bear further discussion, however.

Uterine Leiomyomas

Uterine leiomyomas or fibroids are one of the most common conditions affecting women of reproductive age. They account for approximately one third of all hysterectomies. Symptoms attributable to uterine leiomyomas include excessive menstrual bleeding, dysmenorrhea, pelvic pain, and so-called bulk symptoms, or symptoms related to pressure on adjacent organs such as ureteral obstruction, urinary frequency and urgency, rectal pressure, pelvic pressure, and increasing abdominal girth. Uterine leiomyomas are very common, with some studies estimating that as many as 60% to

Table 29-1

Indications for hysterectomy

Benign Disease	Malignant Disease
Uterine leiomyomas	Cervical cancer
Excessive menstrual bleeding	Endometrial cancer
Pelvic organ prolapse	Ovarian cancer
Endometriosis	Fallopian tube cancer
Adenomyosis	Gestational trophoblastic tumors
Pelvic inflammatory disease*	Rectal or bladder cancer with uterine
Chronic pelvic pain	involvement
Dysmenorrhea	
Obstetric indications†	
Cervical intraepithelial neoplasia (CIN)‡	
Atypical endometrial hyperplasia	

*Hysterectomy may be indicated in some cases of pelvic inflammatory disease that are refractory to medical management or in the case of a ruptured or persistent tubo-ovarian abscess. In patients who desire future fertility, unilateral adnexectomy is often adequate, however.
†Hysterectomy may be required for obstetric emergencies such as uterine rupture, hemorrhage, placenta accreta, or endometritis unresponsive to medical management. Hysterectomy may also be necessary in some cases of cornual or cervical ectopic pregnancy and as a result of complications from therapeutic or septic abortions.
‡In general, CIN is treated conservatively with high success rate. Rarely, hysterectomy may be indicated for cases of CIN III that cannot be completely removed with cervical conization.

Prevalence-corrected probability of hysterectomy across the age span in Utah by cause, 1995–1997. (From Merrill RM: Prevalence corrected hysterectomy rates and probabilities in Utah. Ann Epidemiol 11:127–135, 2001.)

Figure 29-1

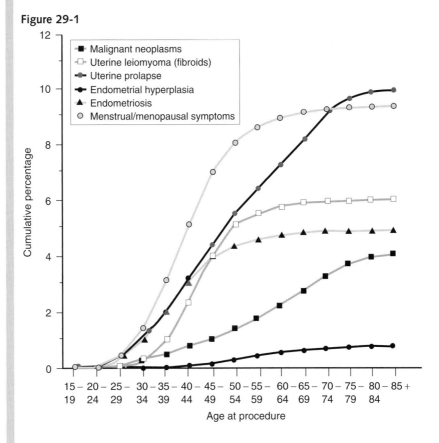

80% of women are affected. However, the majority never develop symptoms or are unaware of their presence. The development of fibroid symptoms largely depends upon the size, number, and location of the tumors. Fibroid growth is associated with the presence of estrogen, so they stop growing and often shrink after menopause. One of the few identified risk factors for uterine fibroids is race. The incidence of uterine fibroids among black women is approximately three times that among white women. In addition, uterine fibroids are diagnosed earlier in black women, who are more likely to undergo both hysterectomy and myomectomy for fibroids. Other known risk factors include obesity and low parity. Smoking tobacco appears to decrease the risk (presumably because of the associated decrease in estrogen levels).

In general, hysterectomy should be reserved for those women with symptomatic fibroids who no longer desire fertility. In the past, gynecologists frequently performed hysterectomies on women with fibroids whose uterine size was greater than 12 weeks, even if they were asymptomatic. The rationale for this included avoidance of future symptoms, concern about increased operative morbidity if the uterus continued to enlarge, and the inability to assess the ovaries during routine pelvic examination if an enlarged uterus was present. Evidence to support this rationale is lacking. Today, hysterectomy in asymptomatic women with uterine fibroids is rarely indicated regardless of uterine size. Exceptions include ureteral obstruction and signs suggesting the possibility of uterine leiomyosarcoma, such as rapid uterine growth or growth after menopause. In postmenopausal women not taking exogenous estrogen, uterine enlargement suggests the possibility of malignancy and hysterectomy is often indicated. In premenopausal women, leiomyosarcoma is exceedingly rare, even in the presence of rapid uterine growth. In one study of women undergoing hysterectomy for rapid uterine growth, the incidence of uterine sarcoma was only 0.27%, bringing this indication for hysterectomy into question.

Hysterectomy should be considered in a woman with symptomatic uterine fibroids who no longer desires fertility, particularly if the severity of symptoms is such that they interfere with her daily life. Before proceeding with a hysterectomy, other sources for the patient's symptoms should be ruled out. Women with excessive or irregular menstrual bleeding should be evaluated with endometrial sampling, hysteroscopy, ultrasound, or a combination of these. In patients with fibroids and pelvic pain, other sources of the pain should be ruled out including other gynecologic diseases and urologic, gastrointestinal, or musculoskeletal disorders. Although many advocate a trial of medical management before proceeding with hysterectomy, the evidence supporting this requirement is lacking in women with uterine fibroids. In spite of this, a trial of medical management is often prudent before considering hysterectomy because of hysterectomy's definitive nature and associated risks.

Alternatives to hysterectomy that should be discussed for women with symptomatic fibroids include myomectomy (which can be performed hysteroscopically, laparoscopically, and abdominally) and uterine fibroid embolization. The need for subsequent hysterectomy after myomectomy because of persistent or recurrent symptoms is 0.5% to 12%, and the need for subsequent medical therapy ranges from 4% to 76%, depending on the technique and length of follow-up. Myomectomy has the obvious advantage of allowing future fertility. Uterine embolization for fibroids was first reported in 1995. A recent prospective nonrandomized study comparing uterine fibroid embolization to hysterectomy found marked improvement in symptoms and quality of life in both groups. Although hysterectomy resulted in an elimination of bleeding symptoms, those who underwent embolization noted a 55% reduction in bleeding and a 33% reduction in uterine size. Hysterectomy also demonstrated an advantage in improving pelvic pain but had a higher long-term complication rate. Uterine fibroid embolization is not recommended for those who desire future fertility. The use of gonadotropin-releasing hormone (GnRH) agonists is not a viable long-term treatment option for uterine fibroids in most women because of fibroid regrowth after treatment cessation and the long-term risks of estrogen deficiency. However, the use of GnRH agonists in perimenopausal women with symptomatic fibroids until they reach menopause has been used effectively.

Excessive Uterine Bleeding

Excessive uterine bleeding is the indication for approximately 20% of hysterectomies. This condition can be broadly classified into *menorrhagia*, or heavy menses that is cyclic and presumed to be ovulatory, and *metrorrhagia*, or intermenstrual bleeding that is noncyclic and presumed to be associated with an ovulatory disturbance. The term *dysfunctional uterine bleeding* refers to abnormal uterine bleeding in which anatomic causes have been ruled out. This is a term that has largely fallen out of favor because of its nonspecificity. Common causes of menorrhagia include leiomyomas, adenomyosis, and coagulopathy. Menorrhagia without an anatomic abnormality such as a fibroid may be related to local production of vasoactive prostanoids; nonsteroidal anti-inflammatory agents have been shown to be effective therapy. Common causes of metrorrhagia include anovulation, endometrial polyps, and leiomyomas. Other causes of abnormal uterine bleeding include pregnancy, gynecologic malignancy, pelvic infection, endometrial hyperplasia, and trauma. In the evaluation of excessive bleeding, underlying causes are sought by endometrial sampling, hysteroscopy, or ultrasound. Evaluation for coagulopathy should also be considered. Treatment is indicated when anemia is present or the bleeding interferes with the patient's quality of life. In cases in which the uterine cavity is normal and malignancy has been ruled out, medical management consisting of oral contraceptives, cyclic progestins, and/or cyclic nonsteroidal anti-inflammatory drugs is usually effective. Hysterectomy is only indicated in women who do not desire fertility and whose conditions have failed to respond to medical management. Endometrial ablation is an alternative to hysterectomy in this situation and is effective in reducing excessive bleeding in 70% to 90% of patients. However, amenorrhea only occurs in 45% and recurrent excessive bleeding occurs in 15% to 25% of cases. Approximately 9% to 34% of patients who receive endometrial ablation will undergo subsequent hysterectomy.

Pelvic Organ Prolapse

Surgical management of pelvic organ prolapse accounts for approximately 15% to 18% of hysterectomies in the United States. Symptoms associated with pelvic organ prolapse include pelvic pressure, vaginal bulging, urinary incontinence, voiding dysfunction, fecal incontinence, defecatory dysfunction, and sexual dysfunction. Surgery is considered in patients with symptomatic prolapse who do not desire to use a pessary or have tried one but failed to respond adequately. In patients who are asymptomatic or are minimally bothered, surgery is rarely indicated regardless of the extent of the prolapse. A hysterectomy is indicated at the time of surgical correction of prolapse when uterine prolapse is present. Uterine prolapse is typically not an isolated event and is often associated with other pelvic support defect. A hysterectomy alone is almost never adequate treatment for prolapse; typically, associated surgical repairs are necessary. Even in the rare cases of isolated uterine prolapse, a vaginal vault suspension is typically required. In cases of isolated anterior or posterior vaginal wall prolapse where the uterus is well supported, a hysterectomy is often unnecessary. Studies have also demonstrated that a hysterectomy is unnecessary at the time of Burch colposuspension for treatment of stress urinary incontinence, unless uterine prolapse is also present. In patients with symptomatic uterine prolapse who still desire fertility, options include use of a pessary or a uterine suspension procedure such as sacral hysteropexy or sacrospinous hysteropexy.

Chronic Pelvic Pain

Chronic pelvic pain is a complex condition with multiple causes. The evaluation of chronic pelvic pain should include an evaluation for urologic, gastrointestinal, musculoskeletal, psychological, and gynecologic sources of the pain. Depression is common in these patients regardless of the cause. The prevalence of sexual abuse in this population is as high as 40% to 60%. A multidisciplinary approach to management is necessary, addressing somatic, psychological, and social issues as well as sleep disturbance and other factors. Hysterectomy should only be performed for chronic pelvic pain in patients whose pain is of uterine origin and does not respond to nonsurgical management.

Endometriosis

Endometriosis is a common gynecologic source of chronic pelvic pain, dysmenorrhea, and dyspareunia. Diagnostic laparoscopy is necessary to diagnose endometriosis; however, some advocate a trial of medical management in those patients with pelvic pain suspected of having endometriosis without definitive laparoscopic diagnosis. Effective medical treatment for pelvic pain resulting from endometriosis includes oral contraceptive pills, progestins, danazol, and GnRH agonists. Conservative surgical treatment of endometriosis involves excision and/or ablation of endometriotic implants, typically by laparoscopy. Hysterectomy should only be considered in patients with pelvic pain from endometriosis if fertility is no longer desired and medical or conservative surgical therapy has proven inadequate. Bilateral oophorectomy is often recommended at the time of hysterectomy for endometriosis. Approximately 20% of hysterectomies in women of reproductive age are performed for pelvic pain resulting from endometriosis.

Dysmenorrhea

Dysmenorrhea, or painful menses, can be idiopathic (primary dysmenorrhea) or the result of an identified underlying condition (secondary dysmenorrhea.) Conditions known to cause secondary dysmenorrhea include endometriosis, adenomyosis, and uterine leiomyomas. Typically, dysmenorrhea can be adequately treated with nonsteroidal anti-inflammatory drugs alone or in combination with oral contraceptives or other hormonal agents. A hysterectomy is indicated only for intractable dysmenorrhea refractory to medical management in patients who no longer desire fertility.

CHOOSING ROUTE OF HYSTERECTOMY

Hysterectomy can be performed vaginally, abdominally, or with laparoscopic assistance. Choice of hysterectomy route should be individualized to the patient and the indication for surgery. In the United States, abdominal hysterectomy is the route chosen in almost two thirds of cases. This is in spite of well-documented evidence that vaginal hysterectomy on average results in fewer complications, decreased postoperative pain, shorter length of stay, speedier return to normal activities, reduced cost, and lower mortality than abdominal hysterectomy. In 1982, the CDC published one of the largest studies evaluating differences in complications between vaginal and abdominal hysterectomies. The study included 1851 patients aged 15 to 44 years in whom hysterectomy was performed for benign gynecologic disorders. In this study, the odds of one or more complications after abdominal hysterectomy was 1.7 times that of vaginal hysterectomy. The rate of febrile morbidity was 1.9 times higher and the risk of transfusion was 2.1 times higher for the abdominal than for the vaginal route. Although certain conditions and patient characteristics necessitate an abdominal approach, several authors have demonstrated that with appropriate treatment guidelines and adequate surgical skill, the proportion of hysterectomies performed vaginally can be increased dramatically. Kovac and colleagues studied the effect of adopting the Society of Pelvic Reconstructive Surgeons Guidelines for choosing route of hysterectomy (Fig. 29-2) in a resident clinic population. They found that resident physicians who followed the guidelines increased the proportion of hysterectomies performed vaginally to over 90% and reduced the ratio of abdominal-to-vaginal hysterectomy from

Figure 29-2

Society of Pelvic Reconstructive Surgeons Guidelines for choosing route of hysterectomy. (From Kovac RS: Clinical opinion: Guidelines for hysterectomy. Am J Obstet Gynecol 191:635–640, 2004.)

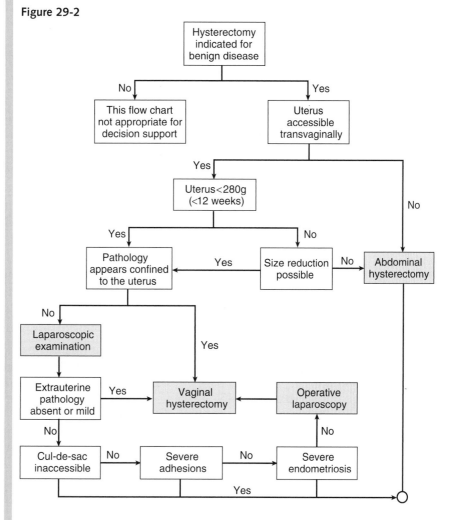

3:1 to 1:11. Use of uterine morcellation or other sophisticated uterine size reduction techniques was only necessary in 11% of cases.

With rare exception, hysterectomy for gynecologic malignancy should be performed abdominally. For benign conditions, route of hysterectomy should largely be determined by the following factors: vaginal accessibility, uterine size and shape, and extent of extrauterine disease. Because of its well-documented advantages, vaginal hysterectomy should be the approach of choice when feasible. Factors that impair vaginal access to the uterus and make vaginal hysterectomy difficult include a narrow pubic arch (<90 degrees), a narrow vagina (narrower than two fingerbreadths, especially at the apex), and an undescended and immobile uterus. When one or more of these factors are present, the laparoscopic or abdominal route should be considered. In spite of its frequent mention, nulliparity in and of itself is not a contraindication to the vaginal route. Many nulliparous women have adequate vaginal caliber to allow successful completion of a vaginal hysterectomy. Even in the case of minimal uterine descent, if the upper vagina allows adequate access for transection of the uterosacral and cardinal ligaments, uterine mobility will improve, making the remainder of the vaginal hysterectomy easier to accomplish.

When vaginal access is adequate and the uterus is less than 12 weeks' gestational size (<280 g), vaginal hysterectomy is the route of choice in the absence of significant extrauterine disease. For uteri larger than 12 weeks' size, vaginal hysterectomy can often be accomplished safely using uterine size reduction techniques such as wedge morcellation, uterine bisection, and intramyometrial coring. Randomized trials comparing the vaginal to the abdominal route for women with enlarged uteri (200 to 1300 g) demonstrate decreased operative time, febrile morbidity, postoperative narcotic use, and hospital stay for those who received vaginal hysterectomy with morcellation without an increase in perioperative morbidity. When considering whether to perform a vaginal hysterectomy in a woman with an enlarged uterus, uterine shape is often more important than actual size. Before beginning any morcellation procedure, the uterine vessels must be ligated bilaterally and the peritoneal cavity must be entered. If the cervix or lower uterine segment is enlarged or contains fibroids that prevent uterine artery ligation or entry into the peritoneal cavity, then the procedure should not be performed vaginally regardless of size. In contrast, if the lower uterine segment is accessible surgically, then even very large uteri (>20 weeks' size) can be removed transvaginally by an appropriately skilled surgeon. However, many would consider 16 weeks the upper limit for a vaginal hysterectomy.

The presence of disease outside the uterus, such as severe endometriosis, severe pelvic adhesions, or adnexal pathology typically precludes vaginal hysterectomy. In these cases, the abdominal or laparoscopic approach is preferred. Additionally, in cases where visualization of the pelvis or abdomen is required diagnostically, such as chronic pelvic pain, the vaginal route is not appropriate. Mild pelvic adhesive disease is not a contraindication for the vaginal route, however; neither is history of previous cesarean section. Several studies have demonstrated that the risk of bladder injury during hysterectomy in a woman with a history of cesarean section is highest when the laparoscopic route is used and is approximately equal for the abdominal or vaginal route, regardless of the number of previous cesarean sections. In situations where the degree of extrauterine pathology is unclear, diagnostic laparoscopy immediately before the hysterectomy can be a useful way to accurately evaluate presumed contraindications to the vaginal approach. In 1990, Kovac and colleagues reported on 46 patients in whom intraoperative laparoscopy was used to evaluate pelvic disease after they had been advised to have abdominal hysterectomy. They found that, in general, uterine size had been overestimated, uterine mobility underestimated, and all 14 patients referred for assessment of adnexal pathology had none. In 91% (42 of 46), vaginal hysterectomy was performed successfully at the same setting as the laparoscopy.

Operative laparoscopy to complete all or part of the hysterectomy is used in approximately 10% of hysterectomies in the United States today. Although first introduced over 15 years ago, there still remains considerable debate about the appropriate indications for laparoscopic hysterectomy. Randomized trials have demonstrated that, compared with vaginal hysterectomy, laparoscopic hysterectomy has a longer operative time and greater cost with similar complication rates and postoperative recovery. Therefore, laparoscopic hysterectomy has no advantages over vaginal hysterectomy. It should instead be considered an alterative for those patients in whom a vaginal hysterectomy is not indicated or is deemed not feasible. Circumstances in which the laparoscopic approach may be helpful include hysterectomy in a patient with documented endometriosis, chronic pelvic pain, known pelvic adhesive disease, or a concurrent adnexal mass that requires removal. Laparoscopic hysterectomy can also be useful in patients with limited vaginal access. Additionally, laparoscopic hysterectomy may be appropriate in some cases of stage 1 endometrial cancer. Although some have suggested that increased uterine size is an appropriate indication for laparoscopic hysterectomy, there is no evidence of any advantage over vaginal hysterectomy with morcellation. Randomized trials comparing laparoscopic hysterectomy to abdominal hysterectomy demonstrate a longer operative time and higher risk of lower urinary tract injury, but less blood loss, fewer wound infections, fewer febrile episodes, a more rapid postoperative recovery, and an earlier return to work for those who receive the laparoscopic approach. Some studies have demonstrated a higher cost with laparoscopic hysterectomy, but others have not.

PREPARATION FOR HYSTERECTOMY

Before undergoing a hysterectomy, a patient should have a complete history and physical examination. The number and severity of a patient's medical comorbidities directly correlates with her operative risk. Therefore, the patient's health care status should be optimized preoperatively to reduce the risk of perioperative morbidity. In most women, the only preoperative laboratory tests necessary are a complete blood count and a blood type and screen. Women of reproductive age should have a pregnancy test, and all women should have a recent Papanicolaou (Pap) smear before undergoing a hysterectomy. Other laboratory tests, imaging studies, or consultations should be ordered based on the patient's medical history, review of systems, and gynecologic condition. Preoperative chest radiography and electrocardiography are not routinely indicated in women without cardiovascular or pulmonary disease.

All patients should undergo a comprehensive informed consent process before surgery. This should include a review of the planned procedure and a discussion of the risks of potential perioperative complications and the anticipated outcome of the surgery, including the likelihood of resolution the patient's symptoms and the risk of developing new symptoms. Alternative treatment options should also be reviewed. Procedures that may be performed in addition to the hysterectomy should also be discussed; in particular, it should be discussed whether the patient desires prophylactic oophorectomy. If a vaginal or laparoscopic approach is planned, the patient should be informed of the potential need for conversion to laparotomy. It is also useful to discuss specific details of the hospital stay and postoperative course including expected length of stay, postoperative limitations, and anticipated time until return to work.

Women with anemia resulting from excessive menstrual bleeding should be given oral iron for several months preoperatively to correct the anemia. Patients whose anemia does not resolve with oral iron should undergo further evaluation to rule out other sources of bleeding, including gastrointestinal causes. In women with uterine fibroids and anemia, GnRH agonists should be considered. A common regimen is leuprolide acetate 3.75 mg given intramuscularly at monthly intervals for 3 months preoperatively. A meta-analysis of 26 randomized trials comparing preoperative GnRH agonists to no treatment or placebo found that patients who received preoperative GnRH agonists increased their hematocrit an average of 3%, decreased their uterine volume an average of two gestational sizes (i.e., from 14 to 12 weeks' size) and decreased intraoperative blood loss an average of 58 mL. Additionally, because of the decrease in uterine volume, women who received preoperative GnRH agonists were both less likely to need a vertical incision at the time of abdominal hysterectomy and more likely to receive a vaginal hysterectomy than those who did not. Preoperative GnRH agonists use does not decrease the blood transfusion rate, however.

Mechanical bowel preparation should be routinely given before laparoscopic hysterectomy or any hysterectomy in which there is a concern for possible bowel injury. In general, bowel preparation is not necessary for vaginal hysterectomies when the uterus is not enlarged.

Deep vein thrombosis and pulmonary embolism are important contributors to morbidity and mortality in patients undergoing hysterectomy. Routine prophylaxis with pneumatic leg compression, low-dose heparin, or low-molecular-weight heparin is indicated in women undergoing hysterectomy who have moderate to high risk of developing thromboembolic disease. This includes all women aged 40 years or older and younger women with other risk factors including history of deep vein thrombosis or pulmonary embolism, cancer, obesity, or an inherited thrombophilia.

All patients undergoing hysterectomy should receive intravenous antibiotics within a 60-minute window before the surgical incision to reduce postoperative infection. Randomized trials have demonstrated a significant reduction in febrile morbidity and infection in both abdominal and vaginal hysterectomy with prophylactic antibiotics. A first-generation cephalosporin, such as cefazolin 1 to 2 g given intravenously, is most often recommended. In patients who are allergic to penicillin or cephalosporin, intravenous clindamycin 900 mg is an acceptable alternative. The antibiotic dose should be repeated intraoperatively if the estimated blood loss exceeds 1000 mL or the operative time exceeds 4 hours. Antibiotic administration need not be extended into the postoperative period because several randomized trials have shown that a single dose of antibiotics given preoperatively decreases the infection rate as well as antibiotics given for 24 hours or more. Patients should be instructed not to shave the operative site before surgery because this has been shown to increase the risk of incisional infection. If necessary, hair at the operative site should be removed just before surgery. Hair clipping is preferable to shaving, as it has been shown to decrease infection.

VAGINAL HYSTERECTOMY

When adequate anesthesia has been attained, the patient should be placed in high dorsal lithotomy position with the hips flexed and legs in almost complete extension using candy-cane or Allen stirrups. The patient's buttocks should be brought to the edge of the table. Care should be made to avoid hyperflexion of the thigh because this can result in femoral neuropathy. The height of the table should be adjusted to a level comfortable to the surgeon and his or her assistants. Adequate padding should be used at potential compression sites. An examination should be performed with the patient under anesthesia to confirm preoperative findings and to ensure the appropriateness of the planned procedure.

A vaginal/perineal preparation should be performed, and the patient should be draped. A Foley catheter is inserted into the bladder and a short weighted speculum is placed in the vagina. The patient is placed in Trendelenburg position to promote retention of the weighted vaginal speculum and to keep the bowel out of the operative field. The cervix is grasped with one or more tenaculum and circumferentially injected with a vasoconstrictive agent; typically 0.5% to 1% lidocaine with epinephrine (1:200,000 concentration), 0.25% bupivacaine with epinephrine, or dilute pitressin (20 units/100 mL of normal saline) (Fig. 29-3). Injection of a vasoconstrictive agent promotes hemostasis at the vaginal cuff during the procedure and assists in identification of dissection planes. Clinical

Figure 29-3

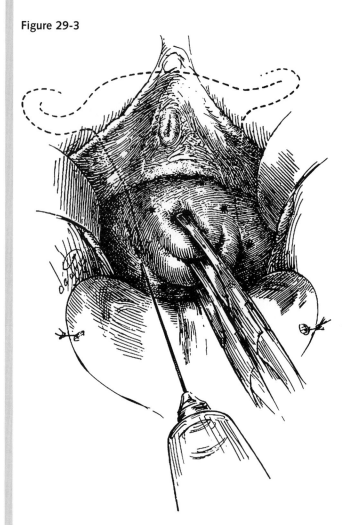

Injection of the para-cervical tissues with a vasoconstrictive agent before the initial incision of a vaginal hysterectomy. (From Nichols DH, Clarke-Pearson DL: Gynecologic, Obstetric, and Related Surgery, 2nd ed. St. Louis, Mosby, 1999.)

trials have demonstrated a decreased blood loss and, in the case of bupivacaine, decreased postoperative pain compared with injection with saline. Early studies suggested an increased risk of infection after injection with vasoconstrictive agents at the time of vaginal hysterectomy, but this does not appear to be the case when used concurrently with prophylactic antibiotics. Figures 29-4 through 29-11 illustrate the basic steps of a vaginal hysterectomy.

After the vaginal hysterectomy is completed, if a salpingo-oophorectomy is to be performed, the ovary is grasped gently with a long Allis clamp and the fimbriated end of the tube with a Kelly clamp allowing for maintenance of the orientation of the ovary and tube. It may be necessary to place a sponge stick or pack into the pelvis to prevent bowel or omentum from obscuring visualization. The mesosalpinx is clamped laterally with a Heaney clamp and a Kelly clamp is placed adjacent to the tube (Fig. 29-12). The lateral mesosalpinx is clamped, cut, and suture ligated sequentially with small 1- to 2-cm bites holding the suture ends long. Subsequent bites continue laterally and cephalad toward the infundibulopelvic ligament, advancing

Figure 29-4

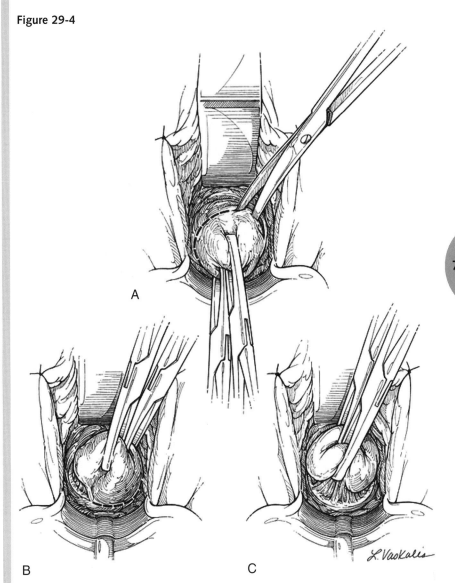

A

B

C

721

the Kelly clamp opposite the Heaney clamp. After the infundibulopelvic ligament is skeletonized, which usually requires two or three clampings of the mesosalpinx, it is clamped transversely with a Heaney clamp close to but not including the ovary (Fig. 29-13). This pedicle is either singly or doubly ligated with absorbable suture. After inspection of the pedicles to ensure hemostasis, the suture ends are cut and a similar procedure is performed on the opposite side as indicated.

In general, a McCall's culdoplasty should be performed routinely after a vaginal hysterectomy to prevent subsequent vaginal vault prolapse. A randomized trial performed by Cruickshank and Kovac compared the McCall's culdoplasty to both simple peritoneal closure and intraperitoneal uterosacral ligament plication for the prevention of enterocele after hysterectomy. Three years after surgery, none of the subjects who received a

Figure 29-5

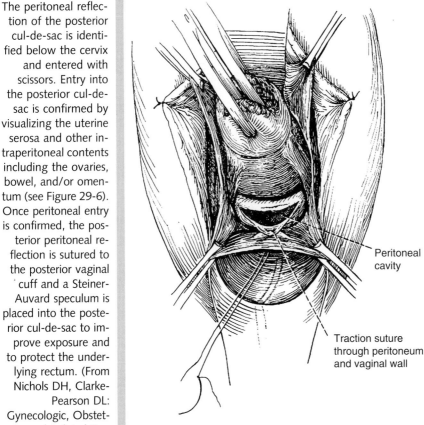

Peritoneal cavity

Traction suture through peritoneum and vaginal wall

The peritoneal reflection of the posterior cul-de-sac is identified below the cervix and entered with scissors. Entry into the posterior cul-de-sac is confirmed by visualizing the uterine serosa and other intraperitoneal contents including the ovaries, bowel, and/or omentum (see Figure 29-6). Once peritoneal entry is confirmed, the posterior peritoneal reflection is sutured to the posterior vaginal cuff and a Steiner-Auvard speculum is placed into the posterior cul-de-sac to improve exposure and to protect the underlying rectum. (From Nichols DH, Clarke-Pearson DL: Gynecologic, Obstetric, and Related Surgery, 2nd ed. St. Louis, Mosby, 1999.)

McCall's culdoplasty developed apical prolapse, compared with 15% of those who received a uterosacral ligament plication and 18% of those who had peritoneal closure alone. Figure 29-14 demonstrates the McCall's culdoplasty technique.

Techniques for Removing the Enlarged Uterus

When the uterus is enlarged from uterine fibroids or adenomyosis, uterine debulking techniques such as wedge morcellation, intramyometrial coring, or uterine bivalving are often necessary to successfully complete the hysterectomy transvaginally. These techniques may be used alone or in combination with each other. As mentioned, the uterine vessels must be ligated bilaterally, and preferably the peritoneal cavity should be entered anteriorly and posteriorly before any morcellation procedure is begun. If the cervix or lower uterine segment is enlarged or contains fibroids that prevent uterine artery ligation or entry into the peritoneal cavity, the procedure should not be performed vaginally regardless of size. Because the uterine vessels have been ligated, the amount of bleeding from any of these techniques is limited.

Before beginning any of the uterine debulking procedures, it is useful to place Heaney clamps or single-tooth tenacula bilaterally on the uterine fundus just above the highest ligated pedicle. This ensures that the pedicles will not be lost, maintains uterine orientation, and provides useful

Figure 29-6

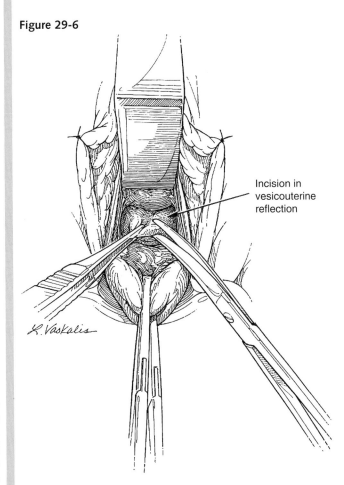

Incision in
vesicouterine
reflection

L. Vaskalis

723

The bladder is dissected off the cervix and lower uterine segment in the midline anteriorly using sharp and blunt dissection. When scarring from previous surgery is present, sharp dissection is preferred. Dissection is carried out in the avascular plane just anterior to the cervix until the anterior peritoneal reflection is identified. The anterior peritoneum is typically located just above the level of the cervicouterine junction and is smooth and slippery to palpation. Once identified, it should be grasped and entered with scissors. Entry into the anterior cul-de-sac is confirmed by visualizing intraperitoneal contents such as the bowel or omentum. A narrow right angle (Heaney-Simon) retractor is then placed into the anterior cul-de-sac under the surgeon's protective finger and used to retract anteriorly. In some cases, anterior peritoneal entry cannot be immediately accomplished. In this case, transection of the uterosacral and lower cardinal ligaments should be performed to improve uterine descensus and to bring the anterior peritoneal reflection closer to the surgical field. (From Nichols DH, Clarke-Pearson DL: Gynecologic, Obstetric, and Related Surgery, 2nd ed. St. Louis, Mosby, 1999.)

lateral landmarks for morcellation. Long vaginal retractors should be in place anteriorly and posteriorly to protect the bladder and rectum. Careful observation for nearby intestines or intestinal adhesions should be made throughout to prevent accidental bowel injury. Wedge morcellation begins by amputating the cervix with a wedged-shaped incision into the uterine corpus (Fig. 29-15). V-shaped pieces of tissue are removed piecemeal from the anterior and posterior uterine walls to centrally debulk the uterus. Uterine myomas are removed as encountered. Morcellation is continued until the round ligament, utero-ovarian ligament, and fallopian tube are accessible and can be clamped, cut, and ligated. Uterine bivalving or hemisection is performed by splitting the uterus in the midline into halves before removal. This allows one half of the uterus to be temporarily displaced into the pelvis, providing greater mobility and visualization for surgical removal other half of the uterus. Bivalving is best performed on mildly enlarged uteri that are symmetric.

Intramyometrial coring facilitates removal of the enlarged uterus by decreasing the uterine width as its length is increased. Using a scalpel or Mayo scissors, the myometrium is incised circumferentially parallel to the long axis of the uterine cavity just below the site of the ligated vessels while firm traction is applied to the cervix (Fig. 29-16). Care must be

Figure 29-7

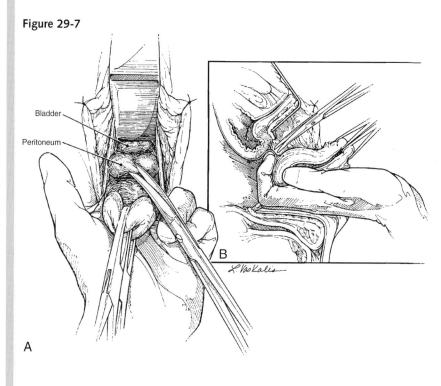

An alternative method of opening the anterior peritoneal fold in women with prolapse. **A,** The fingers of the operator's left hand are inserted through the opening of the posterior cul-de-sac and flexed around the uterine fundus. The anterior vesicouterine peritoneum is identified and distended by the tips of the operator's finger and can be easily opened with scissors or cautery. **B,** Sagittal view. (From Nichols DH, Clarke-Pearson DL: Gynecologic, Obstetric, and Related Surgery, 2nd ed. St. Louis, Mosby, 1999.)

Figure 29-8

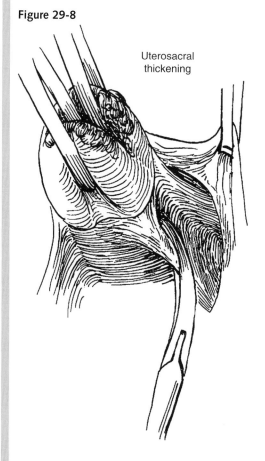

After entry into the anterior and posterior cul-de-sacs, the uterosacral ligament is clamped with a curved Heaney clamp. Heaney clamps should be placed with the tips directed toward the uterus and in such a way so that they roll off the cervix to ensure that the tip is as close to the cervix as possible. (From Nichols DH, Clarke-Pearson DL: Gynecologic, Obstetric, and Related Surgery, 2nd ed. St. Louis, Mosby, 1999.)

Figure 29-9

The uterosacral and cardinal ligaments are sequentially clamped with Heaney clamps, cut, and suture ligated with absorbable sutures. The peritoneum is incorporated into the clamp both anteriorly and posteriorly to ensure inclusion of all vessels into the pedicle. Each clamp should be placed inside the last to avoid ureteral injury. Many surgeons choose to hold the sutured ends of the first pedicle on each side (uterosacral ligaments) rather than cut them to assist with cuff closure and/or culdoplasty at the end of the procedure. (From Nichols DH, Clarke-Pearson DL: Gynecologic, Obstetric, and Related Surgery, 2nd ed. St. Louis, Mosby, 1999.)

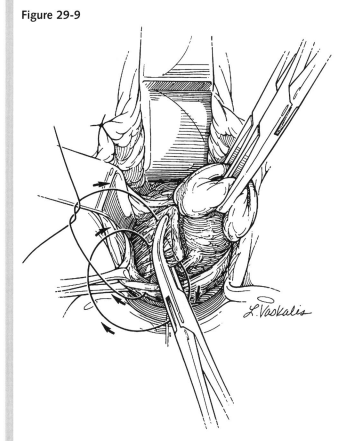

taken to avoid incision through the uterine serosa. As the cervix is pulled, the myometrium is "cored out" so that the endometrial cavity and a layer of myometrium are pulled toward the surgeon, collapsing the bulky uterus and allowing access to the upper pedicles (Fig. 29-17). Coring is most easily performed on symmetrically enlarged uteri without multiple fibroids.

ABDOMINAL HYSTERECTOMY

The patient is placed in the dorsal supine position. After attainment of adequate anesthesia, the patient is placed in frog-leg position and an examination is performed to confirm the preoperative findings. The vagina and perineum are prepared, and an indwelling Foley catheter is placed into the bladder under sterile conditions. The legs are extended to resume dorsal supine position, and the abdomen is prepared and draped. Alternatively, patients can be placed in low lithotomy position with Allen stirrups. This position is particularly useful for hysterectomies that are expected to be challenging because it has the advantage of allowing access to the perineum in case a vaginal or rectal examination and/or cystoscopy is necessary during the case. It also allows a second assistant to stand close to the operative field.

Figure 29-10

The left uterine artery is clamped, cut, and suture ligated. The procedure is repeated on the right side. The spiraling uterine artery can often be visualized in the lower half of the cardinal ligament during the second or third sequential bite. (From Nichols DH, Clarke-Pearson DL: Gynecologic, Obstetric, and Related Surgery, 2nd ed. St. Louis, Mosby, 1999.)

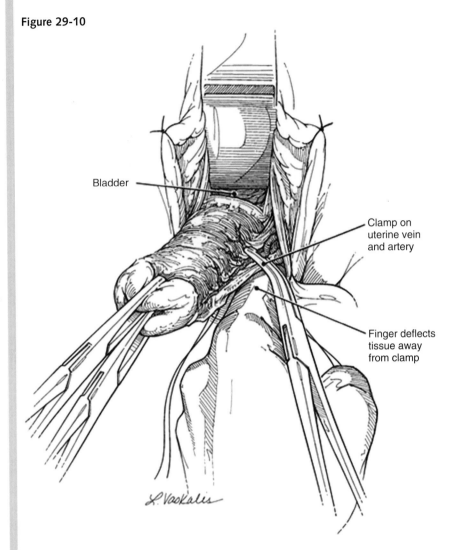

Bladder

Clamp on uterine vein and artery

Finger deflects tissue away from clamp

The type of abdominal incision to be made is determined by a number of factors including the amount of exposure required, the potential need for enlarging the incision, the strength of the healed incision, cosmesis, and the location of the previous surgical scars. The majority of hysterectomies performed for benign disease can be performed via a Pfannenstiel incision. In cases where access to the upper abdomen may be necessary, as in the case of malignancy or a very large uterus, a vertical incision is preferable. In cases where increased pelvic exposure is desired but access to the upper abdomen is not necessary, a Maylard or Cherney incision can be performed.

After the peritoneal cavity is entered, a manual exploration of the pelvis and upper abdomen is performed. If there is concern about potential malignant disease, pelvic washings are obtained. A self-retaining retractor is placed, the patient is placed in Trendelenburg position, and the bowel is packed out of the pelvis. The uterus is elevated via long Kelly clamps placed at each cornua. The hysterectomy is then performed as illustrated in Figures 29-18 through 29-24.

Figure 29-11

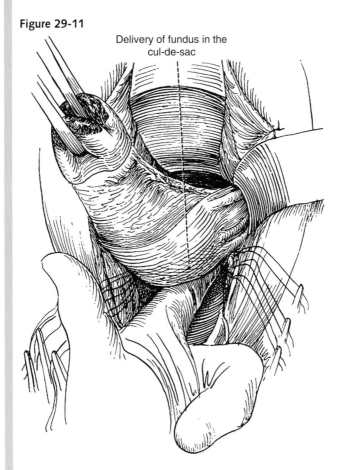

Delivery of fundus in the cul-de-sac

Sequential transection and ligation is carried bilaterally up the uterus through the broad ligaments to the upper pedicle. This last pedicle often includes the round ligament, fallopian tube, and utero-ovarian ligament. Clamping the upper pedicle can often be facilitated by delivering the fundus of the uterus through the posterior cul-de-sac and thereby allowing direct visualization of the pedicle The upper pedicle is then cut and either singly or doubly ligated, depending on surgeon preference. Suture ends of this pedicle are held long to assist in inspection and/or removal of the adnexa. The surgical site is inspected and additional hemostatic sutures are placed as needed. (From Nichols DH, Clarke-Pearson DL: Gynecologic, Obstetric, and Related Surgery, 2nd ed. St. Louis, Mosby, 1999.)

LAPAROSCOPIC HYSTERECTOMY

Laparoscopy can be used at the time of hysterectomy as a diagnostic device or to perform part or all of the procedure. Diagnostic laparoscopy performed before hysterectomy has been advocated as a method to assess whether vaginal hysterectomy is feasible in patients with presumed contraindications to the vaginal approach. It can also be used to survey the pelvis and abdomen in a patient with chronic pelvic pain before proceeding with a vaginal hysterectomy, assuming significant extrauterine pathology is not identified.

The use of operative laparoscopy to perform part or all of the hysterectomy was first described in 1989, and though it has gained wide acceptance, there is still considerable controversy regarding its role and indications. Although numerous terms have been used, including *laparoscopically assisted vaginal hysterectomy, laparoscopic-directed hysterectomy, laparoscopic hysterectomy,* and *laparoscopic-assisted hysterectomy,* it is now commonly accepted that

Figure 29-12

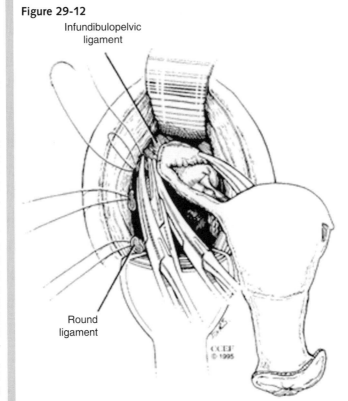

Infundibulopelvic ligament

Round ligament

Method of vaginal oophorectomy. With the adnexal pedicle pulled downward and the round ligament pulled laterally, the mesosalpinx is doubly clamped, cut, and ligated. Subsequent bites continue along the mesosalpinx laterally and cephalad toward the infundibulopelvic ligament. (Reprinted with permission from The Cleveland Clinic Foundation. From Ballard LA, Walters MD: Transvaginal mobilization and removal of ovaries and fallopian tubes after vaginal hysterectomy. Obstet Gynecol 87:35–39, 1996.)

Figure 29-13

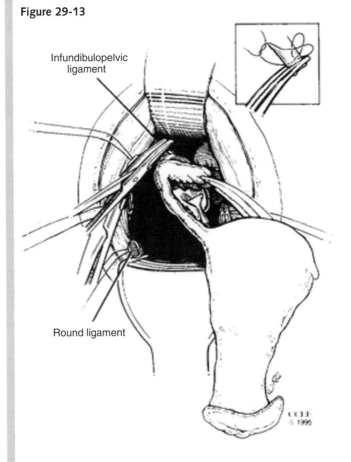

Infundibulopelvic ligament

Round ligament

Method of vaginal oophorectomy. The ovarian vessels are double-clamped above the ovary, cut, and ligated. (From Nichols DH, Clarke-Pearson DL: Gynecologic, Obstetric, and Related Surgery, 2nd ed. St. Louis, Mosby, 1999.)

Figure 29-14

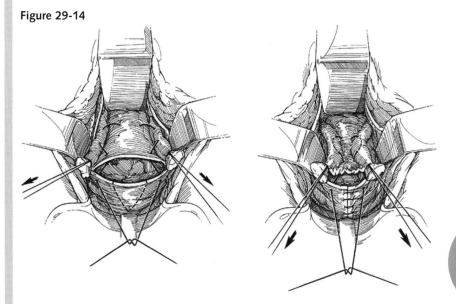

A modified McCall's culdoplasty. A delayed absorbable suture is placed through the full thickness of the posterior vaginal wall at a point where the highest portion of the vaginal vault will be. The patient's right uterosacral ligament pedicle is grasped and the suture passed through. The suture is then reefed across the anterior rectal peritoneum and passed through the left uterosacral ligament. Finally, the needle is passed from inside the posterior cul-de-sac through the vagina full thickness so that it exits next to the original suture placement. The McCall's culdoplasty sutures are then held and not tied until after the vaginal cuff has been closed. The vaginal cuff can be closed in a vertical or horizontal manner using either interrupted sutures or a running closure with absorbable suture. (From Nichols DH, Clarke-Pearson DL: Gynecologic, Obstetric, and Related Surgery, 2nd ed. St. Louis, Mosby, 1999.)

The American Association of Gynecologic Laparoscopists' Classification System for Laparoscopic Hysterectomy

any hysterectomy in which laparoscopy is used to perform any part of the procedure should be called a *laparoscopic hysterectomy*. Since its initial description, a number of laparoscopic hysterectomy techniques have been described, varying primarily by the proportion of the procedure performed laparoscopically versus vaginally. In 2000, the American Association of Gynecologic Laparoscopists published its classification system of laparoscopic hysterectomy to standardize the terminology of this procedure and to improve communication between clinicians and researchers (Table 29-2). In the United States, most laparoscopic hysterectomies involve laparoscopic occlusion of the ovarian and/or utero-ovarian pedicles along with the round ligament and upper broad ligament using bipolar electrocautery or a laparoscopic stapler device, stopping above the uterine

Table 29-2

Type	Laparoscopic Component of Hysterectomy
0	Laparoscopic-directed preparation for vaginal hysterectomy, including adhesiolysis and/or excision of endometriosis
I	Occlusion and division of at least one ovarian pedicle, utero-ovarian ligament, or infundibulopelvic ligament, but not the uterine artery
II	Type I plus occlusion and division of one or both uterine arteries
III	Type II plus a portion, but not all, of the cardinal-uterosacral ligament complex, unilateral or bilateral
IV	Complete detachment of the cardinal-uterosacral complex, unilateral or bilateral, with or without entry into the vagina. Includes total laparoscopic hysterectomy.

Each type of laparoscopic hysterectomy is further stratified into subgroups: subgroup A—cases limited to the division of the pedicle(s) containing ovarian or uterine artery/arteries; subgroup B—cases that include dissection of the bladder; subgroup C—cases that include performance of a posterior colpotomy; subgroup D—cases that include both bladder dissection and a posterior colpotomy; subgroup E—only to type IV laparoscopic hysterectomies, reserved for total laparoscopic hysterectomies.

Figure 29-15

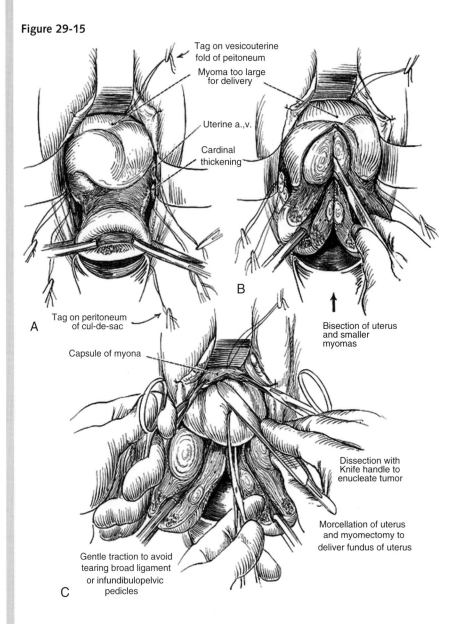

vessels. The remainder of the procedure, including uterine vessel ligation, is performed vaginally (i.e., type I laparoscopic hysterectomy). With advances in laparoscopic technique and increased training in gynecologic laparoscopy, the proportion of laparoscopic hysterectomies that involve more extensive laparoscopic surgery (i.e., types II, III, and IV), including total laparoscopic hysterectomies, is expected to rise.

Laparoscopic hysterectomy is performed with the patient under general anesthesia in the low lithotomy position. After adequate anesthesia is attained, the patient is positioned and an examination is performed to confirm the preoperative findings. The patient is sterilely prepared and draped, and a Foley catheter and uterine manipulator are placed. If a laparoscopic colpotomy is planned, a vaginal occlusive device such as a KOH Colpotomizer with inflatable balloon (Cooper Surgical Instruments; Shelton, CT) or a

Figure 29-16

The Lash intramyometrial coring technique for removal of symmetrically enlarged uteri. (From Nichols DH, Clarke-Pearson DL: Gynecologic, Obstetric, and Related Surgery, 2nd ed. St. Louis, Mosby, 1999.)

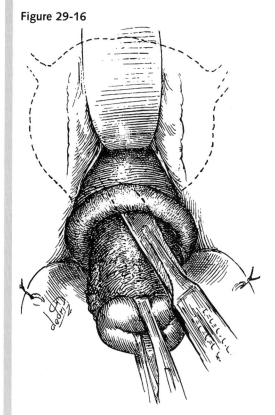

wet Kerlix sponge is placed into the vagina to maintain pneumoperitoneum after the colpotomy is performed. A 5- or 10-mm umbilical port is placed. If the patient has had a previous vertical incision or there is suspicion of periumbilical adhesions, either an open laparoscopic technique or a 5-mm left upper quadrant port should be used instead. Right and left lower quadrant ports are then placed under direct visualization lateral to the epigastric vessels at a level that allows easy access to the ovarian and uterine vessels. The size of these lateral ports will depend on the surgeon's choice of operative laparoscopic instruments. An additional 5-mm left- or right-sided port may be placed at the discretion of the surgeon, so the primary surgeon can operate with both hands. The patient is placed in the Trendelenburg position and the abdomen and pelvis are surveyed. If necessary, adhesiolysis is performed to allow proper visualization of the pelvis. If a left upper quadrant port was used, any periumbilical adhesions should be removed to facilitate umbilical port placement.

Before beginning the hysterectomy, the course of the ureters should be identified. Laparoscopically, the ureters are often easily visualized transperitoneally, crossing the pelvic brim and coursing toward the bladder beneath the infundibulopelvic ligaments. A peritoneal incision made below and parallel to the infundibulopelvic ligament allows entry into the retroperitoneum and visualization of the ureter throughout the case. Alternatively, the retroperitoneum can be entered lateral to the infundibulopelvic ligament and the ureter identified in the same manner as it would for an abdominal

Figure 29-17

Sagittal drawing of intramyometrial coring. (From Nichols DH, Clarke-Pearson DL: Gynecologic, Obstetric, and Related Surgery, 2nd ed. St. Louis, Mosby, 1999.)

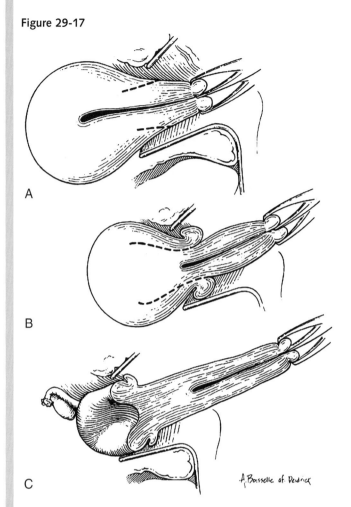

A

B

C

hysterectomy, although this tends to provide inferior visualization of the ureter because of the angle of the laparoscope.

Vascular pedicles can be occluded and divided with bipolar electrocautery and endoscopic scissors, a bipolar cutting device, a harmonic scalpel, or a laparoscopic stapling device. In general, laparoscopic suturing of vascular pedicles should be avoided because this has been associated with a significant increase in operative morbidity compared with bipolar cautery or laparoscopic stapling. If the ovaries are to be conserved, the utero-ovarian ligament and fallopian tube are occluded and divided (Fig. 29-25). If oophorectomy is planned, then the infundibulopelvic ligament is skeletonized and, after safe distance from the ureter is ensured, the ovarian vessels are occluded and divided cephalad to the ovary. The round ligaments are then occluded and divided. An incision is made with monopolar scissors in anterior leaf of the broad ligament from the ligated round ligaments along the vesicouterine fold separating the peritoneal reflection of the bladder from the lower uterine segment. The bladder is separated from the lower uterine segment and cervix using blunt and sharp dissection (Fig. 29-26). This dissection is

Figure 29-18

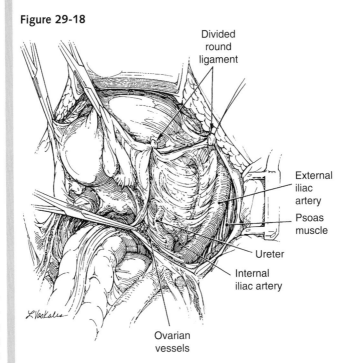

Divided round ligament

External iliac artery

Psoas muscle

Ureter

Internal iliac artery

Ovarian vessels

Identification of retroperitoneal structures. The round ligaments are suture ligated and divided at their mid point and the posterior leaf of the broad ligament is opened parallel and lateral to the infundibulopelvic ligament. The avascular perirectal space is developed to explore the retroperitoneum. The ureter is identified adherent to the medial leaf of the broad ligament below the infundibulopelvic ligament. If the course of the ureter is not readily apparent, the peritoneal incision can be extended to allow the external iliac artery to be followed cephalad to the bifurcation of the common iliac artery. Invariably, the ureter can be identified crossing the common iliac artery to enter the pelvis. (From Nichols DH, Clarke-Pearson DL: Gynecologic, Obstetric, and Related Surgery, 2nd ed. St. Louis, Mosby, 1999.)

carried out in the avascular vesicocervical space and should continue until the bladder is cleanly separated from the cervix and upper vagina.

If the uterus is mobile enough to be removed through the vagina, the surgeon may choose to stop the laparoscopic portion of the procedure at this point and complete the remainder of the hysterectomy vaginally (i.e., type I laparoscopic hysterectomy). In this case, the patient's legs are repositioned into a high lithotomy position and a standard vaginal hysterectomy technique is used. After removal of the uterus and closure of the vaginal cuff, the operative site should be reinspected laparoscopically to ensure hemostasis. If laparoscopic occlusion of the uterine vessels is necessary or desired, they should first be skeletonized as they enter the uterus. After it is ensured that the ureter is safely away, they are occluded and divided bilaterally (Fig. 29-27). Because of the close proximity of the ureter to the uterine artery and the width of laparoscopic stapler devices, many surgeons prefer bipolar electrocautery for occlusion of the uterine vessels. The vessels should be desiccated in several adjacent areas before they are divided. Again, a surgeon may choose to stop the laparoscopic portion of the procedure at this point and complete the hysterectomy vaginally (i.e., type II laparoscopic hysterectomy).

Anterior and posterior colpotomies are facilitated by the KOH Colpotomizer or a similar device (Fig. 29-28). The cervical cup of these devices elevates the vaginal fornices and provides a backstop for monopolar cautery. The inflatable balloon below the cup prevents loss of pneumoperitoneum after entry into the vagina. A monopolar hook or similar device is used to detach the uterus from the vagina. The ureters should be visualized

Figure 29-19

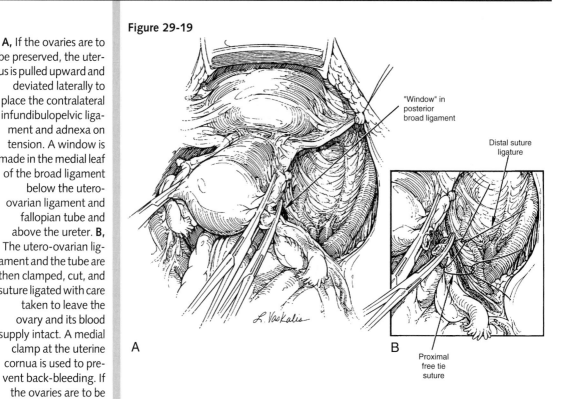

A, If the ovaries are to be preserved, the uterus is pulled upward and deviated laterally to place the contralateral infundibulopelvic ligament and adnexa on tension. A window is made in the medial leaf of the broad ligament below the utero-ovarian ligament and fallopian tube and above the ureter. B, The utero-ovarian ligament and the tube are then clamped, cut, and suture ligated with care taken to leave the ovary and its blood supply intact. A medial clamp at the uterine cornua is used to prevent back-bleeding. If the ovaries are to be removed, a window is made in the medial leaf of the broad ligament below the infundibulopelvic ligament and above the ureter, cephalad to the ovary and tube. The infundibulopelvic ligament is doubly clamped, cut, and ligated. If the ovary is suspicious for malignancy, it can now be removed from its uterine attachments and the specimen sent for frozen-section pathology. (From Nichols DH, Clarke-Pearson DL: Gynecologic, Obstetric, and Related Surgery, 2nd ed. St. Louis, Mosby, 1999.)

throughout to prevent injury. Once the uterus is detached, it can be removed through the vagina and the balloon or a wet Kerlix reinserted to reestablish the pneumoperitoneum. If the uterus is too large to be removed via the vagina, a laparoscopic morcellation should be used for uterine removal. In the case of a total laparoscopic hysterectomy, the vaginal cuff is closed with absorbable suture using laparoscopic suturing techniques.

After the vaginal cuff has been closed, the pelvis should be copiously irrigated with normal saline or lactated Ringer's solution. Additional hemostasis is obtained with electrocautery or suturing as needed. If there is any concern about lower urinary tract or ureteral injury, cystoscopy with administration of intravenous indigo carmine dye is warranted. Lateral trocars are removed under direct visualization. Fascial closure is required for trocar sites 10 mm or greater in diameter. All skin incisions are closed with subcuticular closure and/or Steri-Strips.

SUBTOTAL HYSTERECTOMY

Subtotal (i.e., supracervical) hysterectomies, in which the uterus is removed and the cervix left *in situ*, make up approximately 6% of hysterectomies performed in the United States. In some cases, there is pelvic pathology that makes cervical removal challenging (e.g., obliterated cul-de-sac from

Figure 29-20

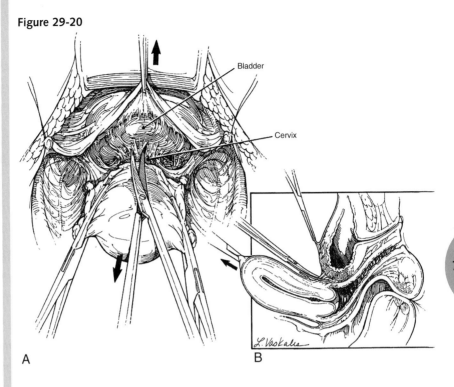

Dissecting the bladder flap. **A,** The pelvic peritoneum is incised by dividing the round ligaments and extending the peritoneal incision cephalad to expose the sidewall retroperitoneal structures. It is then carried along the anterior broad ligament and across the vesicouterine fold. The bladder is then sharply dissected off the lower uterine segment and cervix using Metzenbaum scissors. This dissection is carried out in the vesicocervical space, an avascular plane that exists between the lower uterine section and the bladder, and should continue until the bladder is cleanly separated from the cervix and upper vagina. **B,** Sagittal view. (From Nichols DH, Clarke-Pearson DL: Gynecologic, Obstetric, and Related Surgery, 2nd ed. St. Louis, Mosby, 1999.)

735

endometriosis) and the decision to perform a subtotal hysterectomy is made intraoperatively. In most cases, however, subtotal hysterectomy is performed electively.

There has been considerable debate in both the medical literature and the lay press about the effect of cervical removal at the time of hysterectomy. Advocates of subtotal hysterectomy suggest that cervical removal results in decreased sexual function, adverse bladder function, increased operative time, increased postoperative morbidity, vaginal shortening, and vaginal vault prolapse. Several mechanisms of how cervical removal could adversely affect sexual function and bladder function have been postulated, including disruption of the parasympathetic and sympathetic nerve fibers that pass from the cervix through the Frankenhäuser plexus and pelvic nerves that arise from the second through fourth sacral nerve roots.

Until recently, information about the relative risks and benefits of subtotal hysterectomy has been based on retrospective studies and nonrandomized comparisons. In the last 3 years, however, several well-designed prospective randomized trails comparing total abdominal hysterectomy to subtotal abdominal hysterectomy have been reported. None of these trials demonstrated an advantage of subtotal hysterectomy with regard to sexual function. One trial suggests bladder function is superior in persons who have their cervix removed. Thakar and colleagues performed a multicenter randomized double-blind clinical trial of total and subtotal abdominal hysterectomy in 279 women. They demonstrated an improvement in urinary frequency, nocturia, and stress urinary

Figure 29-21

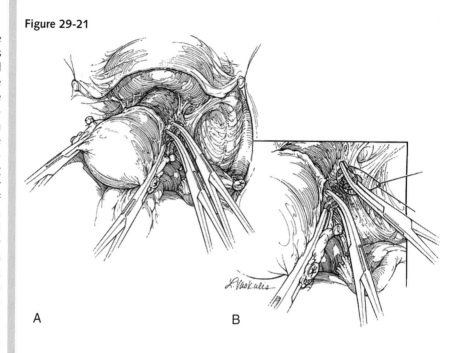

A   B

Clamping the uterine vessels. The uterus is pulled cephalad and deviated to one side of the pelvis to place the contralateral cardinal ligaments on stretch. The uterine vessels are skeletonized by removing the adjacent areolar connective tissue. If necessary, the rectum should be mobilized from the posterior cervix using sharp dissection. **A,** Using a Heaney clamp, the uterine vessels are clamped perpendicularly at the cervicouterine junction (level of the internal cervical os). When placing the clamp, it should roll off the uterus to ensure that the tip is as close to the uterus as possible. A second clamp is placed medially to prevent back-bleeding. The uterine vessels are cut and suture ligated bilaterally. **B,** The vessels are then divided and suture ligated with 0-Vicryl suture. (From Nichols DH, Clarke-Pearson DL: Gynecologic, Obstetric, and Related Surgery, 2nd ed. St. Louis, Mosby, 1999.)

incontinence in both groups, with no difference between the two groups 12 months after surgery. Sexual function and bowel function did not change significantly in either group. Women who received a subtotal abdominal hysterectomy had a shorter operative time, fewer short-term complications, and a shorter hospital stay, but 7% had persistent cyclic bleeding and 2% developed cervical prolapse beyond the introitus. A smaller randomized trial performed in the United States found no significant differences in surgical complications or clinical outcomes between subtotal and total abdominal hysterectomy after 2 years of follow-up. Hysterectomy by either technique led to significant reductions in most symptoms, including pelvic pain, back pain, urinary incontinence, and voiding dysfunction. In contrast, a Danish trial of 319 patients found that women who received a total abdominal hysterectomy were less likely to have urinary incontinence than those who underwent subtotal abdominal hysterectomy 1 year after surgery (9% versus 18%). Additionally, 20% of those who received a subtotal hysterectomy had persistent vaginal bleeding postoperatively. There are no randomized trials comparing laparoscopic hysterectomy to laparoscopic subtotal hysterectomy.

A recent normal Pap smear result is a prerequisite for a subtotal hysterectomy. Patients with cervical dysplasia or other significant cervical pathology are not candidates for this procedure. Patients who desire a subtotal hysterectomy should be informed that Pap smears will need to be continued after surgery at regular intervals and that there is a risk of persistent cyclic bleeding in 3% to 20% of patients. The technique for subtotal abdominal hysterectomy is similar to that of total abdominal hysterectomy until after the uterine vessels have been ligated bilaterally. Once the uterine vessels have been ligated, electrocautery is used to transect the

Figure 29-22

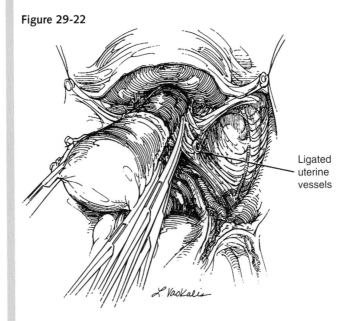

Ligated uterine vessels

The cardinal and uterosacral ligaments are sequentially clamped, cut, and suture ligated using straight Heaney clamps. Each clamp is placed inside the last to prevent ureteral injury. (From Nichols DH, Clarke-Pearson DL: Gynecologic, Obstetric, and Related Surgery, 2nd ed. St. Louis, Mosby, 1999.)

Figure 29-23

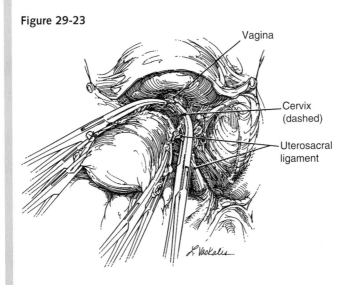

Vagina

Cervix (dashed)

Uterosacral ligament

Cross-clamping the upper vagina and uterosacral ligament complex. When the tip of the cervix is encountered, curved Heaney clamps are placed bilaterally across the uterosacral ligaments and upper vagina just below the cervix. The cervix is then amputated from the upper vagina with scissors. The incision is made as close to the cervix as possible to preserve vaginal depth. (From Nichols DH, Clarke-Pearson DL: Gynecologic, Obstetric, and Related Surgery, 2nd ed. St. Louis, Mosby, 1999.)

uterine fundus from the cervix below the level of the internal os and above the ligated uterine vessels. Wedging the cervix out in a shallow "V" anterior to posterior facilitates cervical stump closure. The endocervical canal is desiccated with monopolar cautery (40 Watts modulated coagulation current) to decrease the risk of persistent endometrial tissue and cyclic bleeding. The cervical stump is closed with several interrupted figure-of-eight delayed absorbable sutures. The technique for laparoscopic subtotal hysterectomy is similar. After the uterine arteries have been occluded and divided, the uterus is amputated at the level of the internal cervical os with a monopolar hook electrode or similar device. The uterine fundus is then removed via colpotomy or laparoscopic uterine morcellation. The endocervical canal is

Figure 29-24

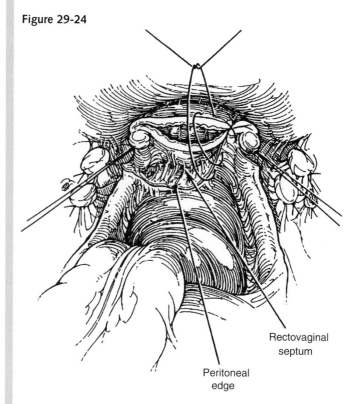

Closing of the vaginal cuff. The edges of the open vaginal cuff are grasped with Allis or Kocher clamps, and the vaginal cuff is closed with a running locked absorbable suture or with interrupted figure-of-eight sutures. The uterosacral ligaments can be incorporated to the vaginal apices using the technique described by Richardson. If the uterus is large and bulky, making visualization difficult, it is often useful to remove the uterine corpus by transecting it from the cervix above the ligated uterine vessels with a scalpel or cautery. The remaining cervix is then grasped with a single tooth tenaculum and removed with improved visualization. (From Nichols DH, Clarke-Pearson DL: Gynecologic, Obstetric, and Related Surgery, 2nd ed. St. Louis, Mosby, 1999.)

Rectovaginal septum

Peritoneal edge

desiccated with monopolar energy, and hemostasis of the cervical stump is ensured by electrocautery and/or laparoscopic suturing.

CONCURRENT PROCEDURES

Prophylactic Oophorectomy

Elective bilateral oophorectomy is performed in 40% to 66% of hysterectomies in women older than 40 years of age, primarily as a prophylaxis for ovarian cancer. Factors that affect the decision to perform a prophylactic oophorectomy at the time of hysterectomy include age, cancer risk, menopausal status, risk of osteoporosis or cardiovascular disease, and the patient's willingness to take estrogen replacement therapy. Prophylactic oophorectomy is effective in preventing ovarian cancer and appears to add minimal additional surgical morbidity when performed with a hysterectomy. In women scheduled for hysterectomy who are postmenopausal, the benefits of prophylactic oophorectomy likely outweigh the risks. In premenopausal and even perimenopausal patients this is less clear, especially given the recent data from the Women's Health Initiative and other studies demonstrating an increased risk of breast cancer and cardiovascular disease in women who take hormone replacement therapy. In women scheduled

Figure 29-25

Ligation of the utero-ovarian ligament during laparoscopic hysterectomy. (From Nichols DH, Clarke-Pearson DL: Gynecologic, Obstetric, and Related Surgery, 2nd ed. St. Louis, Mosby, 1999.)

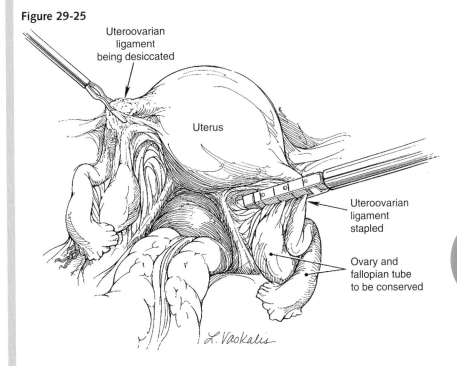

Figure 29-26

Bladder flap dissection during laparoscopic hysterectomy. (From Nichols DH, Clarke-Pearson DL: Gynecologic, Obstetric, and Related Surgery, 2nd ed. St. Louis, Mosby, 1999.)

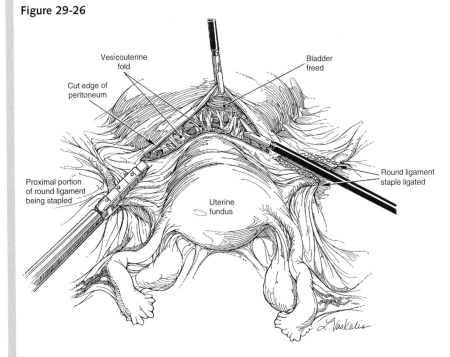

for a hysterectomy who are younger than 45 years old and have not yet undergone menopause, the risks of prophylactic oophorectomy likely outweigh the benefits. One exception to this is a hereditary predisposition to ovarian cancer, such as *BRCA1* mutation, wherein the lifetime risk of ovarian cancer is as high as 16% to 54%. In women older than 45 years of age and women showing signs of perimenopause, it is important to discuss the relative risks and benefits of prophylactic oophorectomy before surgery.

Figure 29-27

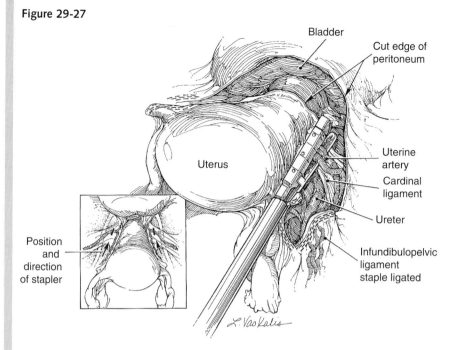

Laparoscopic ligation of the uterine vasculature. (From Nichols DH, Clarke-Pearson DL: Gynecologic, Obstetric, and Related Surgery, 2nd ed. St. Louis, Mosby, 1999.)

Figure 29-28

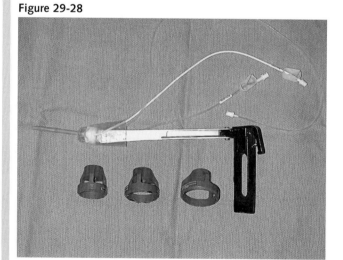

KOH uterine manipulator.

Although prophylactic oophorectomy eliminates the great majority of cancer risk, rare cases of primary peritoneal cancer, which behaves much like ovarian cancer, have been seen in women after ovarian removal. Ovarian cancer is the fourth leading cause of cancer death in American women, with 14,000 deaths annually. Because the majority of patients with ovarian cancer present in advanced stages of the disease and there is currently no reliable screening tool, ovarian cancer prevention has been a point of emphasis. One study estimated that approximately 1000 cases of ovarian cancer can be prevented annually if all women older than 40 years who undergo hysterectomy (approximately 300,000) receive a prophylactic oophorectomy. Another study estimated that 700 prophylactic oophorectomies would have to be performed to prevent one case of ovarian cancer. The exact number of ovarian cancers prevented by the current rate of prophylactic oophorectomy is unknown, however. A secondary benefit of elective oophorectomy at the time of hysterectomy is the potential avoidance of future surgery for benign ovarian disease. One retrospective study of 1200 women who had undergone hysterectomy but retained at least one ovary demonstrated a 4% reoperation rate for benign ovarian disease.

The major risks associated with prophylactic oophorectomy include the potential increased operative risk and the risks associated with premature estrogen deprivation. Studies of abdominal and vaginal hysterectomy demonstrate no increased morbidity when prophylactic oophorectomy is performed. Women who undergo surgical menopause are more likely to experience climacteric symptoms, osteoporosis, and increased cardiovascular disease. Several other risks have been suggested, including increased urinary incontinence and alterations in memory function, but these are less well established. The Maryland Women's Health Study found that performing a bilateral oophorectomy at the time of hysterectomy was associated with significantly poorer outcomes 2 years after surgery. Hormone replacement therapy is effective in treating vasomotor symptoms and preventing osteoporosis but appears to cause a small, but significant, increase in the risk of breast cancer, myocardial infarctions, strokes, and stress urinary incontinence. Preventive measures, other than oophorectomy, that have been shown to reduce the risk of ovarian cancer include use of oral contraceptive pills and hysterectomy alone without oophorectomy. Both have been shown to reduce the risk of ovarian cancer by 40% to 50%. When assessing the risk and benefits of prophylactic oophorectomy, these alternative options should also be considered.

Other Concurrent Procedures

Some surgeons advocate prophylactic appendectomy at the time of hysterectomy to prevent appendicitis and its associated morbidity. Studies have shown that there is no increase in morbidity associated with appendectomy performed at the time of hysterectomy and it adds only 10 minutes to the operative time. However, the peak incidence of appendicitis is between the ages of 20 and 40 years. Because most hysterectomies occur after this time, it is unlikely that prophylactic appendectomy at the time of hysterectomy is an effective prevention strategy. Women who are suspected of having diseased appendix at the time of hysterectomy should undergo concurrent appendectomy.

Gallbladder disease is common among middle-aged women. Studies have shown that cholecystectomy performed at the time of hysterectomy for symptomatic cholelithiasis or cholecystitis does not increase febrile morbidity or length of hospital stay. Similarly, abdominoplasty performed at the time of hysterectomy is associated with a shorter hospital stay, shorter operative time, and lower blood loss than when the two operations are performed separately.

741

COMPLICATIONS

The complication rate of hysterectomy is similar to that of other major abdominal or pelvic surgeries. The mortality rate from hysterectomy is estimated at 0.12 to 0.34 per thousand surgeries. The mortality rate is substantially higher when the hysterectomy is performed for an obstetric indication or for malignancy. The Maryland Women's Health Study, a prospective cohort study of 1299 women undergoing hysterectomy for benign disease, reported that 66.8% had one or more mild complications, 11.1% had one or more moderate complications, and 0.7% had a serious complication. The hospital readmission rate for a reason related to the hysterectomy was 4% during the first year after surgery. The Vaginal Abdominal Laparoscopic Uterine Excision (VALUE) study investigated the complication rate in 37,512 women undergoing hysterectomy for benign disease in United Kingdom and found a 3% risk of severe complications including death, thromboembolic disease, myocardial infarction, stroke, hemorrhage, visceral injury, and end-organ failure. The risk of operative complications in this study increased in women undergoing hysterectomy for fibroids and decreased with increasing age. The lowest complication rate is associated with vaginal hysterectomy. Laparoscopic hysterectomy has the highest rate of intraoperative complications and, like all laparoscopic procedures, has its own set of unique complications related to trocar insertion. The highest-risk groups in the VALUE study were younger women who underwent laparoscopic hysterectomy for fibroids and those with a history of serious comorbidities.

Hemorrhage

The most common intraoperative complications of hysterectomy are hemorrhage and lower urinary tract injury. Although the definition of hemorrhage is somewhat arbitrary, most would consider a blood loss of greater than 1000 mL or need for a blood transfusion as acceptable criteria. Using this definition, the risk of hemorrhage at hysterectomy is approximately 1% to 5%. A systematic review performed by the Cochrane Collaboration found no differences in transfusion rate between the abdominal, vaginal, or laparoscopic approaches. The risk of intraoperative bleeding is increased in the presence of extensive endometriosis, malignancy, a uterus enlarged by fibroids (>500 g), and large pelvic masses that obscure the operative field. A hysterectomy performed for an obstetric indication is also at increased risk of excessive blood loss.

Lower Urinary Tract Injury

Lower urinary tract injury, including bladder injury, ureteral injury, and vesicovaginal fistula occurs in approximately 1% to 3% of hysterectomies. There is an increased risk of lower urinary tract injury in women with previous cesarean sections, severe pelvic adhesive disease, pregnancy, malignancy, and those undergoing concurrent urogynecologic procedures. A systematic review of 27 randomized trials found that laparoscopic hysterectomy has a 2.6 times greater risk of lower urinary tract injury than that of abdominal hysterectomy. Some studies have shown an increased risk of bladder injury with vaginal hysterectomy, whereas others have not. The most commonly reported rate of bladder injury after hysterectomy is 1% to 2%. Every effort should be made to recognize bladder injuries intraoperatively so that they can be immediately repaired. Delayed repair is associated with increased morbidity including fever, prolonged hospital stay, ileus, and vesicovaginal fistula. Bladder injuries should be repaired without tension using two layers of small-caliber absorbable suture, such as 2-0 or 3-0 polyglycolic acid. Closures should be watertight, and the bladder should be drained for 3 to 14 days depending on the size and location of the injury.

The risk of ureteral injury is 0.2% to .08% after abdominal hysterectomy, 0.05% to 0.1% after vaginal hysterectomy, and 0.2% to 3.4% after laparoscopic hysterectomy. The most common location of ureteral injury at the time of hysterectomy is the distal 3 to 4 cm of the ureter as it passes under the uterine artery and travels through the cardinal ligament to enter the bladder. Injury can also occur at or below the infundibulopelvic ligament and along the pelvic sidewall just above the uterosacral ligament. The ability to adequately identify ureteral injuries at the time of the initial operation is of paramount importance. Permanent damage can, in most cases, be avoided if the diagnosis of the ureteral injury is made at the time of surgery. Delay can put the patient at risk of permanent loss of renal function and ureterovaginal fistula. Studies have shown that the intraoperative recognition and repair decreases postoperative morbidity, minimizes loss of kidney function and need for nephrectomy, and decreases the incidence of ureterovaginal fistula development compared with postoperative diagnosis and delayed repair of ureteral injuries. If a ureteral injury is suspected or if the patient is at high risk of a ureteral injury, intraoperative cystoscopy with intravenous indigo carmine dye is an effective method of confirming ureteral patency. In fact, some authors have advocated routine use of intraoperative cystoscopy for all hysterectomies. Visco and colleagues evaluated the cost-effectiveness of this strategy and found that when the risk of ureteral injury was greater than 1.5%, routine cystoscopy at the time of hysterectomy resulted in a cost savings. For abdominal hysterectomies, where the average rate of ureteral injury is 0.5%, 200 cystoscopies would need to be performed to diagnose one ureteral injury intraoperatively, and would cost a total of $16,600 for each ureteral injury diagnosed. The medicolegal costs associated with an unrecognized ureteral injury were not included in this analysis. Based on these data, it seems prudent to perform intraoperative cystoscopy routinely during procedures in which the risk of lower urinary tract injury is high, such as during laparoscopic hysterectomy; those in which the average risk is approximately 1.5%; or during cases involving malignancy, severe adhesions, or distorted anatomy requiring extensive sidewall dissection.

Vesicovaginal Fistulas

Vesicovaginal fistulas are a rare complication of hysterectomy with an incidence of 0.1% to 0.2%; hysterectomy is the most common cause of vesicovaginal fistula in the United States. Although many of the factors listed above increase the risk of fistula development, most posthysterectomy vesicovaginal fistulas occur after an apparently uncomplicated total abdominal hysterectomy for benign disease. Steps to avoid fistula formation include identification of the proper plane between the bladder and cervix; use of sharp dissection to develop the bladder flap rather than blunt dissection or use of electrocautery, ensuring that the bladder is dissected below the level that the cervix will be transected from the vagina; and intraoperative identification of any lower urinary tract injury using the techniques previously outlined. Animal studies suggest that vesicovaginal fistulas result from unrecognized bladder injuries. Unrecognized suture placement into the bladder at the time of cuff closure is unlikely to result in fistula formation in the absence of a concurrent bladder laceration. Patients who develop a vesicovaginal fistula typically have a difficult early postoperative course followed by development of watery drainage from the vagina 10 to 14 days after surgery. If not readily apparent on vaginal examination, the diagnosis can be made by instilling the bladder with dilute methylene blue or indigo carmine dye and placing a tampon into the vagina. If the dye is noted on the tampon, then a fistula is confirmed. If there is no dye apparent, ureterovaginal fistula must be ruled out by intravenous administration of indigo carmine dye or radiologic evaluation of the ureter with an intravenous pyelogram or computed tomography scan. Small fistulas may heal spontaneously after 6 to 12 weeks of continuous bladder drainage. For those that do not heal spontaneously, surgical repair is required.

Bowel Injury

Bowel injury occurs in 0.1% to 1% of hysterectomies. Injury to the small intestines occurs most commonly during entry into the abdomen at the time of abdominal or laparoscopic hysterectomy, typically in patients with abdominal wall adhesions. Small lacerations can be closed in two layers with small-caliber sutures. For the first layer, 3-0 absorbable suture is used to approximate the mucosa. For the second layer, interrupted 3-0 suture, often silk, is used to reinforce the serosa. Lacerations should be closed transversely in relation to the bowel lumen to avoid narrowing. Large lacerations or evidence of devascularization require small bowel resection. Rectal injuries occur most often at the time vaginal hysterectomy or in cases of an obliterated posterior cul-de-sac from malignancy or endometriosis. In a patient who has had an adequate bowel preparation, small lacerations can be repaired with a two-layer closures. Large lacerations may require rectal resection or diverting colostomy.

Febrile Morbidity

The most common postoperative complication of hysterectomy is febrile morbidity, which occurs in 10% to 20% of women. Women undergoing abdominal hysterectomy have approximately 2.5 times the risk of postoperative fever as those undergoing vaginal or laparoscopic hysterectomy. Excessive blood loss during the hysterectomy is also a strong predictor of postoperative febrile morbidity. Fevers after hysterectomy can occur for the following reasons: (1) an operative site infection such as a vaginal cuff cellulitis, pelvic abscess, or abdominal wound infection; (2) an infection remote from the operative site, such as a pneumonia or urinary tract infection; or (3) the fever may be unexplained and resolve without consequence (50% of all posthysterectomy fevers). In the past, such unexplained fevers after pelvic surgery were often attributed to pulmonary atelectasis. However, recent evidence suggests that most unexplained postoperative fevers are the result of an increase in interleukins and cytokines rather than being pulmonary in origin. Regardless of the cause, a postoperative fever after hysterectomy increases the hospital stay an average of 1 to 2 days. Infections with an associated abscess or fluid collection such as an abdominal wound infection or pelvic abscess require surgical drainage. In the case of the posthysterectomy pelvic abscess, this can often be accomplished transvaginally; however, computed tomography–guided drainage or surgical exploration is sometimes required. Pelvic abscesses also require a course of intravenous broad-spectrum antibiotics followed by 10 to 14 days of oral antibiotics when the fevers resolve. Vaginal cuff cellulitis is diagnosed in patients who have persistent postoperative fever, vaginal cuff induration, and purulent discharge, without evidence of abscess. Antibiotics are usually adequate therapy. Abdominal wound infections often do not require antibiotics unless there is an associated skin cellulitis. Urinary tract infections are relatively common after hysterectomy; however, they are rarely a source of fever unless the upper urinary tract is involved.

Fallopian Tube Prolapse

Fallopian tube prolapse is a rare but unique complication of hysterectomy. Patients present with vaginal spotting, postcoital bleeding, and occasionally pelvic pain or dyspareunia. On examination, fallopian tube prolapse is often confused with granulation tissue at the vaginal cuff. In patients who have vaginal cuff granulation tissue that does not resolve after repeated efforts of cauterization or removal and in patients in whom the diagnosis is unclear, a biopsy should be performed. Fallopian tube prolapse is easily treated by transvaginal excision in the operating room.

OUTCOMES OF HYSTERECTOMY

In general, hysterectomy is a highly effective treatment for many gynecologic disorders. The Maryland Women's Health Study reported that preoperative symptoms resolved completely or mostly in 95.8% and 96% of women, respectively, 12 and 24 months after hysterectomy. An overall improvement in health was seen in 85.3% and 81.6% of women 12 and 24 months after surgery, respectively. Other studies have confirmed these findings, suggesting that hysterectomy significantly reduces the symptoms of abnormal menstrual bleeding, pelvic pain, dyspareunia, and urinary symptoms. Significant improvement in mood states (such as depression and anxiety) and overall quality of life have been consistently demonstrated after hysterectomy. However, new pelvic or psychological symptoms develop in 4% to 12% of patients after hysterectomy, with menopausal symptoms being most common. Preoperative depression and pelvic pain appear to increase the risk of poor outcome after hysterectomy, especially when they coexist. The majority of patients with these conditions still show substantial improvements in symptoms, however. Low socioeconomic status and concurrent bilateral oophorectomy have also been shown to increase the risk of adverse outcome in some studies.

Bleeding

Hysterectomy always provides a definitive cure of irregular or excessive menstrual bleeding. The exception is subtotal hysterectomy, in which cyclic bleeding can be seen in 3% to 20% of patients postoperatively. Hysterectomy should be considered a second-line therapy in most cases of abnormal menstrual bleeding because it results in permanent loss of fertility and has greater risk, higher cost, and longer recovery time than most alternative treatments. Hormonal therapies (such as oral contraceptive pills and oral or intramuscular medroxyprogesterone acetate) and nonsteroidal anti-inflammatory medications (particularly mefenamic acid and naproxen sodium) effectively treat abnormal menstrual bleeding in many patients. However, a significant proportion of patients eventually require further treatment including hysterectomy. The Maine Women's Health Study prospectively evaluated a cohort of women with abnormal uterine bleeding over a 1-year period treated medically. Overall, they had a significant improvement in symptoms and quality of life. However, 23% underwent a hysterectomy in the 12-month follow-up period.

Few randomized clinical trials comparing medical therapy to hysterectomy for treatment of abnormal menstrual bleeding exist. One study randomly assigned 63 premenopausal women who had failed previous treatment with medroxyprogesterone acetate for excessive menstrual bleeding to receive either hysterectomy or expanded medical therapy, typically oral contraceptive pills with or without nonsteroidal anti-inflammatory drugs. During the 2 years of follow-up, 53% of those who received expanded medical treatment eventually underwent hysterectomy. Those who received hysterectomy had greater improvement in their symptoms and quality of life. A large randomized trial of 236 women aged 35 to 49 years with excessive menstrual bleeding compared hysterectomy to a levonorgestrel-releasing intrauterine system (LG-IUS). After 5 years of follow-up, both groups reported high (>90%) satisfaction with treatment. In those who received the LG-IUS, 75% reported amenorrhea or minimal spotting; however, 42% of subjects eventually underwent a hysterectomy during the follow-up period.

Endometrial ablation is an effective alternative to hysterectomy for treatment of excessive menstrual bleeding. To date, there have been five randomized trials with a total of 752 participants comparing either abdominal or vaginal hysterectomy to endometrial ablation in women with abnormal uterine bleeding. Compared with hysterectomy, endometrial ablation is associated with a shorter operative time, shorter recovery period, and lower postoperative complication rate. However, whereas hysterectomy eliminates menstrual bleeding, endometrial ablation results in amenorrhea in only in 45% of patients and recurrent excessive bleeding is seen in 15% to 25% of cases. Approximately 9% to 34% of patients who receive endometrial ablation subsequently undergo hysterectomy. A systematic review performed by the Cochrane Collaboration found that hysterectomy had a significant advantage over endometrial ablation for the improvement in anemia as well as overall satisfaction and general health up to 4 years after surgery. The overall cost of endometrial ablation was lower than that of hysterectomy, but the cost differences narrow over time because of the need for retreatment or eventual hysterectomy in a proportion of those who receive ablation. Alternatives to hysterectomy for treatment of abnormal bleeding in women with uterine fibroids include uterine fibroid embolization and myomectomy. The relative advantages and disadvantages of these therapies were discussed earlier in this chapter. Randomized trials comparing these therapies with hysterectomy do not yet exist.

Pelvic Pain

Hysterectomy is an effective therapy for carefully selected patients with chronic pelvic pain. However, unlike abnormal menstrual bleeding, symptom relief is not guaranteed, with as many as 22% of patients having persistent pelvic pain after surgery. Medical management of chronic pelvic pain, including oral contraceptive pills, anti-inflammatory drugs, and analgesics result in a significant improvement in pain and quality of life. However, after 1 year of therapy, approximately half will still report significant pelvic pain and almost one quarter will undergo a hysterectomy. Hysterectomy provides an effective therapy for many women with pelvic pain whose conditions fail to respond to nonsurgical management. In the Maine Women's Health Study, 65% of subjects reported some degree of pelvic pain before hysterectomy. Twelve months after surgery, only 5% of these had persistent pelvic pain. Back pain, dyspareunia, and abdominal bloating also improved significantly after hysterectomy. Three percent of patients in this study developed new pelvic pain during the 1-year follow-up period. Similarly, the Maryland Women's Health Study found that 88.5% and 89.4% of women with pelvic pain who underwent hysterectomy were relieved of pain at 1 and 2 years after surgery, respectively. Fewer than 4% of patients acquired new pelvic pain during the 2-year study period. In this study, women with pelvic pain fared less well after hysterectomy than those who had hysterectomy for other reasons, particularly if they also had depression. However, substantial improvements in symptoms and quality of life were still seen in this patient group. Two randomized trials comparing total abdominal hysterectomy to subtotal abdominal hysterectomy also demonstrated a substantial improvement in pelvic pain postoperatively, with no difference between groups. In contrast, the trial by Thakar et al. had very few patients with pelvic pain at baseline but found a significant increase in general pain scores in both groups 1 year after surgery.

In patients who undergo hysterectomy for pelvic pain and endometriosis, concomitant removal of the ovaries is an important predictor of satisfactory pain relief. A retrospective study of 138 patients who had a hysterectomy for pelvic pain and endometriosis at Johns Hopkins University found that in women that had a hysterectomy with bilateral oophorectomy only 10% had persistent or recurrent pelvic pain and 3.7% required reoperation. In contrast, those who underwent hysterectomy with ovarian conservation had 6.1 times greater risk of developing recurrent pain and 8.1 times greater risk of reoperation. Use of hormone replacement after total abdominal hysterectomy with bilateral oophorectomy for pelvic pain and endometriosis is associated with a very low risk of recurrent pelvic pain (0.9% per year).

Sexual Function

Although there has been considerable debate about the effect of hysterectomy on sexual function, current evidence suggests that hysterectomy results in improved or unchanged sexual function in the majority of women in the first 1 to 2 years after surgery. Only a small proportion of women will have a decline in sexual function after hysterectomy during this time period. Available research provides information about the short-term effect of hysterectomy on dyspareunia, frequency of intercourse, orgasm, libido/sexual interest, vaginal dryness, and overall sexual function. The long-term effect of hysterectomy on sexual function is largely unknown.

Studies that address the effect of hysterectomy on dyspareunia demonstrate either no change or an improvement in this symptom in the majority of women. The Maryland Women's Health Study demonstrated a significant decline in the number of women who reported dyspareunia 12 and 24 months after hysterectomy compared with the preoperative period. Eighty-one percent of the women in this study who experienced frequent dyspareunia preoperatively had an improvement in this symptom at 24 months after hysterectomy, whereas only 1.9% of women without preoperative dyspareunia developed it by 24 months after surgery. In the Maine Women's Health Study, 39% of women reported dyspareunia preoperatively, whereas only 8% had this complaint 12 months after hysterectomy. By comparison, women in this study who were managed nonsurgically showed no decline in the mean frequency of dyspareunia.

Hysterectomy appears to have little impact on the frequency of intercourse. In the Maryland Women's Health Study, the mean number of sexual relations per month increased from 2.3 per month preoperatively to 2.9 per month 24 months after hysterectomy. Another study found that 56% of the subjects in their study reported an increase in sexual frequency 18 months after hysterectomy, whereas 27% reported no change and 17% had a decrease in frequency. Similarly, most well-designed studies that have evaluated libido or sexual interest have demonstrated either no change or an improvement after hysterectomy. In the Maryland Women's Health Study, 70.8% of women with low libido preoperatively were improved 12 months after hysterectomy, whereas only 4.3% of women who had normal libido preoperatively had developed low libido at 12 months after surgery. In the Maine Women's Health Study, 36% of women had decreased sexual interest preoperatively, whereas 8% had this problem 12 months after hysterectomy. The proportion of women who experienced decreased sexual interest as a new symptom postoperatively was not significantly different from the proportion of women with this symptom in a group that was managed nonsurgically.

There is disagreement in the literature on the effect hysterectomy has on postoperative orgasmic function. The Maryland Women's Health Study demonstrated a significant increase in the proportion of women who experienced orgasms after hysterectomy, from 62.8% before surgery to 71.5% 24 months after hysterectomy. However, three smaller prospective cohort studies demonstrated no change in orgasmic function after hysterectomy. Vaginal dryness appears to improve in a small proportion of women after hysterectomy, but most women with preoperative vaginal dryness continue to have this symptom postoperatively. Development of vaginal dryness after hysterectomy when it did not exist preoperatively largely depends on postoperative hormonal status.

As mentioned earlier, randomized trials comparing total abdominal hysterectomy with subtotal hysterectomy have found no advantage of cervical preservation at the time of hysterectomy with regard to sexual function. Similarly, a prospective cohort of 413 women undergoing either vaginal hysterectomy, subtotal abdominal hysterectomy, or total abdominal hysterectomy found significant improvements in sexual pleasure 6 months after surgery in all groups. The persistence and development of bothersome problems during sexual activity were similar for all three techniques. The 2004 *V*aginal *A*bdominal and *L*aparoscopic hysterectomy (eVALuate) study involved two parallel randomized trials—one comparing laparoscopic with abdominal hysterectomy and the other comparing laparoscopic with vaginal hysterectomy. Body image and sexual function were improved in all groups 4 months and 1 year after surgery, with no differences between the three routes of hysterectomy.

Bladder Function

Many studies have demonstrated an adverse effect on bladder function after radical hysterectomy for cervical cancer. The effect of simple or nonradical hysterectomy on lower urinary tract function is less clear, however. A systematic review of the literature published in 2000 relying heavily on observational studies concluded that hysterectomy increased the odds of urinary incontinence by 60% in women older than 60 years. No increased risk was found in younger women. In contrast, the majority of prospective cohort studies that subjectively evaluate lower urinary tract symptoms before and after hysterectomy demonstrate either a significant improvement or no change in bladder symptoms 3 months to 2 years after surgery. The Maine Women's Health Study demonstrated a significant reduction in urinary incontinence, urinary urgency, and urinary frequency 12 months after hysterectomy. In contrast, no significant change in urinary symptoms was seen in the nonsurgically managed population of this cohort. A randomized trial comparing hysterectomy to endometrial ablation found no difference in bladder function 2 years after the procedure.

One randomized trial of total abdominal hysterectomy versus subtotal hysterectomy found urinary symptoms and incontinence were reduced by 44% to 88% from baseline 2 years after surgery, with no differences between groups, whereas another demonstrated a significant reduction in urinary incontinence in the total abdominal hysterectomy group but no reduction in those who received a subtotal hysterectomy. Thakar et al. found that significantly fewer women had stress incontinence, urinary urgency, frequency, nocturia, interrupted stream, and incomplete bladder emptying 1 year after both total and subtotal abdominal hysterectomy, with no difference between groups.

Bowel Function

The effect of hysterectomy on postoperative bowel dysfunction is controversial. In a population-based cross-sectional study of 1058 women, self-reported constipation was significantly more common in subjects with a prior hysterectomy than women without prior hysterectomy (22% and 9%, respectively), as was straining at defecation and a feeling of incomplete emptying. Similarly, a case-control study found that women who had a hysterectomy 2 to 8 years prior were significantly more likely to have decreased bowel frequency than control subjects. In contrast, several prospective cohort studies that evaluated women before and 3 to 12 months after hysterectomy found either no change or an improvement in bowel function postoperatively. The Maine Women's Health Study is the only prospective study to examine this issue that includes a control group of women who did not get a hysterectomy. This study found that 9% of women who received a hysterectomy developed new-onset constipation by 12 months after surgery compared with 1% of women who received nonsurgical management. Randomized comparisons of total and subtotal hysterectomy demonstrate no change in constipation after surgery and no differences between groups.

Pelvic Organ Prolapse

Hysterectomy appears to increase the risk of subsequent pelvic organ prolapse; however, the development of symptomatic prolapse typically occurs many years after the hysterectomy. In a consecutive series of 693 patients who presented to the Mayo Clinic for surgical management of posthysterectomy vaginal vault prolapse, the median time from hysterectomy to prolapse repair was 15.8 years. A retrospective cohort study of 149,554 women aged 20 years and older found that in women who developed pelvic organ prolapse or urinary incontinence, the mean interval between hysterectomy and surgery for prolapse was 19.3 years. The Oxford Family Planning Association study followed up with 17,032 women aged 25 to 39 years for an average of 17 years. The annual incidence of surgery for pelvic organ prolapse was 0.162% per year. In women who had undergone hysterectomy for reasons other than prolapse, surgical incidence rate increased to 0.290% per year. The cumulative risk of prolapse surgery for rose from 1% at 3 years after hysterectomy to 5% 15 years after hysterectomy. Surgical technique at the time of hysterectomy, including the performance of prophylactic culdoplasty, can decrease development of subsequent pelvic organ prolapse as demonstrated in the trial by Cruikshank and Kovac.

Quality of Life and Psychosocial Function

Hysterectomy results in an increased health-related quality of life (HRQOL), improved general health perception, and improved psychological outcomes in a majority of women. A small proportion of women will have decline in quality of life or a worsening of psychological symptoms after undergoing hysterectomy. Both the Maine and Maryland Women's Health studies demonstrated significant improvement in all aspects of HRQOL as well as decreased anxiety and depression 12 to 24 months after hysterectomy. In the Maryland study, nearly three quarters of patients with preoperative depression and two thirds of women with preoperative anxiety no longer had the psychological condition 12 months after their hysterectomy. However, 3% to 12% of patients in the Maine study developed new-onset depression, anxiety, or negative feelings about themselves as women after the hysterectomy. The presence of depression before the hysterectomy appears to be the most important predictor of postoperative depression after surgery. Women younger than the age of 40 years, less-educated women, those with conflicted feelings about childbearing, and those undergoing oophorectomy may also be at higher risk of depression after hysterectomy.

There appears to be no difference in HRQOL improvement with different types of hysterectomy. Trials comparing total and subtotal hysterectomy demonstrate improved HRQOL in both groups. The trial by Thakar et al. also found improvements in anxiety, depression, and social dysfunction 6 and 12 month after surgery, with no difference between those who had their cervix removed and those whose cervix was left *in situ.* Similarly, vaginal, abdominal, and laparoscopic hysterectomy each appear to result in similar improvements in HRQOL, as recently demonstrated in the eVALuate study.

CONCLUSION

In spite of a considerable increase in conservative therapies for benign gynecologic complaints, hysterectomy remains an important and highly effective option for appropriately selected patients. In patients with symptomatic uterine fibroids, excessive menstrual bleeding, chronic pelvic pain, endometriosis, and a variety of other gynecologic conditions, hysterectomy is the treatment of choice for those whose conditions have failed to respond to conservative management. Several recent high-quality studies confirm that hysterectomy not only successfully alleviates the symptoms of these conditions in the majority of women, but also significantly improves quality of life without compromising bowel, bladder, or sexual function.

KEY POINTS

1. Hysterectomy is the second most frequent major operation performed on women in the United States, following only cesarean section. Approximately 42% of women will undergo a hysterectomy during their lifetime.

2. Uterine leiomyomas, uterine prolapse, and endometriosis are the most frequent indications for hysterectomy, accounting for as many as 73% of hysterectomies.

3. In women with uterine leiomyomas, hysterectomy should be reserved for those who are symptomatic and have completed childbearing. Hysterectomy for asymptomatic women with uterine fibroids is rarely indicated regardless of uterine size.

4. In women with excessive uterine bleeding, treatment is indicated when anemia is present or the bleeding interferes with the patient's quality of life. Hysterectomy is only indicated in women who do not desire fertility and have failed a trial of medical management.

5. Uterine prolapse is typically not an isolated event and is often associated with other pelvic support defects. A hysterectomy alone is almost never adequate treatment for prolapse; concurrent surgical prolapse repairs are necessary.

6. In women with chronic pelvic pain, hysterectomy should only be performed if the pain is thought to be of uterine origin and does not respond to nonsurgical management.

7. For benign conditions, route of hysterectomy should largely be determined by vaginal accessibility, uterine size and shape, and the extent of extrauterine disease.

8. Vaginal hysterectomy is associated with fewer complications, decreased postoperative pain, shorter length of stay, speedier return to normal activities, reduced cost, and lower mortality than abdominal hysterectomy. When feasible, vaginal hysterectomy should be the approach of choice.

9. Laparoscopic hysterectomy offers no advantage over vaginal hysterectomy. It should only be considered in patients who are not candidates for vaginal hysterectomy.

10. Laparoscopic hysterectomy is associated with longer operative time and higher risk of urinary tract injury, but less blood loss, fewer wound infections, fewer febrile episodes, and a more rapid postoperative recovery than abdominal hysterectomy.

11. Gonadotropin-releasing hormone agonists given for 3 months prior to hysterectomy should be considered in patients with both uterine fibroids and anemia.

12. All patients undergoing hysterectomy should receive intravenous antibiotics within a 60-minute window before the surgical incision to reduce the risk of postoperative infection.

13. A McCall's culdoplasty should be performed routinely at the time of vaginal hysterectomy to prevent subsequent vaginal vault prolapse.

752

Continued

KEY POINTS—CONT'D

14. Uterine morcellation and intramyometrial coring allow the removal of enlarged uteri through the vagina.

15. There is no advantage of subtotal hysterectomy over total abdominal hysterectomy with regard to sexual function. Patients who undergo subtotal hysterectomy should be counseled about a 3% to 20% risk of cyclic bleeding after surgery.

16. The most common intraoperative complications of hysterectomy are hemorrhage and lower urinary tract injury. The most common postoperative complication is febrile morbidity and infection.

17. When lower urinary tract injury is suspected or the patient is at high risk for lower urinary tract injury, intraoperative cystoscopy should be performed after the administration of intravenous indigo carmine dye.

18. Hysterectomy significantly reduces symptoms of abnormal menstrual bleeding, pelvic pain, and dyspareunia. Significant improvements in mood states such as depression and anxiety and in overall quality of life have been consistently demonstrated after hysterectomy.

19. Hysterectomy results in improved or unchanged sexual function in the majority of women, at least in the short term. The long-term effects of hysterectomy on sexual function are less clear.

20. Preoperative depression and pelvic pain appear to increase the risk of poor outcomes after hysterectomy, especially when they coexist. However, the majority of these patients still show a substantial improvement in symptoms.

SUGGESTED READING

Ballard LA, Walters MD: Transvaginal mobilization and removal of ovaries and fallopian tubes after vaginal hysterectomy. Obstet Gynecol 87:35–39, 1996.

Brown JS, Sawaya G, Thom DH, Grady D: Hysterectomy and urinary incontinence: A systematic review. Lancet 356:535–539, 2000.

Carlson KJ, Miller BA, Fowler FJ: The Maine Women's Heath Study: I. Outcomes of hysterectomy. Obstet Gynecol 83:556–565, 1994.

Carlson KJ, Miller BA, Fowler FJ: The Maine Women's Health Study: II. Outcomes of nonsurgical management of leiomyomas, abnormal bleeding and chronic pelvic pain. Obstet Gynecol 83:566–572, 1994.

Carlson KJ, Nichols DH, Schiff I: Current concepts: Indications for hysterectomy. N Engl J Med 328:856–860, 1993.

Cruikshank SH, Kovac S: Randomized comparison of three surgical methods used at the time of vaginal hysterectomy to prevent posterior enterocele. Am J Obstet Gynecol 180:859–865, 1999.

Dicker RC, Greenspan JR, Strauss LT, et al: Complications of abdominal and vaginal hysterectomy among women of reproductive age in the United States: The collaborative review of sterilization. Am J Obstet Gynecol 144:841–848, 1982.

Garry R, Fountain J, Mason S, et al: The eVALuate study: Two parallel randomized trails, one comparing laparoscopic with abdominal hysterectomy, the other comparing laparoscopic with vaginal hysterectomy. BMJ 328:129–133, 2004.

Hartmann KE, Ma C, Lamvu GM, et al: Quality of life and sexual function after hysterectomy in women with preoperative pain and depression. Obstet Gynecol 104:701–709, 2004.

Heaney NS: A report of 565 vaginal hysterectomies performed for benign pelvic disease. Am J Obstet Gynecol 28:751–755, 1934.

Johnson N, Barlow D, Lethaby A, et al: Surgical approach to hysterectomy for benign disease. Cochrane Database of Systematic Reviews, Vol 1, 2005.

Kjerulff KH, Langenberg PW, Rhodes JC, et al: Effectiveness of hysterectomy. Obstet Gynecol 95:319–326, 2000.

Kovac SR, Barhan S, Lister M, et al: Guidelines for the selection of the route of hysterectomy: Application in a resident clinic population. Am J Obstet Gynecol 187:1521–1527, 2002.

Kuppermann M, Varner RE, Summitt RL, et al: Effect of hysterectomy vs. medical treatment on health-related quality of life and sexual functioning: The Medicine or Surgery (Ms) Randomized Trial. JAMA 291:1447–1455, 2004.

Lethaby A, Vollenhoven B, Sowter M: Preoperative GnRH analogue therapy before hysterectomy or myomectomy for uterine fibroids. Cochrane Database of Systematic Reviews, Vol 4. 2004.

McPherson K, Metcalfe MA, Herbert A, et al: Severe complications of hysterectomy: The VALUE study. BJOG 111:688–694, 2004.

Myers ER, Barber MD, Gustilo-Ashby T, et al: Management of uterine leiomyomata: What do we really know? Obstet Gynecol 100:8–17, 2002.

Parker WH, Fu YS, Berek JS: Uterine sarcoma in patients operated on for presumed leiomyoma and rapidly growing leiomyoma. Obstet Gynecol 83:414–418, 1994.

Rhodes JC, Kjerulff KH, Langenberg PW, Guzinski GM: Hysterectomy and sexual function. JAMA 282:1934–1941, 1999.

Richardson EH: A simplified technique for abdominal panhysterectomy. Surg Gynecol Obstet 48:248, 1929.

Spies JB, Cooper JM, Worthington-Kirsch R, et al: Outcomes of uterine embolization and hysterectomy for leiomyomas: Results of a multicenter study. Am J Obstet Gynecol 191:22–31, 2004.

Stovall TG, Ling FW, Crawford DA: Hysterectomy for chronic pelvic pain of presumed uterine etiology. Obstet Gynecol 75:676–679, 1990.

Thakar R, Ayers S, Clarkson P, et al: Outcomes after total versus subtotal abdominal hysterectomy. N Engl J Med 347:1318–1325, 2002.

Thakar R, Ayers S, Georgakapolou A, et al: Hysterectomy improves quality of life and decreases psychiatric symptoms: A prospective and randomized comparison of total versus subtotal hysterectomy. BJOG 111:1115–1120, 2004.

Visco A, Taber K, Weidner A, et al: Cost-effectiveness analysis of universal cystoscopy at the time of hysterectomy. Obstet Gynecol 97:685–692, 2001.

Weber AM, Walters MD, Schover LR, et al: Functional outcomes and satisfaction after abdominal hysterectomy. Am J Obstet Gynecol 181:530–535, 1999.

30

ENDOSCOPIC APPROACHES TO GYNECOLOGIC DISEASE

Magdy Milad, Frank Tu, Lee Epstein, and Linda D. Bradley

INTRODUCTION

Over the past 25 years, the role of gynecologic endoscopy has evolved from limited diagnostic procedures to a major surgical tool used to treat a multitude of gynecologic indications. Laparoscopy, hysteroscopy, and cystoscopy have become common surgical instruments used by gynecologists. Endoscopic surgery requires familiarity with instrumentation, a fundamental knowledge of how the equipment works, and the ability to troubleshoot and complete the procedure in an efficient and safe manner. Endoscopic surgeons must overcome the loss of depth, tactile perception, and optical idiosyncrasies. However, there are inherent benefits of endoscopes including magnification and the ability to overcome angles. Endoscopic technology has advanced with the innovation of video cameras and improved optical lenses coupled with improved instrumentation. There is also increasing pressure from patients to offer endoscopic therapies for both benign and possibly malignant disease.

LAPAROSCOPY

History Laparoscopy was first performed in animals in the early 1900s, and the Swedish surgeon Jacobaeus coined the term *laparoscopy (laparothorakoskopie)* in 1901. In 1929, Heinz Kalk, a German gastroenterologist, founded the German School of Laparoscopy. Kalk developed a 135-degree lens system and a dual-trocar approach. He used laparoscopy as a diagnostic method for liver and gallbladder disease. In 1939, he published his experience of 2000 liver biopsies performed using local anesthesia without mortality. By the 1960s, better techniques developed and laparoscopy was accepted as a safe and valuable procedure. In the late 1970s, laparoscopy was being applied to the treatment of ectopic pregnancies and endometriosis. Now, technology and equipment have advanced to include the use of laparoscopy in total and subtotal hysterectomies, complex anti-incontinence procedures, and operations for gynecologic malignancies.

Principles of Electrosurgery

Electricity has multiple applications in endoscopic surgery; an array of electrosurgical instruments is available to the endoscopic surgeon. It is therefore important for endoscopic surgeons to understand the properties of electricity and the instruments that use it as an energy source.

Physics

Electricity refers to the flow of electrons within an electric circuit. A circuit is a pathway for electrons to flow from a source of electrons (anode) to a reservoir that collects them (cathode or ground). The electrons can only move if the circuit is complete. The difference between electrocautery and electrosurgery is commonly misunderstood. *Electrocautery* is defined as direct electric current (electrons flow in one direction) traveling in an unbroken circuit. A wire gets heated by this current and is used for cauterization of tissue. The patient is not part of the circuit, and all tissue effect is a result of the heat of the wire itself. Electrocautery is not commonly used in the modern surgical suite. During electrosurgery, alternating electric current is used (electrons flow in both directions) along a circuit that is completed by the patient. In alternating current, the electrons move both forward and backward along a circuit in a distinct wave pattern (Fig. 30-1). This alternating current is characterized by its frequency, which is the number of cycles per second, with 1 cycle per second defined as 1 Hertz (Hz). Both monopolar and bipolar electric devices use an alternating current.

The electric energy used in electrosurgery causes rapid movement of the ions within a cell. This rapid movement leads to heat formation and ultimate tissue effect. By changing the waveform of energy applied to the tissue, both the rate of temperature change as well as the final temperature reached can be manipulated. It is these factors, the rate of temperature change

Figure 30-1

Anatomy of alternating current. (From Hulka JF, Reich H: Textbook of Laparoscopy, 3rd ed. Philadelphia, W.B. Saunders, 1998.)

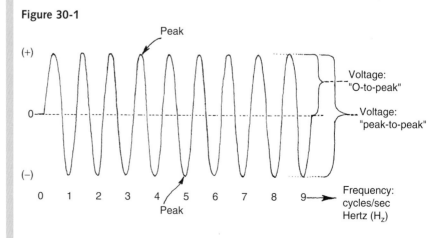

and the final temperature achieved, that determine tissue effect. Since the neuromuscular junction will depolarize with electric stimulation below 10,000 Hz, it is important to operate with a frequency high enough to bypass this effect. Because of this, electrosurgical generators convert household 60-Hz current into 300-kHz to 2.5-mHz current, with no clear benefit in using frequencies over 300 kHz. These frequencies are in the radiofrequency range and, therefore, electrosurgery is sometimes referred to as *radiofrequency surgery.*

Waveforms

The waveforms of energy used include nonmodulated current (cutting), modulated current (coagulation), and blended current. The tissue effects include desiccation, fulguration, and vaporization. It is unfortunate that the manufacturers of electrosurgical devices have coined the terms *cut* and *coag* to describe electrosurgical waveforms. To the electrosurgical novice, it creates confusion between desired tissue effect and desired waveform of energy to use. We will now clarify the distinction between energy waveforms (cut and coag) and desired tissue effect (desiccation, fulguration, and vaporization).

757

Nonmodulated Current

In nonmodulated current (cutting), there is a constant sine wave of high frequency but relatively low-voltage current. This waveform has a higher current density than other waveforms, allowing the overall voltage to be lower than either modulated or blended currents without sacrificing power. The constant nature of this current allows the formation of a plasma pocket between the electrode and the tissue, creating a low-resistance pathway on which energy can travel. This low-resistance pathway allows the deposit of large amounts of energy in a single place (high current density) resulting in superheating of the tissue with intracellular steam formation and cell lysis. This tissue effect is called *vaporization* and is only possible with nonmodulated current.

Modulated Current

A modulated current (coagulating) consists of bursts of high-voltage current that are only "on" 6% of the time. These bursts of high-voltage current cause less heat to build up within the tissue since the tissue has time to cool between bursts. This encourages formation of a coagulum. The high voltages used in modulated current also carry with them a higher risk of sparking and short circuit formation.

Blended Current

Blended current is not a true blend of nonmodulated and modulated current. In blend mode, the generator produces longer bursts of energy at a lower voltage than with simple modulated current. In the blend mode, the current is activated between 50% and 80% of the time. Tissue effects similarly fall in between those of the modulated and nonmodulated currents. See Figure 30-2 for a demonstration of this concept. Note that as the burst time decreases the voltage applied increases. Tables 30-1 and 30-2 compare the tissue effects and factors affecting the biologic effect of applied currents.

Figure 30-2

Clinical currents.
(From Hulka JF, Reich
H: Textbook of
Laparoscopy, 3rd ed.
Philadelphia, W.B.
Saunders, 1998.)

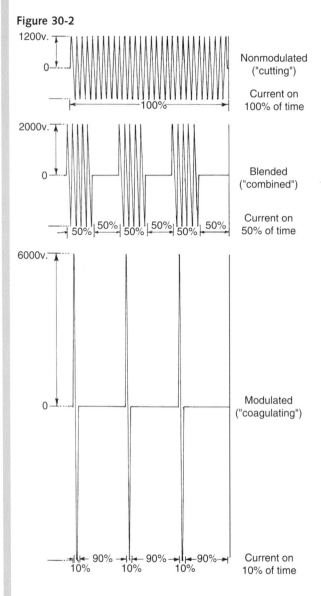

Nonmodulated
("cutting")

Current on
100% of time

Blended
("combined")

Current on
50% of time

Modulated
("coagulating")

Current on
10% of time

Table 30-1

Tissue Effects of
Electrosurgery

Tissue Effect	Explanation
Desiccation	When tissue is slowly heated above 100°C, the water content within the cell evaporates.
Fulguration	Electric arcs striking the tissue at divergent locations cause a surface charring effect. The rapid but superficial rise in tissue temperature leads to carbonization. This is caused by high-voltage current, an effective means of attaining surface hemostasis.
Vaporization	''Cut'' current is applied to tissue without direct contact using a fine-tipped electrode, resulting in ionization of the air pocket between electrode and tissue, resulting in a plasma pocket (ionized gas). The tissue is superheated in a very short time, causing boiling of intracellular water and cell lysis.

758

Table 30-2

Factor	Comment
Tissue type	The resistance of the tissue (related to water content) affects the ability of the current to pass. Increases in resistance cause a buildup of heat and an increase in the lateral thermal spread of energy. In general, muscle has relatively low resistance and fatty tissue has a high inherent resistance.
Electrode size or current density	A larger electrode, like a ball-tipped electrode, will distribute electric current to a larger area of tissue than an electrode with a smaller needle tip.
Contact time	The longer the active electrode is on, the more heat is generated. As heat increases, so does the lateral thermal spread of energy.
Initiation of current	To fulgurate or vaporize tissue, the electrode must be activated without touching the tissue itself, otherwise desiccation will occur.

Monopolar and Bipolar Electrosurgery

Monopolar electrosurgery is defined as electric current traveling from the surgical handpiece, through the patient, to the larger return electrode (usually located on the thigh). Because of the size discrepancy between the surgical handpiece and the return electrode, the intended effect will occur at the area of highest current density close to the handpiece. The larger return electrode has a much lower current density. This allows the return electrode to collect current without causing tissue damage, although thermal studies have shown a mild increase in skin temperature directly under the return electrode. These systems require a significant amount of voltage (1200 volts) to pass current from the surgical handpiece through the patient to the return electrode. These high voltages carry with them an increased risk of inadvertent tissue damage. Electric current using a monopolar circuit will always travel down the path of least resistance to the return electrode. Therefore, if the surgical handpiece contacts another conductor with less resistance than the intended tissue, such as a metal trocar, the current will preferentially conduct to the trocar and any tissue touching it. This is particularly important in laparoscopic surgery, when the field of vision may exclude portions of the surgical handpiece. The tissue effects of fulguration and vaporization are only possible using monopolar surgery in the noncontact mode.

Bipolar electrosurgery was first described by Greenwood in 1940. Using two equally sized electrodes on the handpiece, alternating current is passed from one electrode through the tissue to the other electrode (Fig. 30-3). Since a much smaller amount of tissue is involved (only the tissue in between the handpiece electrodes) a significantly lower voltage (120 volts) can be used with the same effect. This smaller isolated circuit also significantly decreases the risk of inadvertent tissue damage and capacitance (charge buildup). Although both nonmodulated and modulated waveforms of current can be used, nonmodulated (cutting) is preferred

Figure 30-3

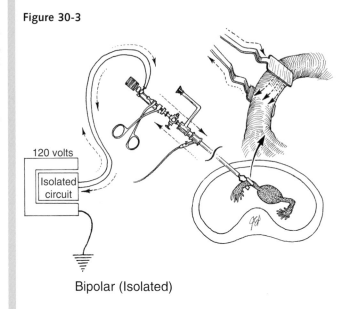

120 volts

Isolated circuit

Bipolar (Isolated)

since it uses lower voltage and is less likely to cause a superficial tissue char impeding complete tissue desiccation.

Preoperative Considerations

Before laparoscopic surgery, it is important to discuss patient expectations as well as the risks associated with surgery. These concerns must be individualized based on the procedure planned and the physiologic state of the patient. To patients, laparoscopic procedures are often considered minor surgery because of the small incisions, decreased postoperative pain, and shorter convalescent period. However, laparoscopy is an intra-abdominal surgery carrying the same risks and complications as a laparotomy. These include the risks of infection, bleeding, and injury to adjacent intra-abdominal structures. Not surprisingly, laparoscopic procedures have unique risks, primarily related to the method of initial entry. Although visceral injury can occur with any method of access, major vascular injury is somewhat limited to laparoscopy. In addition, increased intra-abdominal pressures associated with laparoscopy increase anesthesia-related risks such as aspiration and increased difficulty ventilating the patient. Informed consent should include the risks of unintended laparotomy if a complication occurs, if severe adhesions prevent completion of the procedure, or if undiagnosed cancer is identified.

Preoperative Checklist
The complications of laparoscopic surgery can often be avoided with careful preoperative planning. Patients undergoing elective laparoscopy should typically be NPO (nothing per mouth) for at least 6 hours before surgery. A bowel preparation should be considered in any patient at risk of bowel injury to ensure that the gas and fecal material in the gastrointestinal tract has

been evacuated. This may include patients suspected of endometriosis or adhesions. Four liters of polyethylene glycol electrolyte solution (GoLYTELY, Braintree Laboratories, Braintree, MA) by mouth or sodium phosphate and biphosphate (Fleets Phospho Soda, C.B. Fleet Company, Lynchburg, VA) work equally well to decompress the intestines. Magnesium citrate is also useful for bowel preparation in high-risk patients.

Laboratory studies, electrocardiogram, and other preoperative workup elements should be performed on an individualized basis. In a young, otherwise healthy female patient, a complete blood count is often all that is ordered. Many surgeons recommend routine pregnancy tests for all patients of reproductive age before elective surgery. For some laparoscopic procedures, a blood type and screen is also obtained so that blood is readily available in the rare event it should be needed.

Operating room personnel should be contacted well in advance of the planned procedure to confirm that the needed equipment is available. This might include disposable equipment such as endoscopic loops or bags, as well as specialized instruments such as laparoscopic needle holders or a morcellator.

Before the initial incision, the patient should be positioned, prepared, and draped and the bladder and stomach emptied. A uterine (not cervical) manipulator should be considered to facilitate laparoscopic evaluation and procedures in the posterior cul-de-sac. Attention is then turned to the abdomen. If the patient has risk factors for intra-abdominal adhesions, an alternative site for initial entry should be considered, including the left or right upper quadrant. The operating table should be positioned flat during the initial entry. All methods of entry require an understanding of the tissue layers and an appreciation of the distance from skin to peritoneum. In most women, the umbilical thickness ranges from 1 to 3 cm. However, even among obese patients, the distance to the pocket of gas after insufflation at either entry site rarely exceeds 4 cm. The thickness of the abdominal wall at both the umbilicus and left upper quadrant correlates well with both body mass index and weight (Fig. 30-4).

Figure 30-4

Correlation between body mass index (BMI) and umbilical thickness. Umbilical thickness was measured by the distance the needle traversed from skin edge before an aspirating syringe encountered pneumoperitoneum.

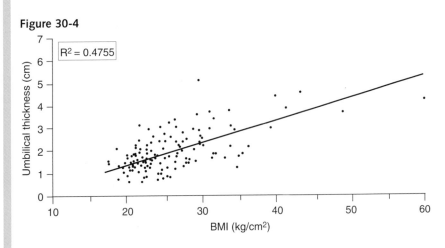

Laparoscopic Equipment

Telescopes/Light Sources/Cameras

Visualization

The most critical feature of pelvic laparoscopy is the ability to visualize the peritoneal cavity despite the limitations of a minimal-access surgical field. A wide variety of narrow-bore telescopes (ranging generally from 2 to 10 mm in diameter) are available to overcome this obstacle (Fig. 30-5). Most cases are performed using a 0-degree telescope, but a 30-degree configuration may be more helpful in certain circumstances. Telescopes featuring an operative port are also available for simple procedures, allowing for single-incision tubal ligation, for example; some also feature an operating laser channel.

Although the surgeon historically placed the telescope lens directly against her eye to inspect the abdominal cavity, modern operative video cameras attach directly to the telescope head to comfortably display the

Figure 30-5

Endoscopes used in gynecologic laparoscopy. (From Bieber EJ, Sanfilippo JS: Laparoscopic instrumentation. In Gershonsen DM, DeCherney AH, Curry SL, Brubaker L [eds]: Operative Gynecology, 2nd ed. Philadelphia, W.B. Saunders, 2001, pp 157–170.)

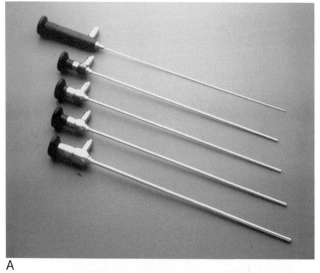

A

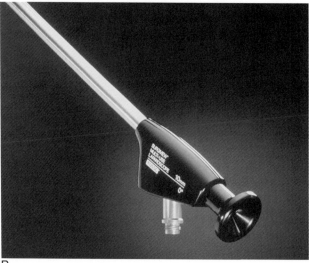

B

operative field on external video monitors; this also allows an assistant to free one of the surgeon's hands for retraction. Overhead flat-top screens flanking each surgeon are ideal because they allow an unencumbered view of the operative field. Illumination of the abdominal cavity is provided via a fiberoptic cable to the telescope. The cables and telescopes must be handled with care because repetitive trauma will inevitably degrade the picture quality afforded with these instruments, as lens and small optic fibers are cracked. Along with the camera head, these should be routinely checked before use to confirm that the optical connections are clear of smudges or fluid, maximizing the clarity of the operative view.

Entry Techniques

Initial Trocar Placement

Nearly all of the well-performed prospective studies on the topic demonstrate that approximately 50% of all major vascular complications and nearly 50% of all bowel injuries occur during the initial entry. This highlights the importance of planning and performing the initial trocar placement. Reducing major vascular injury requires awareness of the short distance from skin to peritoneum, controlled entry during initial penetration, and minimal axial tenting of the anterior abdominal wall during entry.

Numerous techniques exist for placing the initial laparoscopic port into the abdomen. Five common approaches are (1) classic entry with Veres needle insertion followed by primary trocar insertion, (2) direct trocar insertion, (3) open laparoscopy, (4) trocar placement that is radially dilated, and (5) optical trocar insertion. Physician experience significantly contributes to the safety of the individual technique. Both reusable and disposable instruments are available for all types of entry. The choice of instrumentation should take into account the condition of the available reusable equipment and the cost of the disposable equipment.

Veres Needle/Trocar Entry

The umbilicus provides the optimal location for inserting the Veres needle and for the primary trocar. At the level of the umbilicus, the skin of the anterior wall is attached to the fascial layer and anterior parietal peritoneum without any intervening subcutaneous fat or muscle. Therefore, the intraumbilical approach offers the shortest distance between the skin and the peritoneal cavity and can be successfully used even in very obese patients (Fig. 30-6).

The patient should always be in a flat position (not Trendelenburg) during initial trocar insertion to reduce the risk of major vascular injury. During the initial incision, the skin is elevated and a No. 15 blade is used. Injuries have been reported in thin patients with the scalpel at the initial incision. The abdominal wall is then elevated by manually grasping the skin and subcutaneous tissue to maximize the distance between the umbilicus and the retroperitoneal vessels. An alternative method for elevation is to place penetrating towel clips at the base of the umbilicus.

In patients of average weight, the Veres needle is inserted toward the hollow of the sacrum at a 45-degree angle, with the direction described as prouterine. In a very thin patient, the vital structures are much closer

Figure 30-6

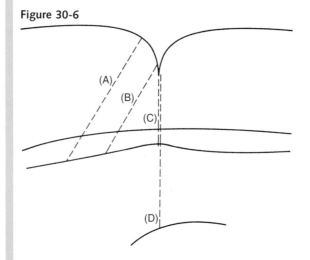

The umbilicus through the sagittal plane shows the much shortened distance from the skin to parietal peritoneum when going straight through the umbilicus (C) compared with the increased distances when the Veres needle is directed in an angle toward the lower pelvis (A and B). Obesity increases this distance for A and B, but not for C. (From Lin P, Grow DR: Complications of laparoscopy: Strategies for prevention and cure. Obstet Gynecol Clin North Am 26:23–38, 1999. Original citation from Hurd WW, Bude RO, DeLancey JOH, et al: Abdominal wall characteristics by MRI and CT imaging: The effect of obesity on laparoscopic approach. J Reprod Med 36:473–476, 1992.)

to the abdominal wall and the margin for error is reduced, with sometimes as little as 4 cm between the skin and large retroperitoneal vessels. In patients who are obese (>200 lb), a more vertical approach, approximately 70 to 80 degrees, is required because of the increased thickness of the abdominal wall. Without the vertical insertion, the trocar would not be long enough to penetrate the layers and enter the peritoneal cavity.

A number of techniques have been described to confirm the proper placement of the Veres needle. These include the following: (1) low "opening" pressures, (2) hanging drop test, (3) injection and aspiration of fluid through the Veres needle, (4) loss of liver dullness early in insufflation, (5) negative pressure associated with elevation of the abdominal wall, and (6) free flow of gas through the Veres needle and observation of the fluctuation of pressure gauge needle with inspiratory and expiratory diaphragmatic motions. However, none of these techniques has been validated, and many surgeons rely on more than one technique in confirming placement.

If umbilical adhesions are suspected or a large pelvic mass has grown above the level of the umbilicus, the initial trocar and Veres needle can be placed in the left upper quadrant in the midclavicular line, at a point halfway between the middle of the costal margin and the umbilicus. This landmark is known as *Palmer's point* and has been shown to be a safe area of entry in patients at high risk of periumbilical adhesions. Surgeons frequently insufflate through this site, then place a 5-mm port and introduce a 5-mm laparoscope to confirm placement and to help safely direct the umbilical port.

Careful technique should be used when placing the Veres needle because the largest number of injuries during laparoscopic surgery occurs during this portion of the procedure. During placement, the Veres needle should be grasped below the hub. Counter-traction should be applied by elevating the anterior abdominal wall by grasping the skin and fat of the lower abdomen, by pulling on an Allis clamp holding the base of the umbilicus, or by elevating two towel clips placed 2 to 3 cm laterally to the incision. The Veres needle is then carefully advanced into the peritoneal cavity without deviating laterally. During advancement of the Veres needle, the surgeon typically feels two "pops"—once as the needle penetrates the fascia, and again when the spring-loaded inner sheath springs out as the peritoneal cavity is entered.

Once the Veres needle has been placed, insufflation should proceed to 15 to 18 mm Hg of pressure. Using volume as an end point may prevent full distension and result in more tenting during initial trocar placement. Some authors advocate hyperinsufflation (25 to 30 mm Hg of pressure) to minimize tenting and more effectively counteract the axial force during initial placement. If higher pressures are initially pursued, the anesthetist should be notified and pressures should be reduced once all ports are in position.

During placement, the initial trocar is "palmed" and an extended finger acts to prevent the sharp trocar tip from thrusting too deeply and causing intra-abdominal injury. An alternative approach is to use two hands to hold the initial trocar, the assisting hand placed at the base of the trocar to prevent overinsertion. The trocar is rotated in a semicircular fashion with its long axis while controlled, firm, downward pressure is being applied. After the port and laparoscope are placed, a three-point check should confirm (1) no bleeding at the site of entry, (2) no omental insufflation, and (3) no evidence of bowel injury.

Direct Trocar Insertion

Direct trocar insertion is insertion of the primary trocar without having previously inserted the Veres needle and insufflated the abdomen with carbon dioxide. The primary trocar is inserted in a manner similar to the Veres needle. The sleeve from the trocar is then used to insufflate the abdomen with carbon dioxide. Although most studies comparing direct to Veres needle entry are underpowered to show differences in safety, a meta-analysis showed that direct trocar insertion has a similar rate of major vascular and visceral injury and may have a decreased rate of minor injuries (mainly related to preperitoneal insufflation) compared with the Veres needle followed by trocar insertion.

Open Laparoscopy

Open laparoscopy involves incising the anterior rectus fascia and bluntly entering the peritoneal cavity under direct visualization. A blunt-tipped trocar with sleeve is then placed into the peritoneal cavity. For the Hasson technique, sutures used on the fascia hold the sleeve in place and anchor the sleeve to help maintain a pneumoperitoneum. Some laparoscopists use this approach exclusively because they believe the risk of major vascular injury is significantly reduced. Additionally, many laparoscopists use this method for patients with risk of abdominal adhesions, although data suggesting that open laparoscopy reduces bowel injury are lacking. In the only systematic review available in the literature, no statistically significant differences in the rates of major vascular or visceral injuries were found between open and "closed" access techniques.

Radially Expanding Access Cannulas

Conventional trocars can cut or tear tissue and require substantial axial force to penetrate the abdominal wall. Excess axial force may cause tenting and disruption of the underlying viscera and vasculature. The Versa-Step (United States Surgical, Norwalk, CT) is designed as a radially expanding cannula. This technique involves the placement of a Veres needle through an expandable sheath for insufflation. After the peritoneal cavity is insufflated, the Veres needle is removed and a 5- to 12-mm blunt trocar is introduced into the expandable sleeve to accommodate a laparoscope or instrument. The stated advantages include the absence of a pyramidal trocar tip during initial entry, a self-anchoring sleeve, tamponade of superficial vessels, and wounds that are approximately half the size of those created by comparably sized trocars. Some retrospective studies suggest a lower postoperative hernia rate with radially expanding trocars.

Optical Trocar Technique

In response to injuries associated with Veres needle entry techniques, optical-access trocars were developed. These trocars were designed to decrease the risk of injury to intra-abdominal structures by allowing the surgeon to visualize abdominal wall layers during placement. Two optical-access trocars are available: one uses a blade that sequentially scores the layers under laparoscopic visualization (Visiport, United States Surgical, Norwalk, CT); the other system has a conical clear tip that is rotated under laparoscopic vision as it penetrates the layers (Optiview, Ethicon Endo-Surgery, Cincinnati, OH). It is unlikely that large studies will have the power to demonstrate which technique is safer. However, 79 serious complications were collected from the U.S. Food and Drug Administration (FDA)'s Medical Device Reporting and the Manufacturer and User Facility Device Experience databases, including four deaths. The Endoscopic Threaded Imaging Port (ENDOTIP, Storz Endoscopy, Germany) is a second-generation trocar with a single thread winding diagonally on its outer surface, terminating with a blunt end. It is a visual trocar that can be used during closed or open laparoscopy.

Ancillary Ports

The accessory trocars are usually placed under the direct visualization of the laparoscope. The inferior epigastric vessels invariably run medial to the deep inguinal ring and lateral to the medial umbilical ligaments. If the surgeon keeps the trocar 8 cm lateral to the midline, injury to the inferior epigastric vessels should be avoided. Transillumination of the abdominal wall with the laparoscope can also help identify the superficial epigastric vessels as they run lateral up the anterior abdominal wall. To avoid trauma to the abdominal structures, secondary ports should be placed with the same caution as the primary trocar.

Operative Instrumentation

Much of the attention in laparoscopic instrumentation focuses on the ever-increasing armamentarium or dissecting and ligating instruments. Perhaps the most critical need, however, is to be able to optimize visualization of the surgical field. Fortunately, the laparoscopist can choose from a wide variety of laparoscopic retractors and graspers. Blunt and sharp graspers are helpful for some of the most challenging dissections: freeing the planes of a myoma bed, peeling off an adherent endometriotic ovarian cyst wall, or dissecting open the paravesical space in stage IV endometriosis. Obviously, a description of all available instruments in this category is impractical, but perusal of the various equipment vendor catalogs is a worthwhile endeavor. For example, right-angle clamps are available that can markedly facilitate dissection of the infundibulopelvic ligament away from the pelvic sidewall. Similarly, fan retractors (both in 5- and 10-mm varieties) can sweep the rectosigmoid safely away to operate within the ovarian fossa.

For advanced procedures such as myomectomy or hysterectomy, a properly fit uterine manipulator that allows mobilization of the uterus may prove critical. Placing a sponge stick into the vagina or inserting specially designed colpotomy rings that distend the vaginal fornix is extremely helpful in freeing a scarred bladder from the lower uterine segment. Finally, just as in open procedures, a functioning suction aspirator or the introduction of gauze sponges through a 10-mm port should be used to clear blood from the operative field. Obviously, any sponges introduced into the abdomen should be systematically tracked to avoid inadvertently leaving them behind.

The design of dissecting and ligating instruments has progressed markedly, allowing for the successful completion of more complicated gynecologic endoscopic procedures. Although traditional monopolar and bipolar electrosurgical instruments are still widely used, current technology includes a number of features that may improve outcomes. One of the most important considerations in using energy sources for tissue dissection is the lateral spread of energy, which can injure adjacent pelvic structures (such as the intestines or ureters).

Bipolar dissecting and vessel-ligating instruments are now available that minimize lateral spread to 3.6 mm; they feature microchip sensors that interpret the return current from tissue, allowing for responsive alterations in the amount of wattage applied to the tissue. Ultrasonic cutting shears, which feature an active element that vibrates 55,000 times per second, are effective hemostatic tissue dissectors; in addition they are FDA approved to ligate vessels up to 5 mm in size while minimizing lateral spread to 2 mm. Operative lasers, including carbon dioxide, argon, or neodymium:yttrium-aluminum-garnet (Nd:YAG) models, work by depositing focused energy in the form of photons to the target tissue. The resulting temperature rise causes tissue dissection and hemostasis by either denaturization of the tissue proteins or vaporization of the tissue water. Lateral tissue effect is dependent on the surface area of the beam and the time activated.

Traditional mechanical approaches to hemostasis can also be used with current laparoscopic instruments. A number of clip or band options have been used to occlude the fallopian tubes for sterilization. Staplers come in a variety of sizes for either vascular or visceral indications but require a

12-mm operating port. For traditional suturing such as closure of the vaginal cuff, placement of retropubic urethropexy stitches, or reapproximation of a serosal intestinal injury, laparoscopic needle drivers and knot pushers allow the use of conventional needles. Suture-assist devices, such as those that feature toggled needle passers, are helpful for surgeons who are less comfortable with intracorporeal needle-handling and knot-tying; dissolvable suture clips can be used in place of knots in some cases.

Specimen Removal

Once the specimen has been dissected free of its attachments, several options exist for its removal from the abdomen. If intact removal is desired (potential ovarian carcinoma), use of endoscopic specimen bags is ideal, with morcellation of the specimen within the bag after it has been exteriorized from the port (Fig. 30-7). Benign tissue can be removed directly through instrument ports if small enough, or by use of electromechanical tissue morcellators, which generally feature a rotary blade traversing several hundred rotations per minute. Alternatively, the abdominal incision can be enlarged slightly to accommodate slightly larger specimens, or the surgeon may choose to incise a posterior colpotomy to deliver the specimen vaginally. The latter option is particularly helpful for draining ovarian teratomas to avoid a chemical peritonitis from spillage.

Robotic Laparoscopy

The development of robotic surgery was intended to improve the limitations of a two-dimensional operative field and the restricted dexterity imposed by straight, nonarticulating laparoscopic instruments. Current robots feature three-dimensional telescopes with three to four instrument arms (Fig. 30-8). Notably, the instruments provide seven degrees of freedom, similar to the human wrist (Fig. 30-9). The surgeon controls these instruments using a remote console. With robotic technology, complex laparoscopic tasks such as laparoscopic suturing can be simplified due to closer resemblance to the dexterity provided in open surgery. As such, these surgical robots have been used in laparoscopic myomectomy, hysterectomy, tubal reanastomosis, and pelvic lymphadenectomy. Data supporting the use of such systems are

Figure 30-7

Specimen bags used in laparoscopic surgery. (From Bieber EJ, Sanfilippo JS: Laparoscopic instrumentation. In Gershonsen DM, DeCherney AH, Curry SL, Brubaker L [eds]: Operative Gynecology, 2nd ed. Philadelphia, W.B. Saunders, 2001, pp 157–170.)

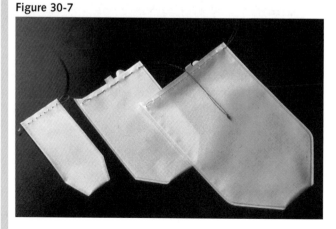

Figure 30-8

Patient side-cart with telerobotic arms for laparoscopic surgery. (From Advincula AP, Falcone T: Laparoscopic robotic gynecologic surgery. Obstet Gynecol Clin North Am 31:599–609, 2004.)

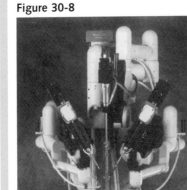

Figure 30-9

EndoWrist instruments used in robotic surgery. (From Advincula AP, Falcone T: Laparoscopic robotic gynecologic surgery. Obstet Gynecol Clin North Am 31: 599–609, 2004.)

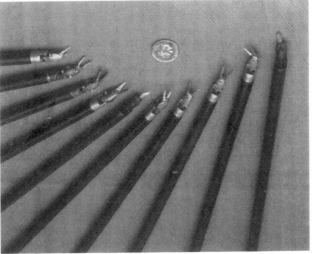

available for laparoscopic prostatectomies, but the ultimate role in gynecology awaits clinical trials.

Complication Prevention

Indications/Contraindications

With improvements in surgical equipment and surgeon skill, procedures encompassing the whole gamut of gynecology have been successfully performed with laparoscopy, including radical hysterectomy. Whether such approaches should be the standard of care remains to be seen. For example, Cochrane reviews of the efficacy of laparoscopy for colposuspension or treatment of infertility were unable to conclude a clear benefit, mainly due to the limited number of well-designed studies. Because of the increased length of time associated with many laparoscopic procedures, a more useful approach for determining which patients are candidates for laparoscopy is to consider a list of contraindications. None is an absolute rule; rather, these are meant to provoke thoughtful consideration on a case-by-case basis (Box 30-1).

Intraoperative Checklist

During positioning of the patient for surgery, common nerve compression points should be padded. Surgical sheets or gown should not be bunched up underneath the back because pressure ulcerations can result. When possible, both arms should be tucked alongside the patient's body. This facilitates surgical access and eliminates the risk of injury to the upper limb resting on an arm board. Often, sheets of foam or other padding coupled with "toboggan-shaped" protectors can be used to facilitate arm placement in obese patients for whom this position would otherwise be difficult. Allen-type stirrups (Allen Medical, Systems, Acton, MA) are preferred over "candy-cane" stirrups for laparoscopic surgery to reduce the risk of nerve compression injury to the lower extremities (Fig. 30-10). An orogastric or nasogastric tube is generally placed before the initial incision to decompress the stomach. A Foley catheter should be placed to evacuate the bladder, even if a short procedure is anticipated. The electrosurgical return electrode should be placed on a site close to the operative field over muscle (e.g., thigh). Care should be taken to ensure that the pad does not get wet during skin preparation.

Prophylactic antibiotics should be administered for all clean-contaminated or possibly contaminated cases (such as bowel surgery or high risk of enterotomy). If antibiotics are given, they are commonly administered intravenously approximately 30 minutes before the initial incision. Sequential compression devices should be applied to the lower extremities for deep vein thrombosis prophylaxis when long surgical times are anticipated.

Pneumo-
peritoneum
Complications

Increased intra-abdominal pressure may not be tolerated in patients with underlying pulmonary disease. The excursion of the diaphragm is necessarily limited, with decreases in pulmonary compliance, vital capacity, and functional residual capacity, while alveolar dead space is increased. Pulmonary shunting is the end result of these changes. Carbon dioxide

---

Box 30-1   Relative and Absolute Contraindications to Laparoscopic Surgery

Lack of surgeon familiarity with laparoscopic approach
Patient with unstable condition
Morbid obesity (body mass index > 35)
Inability to tolerate Trendelenburg position
History of dense bowel adhesions
Metastatic abdominal malignancies

Figure 30-10

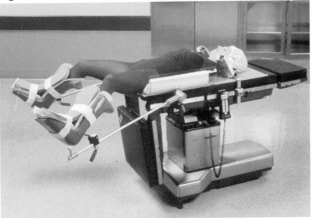

Standard placement of stirrups with minimal knee elevation above the body. (From Bieber EJ, Sanfilippo JS: Laparoscopic instrumentation. In Gershonsen DM, DeCherney AH, Curry SL, Brubaker L [eds]: Operative Gynecology, 2nd ed. Philadelphia, W.B. Saunders, 2001, pp 157–170.)

771

absorption must be monitored to avoid the induction of respiratory acidosis. A full description of the effects of pneumoperitoneum on various organ systems is presented in Table 30-3. Small studies suggest that gasless laparoscopy may be an option for patients who are unable to tolerate the pulmonary compromise of a pneumoperitoneum, either by using commercially available abdominal wall "lift" retractors, or by placing a large Foley catheter through a suprapubic port and using it to pull up on the abdominal wall. The practical utility of this approach awaits larger studies.

Electrosurgical Complications

There are some effects that are somewhat unique to monopolar laparoscopy and should be discussed. These include direct coupling and capacitive coupling. Coupling is the inadvertent passage of electric current to an unintended tissue. Capacitive coupling occurs in monopolar surgery when the unidirectional electric current in the surgical handpiece induces an electromagnetic field. This electromagnetic field then causes the buildup of a static electric charge in a surrounding conductor like a trocar sleeve (Fig. 30-11). The effect of this electric charge varies depending on the trocar sleeve material as well as the surrounding tissue. If the insulating trocar is metal, the charge generated by capacitance will be distributed over a relatively large conductive area and discharged gradually to the skin without ill effect. However, if the metal trocar is isolated from the skin by a plastic "grip" or sleeve, then the charge generated by capacitance can build up (i.e., act like an electric capacitor) and discharge to any surrounding conductor, including the bowel. Although the true incidence of bowel injury as a result of capacitance is unknown, the effect has been replicated in the laboratory. Despite the possibility of this complication, case reports with proven capacitive damage to surrounding organs are rare.

Direct coupling occurs when an activated electrosurgical device comes in contact with another conductive instrument and inadvertently creates a low-resistance pathway for the electric current. Any tissue that is in contact with this unintended pathway is therefore subject to an electric burn (Fig. 30-12).

Table 30-3

Organ System	Physiologic Effects	Potential Outcomes
Pulmonary	↑ peak airway pressures	Barotrauma/ pneumothorax
	↓ pulmonary compliance and vital capacity	↑ PCO_2 and/or ↓ PO_2
	Superior displacement of the diaphragm	↑ PCO_2 and/or ↓ PO_2
	↑ end-tidal CO_2	Acidosis
Circulatory	Direct effects—increased CVP, CWP, SVR, MAP	↑ cardiac work; effects on cardiac output dependent on volume status
	Indirect effects of CO_2—arteriolar dilation and myocardial depression	↓ blood pressure
	Indirect effects on the sympathetic system, renin-angiotensin system, and vasopressin	↑ blood pressure and cardiac output ↓ urine output
Renal	↓ renal blood flow	↓ urine output
Coagulation	Lower extremity venous stasis	DVT and PE
Immunity and inflammation	Preserved systemic immunity	Greater resistance to infection and tumor seeding
	Impaired local immunity	↓ resistance to infection or tumor seeding
Central nervous system	↑ ICP	↓ central perfusion pressure
Intestinal	Attenuated sympathetic response	Less ileus

CVP, central venous pressure; CWP, capillary wedge pressure; SVR, systemic vascular resistance; MAP, mean arterial pressure; DVT, deep venous pressure; PE, pulmonary embolus; ICP, intracranial pressure.
From Chang C, Rege RV: Minimally invasive surgery. In Townsend C, Beauchamp RD, Evers BM, Mattox K (eds): Sabiston Textbook of Surgery, 17th ed. Philadelphia, Elsevier, 2004, pp 445–464, with permission.

Complications/ Postoperative Considerations

General Considerations

Data on the incidence of intraoperative complications during gynecologic laparoscopy come from a handful of sources. In a 1993 survey of the American Association of Gynecologic Laparoscopists, a complication rate of 5 in 1000 cases was found for 45,042 reported operative laparoscopies. The most frequent types encountered were prolonged hospitalization, vascular injury, unintended laparotomy, and gastrointestinal or urologic injury. Notably, these studies likely underestimate the true incidence because the reporting was voluntary and only came from members. Data from a Finnish national database provide a more comprehensive source. In data from 1990 to 1994, a complication rate of 6 per 1000 was identified for operative laparoscopy. Diagnostic laparoscopy had a much lower

Figure 30-11

Unipolar induction of capacitance. (From Hulka JF, Reich H: Textbook of Laparoscopy, 3rd ed. Philadelphia, W.B. Saunders, 1998.)

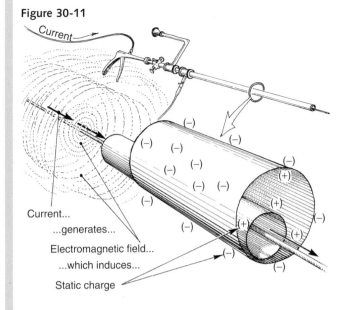

Current...
...generates...
Electromagnetic field...
...which induces...
Static charge

773

Figure 30-12

Direct coupling resulting in inadvertent bowel injury. (From Odell R: Electrosurgery. In Sutton C, Diamond MP [eds]: Endoscopic Surgery from Gynecologists, 2nd ed. Philadelphia, W.B. Saunders, 1998, pp 83–92.)

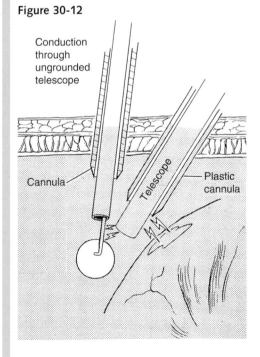

Conduction through ungrounded telescope

Cannula

Telescope

Plastic cannula

rate of complications at 0.3 per 1000. Factors that appear to influence the likelihood of complications include patient obesity, physician experience, smoking, previous abdominal surgery, and the performance of major gynecologic procedures.

After any gynecologic laparoscopic procedure, progressive resolution of symptoms is to be expected 3 to 14 days postoperatively. With major procedures, a return to completely normal bowel function may take several days. For any procedure, pain may be perceived as slightly worse on the day after the procedure but should improve after this point. Likewise, the incision should appear healthy and become almost painless within the first week. Patients are commonly counseled on the natural postoperative course of events, and patients should be instructed to contact their physician if any deviation from this course occurs. A natural tendency may be to reassure a patient who calls that their postoperative discomfort is within the normal range. However, this reassurance should be offered with caution because delaying appropriate care can often compound the effects of complications and may be fatal. Any deviation from progressive recovery should be thoroughly investigated.

Probably the most concerning postoperative symptom is worsening abdominal pain, especially in the presence of distension. Signs of an occult injury of bowel or bladder may take hours or days to develop. Any patient with worsening abdominal pain after laparoscopy should be advised to come in for an evaluation by someone experienced in recognizing postoperative complications. In general, a patient's condition should improve every day after endoscopic surgery. If a patient calls more than once about questions regarding her postoperative course, she should be advised to come in for evaluation.

Gastrointestinal Complications

Finnish national data suggest an incidence rate of 2.1 per 1000 for injuries to the gastrointestinal tract during operative gynecologic laparoscopy. These can occur as a result of blunt trauma during retraction, sharp injury during trocar insertion or intraoperative dissection, or direct tissue damage from use of energy sources. Prompt recognition of these problems intraoperatively can prevent serious sequelae such as intra-abdominal infection and sepsis. Postoperative worsening pain, fever, nausea, vomiting, and distension should prompt an immediate evaluation of bowel injury. Clinical examination and awareness of the nature of the procedure should guide interpretation of serum studies and imaging results. When approaching bowel adhesions, sharp dissection can help limit the risk of lateral spread of thermal injury. Keeping the length of instrument sleeves under visualization and away from adjacent bowel when using monopolar energy sources can minimize problems from unexpected sleeve insulation failures. If intraoperative injury is suspected, the bowel should be run across its entire length. Rectosigmoid injuries can be detected by filling the cul-de-sac with sterile saline, insufflating the rectum with a wide-bore syringe (or with a rigid proctoscope) while an assistant compresses the proximal rectosigmoid against the sacral promontory or with a laparoscopic bowel grasper. The observation of bubbles in the cul-de-sac fluid during bowel insufflation signifies the presence of a rectosigmoid injury.

Treatment of such complications depends on the nature of the injury and the skill of the surgeon. Small Veres needle injuries to the gastrointestinal tract may respond well to observation in the hospital overnight with consideration of broad-spectrum antibiotics. Larger defects or electrothermal injuries are generally best managed in consultation with a general or colorectal surgeon. Some bowel injuries can be repaired through a minilaparotomy incision or laparoscopically, depending on the experience of the surgical team. Optimal repair of injuries to the uncleansed colon remains controversial, but some colorectal surgeons advocate offering a primary repair for small confined injuries. With delayed presentation of these injuries, where the patient likely has significant intraperitoneal inflammation and infection, immediate laparotomy is generally ideal.

An unusual cause of abdominal pain after laparoscopic surgery is an entrapped incisional hernia through one of the laparoscopic port sites. Herniation is rare at the site where the laparoscope is placed through the umbilicus. However, bowel herniation has been reported to occur when larger trocars (>5 mm) are used in locations lateral to the midline. Hernia can occur either through the fascia or peritoneum, with entrapment of bowel into the preperitoneal space. After laparoscopy, herniation may manifest as severe abdominal pain accompanied by signs of bowel obstruction. Although incisional hernias should always be considered as a cause of abdominal pain after laparoscopic surgery, they are relatively infrequent. Thus, other intra-abdominal processes should also be considered.

Practical approaches to minimizing gastrointestinal injury should be considered for all cases. Preoperative bowel preparation has not been formally evaluated to prevent such complications, but the decompressed bowel will be easier to retract out of the surgical field. In patients with a history of extensive bowel surgery, laparoscopy may not be the ideal approach depending on a surgeon's skill; alternatively, open umbilical access or left upper quadrant entry should be considered. As with the genitourinary structures, when adjacent structures are dissected using energy sources or using electric morcellators intra-abdominally, the location of the intestines must be certain. Gentle tissue handling when retracting bowel is also helpful; a variety of atraumatic graspers are available for this purpose.

Genitourinary Complications

Gynecologic surgery is the most common cause of urologic injuries. In the Finnish study, an incidence of 3 in 1000 cases of bladder or ureteral injury was identified among operative laparoscopic cases. Bladder injury is most likely to occur during either insertion of a suprapubic trocar or when exposing the lower uterine segment at time of hysterectomy. The most common sites of ureteral injury are likely to be at the pelvic brim during ligation of the infundibulopelvic ligament and near the uterosacral ligament during ligation of the uterine vessels. Careful skeletonization of the broad ligament can help prevent inadvertent injury, particularly when attempting to control persistent bleeding after ligation of these pedicles.

When such injuries are suspected, simple tests can identify the site of injury, allowing for primary treatment. Intravenous indigo carmine dye will appear in the bladder within 5 minutes of injection; any spill into the peritoneal cavity will be diagnostic. Cystoscopy can help identify a site of bladder injury. If trained in stent placement, the surgeon may consider placement of temporary stents to confirm the ureters have not been ligated if indigo carmine spill is not seen during cystoscopy. Once a bladder or ureteral injury is identified, intraoperative consultation with a urologist may help in determining the best approach for treatment. Small bladder injuries (<2 cm) in the dome of the bladder often respond to prolonged gravity drainage. However, two-layer closure should be considered for larger defects; skilled laparoscopic teams may elect to repair these laparoscopically. In situations with delayed recognition of injury, intravenous pyelogram or computed tomography will likely demonstrate the presence of a urinoma. Depending on the site of ureteral injury, management may only require prolonged double-J stent placement, but complex injuries may require ureteral reanastomosis, reimplantation of the ureter into the bladder, transureteral ureterostomy, or bladder mobilization.

Prevention depends on an awareness of the urinary structures during all aspects of gynecologic surgery. Trocar injuries are less likely with the bladder decompressed; in the setting of multiple previous cesarean sections, retrograde distension of the bladder intraoperatively may aid in defining the upper border. Ideally, preoperative placement of stents might aid in avoidance of ureteral injury in difficult dissections, but studies still report injury even with this preventive strategy.

Vascular Complications

As in open surgery, vascular injury can occur at numerous steps during laparoscopy. During initial entry, port placement, and dissection, a surgeon may encounter unanticipated bleeding, most often from the epigastric vessels of the abdominal wall. In general, vascular injury, particularly major vascular injury, has not been commonly reported. The Finnish registry noted a 0.4 per 1000 risk of major vascular complications based on 11,000 operative laparoscopic cases. Because vascular injuries are frequently related to the initial placement of the insufflation needle, some surgeons advocate open entry into the abdomen for all laparoscopic cases. However, randomized controlled trials have failed to show a clear benefit of open access techniques.

Evidence for vascular injury is usually immediate, often following difficulty in gaining initial peritoneal access. Signs may include frank blood from the insufflation needle, large amounts of unexpected intraperitoneal blood, swelling and dark bruising of the retroperitoneum, or sudden hypotension. Management of such serious complications should be individualized, but immediate laparotomy should be performed in unstable patients. This allows manual compression of the bleeding site and subsequent exploration and ligation of the bleeding vessel(s), along with notification of anesthesia, coordination of transfusion services with the blood bank, and consultation with the vascular surgery service. If a stable hematoma is noted in the retroperitoneum, it may be best to observe it under pneumoperitoneum to allow tamponade, but preparation for open surgery and admission to the intensive care unit should still be made. In the event of sudden return of blood after needle insertion, some surgeons advocate leaving the insufflation needle in place while performing laparotomy to facilitate identification of the injury site.

Reproductive Tract Injury

Although not mentioned generally in larger reports from databases, injury to the uterus does occur with laparoscopy—most commonly with the use of a uterine manipulator. Uterine injuries to the fundus generally can be repaired laparoscopically if the surgeon is comfortable with intracorporeal suturing. With broad ligament perforation, observation under pneumoperitoneum may allow the bleeding to be contained without intervention; after a period of waiting, the abdominal pressure can be decreased to assess hemostasis. In general, leaving the hematoma undisturbed is best because the small branching vessels within the ligament may be very difficult to isolate.

HYSTEROSCOPY

History

Although hysteroscopic procedures were first described by Pantaleoni in the late 1860s, they did not gain popularity until the late 1970s, with increasing interest for the use of hysteroscopy in the diagnosis of causes of abnormal uterine bleeding. Fiberoptic lighting and advances in instrumentation have helped make hysteroscopy the gold standard for the evaluation of abnormal uterine bleeding and have greatly expanded the applications for diagnostic and operative hysteroscopy. Many of these procedures can be performed in the physician's office with little or no anesthesia, particularly with the development of flexible hysteroscopes (Fig. 30-13). However, treatment of significant pathology, such as resection of submucosal leiomyoma or global endometrial ablation, is still often performed in the hospital outpatient setting.

Equipment

The basic components of a hysteroscope include the telescope (with straight or angled lenses), a sheath through which fluid and instruments can be introduced, and a light source. Additionally, a camera system can be attached to the telescope head to allow viewing on a monitor.

Figure 30-13

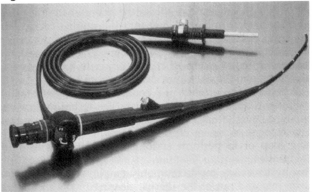

Flexible hysteroscope suitable for office diagnostic procedures. (From Cooper JM, Brady RM: Hysteroscopy in the management of abnormal uterine bleeding. Obstet Gynecol Clin North Am 26[1]:217–236, 1999.)

The basic system is similar to that used in cystoscopy (see further discussion). Hysteroscopes may be either rigid or flexible; they vary in diameter, with sheath sizes increasing to accommodate operating channels.

Distension Media

Operative hysteroscopy must be performed in a fluid medium (diagnostic hysteroscopy can be performed with carbon dioxide distension). The type of fluid depends on the surgeon's preference, instruments utilized, and type of electric generator used, but any fluid can be associated with complications. Fluid choices with monopolar instruments include glycine 1.5%, a mixture of sorbitol 3% and mannitol 0.54%, and 5% mannitol. These fluids are frequently used with the continuous-flow resectoscope. Bipolar operative hysteroscopy can be performed using saline.

Among the options for distension media in operative and diagnostic hysteroscopy are high-viscosity dextran 70 and low-viscosity fluids such as hypotonic, electrolyte-free and isotonic, electrolyte-containing solutions. The popularity of dextran 70 is waning, however. Although it is immiscible with blood, significant complications have been reported. Signs of anaphylactic reactions to dextran 70 include acute hypotension, hypoxia, pulmonary edema, fluid overload, fulminant coagulopathies, and anemia. When using dextran 70, the surgeon must operate quickly, minimize unnecessary endometrial trauma, use continuous pulse oximetry, and perform a preoperative coagulation panel of tests. Dextran 70 also can ruin operative hysteroscopes if they are not cleaned promptly and thoroughly after each use.

Hypotonic, Electrolyte-Free Solutions
With hypotonic, electrolyte-free solutions such as glycine 1.5%, early recognition of possible complications, including hyponatremic hypervolemia, is vital. For example, when glycine and sorbitol are metabolized, free water accumulates and the body attempts to achieve homeostasis through compensatory mechanisms including osmosis, which moves free water into extracellular and intracellular spaces. This can lead to increased free water in the brain, resulting in cerebral edema, rising intracranial pressure, and cellular necrosis.

The cerebral cation pump normally pumps osmotically active cations into the extracellular space, thereby minimizing cerebral edema. However, this pump is inhibited by estrogen, so the compensatory mechanism is diminished.

Classic clinical features of hyponatremic hypervolemia include apprehension, confusion, fatigue, headache, mental agitation, nausea, visual disturbances (including blindness), vomiting, and weakness. These complications are more readily recognized when regional anesthesia is used rather than general anesthesia.

If hyponatremic hypervolemia goes unrecognized, bradycardia and hypertension can ensue, followed rapidly by cerebral and pulmonary edema and cardiovascular collapse. In addition, glycine 1.5% is metabolized to glycolic acid and ammonia. Free ammonia is associated with central nervous system disorders. Recognition and prompt treatment by an intensi-vist may prevent permanent neurologic sequelae and death.

Isotonic Solutions

Mannitol 5% is electrolyte poor but isotonic, creating less risk for hypo-osmolality. However, dilutional hyponatremia can still occur. Normal sa-line and lactated Ringer's solution are isotonic, electrolyte-containing fluids that can be used with bipolar instrumentation. They are considered one the safest media for distension. With all distension media, complica-tions can generally be avoided with vigilant fluid monitoring and proper fluid documentation. If fluid overload occurs, comanagement and consul-tation with an intensive care specialist is advised.

Advantages of Bipolar Instruments

To minimize complications from hypotonic, electrolyte-free solutions, manufacturers have developed operative hysteroscopes that can function in a bipolar environment. Bipolar instruments can operate in an isotonic, physiologic, electrolyte-containing media. Although fluid overload can oc-cur with normal saline or lactated Ringer's solution, hyponatremia and hypo-osmolality cannot. Fluid overload with saline can cause pulmonary edema and congestive heart failure, however. Hence, fluid monitoring is still necessary.

779

The amount of fluid absorbed depends on factors including surface area of the surgical field, duration of surgery, opened venous channels, type of irrigation fluid used, and pressure of the delivery system. Modern gyneco-logic suites use fluid irrigation systems that continuously measure input and output, with audible or visual alarms that signal a predetermined flu-id deficit. The alarm indicates the need to halt the procedure and quickly evaluate the patient. Careful attention to the fluid management will lead to fewer complications.

Procedural Complications

In a retrospective investigation, Propst evaluated the rate of complications associated with specific hysteroscopic procedures. Demographic data and medical histories were collected for 925 women who underwent operative hysteroscopy in 1995 and 1996. The overall complication rate was 2.7%. Myomectomy and resection of uterine septa carried the greatest odds of complications, and polypectomy and endometrial ablation had the lowest odds. Preoperative treatment with a gonadotropin-releasing hormone (GnRH) agonist increased the odds of operative complications by a factor of four to seven. Women younger than 50 years of age were more likely to experience complications than older than 50 years.

In a 2000 study by Jansen and colleagues, 38 complications occurred in 13,600 procedures—a rate of 0.28%. The greatest risk of complications occurred with adhesiolysis (4.48%), followed by endometrial resection (0.81%), myomectomy (0.75%), and polypectomy (0.38%). Risk factors for uterine perforation include nulliparity, menopause, use of GnRH ago-nists, prior cone biopsy, markedly retroverted uterus, and undue force during the procedure.

Signs of Perforation

Patients who sustain a perforation of the uterus with subsequent intraperitoneal bleeding often experience abdominal pain, shoulder pain, and hemodynamic instability. A quick survey of the abdomen with sonography demonstrates free intraperitoneal fluid. It is rare for large amounts of intraperitoneal fluid to accumulate by transtubal regurgitation during operative hysteroscopy because most fluid is absorbed intravascularly.

If perforation is suspected, laparoscopy or laparotomy is necessary to clarify the cause of pain, unstable vital signs, or free fluid visualized by ultrasound. Extra care and precautions must be undertaken in women who have had a prior cesarean section, myomectomy, or uterine perforation. Complete visualization of uterine landmarks during operative hysteroscopy must be undertaken to detect uterine dehiscence, sacculation, or perforation. Prior uterine surgery leads to myometrial weakness and possible perforation. Surgeons should abandon the procedure and avoid activation of electric energy if perforation is detected. If uterine perforation occurs with an activated electrode, serious injury to abdominal viscera including bladder, bowel, and even ureteral injury has been reported. Strict visualization of uterine anatomy at all times is necessary to avoid bowel and bladder burns. If visualization is compromised, then operative hysteroscopy should be abandoned.

Postoperative Complications

Some complications of hysteroscopy may not become clinically evident for months or even years. The most common are complications of hysteroscopic endometrial ablation including unplanned pregnancy, postablation tubal sterilization syndrome, new or worsening dysmenorrhea, hematometra, endometrial cancer, and failure to completely treat symptoms.

Patients scheduled to undergo hysteroscopy must be informed of potential delayed risks of the procedure. In addition, all women of reproductive age should be advised that pregnancy is possible after endometrial ablation or operative removal of an intracavitary mass, and therefore contraception is crucial. The endometrial tissue is quite resilient and may regenerate after ablation.

Hematometra is an infrequent late complication of operative hysteroscopy. If cyclic or chronic lower pelvic pain occurs after surgery in menstruating women or among women taking hormone replacement therapy, scarring or narrowing of the endometrial cavity may be the cause. Approximately 1% to 2% of women who undergo operative hysteroscopy experience this phenomenon. In most cases, it can be treated successfully with cervical dilation alone.

Pregnancy Complications

Uterine dehiscence and sacculation may result from an extremely thin myometrium after uterine adhesiolysis, uterine perforation, or myoma resections. A high index of suspicion is vital when a gravida presents with pelvic pain, decreased fetal movement, vaginal bleeding, or abnormal uterine masses detected ultrasonographically.

Patients who experience intraoperative complications during metroplasty or deep resection of intramural fibroids should be informed of the risk of uterine rupture so they can consider elective cesarean section. Regardless of the mode of delivery, prompt attention is vital if fetal distress is suspected. Hysteroscopic technique is discussed in Chapter 19, Leiomyomas.

CYSTOSCOPY

History

The first documented cystoscope was developed and used by Bozini in the 1800s. This instrument involved a combination of angled mirrors, a cone-shaped funnel, and a candle for a light source. Although this represented an advance in the evaluation of the bladder, technical difficulties prevented it from becoming a widespread diagnostic tool; operators would frequently get burned after tipping the candle over. In the late 1800s, Kelly introduced the knee-chest position as an easy way to visualize the bladder. Using electric lighting and a hollow tube, cystoscopy became widespread and available to the general practitioner. Since then, the introduction of fiberoptic lens systems, operative cystoscopic bridges, and flexible cystoscopes has revolutionized the field.

781

Equipment

The modern rigid cystoscope is composed of four pieces: light source, telescope, bridge, and sheath. A high-intensity (xenon) light source is usually recommended for adequate visualization and attaches to the telescope via a flexible fiberoptic cable. The telescope itself uses a rod lens system to transmit both light and imagery to the viewer and is available in many viewing angles from 0 (straight) to 120 degrees (retro view). It is generally advisable to use a 0-degree telescope to visualize the urethra, a 30-degree telescope to visualize the bladder dome and walls, and a 70-degree telescope to visualize the ureteric ridge and ureteral openings. The angled telescopes will have a black notch just outside the visual field to assist in orientation. This notch will be on the opposite side from the angle of deflection. The 120-degree telescope is not used in routine gynecology.

The bridge serves as a watertight spacer between the telescope and the sheath and may have ports for the introduction of instruments into the visual field. The sheath is an outer covering for the rigid cystoscope and allows for influx and efflux of distension media. Flexible cystoscopes are also available but are seldom needed in gynecologic patients because of the short length of the female urethra. Urethroscopes are also available, and these have a 0-degree telescope and a shorter overall length. However, a cystoscope with a 0-degree telescope can usually be used in its place. The diameter of the cystoscope sheath also varies, with larger-diameter sheaths used for operative procedures and smaller-diameter sheaths for diagnostic purposes.

General Cystoscopic Technique

The cystoscope should be completely assembled and flushed with normal saline before insertion in the urethra. The distension media should be gently flowing as the cystoscope is inserted, and topical anesthetic can be placed on the outside of the sheath to decrease discomfort with manipulation. In general, the distension media used is sterile water or normal saline and is delivered using gravity alone with the reservoir bag 100 cm above the patient's pelvis. Once the cystoscope is in the bladder, a systematic evaluation of the entire bladder and trigone should be performed. This can be done by performing 12 sweeps of the bladder going from the superior dome to the urethrovesical junction (Fig. 30-14). After the bladder mucosa has been examined, a 70-degree telescope can be used to evaluate the bladder trigone and assess the ureteral orifices. Ureteral patency can be assessed by giving the patient 2.5 to 5 mL of indigo carmine dye intravenously and then looking for efflux of dye from the ureteral openings in the bladder. This technique is usually used to assess patency after surgery that may affect the ureters, such as hysterectomy or reconstructive surgery. The operator should always pay attention to how much distension media has been infused during cystoscopy; 250 to 300 mL should be adequate for complete evaluation of the bladder.

Practical Uses of Cystoscopy in Gynecology

The indications for cystoscopy in gynecology are fairly broad, including evaluation of hematuria and diagnosis of interstitial cystitis. However, one of the most practical uses of cystoscopy for general practitioners is to evaluate the bladder and ureters for operative injury. The reported incidence of lower urinary tract injury during gynecologic surgery varies between 0.16% and 3%, depending on the type of operation. Intraoperative cystoscopy, performed while the patient is still anesthetized in the operating room, provides a powerful tool for the evaluation of possible lower urinary tract injuries. An analysis of 22 publications reported that

Figure 30-14

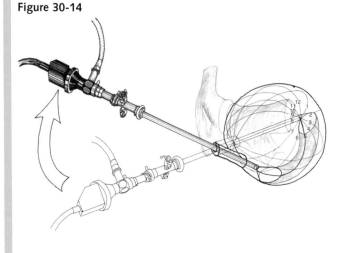

Diagnostic cystoscopy. A survey of the vesical cavity is made by making 12 sweeps from the superior bladder to the urethrovesical junction. The 5-o'clock sweep is demonstrated. (From Cundiff GW, Bent AE: Endoscopic evaluation of the lower urinary tract. In Walters MD, Karram MM [eds]: Urogynecology and Reconstructive Pelvic Surgery, 2nd ed. St. Louis, Mosby, 1999, pp 111–121.)

782

intraoperative cystoscopy identified 90% of unsuspected ureteral and 85% of unsuspected bladder injuries. This is especially important in pelvic reconstructive and procedures, in which the incidence of ureteral injury may be four-fold higher than with general gynecologic surgeries.

VAGINOSCOPY

A brief mention of the use of cystoscopes or hysteroscopes in the evaluation of the vaginal canal is warranted, primarily with regard to pediatric gynecologic examination. Indications include recurrent vulvar infection, presence of a foreign body or neoplasm, abnormal bleeding, and congenital anomaly. The knee-chest position is generally favored for vaginoscopy. Topical application of local anesthetic to the vestibule before the procedure may facilitate the examination. Gentle lavage of the canal assists in performance of this evaluation by providing mild distension of the vaginal walls. As with examination of all pediatric patients, patience and assistance from the nurse and family will reduce the natural discomfort associated with this evaluation. In some circumstances, sedation may be necessary.

783

KEY POINTS

1. Operative endoscopy allows many gynecologic conditions to be treated with less patient discomfort and shorter hospital stays.
2. Clear visualization of the operative field at all times is needed to safely perform laparoscopic surgery.
3. Trocar placement must be performed by a clinician with a thorough knowledge of the vascular anatomy of the anterior abdominal wall and adjacent retroperitoneum.
4. Surgeons must maintain familiarity with constantly evolving surgical instruments to facilitate endoscopic procedures.
5. Patients with dense intra-abdominal adhesions, inability to tolerate the Trendelenburg position, metastatic intra-abdominal malignancies, unstable hemodynamic or cardiovascular status, and gross obesity may not be ideal candidates for laparoscopic surgery.
6. Serious complications of laparoscopy are uncommon, but a high clinical suspicion must be maintained in patients not exhibiting a typical recovery trajectory.
7. Careful fluid monitoring is an important component to the success of operative hysteroscopy; consideration should be made for completing the procedure when a 1000- to 1500-mL fluid deficit with occurs with isotonic solutions. Hypotonic solutions should be used with great care.
8. Cystoscopic evaluation should be considered whenever urinary tract injury is suspected during gynecologic surgery.

SUGGESTED READING

Advincula AP, Falcone T: Laparoscopic robotic gynecologic surgery. Obstet Gynecol Clin North Am 31:599–609, 2004.

Al-Fozan H, Tulandi T: Safety and risks of laparoscopy in pregnancy. Curr Opin Obstet Gynecol 14(4):375–379, 2002.

Baggish M, Barbot J, Valle R: Diagnostic and Operative Hysteroscopy: A Text and Atlas. 2nd ed. St. Louis, Mosby, 1999.

Bettocchi S, Nappi L, Ceci O, Selvaggi L: Office hysteroscopy. Obstet Gynecol Clin North Am 31:641–654, 2004.

Chapron C, Fauconnier A, Goffinet F, et al: Laparoscopic surgery is not inherently dangerous for patients presenting with benign gynaecologic pathology: Results of a meta-analysis. Hum Reprod 17:1334–1342, 2002.

Cundiff G: Endoscopy. In Cardozo L, Staskin D (eds): Textbook of Female Urology and Urogynaecology. London, Martin Dunitz, 2002 pp 314–322.

Cundiff GW, Bent AE: Cystourethroscopy. In Cundiff GW, Bent AE, Ostergard DR, Swift SE (eds): Ostergard's Urogynecology and Pelvic Floor Dysfunction, 5th ed. Philadelphia, Lippincott Williams & Wilkins, 2003, pp 141–153.

Garry R, Fountain J, Mason S, et al: The eVALuate study: Two parallel randomised trials, one comparing laparoscopic with abdominal hysterectomy, the other comparing laparoscopic with vaginal hysterectomy [online]. BMJ 328:129, 2004.

Hammoud A, Gago LA, Diamond MP: Adhesions in patients with chronic pelvic pain: A role for adhesiolysis? Fertil Steril 82:1483–1491, 2004.

Harkki-Siren P, Kurki T: A nationwide analysis of laparoscopic complications. Obstet Gynecol 89:108–112, 1997.

Harkki-Siren P, Sjoberg J, Makinen J, et al: Finnish national register of laparoscopic hysterectomies: A review and complications of 1165 operations. Am J Obstet Gynecol 176:118–122, 1997.

Hulka J and Reich H (eds): Textbook of Laparoscopy, 3rd ed. Philadelphia, W.B. Saunders, 1998.

Jacobson TZ, Barlow DH, Koninckx PR, et al: Laparoscopic surgery for subfertility associated with endometriosis. Cochrane Database Syst Rev 4: CD001398, 2002.

Jansen FW, Vredevoogd CB, Ulzen K, et al: Complications of hysteroscopy: A prospective, multicenter study. Obstet Gynecol 96:266–270, 2000.

Lamvu G, Tu F, As-Sanie S, et al: The role of laparoscopy in the diagnosis and treatment of conditions associated with chronic pelvic pain. Obstet Gynecol Clin North Am 31:619–630, 2004.

Lamvu G, Zolnoun D, Boggess J, Steege JF: Obesity: Physiologic changes and challenges during laparoscopy. Am J Obstet Gynecol 191:669–674, 2004.

Mansuria SM, Sanfilippo JS: Laparoscopy in the pediatric and adolescent population. Obstet Gynecol Clin North Am 31:469–483, 2004.

Moehrer B, Carey M, Wilson D: Laparoscopic colposuspension: A systematic review. BJOG 110:230–235, 2003.

Nezhat CR, Siegler AM, Nezhat FR, Seldman DS: Operative Gynecologic Laparoscopy: Principles and Techniques, 2nd ed. New York, McGraw-Hill, 2000.

Ostrzenski A, Radolinski B, Ostrzenska KM: A review of laparoscopic ureteral injury in pelvic surgery. Obstet Gynecol Surv 58:794–799, 2003.

Paraiso MF, Walters MD: Laparoscopic pelvic reconstructive surgery. Clin Obstet Gynecol 43:594–603, 2000.

Peterson HB, Xia Z, Hughes JM, et al: The risk of ectopic pregnancy after tubal sterilization. U.S. Collaborative Review of Sterilization Working Group. N Engl J Med 336:762–767, 1997.

Peterson HB, Xia Z, Hughes JM, et al: The risk of pregnancy after tubal sterilization: Findings from the U.S. Collaborative Review of Sterilization. Am J Obstet Gynecol 174:1161–1168, 1996.

Propst AM, Liberman RF, Harlow BL, Ginsburg ES: Complications of hysteroscopic surgery: Predicting patients at risk. Obstet Gynecol 96:517–520, 2000.

Ramsay IN: The treatment of stress incontinence—Is there a role for laparoscopy? BJOG 111:49–52, 2004.

Swank DJ, Swank-Bordewijk SC, Hop WC, et al: Laparoscopic adhesiolysis in patients with chronic abdominal pain: A blinded randomised controlled multi-centre trial. Lancet 361:1247–1251, 2003.

Tu FF, Lamvu GM, Hartmann KE, Steege JF: Preoperative ultrasound to predict infraumbilical adhesions: A study of diagnostic accuracy. Am J Obstet Gynecol 192:74–79, 2005.

Tulikangas PK, Robinson DS, Falcone T: Left upper quadrant cannula insertion. Fertil Steril 79:411–412, 2003.

INDEX

Note: Page numbers followed by f refer to figures; page numbers followed by t refer to tables; page numbers followed by b refer to boxes.

A

Abdominal aorta, 77, 77f
Abdominal ectopic pregnancy,
  280–281
Abdominal hysterectomy,
  725–727f, 733–740f
Abdominal pain, causes of,
  104, 106b
Abdominal sacrocolpopexy, for
  uterine/vaginal vault
  prolapse, 567–569, 568f
Abdominal wall, anterior, nerves
  of, 77–83, 77f, 80f
Abembryonic abortion, 225
Abnormal uterine bleeding
  in adolescence, 201–202,
    202b, 203b, 353, 353b
  diagnosis of, 349–352,
    351b, 355b
  endometrial cancer, 355, 356b
  endometrial hyperplasia, 355,
    356b
  intrauterine device and, 170
  menopausal bleeding,
    354–355, 355b
  oral contraceptives for, 354
  outcomes of, 364
  pathophysiology of, 348–349,
    349b
  perimenopause, 353–354
  in premenarchal girls, 353
  prevalence of, 348
  signs of, 349
  symptoms of, 349
  therapy for, 358–363
    medical, 358–360
      Danazol, 359
      gonadotropin-releasing
        hormone, 359–360

Abnormal uterine bleeding
  (Continued)
  therapy for (Continued)
    medical (Continued)
      intravenous conjugated
        equine estrogen, 359
      levonorgestrel intrauterine
        device, 360
      nonsteroidal anti-
        inflammatory
        drugs, 358
      oral contraceptive
        pills, 358
      progesterone, 359
    surgical, 360–363
      dilation and curettage, 362
      endometrial ablation, 362,
        363t
      hysterectomy, 361
      management of,
        362–363
      myomectomy, 361
      operative hysteroscopy,
        360–361
      uterine fibroid
        embolization, 361
    von Willebrand's disease,
      352–353
Abortion, 225–226 See also
  Pregnancy loss; See also
  Pregnancy termination
  tubal, ectopic pregnancy and,
    262–263
Accessory glands, ostia of, 83, 84f
Acetic acid visual inspection,
  for cervical cancer,
  447–448, 448f
Acquired gene mutations, 52–53
Acrosome reaction, 3

ACTH. See Adrenocorticotropic
  hormone
Adenocarcinoma, 2001
  Bethesda System and,
    435–436
Adenomyosis
  clinical diagnosis of, 342–343
    imaging, 343
    signs, 343
    symptoms, 342
  management of, 343
  pathogenesis of, 341–342
  pathology of, 342
ADH. See Antidiuretic hormone
Adnexal masses, in adolescence,
  485–487, 486f, 492f, 482b
Adolescence
  intrauterine device and, 170
  menorrhagia in, 201–202,
    202b, 203b
  ovarian cysts in, 192–193
  pelvic mass in, 482–487, 482b
    adnexal masses, 485–487,
      486f, 492f, 482b
    congenital obstructive
      lesions, 483
    functional ovarian cysts,
      483–485, 484f
    ovarian masses, 483
    ovarian neoplasms, 485
  pelvic pain in, 198–199, 199b
  problems in, 193–194
    abnormal uterine bleeding,
      201–202, 202b,
      203b, 353, 353b
    androgen insensitivity
      syndrome, 196
    chemotherapy, 195–196
    chronic disease, 195

Adolescence *(Continued)*
  problems in *(Continued)*
    delayed puberty, 193–194,
      194b, 196, 196f
    eating disorders, 194
    endocrine disease, 195
    endometriosis, 199–200
    hypergonadotropic
      hypogonadism, 195
    hypogonadotropic
      hypogonadism, 195
    menorrhagia, 201–202,
      202b, 203b
    ovarian cysts, 192–193
    pelvic pain, 198–199, 199b
    primary amenorrhea,
      193–194, 196, 196f
    secondary amenorrhea, 193,
      196f, 196
    uterovaginal anomalies,
      200–201
Adrenal suppression, gynecologic
  surgery and, 691
Adrenocorticotropic hormone
  (ACTH), 24
Alcohol, decrease in, menopause
  and, 402
Allantois, 19f, 20
Allergies, gynecologic surgery
  and, 692
Ambiguous genitalia, in
  newborns, 205–208, 206f,
  206b, 207b
  management of, 207–208
Amenorrhea, 347
  primary, 193–194, 196, 196f,
    369–372, 369b
    anatomic abnormalities, 371
    androgen insensitivity
      syndrome, 371
    evaluation of, 371–372
    gonadal dysfunction, 373
    hypothalamic dysfunction,
      370
    pituitary dysfunction, 370
    treatment of, 371–372
  secondary, 193, 196f, 196,
    372–375
    evaluation of, 374–375
    gonadal dysfunction, 373
    hypothalamic dysfunction,
      372–373

Amenorrhea *(Continued)*
  secondary *(Continued)*
    pituitary dysfunction,
      372–373
    treatment of, 374–375
    uterine dysfunction,
      373–374
  therapeutic, 376–377
Amsterdam criteria, 64, 65b
Anal fissure, 626–627
Anal fistula, 628–630,
  629f, 630b
Anal intraepithelial
  neoplasia, 635
Anal margin, 610
Anal neoplasia, 634–636
  anal intraepithelial neoplasia,
    635
  Bowen's disease, 635–636, 635f
  invasive anal carcinoma, 636
  Paget's disease, 636
Anal stenosis, 627–628, 628f
Anal transition zone, 609
Ancillary ports, for laparoscopy,
  766
Androgen insensitivity
  syndrome, 196
  amenorrhea and, 371
Androgens, ovaries and, 27, 30
Anomalous obturator artery, 79
Anorectal disease, benign, bowel
  disorders, 620–630
  anal fissure, 626–627
  anal fistula, 628–630, 629f, 630b
  anal stenosis, 627–628, 628f
  fecal incontinence, 620–626,
    620b, 621b, 621f
  hemorrhoidal disease,
    624–626, 625b, 626b
  rectal prolapse, 622–624,
    623b, 624f
Anorectal ring, anatomy of,
  609–610
Anorexia nervosa, diagnosis
  criteria for, 115b
Anterior colporrhaphy, for anterior
  vaginal wall prolapse,
  571–572, 572–574f
Anterior vaginal wall prolapse,
  surgical repair techniques of
  anterior colporrhaphy,
  571–572, 572–574f

Anterior vaginal wall prolapse,
  surgical repair techniques of
  (Continued)
  paravaginal defect repair,
    572, 575
Antiangiogenesis, for
  endometriosis, 340
Antidiuretic hormone (ADH), 26
Antiprogestins, for endometriosis,
  332t, 334
Anus
  carcinoma of, invasive, 636
  gynecologic assessment of,
    116–118
Anxiety disorders, 114–115
Appendectomy, prophylactic,
  hysterectomy and, 741
Appendix of the testis, 15
Arcus tendineus levator ani, 76
Arias-Stella reaction, 4
Aromatase inhibitors, for
  endometriosis, 340
Arteries, of pelvis, 77–79, 77–79f
Asherman's syndrome, 362
Aspirin, cardiovascular disease
  and, 137–138
Ataxia-telangiectasia, 58
Atrophic vaginitis, menopause
  and, 388–389, 389b, 389t
Autosomal dominant, family
  history, cancer risk
  assessment and, 46
Autosomal recessive, family
  history, cancer risk
  assessment and, 46

B
Bacterial endocarditis prevention,
  gynecologic surgery
  and, 690
Baden-Walker halfway
  system, 121
Barrier method contraceptives,
  176–177
  cervical cap, 177
  condoms, 176
  diaphragm, 177
  sponge, 177
Bartholin's abscess,
  426–427
Bartholin's gland carcinoma,
  426, 426b

Basal cell carcinoma, of vulva, 426, 426b

Beecham system, 121

Behçet's disease, of vulva, 419

Bethesda criteria 64, 65b *See also* 2001 Bethesda System

Bicornuate uterus, 213–214, 214f

Bilaminar germ disc, 5

BIRADS. *See* Breast Imaging Reporting and Data System atlas

Bisphosphonates, menopause and, 399–400

Bladder, 19f, 20

Blastocele, 3

Blastocyst, 3, 4f

Blastomeres, 3

Bleeding, abnormal uterine
in adolescence, 201–202, 202b, 203b, 353, 353b
diagnosis of, 349–352, 351b, 355b
endometrial cancer, 355, 356b
endometrial hyperplasia, 355, 356b
intrauterine device and, 170
menopausal bleeding, 354–355, 355b
oral contraceptives for, 354
outcomes of, 364
pathophysiology of, 348–349, 349b
perimenopause, 353–354
premenarchal girls, 353
prevalence of, 348
signs of, 349
symptoms of, 349
therapy for, 358–363
medical, 358–360
Danazol, 359
gonadotropin-releasing hormone, 359–360
intravenous conjugated equine estrogen, 359
levonorgestrel intrauterine device, 360
nonsteroidal anti-inflammatory drugs, 358
oral contraceptive pills, 358
progesterone, 359
surgical, 360–363

Bleeding, abnormal uterine (*Continued*)
therapy for (*Continued*)
surgical (*Continued*)
dilation and curettage, 362
endometrial ablation, 362, 363t
hysterectomy, 361
management of, 362–363
myomectomy, 361
operative hysteroscopy, 360–361
uterine fibroid embolization, 361
von Willebrand's disease, 352–353

Blighted ovum, 226

Blood pressure, classification of, hypertension and, 128t

Bloom syndrome, 58

Bone mineral density, testing of, 109b

Bones, of pelvis, 73–75, 74f

Bowel disorders
benign diseases, 612–630
benign anorectal disease, 620–621
anal fissure, 626–627
anal fistula, 628–630, 629f, 630b
anal stenosis, 627–628, 628f
fecal incontinence, 620–626, 620b, 621b, 621f
hemorrhoidal disease, 624–626, 625b, 626b
rectal prolapse, 622–624, 623b, 624f
colonic diseases, 612–620
constipation, 618–619
Crohn's disease, 616–618, 617b
defecatory disorders, 618–619
diverticular disease, 612–614, 613f
inflammatory bowel disease, 614–616, 615b, 616f

Bowel disorders (*Continued*)
benign diseases (*Continued*)
colonic diseases (*Continued*)
mucosal ulcerative colitis, 614–616, 615b, 616f
rectocele, 619–620
cancer screening guidelines, 612b
diagnostic tests for, 611–612, 613f
history of, 610–611
malignant diseases, 630–636
anal neoplasia, 634–635
anal intraepithelial neoplasia, 635
Bowen's disease, 635–636, 635f
invasive anal carcinoma, 636
Paget's disease, 636
colorectal cancer, 630–636, 631f, 633–634b, 634f
physical examination for, 610–611
polypoid lesion, 611f
prolapsing hemorrhoids, 610f

Bowen's disease, 635–636, 635f

BRCA1, hereditary cancer syndromes, 58–60, 57t

BRCA2, hereditary cancer syndromes, 58–60, 57t

Breast Imaging Reporting and Data System atlas (BIRADS), 507, 508t

Breasts
anatomy of, 497–498
adult, 498
embryology, 497
microscopic, 498
nerves, 498
assessment of, well-woman exam and, 113–114
breast cancer, 113
fibroadenoma, 113
fibrocystic changes, 113
benign disease of, 499–506
breast malformation, 505–506
fat necrosis, 504–505
fibroadenoma, 501–502
fibrocystic changes, 499–501
cancer association, 501, 501b

Breasts (Continued)
  benign disease of (Continued)
    fibrocystic changes
        (Continued)
      mastalgia, 499
      treatment, 499–501
    infections, 502–503
      lactational mastitis, 502
      nonlactational (subareolar)
          abscess, 502–503
    nipple discharge, 503–504
      end-organ lesions, 504
      galactorrhea, 503–504,
          503b
  cancer of, 113
    clinical detection of, 506–507
    early detection of, 507–509,
        508t
    future directions for, 519
    hereditary, 518–519
    pathology of, 509–510
    post-treatment follow-up,
        516–517
    pregnancy-associated,
        517–518
    prognosis of, 516
    risk factors for, 506b
    screening for, 141, 145
      hereditary, 58
    staging of, 510, 511t
    treatment of, 510–516
      chemotherapy, 513–514
      hormonal therapy, 514
      neoadjuvant
          chemotherapy,
          514–515
      radiation therapy,
          515–516
      surgical, 510–511
      surgical technique,
          511–512
      systemic therapy, 512
  fibroadenoma of, 113,
      501–502
  fibrocystic changes of, 113
  gynecologic assessment of, 116
  hereditary cancer syndrome,
      57–67
    BRCA1, 58–60, 57t
    BRCA2, 58–60, 57t
    cancer screening, 60–61

Breasts (Continued)
  hereditary cancer syndrome
      (Continued)
    chemoprevention, 63
    mastectomy, prophylactic, 62
  puberty and, 38–39, 39t
Bulimia, diagnosis criteria for,
    115b
Bulk enhancing agent injection,
    for urinary incontinence,
    605–606
  complications of, 605–606
  outcomes of, 606
  periurethral technique, 605
  transurethral technique, 605
Burch colosuspension, 599, 600f
Burnham, Walter, 707

C
Caffeine, decrease of, menopause
    and, 402
CAGE Questionnaire, 153b
CAGE-AID Questionnaire, 153b
CAH. See Congenital adrenal
    hyperplasia
Calcitonin-salmon, menopause
    and, 401
Calcium supplements, menopause
    and, 401
Cancer
  of anus, invasive, 636
  of breasts, 113
    clinical detection of,
        506–507
    early detection of, 507–509,
        508t
    future directions for, 519
    hereditary, 518–519
    pathology of, 509–510
    post-treatment follow-up,
        516–517
    pregnancy-associated,
        517–518
    prognosis of, 516
    risk factors for, 506b
    screening for, 141, 145
      hereditary, 58
    staging of, 501, 511b
    treatment of, 510–516
      chemotherapy, 513–514
      hormonal therapy, 514

Cancer (Continued)
  of breasts (Continued)
    treatment of (Continued)
      neoadjuvant
          chemotherapy,
          514–515
      radiation therapy,
          515–516
      surgical, 510–511
      surgical technique,
          511–512
      systemic therapy, 512
  cell cycle control and, 52–57
    acquired gene mutations,
        52–53
    DNA alteration types, 53–54
    inherited gene mutations,
        52–53
    mutated gene classes, 54–56
  cervical epidemiology of, 420
    evaluation techniques for,
        447–451
      acetic acid visual
          inspection, 447–448,
          448f
      cervicography, 448
      colposcopy, 448–451,
          450f, 450t
      optical biopsy diagnosis,
          448, 449f
    risk factors for, 431–435,
        432b
      cigarette smoking, 434
      herpes simplex virus, 435
      human papillomavirus,
          431–435, 432b
      immunosuppression, 435
    screening for, 145–146
  colorectal, 630–634, 631f,
      633–634b, 634f
    screening for, 146, 147t
    staging of, 633–634b
  genetic counseling, 44
  lung
    risk factors for, 103b
    screening for, 146
  ovarian, screening for, 145
  risk assessment, 44–45, 45b
    family history, 45–47
    process of, 47–52, 48b
  screening

Cancer *(Continued)*
  screening *(Continued)*
    bowel disorder guidelines, 612b
    of breasts, 141, 145
      hereditary, 58
    of cervix, 145–146
    colorectal, 146, 147t
    of lungs, 146
    during menopause, 405, 405t
    of ovaries, 145
    of skin, 146, 148
    skin, screening for, 146, 148
Cancer risk assessment
  familial, 48
  family history, 45–47
  inherited cancer syndrome, 49
  process of, 47–52, 48b
    determination, 47–49, 48f
    genetic testing, 49–52, 49b
  sporadic disease, 48
Candida albicans, 411
Candidiasis, of vulva, 413–414
Capacitation reaction, 3
Carcinogenesis multistep process, genetic testing, cancer risk assessment and, 56
Cardiogenic area, 8
Cardiovascular disease
  gynecologic surgery and, 689–690
  menopause and, 402–404, 404b, 403t
  prevention health care, 126–138
    aspirin and, 137–138
    diabetes, 133–134, 134t, 135b, 136t, 137t
    dyslipidemia, 130–133, 132t, 133t
    exercise, 137
    HRT and, 137–138
    hypertension, 127–130, 128t, 129t, 130t
    prevention of, 137–138
    risk factor assessment, 126–127, 127b
    smoking, 135, 137
Cardiovascular system, well-woman exam and, 101–102, 101b

Catecholamines, 24
Caudal dysgenesis, 10, 11f
Cell cycle control, cancer and, 52–57
  acquired gene mutations, 52–53
  DNA alteration types, 53–54
  inherited gene mutations, 52–53
  mutated gene classes, 54–56
Cervical agenesis, 217–218, 217f
Cervical cap, 177
Cervical cytology, history of, 429–430, 430f
Cervical ectopic pregnancy, 281–282
Cervical intraepithelial neoplasia (CIN), 430, 435, 436f
Cervicitis, 531–532
  chlamydia, 531–532, 532b
  gonorrhea, 532, 533b
Cervicography, for cervical cancer, 448
Cervix
  anatomy of, 430–431
  cancer of
    epidemiology of, 431
    evaluation techniques for, 447–451
      acetic acid visual inspection, 447–448, 448f
      cervicography, 448
      colposcopy, 449–451, 450f, 450t
      optical biopsy diagnosis, 448, 449f
    risk factors for, 431–435, 432b
      cigarette smoking, 434
      herpes simplex virus, 435
      human papillomavirus, 431–435, 432b
      immunosuppression, 435
    screening for, 145–146
  gynecologic assessment of, 116
  intraepithelial lesions of, treatment of, 451–455, 451f, 455f, 452t
    cold-knife conization, 454
    cryosurgery, 452–453

Cervix *(Continued)*
  intraepithelial lesions of, treatment of *(Continued)*
    hysterectomy, 454–455
    laser vaporization, 453
    loop electrosurgical excision procedure, 453–454, 454b, 454f
  neoplasia of, screening for, 442–447
    cervical sampling, 443, 443b
    HPV DNA adjunct to, 444
    liquid-based cytology, 443–444
    modern recommendations, 445–447, 446f, 446t, 447b
    negative, 444–445
  preinvasive disease pathology of, 435–442
    2001 Bethesda System, 436–442
      adenocarcinoma, 441, 442
      endometrial cells, 437
      glandular cell abnormalities, 440–441, 440b, 441f
      negative intraepithelial lesion, 437
      negative malignancy, 437
      specimen adequacy, 437
      squamous cell abnormalities, 437–440, 438–440, 439f
    cervical intraepithelial neoplasia, 435, 436f
Chancroid, 527, 527b
CHD. *See* Coronary heart disease
Chemoprevention
  for hereditary breast cancer, 58
  in nonpolyposis colorectal, 64
Chemotherapy
  adolescence and, 197
  for breast cancer, 513–514
    neoadjuvant, 514–515
Children, pelvic mass of, 481–482, 482b
Chlamydia trachomatis, 411, 531–532, 532b

Cholecystectomy, hysterectomy and, 741

Chorionic activity, 6

Chromosomal, family history, cancer risk assessment and, 47

Chromosomes, DNA alterations, in cancer cells, 53

Chronic pelvic pain, 679
diagnosis of, 683
differential diagnosis of, 680–683, 680b
treatment of, 683–684

Cigarette smoking. *See* Smoking

CIN. *See* Cervical intraepithelial neoplasia

Cleavage, 3
of clitoris, 215

Clitoris, 15, 17f, 18t, 83, 84f
anomalies of, 219–220, 219f
cleavage, 220
clitoromegaly, 219–220, 219f
splitting, 220

Clitoromegaly, 219–220, 219f

Clomid, infertility and, 303–304

Clomiphene citrate, infertility and, 312

Coccygeus muscles, 75–76, 75f, 76f

Coccyx, 73, 74f

Coelomic metaplasia theory, 322–323

Cold-knife conization, for cervical intraepithelial lesions, 434

Collecting tubules, 19

Colonic diseases, bowel disorders, 612–614
constipation, 618–619
Crohn's disease, 616–618, 617b
defecatory disorders, 618–619
diverticular disease, 612–614, 613f
inflammatory bowel disease, 614–616, 615b, 616f
mucosal ulcerative colitis, 614–616, 615b, 616f
rectocele, 619–620

Colorectal cancer, 630–636, 631f, 633–634b, 634f

Colorectal cancer *(Continued)*
screening for, 146, 147t
staging of, 633–634b

Colpectomy, pelvic organ prolapse and, 571

Colpocleisis, pelvic organ prolapse and, 571

Colporrhaphy, anterior, for anterior vaginal wall prolapse, 571–572, 572–573f

Colposcopy, for cervical cancer, 448–450, 450f, 450t

Combined oral contraceptives, 162–167, 162b, 163t, 164t, 166b
action mechanisms of, 162
contraindications of, 162–163, 162b, 163t
noncontraceptive benefits, 165, 166b
preparations for, 166–167
prescription guidelines for, 163–164t
risks of, 163–165
side effects of, 163–165

Common iliac arteries, 77, 78f

Condoms, 176

Congenital adrenal hyperplasia (CAH), 205

Congenital obstructive lesions, in adolescence, 483

Constipation, 618–619

Contraceptive patch, 168

Contraceptives
barrier methods, 176–177
cervical cap, 177
condoms, 176
diaphragm, 177
sponge, 177
development of, 157–159
effectiveness of, 158–159, 160–161t
provision requirements of, 159
diabetes and, 184
emergency, 181–182
epilepsy and, 184–185
failed, ectopic pregnancy and, 261
hypertension and, 183
implants, 169–170

Contraceptives *(Continued)*
injectable, 168–169
intrauterine device, 170–176
lactation and, 182
medical conditions and, 183–185
diabetes, 184
epilepsy, 184–185
hypertension, 183
sickle cell disease, 184
microbicides, 181–182
natural, 178
Nuva Ring, 167
oral
for abnormal uterine bleeding, 358
combined, 162–167, 162b, 163t, 164t
action mechanisms of, 162
contraindications of, 162–163, 162b, 163t
noncontraceptive benefits, 165, 166b
preparations for, 166–167
prescription guidelines for, 163–164t
risks of, 163–165
side effects of, 163–165
for endometriosis, 332t, 334
leiomyomas, 469
Ortho Evra, 168
patch, 168
perimenopause and, 183
postpartum period and, 182
sickle cell disease and, 184
spermicides, 177–178
sterilization, 178–181
systemic hormonal, 159, 162–170
combined oral, 162, 162b, 163t, 164t, 166b
contraceptive patch, 168
implants, 169–170
injectables, 168–169
progestin-only pill, 168
vaginal ring, 167

Controlled ovarian hyperstimulation, infertility and, 312

Cooper's ligament, 75
Coronary heart disease (CHD), 130–131
Cortical cords, 13f, 14
Corticotropin-releasing hormone (CRH), 24–25
Cowden Syndrome, 58
Coxal bones, 73, 74f
CRH. *See* Corticotropin-releasing hormone
Crohn's disease, 616–618, 617b
Cryosurgery, for cervical intraepithelial lesions, 452–453
Culdocentesis, ectopic pregnancy and, 269, 271
Cystoscopy, hysterectomy, 781–783
  equipment of, 781
  history of, 781
  practical uses of, 782–783
  technique of, 782, 782f
Cysts
  ovarian
    in adolescence, 198
    functional, 483–485, 484f
    in prepuberty patients, 192–193
  paraovarian, 15
  peritoneal inclusion, in reproductive-age women, 493–494, 493f
Cytotrophoblast, 4

D

Danazol
  for abnormal uterine bleeding, 359
  for endometriosis, 331, 332t, 333
Defecatory disorders, 618–619
Definitive oocyte, 3
Definitive placental villous, 8, 9f
Dementia, 150, 149b
  menopause and, 392–393
Depot medroxyprogesterone acetate (DMPA), 168–169
Depression, 148–149
  Diagnostic and Statistical Manual for diagnosis of, 149b

Depression *(Continued)*
  presentation of, 149b
Dermatitis, of vulva, 412–413
Dermatologic conditions, of vulva, pruritus, 414–416
  lichen sclerosus, 414–415
  lichen simplex chronicus, 415–416
  psoriasis, 416
DEXA. *See* Dual energy x-ray absorptiometry
Diabetes, 106–107, 108b
  cardiovascular disease and, 133–134, 134t, 135b, 136t, 137t
  contraceptives and, 184
  gynecologic surgery and, 691
  National Institute of Diabetes and Digestive and Kidney Diseases, 667, 668b
  preoperative evaluation of, for gynecologic surgery, 691
Diabetes mellitus (DM), 133–134, 134t, 135b, 136t, 137t
Diagnostic and Statistical Manual, depression, diagnosis of, 149b
Diaphragm, 177
Didelphic uterus, 214–215, 214f
Dilation and curettage, for abnormal uterine bleeding, 362
Diplotene stage, 1–2
Direct implantation theory, 324
Direct trocar insertion, for laparoscopy, 765
Discrete rectovaginal fascia defect repair, for posterior vaginal wall prolapse, 576–579, 577f, 578f
Diverticular disease, 612–614, 613f
DM. *See* Diabetes mellitus
DMPA. *See* Depot medroxyprogesterone acetate
DNA alterations, in cancer cells, types of, 53–54
  chromosomes, 53
  genes, 53
  viruses, 53–54

DNA repair genes, 56
Domestic violence, 150–152
  risk factors for, 151b
  warning signs of, 152b
Dual energy x-ray absorptiometry (DEXA), 395
DUB. *See* Dysfunctional uterine bleeding
Ductus deferens, 15
Dysfunctional uterine bleeding (DUB). *See* Abnormal uterine bleeding
Dyslipidemia, cardiovascular disease and, 130–133, 132t, 133t
Dysmenorrhea, 377–378, 714
Dyspepsia, 104

E

Eating disorders, 114, 114b
  in adolescence, 194
  signs/symptoms of, 114b
Ectoderm, 7, 7f, 10
Ectopic pregnancy (EP)
  assisted reproduction and, 261
  clinical presentation of, 262–265
  diagnostic modalities in, 265–271
    culdocentesis, 269, 271
    laboratory tests, 265–266
    quantitative serum hCG, ultrasonography plus, 268–269, 269f
    ultrasonography, 266–268, 267f, 268t, 269f, 270t
    quantitative serum hCG plus, 268–269, 269f
    uterine curettage, 271
  epidemiology of, 257–259
    incidence of, 257, 258f
    mortality, 258–259, 258f
  failed contraception, 261
  functional factors in, 260–261
  infertility, 261
  location of, 262, 263f
  medical management of, 274–278
    direct injection methotrexate, 278

Ectopic pregnancy (EP)
      (*Continued*)
   medical management of
         (*Continued*)
      multidose systemic
            methotrexate,
            274–275, 275t
      patient counseling in, 277,
            277b
      patient monitoring in,
            276–277
      patient safety in, 277–278
      patient selection in, 276,
            276b
      single-dose systemic
            methotrexate, 275
   natural history of, 262–265
   pathogenesis of, 259–262
   reproductive performance
         after, 283–284, 283b
   Rh sensitization, 279
   risk factors of, 259–262, 259t
   salpingitis, 259–260
   signs of, 264–265, 264t
   sterilization, 261
   surgical management of,
         271–274
      conservative surgery,
            272–273, 273f
      laparotomy *vs.* laparoscopy,
            271–272
      persistent, 273–274, 274b
      radical surgery, 272
   symptoms of, 264–265, 264t
   treatment of, medical *vs.*
         surgical, 278–279
      efficacy, 278–279
      expectant management, 279
      safety, 278–279
   tubal abortion, 262–263
   tubal injury in, 259–260, 260f
   tubal rupture, 263–264, 264f
   tubal surgery, 261
   types of, uncommon, 279–282
      abdominal, 280–281
      cervical, 281–282
      heterotopic, 282
      interstitial, 279–280, 280f
      ovarian, 281
Efferent ducts, 15
Ejaculatory ducts, 15, 18f, 20

Electrosurgery, principles,
      laparoscopy, 756–760
   bipolar electrosurgery,
         759–760, 760f
   monopolar electrosurgery,
         759–760
   physics, 756–757, 756f
   waveforms, 757
      blended current, 757, 758f,
            758t, 759t
      modulated current, 757
      nonmodulated, 757
Embryoblast, 4, 5, 6f
Embryology
   development in
      second week, 5–6
      third week, 6–8
   fertilization, 1, 3–5
   fetal-maternal circulation,
         8–10, 9f
   muscular system, 8
   neural tube formation in, 8
   skeletal system, 8
   urogenital system in, 10–20
      external genitalia, 15
      genetic sex, 11
      genital ducts, 14–15
      gonadal sex, 11
      gonads, 12–14, 13f
      phenotypical sex, 11
      sexual differentiation, 11
      urinary system, 16–20
         allantois, 19f, 20
         bladder, 19f, 20
         collecting tubules, 19
         ejaculatory ducts, 18t, 20
         median umbilical
               ligament, 20
         membranous urethra,
               19f, 20
         mesonephric duct, 17
         mesonephros, 16, 17
         metanephric mesoderm,
               17
         metanephros, 16
         nephrons, 19, 19f
         penile urethra, 17f, 20
         pronephros, 16
         prostatic urethra, 19f, 20
         urachus, 19f, 20
         ureter, 19f, 20

Embryology (*Continued*)
   urogenital system in
         (*Continued*)
      urinary system (*Continued*)
         ureteric buds, 17, 19f
         urethra, 19f, 20
         urogenital sinus, 19–20
         vestibule of the vagina,
               19f, 20
Embryonic demise, 225
Embryonic rest theory, 324
Emsel's criteria, 530b
Endocrine disease, in adolescence,
      195
Endocrine system, well-woman
      exam and, 106–109
Endoderm, 7, 7f, 10
Endometrial cells, 2001 Bethesda
      System and, 436
Endometrioma, in reproductive-
      age women, 491
Endometriosis, 199–200
   in adolescence, 199–200
   assisted reproduction and, 341
   clinical diagnosis of, 325–329
      imaging, 329
      laparoscopic, 327–329,
            328f, 329f
      serum markers, 329
      signs, 327
      symptoms, 325–327, 325t,
            326b, 327b
   differential diagnosis of, 330
   etiology of, 322–324, 322b
      coelomic metaplasia theory,
            322–323
      direct implantation theory,
            324
      embryonic rest theory, 324
      genetic theory, 323
      immunologic theory, 323
      lymphatic/vascular
            metastasis theory, 323
      retrograde menstruation
            theory, 322
   hysterectomy and, 708
   management of, 330–340
      decision making/therapy
            selection, 337, 338t
      at gastrointestinal tract,
            338–339

Endometriosis *(Continued)*
  management of *(Continued)*
    medical therapy, 331–335,
      332t
      antiprogestins, 332t, 334
      Danazol, 331, 332t, 333
      gestrinone, 335
      GnRH agonists, 332t, 333
      GnRH antagonists, 335
      nonsteroidal
        antiinflammatory
        drugs, 335
      oral contraceptives, 338t,
        334
      progestins, 332t, 334
    plan, 330
    surgical therapy, 335
      approach, 335
      combined, 337
      conservative interventions,
        336–337, 337b
      definitive interventions, 337
    at uterine tract, 339, 339f
  pathology of, 324–325
    anatomic sites of, 324, 324t
    gross, 325
    microscopic, 325
  treatment of, future, 339
    antiangiogenesis, 340
    aromatase inhibitors, 340
    immune system modulators,
      340
    matrix metalloproteinases
      inhibition, 340
Endometrium, 35–38
  ablation of, for abnormal uterine
    bleeding, 362, 363t
  abnormal uterine bleeding and
    ablation, 362, 363t
  cancer of, 355, 356b
  hyperplasia, 355, 356b
  anatomy of, 35
  breakdown of, 37–38
  cancer of, abnormal uterine
    bleeding in, 355, 356b
  evaluation of, tools for,
    356–358
    biopsy, 356
    hysteroscopy, 357–358
    magnetic resonance
      imaging, 358

Endometrium *(Continued)*
  evaluation of, tools for
    (Continued)
    saline infusion sonography,
      357, 357b
    transvaginal ultrasound,
      356–357
  hyperplasia of, abnormal
    uterine bleeding and, 355,
    356b
  proliferative phase of, 35, 36f
  reproductive cycle, 35–38
    anatomy of, 35
    breakdown of, 37–38
    proliferative phase of,
      35–36, 36f
    secretory phase of, 36–37,
      37f
  secretory phase of, 36–37, 37f
End-organ lesions, of breasts, 504
Enterobius vermicularis. *See*
  Pinworms
EP. *See* Ectopic pregnancy
Epiblast, 5
Epididymis, 15
Epilepsy, contraceptives and,
  184–185
Epoophoron, 15
Equipment
  for cystoscopy, 781–783
  for hysterectomy, 777–778,
    777f
  for laparoscopy, 762–763
    ancillary ports, 766
    classic entry, 763–66, 764f
    direct trocar insertion, 765
    initial entry, 763, 764f
    initial trocar placement, 763
    open laparoscopy, 765
    optical trocar technique, 766
    radial expanding access
      cannulas, 766
    visualization, 762–763,
      762f
Estrogen, ovaries and, 29–30, 30t
Ethanol abuse,
  holoprosencephaly and, 10,
  12f
Exercise, cardiovascular disease
  and, 137
External genitalia, 15

External genitalia *(Continued)*
  anomalies of, 219–222
    clitoris, 219–220, 219f
    hymen, 220–221, 221f
    labia minora, 220
  gynecologic assessment of,
    118–119
External iliac arteries, 77, 78f

F
Fallopian tubes
  genital ducts, female, 14, 17f
  prolapse of, hysterectomy and,
    745
  reproductive organs, 87f, 88
  tubal abortion, 262–263
  tubal injury in, 259–260, 260f
  tubal rupture, 263–264, 264f
  tubal surgery, 261
Family history, cancer risk
  assessment and, 45–47
  inheritance modes, 46–47
    autosomal dominant, 46
    autosomal recessive, 46
    chromosomal, 47
    mitochondrial, 47
    multifactorial, 47
    x-linked dominant/recessive,
      46–47
Family planning. *See*
  Contraceptives
Febrile morbidity, hysterectomy
  and, 744–745
Fecal incontinence, 620–622,
  620b, 621b, 621f
Fecal incontinence score (FIS),
  620–621, 621b
Fecundability, 287
Fecundity, 287
Female pronucleus, 3
Female sexual dysfunction,
  387–388
Fertilization, 1, 3–5
  acrosome reaction, 3
  blastocele, 3
  blastocyte, 3, 4f
  blastomeres, 3
  capacitation reaction, 3
  cleavage, 3
  definitive oocyte, 3
  embryoblast, 4

793

Fertilization (Continued)
  female pronucleus, 3
  implantation, 4, 5t
    Arias-Stella reaction, 4
    cytotrophoblast, 4
    syncytiotrophoblast, 4
  male pronucleus, 3
  morula, 3
  one-cell embryo, 3, 4f
  trophectoderm, 3
  trophoblast, 4
Fetal-maternal circulation, 8–10, 9f
Fever, gynecologic surgery and, 697–698
Fibroadenoma, of breasts, 113, 501–502
Fibroids. See Leiomyomas
Fimbria, 14, 13f
First-trimester pregnancy termination, 232–233, 232–239, 234t, 235t
  complication incidence, 238–239
  complication management, 238–239
  gestational age determination, 232–233, 233t, 234t
  pain management, 236–238
  pregnancy diagnosis, 232–233, 233t, 234t
  preoperative evaluation, 234, 235t
  products of conception examination, 238
  surgical technique, 234–236
Follicle-stimulating hormone (FSH), 21, 25, 30, 31–32, 33–34
Follicular cells, 14, 14f
Framingham Scoring System, 132t, 133t
Freund, W. A., 707
FSH. See Follicle-stimulating hormone

G
Galactorrhea, of breasts, 503–504
Gametes, 1
Gametogenesis, 1–3
Gartner cysts, 13f, 15

Gastroesophageal reflux disease (GERD), 102–103
Gastrointestinal system, well-woman exam and, 103–106, 105b
Gastrointestinal tract, endometriosis at, 338–339
Gene expression profiling, genetic testing, cancer risk assessment and, 56–57
Genes
  DNA alterations, in cancer cells, 53
  mutations of, 52–53
    classes of, 54–56
      DNA repair genes, 56
      proto-oncogenes, 54, 55
      tumor suppressions, 54–56, 57t
Genetic counseling, 44
Genetic sex, 11
Genetic testing, cancer risk assessment and, 49–52
  algorithm for, 49–50, 49b
  carcinogenesis multistep process, 56
  gene expression profiling, 56–57
  informed consent, 52
  post-test counseling, 52
  pretest counseling, 50–52
Genetic theory, 323
Genital ducts, 14–15
  female, 14–15
    epoophoron, 15
    fallopian tubes, 14, 16f
    fimbria, 14, 13f
    Gartner cysts, 13f, 15
    hydatid cysts of Morgagni, 15
    hymen, 14
    müllerian tubercle, 14
    paraovarian cysts, 15
    paroophoron, 15
    Rokitansky syndrome, 15
    uterine canal, 14
    vagina, 14
    vaginal plate, 14
  male
    appendix of the testis, 15
    ductus deferens, 15
    efferent ducts, 15

Genital ducts (Continued)
  male (Continued)
    ejaculatory duct, 15
    epididymis, 15
    prostatic utricle, 15
    seminal vesicle, 15
Genital ridge, 12–13
Genital tract fistulas
  complications of, 660
  diagnosis of, 653–654, 653f
  epidemiology of, 651–652, 652b
  etiology of, 651–652, 652b
  further investigation of, 654–655
  presentation of, 652–653
  treatment of, 655–660
    conservative management of, 655–656
    interposition flaps, 660
    postoperative care, 660
    preoperative management of, 657
    repair timing, 656, 656b
    surgical approach in, 657–659
      abdominal, 659–660
      vaginal, 657–659, 658f, 659f
    surgical management of, 656, 657
Genital tubercle, 15
Genitalia, external, 83–86, 84f
  anal membrane, 15, 17f, 18t
  female, 15–16, 18t
    clitoris, 15, 17f, 18t
    labia majora, 16, 17f, 18t
    labia minora, 15, 17f, 18t
    mons pubis, 16, 17f, 18t
  genital tubercle, 15, 17f, 18t
  labioscrotal swelling, 15, 17f, 18t
  male, 15, 18t
    penile urethra, 15, 17f, 18t
    penoscrotal hypospadias, 15, 18f, 18t
    phallus, 15, 17f, 18t
    scrotum, 15, 17f, 18t
  urethral groove, 15, 17f, 18t
  urogenital fold, 15, 17f, 18t
Genitals
  ulcerative disease of, 525–529

Genitals *(Continued)*
    ulcerative disease of
        (Continued)
        chancroid, 527, 527b
        granuloma inguinale, 528
        herpes, 515, 526b
        lymphogranuloma
            venereum, 527–528
        syphilis, 525–527
        tuberculosis, 528–529
    upper, infections of, 532–537
        endometritis, 532–533
        human immunodeficiency
            virus, 536–537
        pelvic inflammatory disease,
            533–535, 535b, 536b
        tubo-ovarian abscess,
            535–536
        viral hepatitis, 537
GERD. *See* Gastroesophageal
    reflux disease
Germinal epithelium, 87
Gestrinone, for endometriosis,
    335
GHRF. *See* Growth hormone-
    releasing factor
Glucose values, 134t
GnRH. *See* Gonadotropin
    releasing hormone
Gonad, dysfunction of
    primary amenorrhea and, 370
    secondary amenorrhea and,
        370
Gonadal sex, 11
Gonadotropin-releasing
    hormone (GnRH), 21–23,
        193–194
    abnormal uterine bleeding and,
        359–360
    for endometriosis agonists,
        332t, 333
    antagonists, 335
    leiomyomas and, 470
Gonadotropins, infertility and,
    305–306
Gonads, 12–14, 13f
    embryology and,
        12–14, 13f
Gonorrhea, 532, 532b
Graft reconstructive, pelvic organ
    prolapse and, 579

Granuloma inguinale, 528
Growth hormone-releasing factor
    (GHRF), 24–25
Gynecologic assessment
    anus examination, 119–120
    breast assessment, 118
    cervical assessment, 120
    diagnosis testing, 118–121
    examination, 118–121
    external genitalia assessment,
        118–119
    history, 116–118
    pelvic organ prolapse
        assessment, 121
    perineal body examination,
        119–120
    upper genital tract assessment,
        121
    urethral examination, 119
    vaginal assessment, 120
    vulvar examination, 119
Gynecologic surgery
    postoperative care, 697–704
        fever, 697–698
        ileus, 703–704
        infection, 701–702
        neurologic injury, 704
        respiratory complications,
            698–699
        thromboembolic
            complications,
            699–701
        urinary retention, 702
        wound care, 701–702
    preoperative evaluation of,
        687–697
        adrenal suppression, 691
        age, 688
        allergies, 692
        asthma, 690–691
        bacterial endocarditis
            prevention, 690
        bowel preparation,
            695–696, 696b
        cardiac disease, 689–690
        cardiovascular disease,
            689–690
        consultation, 688
        diabetes, 691
        exercise tolerance, 688–689
        hypertension, 690

Gynecologic surgery *(Continued)*
    preoperative evaluation of
        (Continued)
        imaging studies, 693
        informed consent, 694
        laboratory tests, 693
        medical comorbidities,
            689–690
        medications, 691–692, 692b
        patient positioning,
            696–697
        prior surgery, 692–693
        substance abuse, 692
        surgical risk, 689
        surgical site infection
            prophylaxis, 694–695
        total joint replacement,
            691
    preparation for, 687–697

H
Haemophilus ducreyi, 411
HBOC. *See* Hereditary breast and
    ovarian cancer
HDLs. *See* High-density
    lipoproteins
Headaches, menopause and, 391
Heaney, N. S., 708
Helicobacter pylori, 104–106
Hematochezia, 105
Hematuria
    differential diagnosis of, 10,
        111b
    evaluation of, 111b
Hemorrhage, hysterectomy
    and, 742
Hemorrhoidal disease, 624–626,
    625b, 626b
    benign anorectal disease,
        620–630, 620b, 621b
    prolapsing, 610f
    thrombosed, 625
Hereditary breast and ovarian
    cancer (HBOC), 58–64
Hereditary cancer syndromes,
    57–67, 57t
    breast, 58–64
        BRCA1, 58–59, 57t
        BRCA2, 58–59, 57t
        cancer screening, 60–61
        chemoprevention, 63

Hereditary cancer syndromes
 (Continued)
 breast (Continued)
  mastectomy, prophylactic,
   62
  nonpolyposis colorectal,
   64–67
   chemoprevention in, 67
   clinical manifestations of,
    64, 65b, 65f
   genetic testing in, 64–66
   management of, 66
   surgical strategies for, 67
   surveillance of, 66
 ovarian, 58–64
  cancer screening, 61–62
  oophorectomy, prophylactic,
   62–63
  risk reduction of, 63–64
Hereditary nonpolyposis
 colorectal cancer (HNPCC),
 46, 64–67
 chemoprevention in, 67
 clinical manifestations of, 64,
  65b, 65f
 genetic testing in, 64–66
 management of, 66
 surgical strategies for, 67
 surveillance of, 66
Herpes, of genitals, 525, 526b
Herpes simplex virus
 cervical cancer and, 435
 of vulva, 416–418, 418t
Heterotopic ectopic pregnancy,
 282
Hidradenitis suppurativa, 426–427
High recurrent mutation rates,
 46
High-density lipoproteins (HDLs),
 131
Hip protector pads, menopause
 and, 402
HIV. See Human
 immunodeficiency virus
HNPCC. See Hereditary
 nonpolyposis colorectal
Holoprosencephaly, 10, 12f
Hormonal therapy
 for breast cancer, 514
 menopause and, 396,
  398–399

Hot flashes, 386b
HPV. See Human papillomavirus
HRT, cardiovascular disease and,
 137–138
Human immunodeficiency virus
 (HIV), 536–537
Human papillomavirus (HPV),
 423–425, 424t
 cervical cancer and, 431–434,
  432b
 DNA adjunct to, for cervical
  neoplasia, 444
Hunner's ulcers, 663
Huntington's disease, 46
Hydatid cysts of Morgagni, 15
Hymen, 14
 anomalies of, 220, 221f
 cribriform, 221
 imperforate, 220–221
 microperforate,
  221, 221f
 septate, 221, 221f
Hypergonadotropic
 hypogonadism, 195
Hypertension, 127–130
 blood pressure classification,
  128t
 cardiovascular disease and,
  126–138, 128t, 129t, 130t
 causes of, 129t
 contraceptives and, 183
 end-organ damage evaluation,
  130t
 gynecologic surgery
  and, 690
 management of, 130t
 prevention of, 130t
Hyperthyroidism, 106–107,
 107b
Hypoblast, 5
Hypogonadotropic
 hypogonadism, 190–195
Hypophyseal portal circulation,
 23f
Hypothalamic axis, regulation of,
 reproductive cycle,
 23–24
Hypothalamus, 21–25
 adrenocorticotropic hormone,
  24
 catecholamines, 24

Hypothalamus (Continued)
 circulation, 23f
 corticotropin-releasing
  hormone, 24–25
 dysfunction of
  primary amenorrhea and,
   369–370
  secondary amenorrhea and,
   372–373
 gonadotropin-releasing
  hormone, 21–23
 growth hormone-releasing
  factor, 24–25
 somatostatin, 24–25
 thyroid-stimulating hormone,
  24–25
 thyrotropin-releasing
  hormone, 24–25
Hypothyroidism, 106, 107b
Hypotonic electrolyte-free
 solutions, hysteroscopy and,
 778–779
Hysterectomy
 abdominal, 725–727,
  728–739f
 for abnormal uterine bleeding,
  361
 for cervical intraepithelial
  lesions, 454–455
 complications of,
  742–745
  bowel injury, 744
  fallopian tube prolapse, 745
  febrile morbidity,
   744–745
  hemorrhage, 742
  lower urinary tract injury,
   742–743
  vesicovaginal fistulas,
   743–744
 concurrent procedures,
  738–741
  cholecystectomy, 735
  prophylactic appendectomy,
   741
  prophylactic oophorectomy,
   738–741
 cystoscopy, 781–783
  equipment of, 781
  history of, 777
  practical uses of, 782–783

Hysterectomy (Continued)
  cystoscopy (Continued)
    technique of, 782, 782f
  epidemiology of, 709
  historical perspective of,
    707–708
  hysteroscopy, 777–780
    bipolar instrument
      advantages, 779
    distension media,
      778–779
    hypotonic electrolyte-free
      solutions, 778–779
    isotonic solutions, 779
    equipment for, 777, 777f
    history of, 777
    postoperative complications,
      780–781
    pregnancy complications,
      780–781
    procedural complications,
      779–780
    perforation, 780
  indications for, 709–714,
    710t, 711f
    chronic pelvic pain, 714
    dysmenorrhea, 714
    endometriosis, 714
    excessive uterine bleeding,
      712–713
    pelvic organ prolapse, 713
    uterine leiomyomas,
      710–712
  laparoscopic, 727, 729–724,
    729t, 728–729f
  outcomes of, 745–751
    bladder function, 749–750
    bleeding, 746–747
    bowel function, 750
    pelvic organ prolapse,
      750–751
    pelvic pain, 747–748
    psychosocial function, 751
    quality of life, 751
    sexual function, 748–749
  preparation for, 717–719
  route of, 714–715,
    715f, 709f
  subtotal, 734–738
  for uterine/vaginal vault
    prolapse, 561

Hysterectomy (Continued)
  vaginal, 719–725,
    720–725f
    enlarged uterus removal,
      722–725
    vaginoscopy, 783
Hysterosalpingography, 466,
  467f
  infertility and, 300–301
Hysteroscopy
  endometrium and, 356–358
  hysterectomy, 777–781
    bipolar instrument
      advantages, 779
    distension media, 778–779
      hypotonic electrolyte-free
        solutions, 778–779
    isotonic solutions, 779
    equipment for, 777, 777f
    history of, 777
    postoperative complications,
      780–781
    pregnancy complications,
      780–781
    procedural complications,
      779–780
    perforation, 780
  leiomyomas and, 466–469,
    468f
Hysteroscopy, operative, for
  abnormal uterine bleeding,
  360–361

I

IBS. See Irritable bowel syndrome
Ileus, gynecologic surgery and,
  703–704
Iliococcygeus fascia suspension,
  for uterine/vaginal vault
  prolapse, 565–567, 566f
Iliolumbar artery, 77–79, 78f
Ilium, 79, 80f
Immune system modulators, for
  endometriosis, 340
Immunizations, preventive health
  care and, 141, 142–144t
Immunologic theory, 323
Immunosuppression, cervical
  cancer and, 435
Implantation, 4, 5t
  Arias-Stella reaction, 4

Implantation (Continued)
  cytotrophoblast, 4
  syncytiotrophoblast, 4
Implants, contraceptive,
  169–170
In vitro fertilization, infertility
  and, 312–315, 314f
Incomplete abortion, 225
Inevitable abortion, 225
Infection, gynecologic surgery
  and, 701–702
Inferior gluteal artery, 77, 78f
Infertility, 281
  ectopic pregnancy and, 261
  evaluation of, 294–302, 294t
    endometrial biopsy,
      296–297
    hysterosalpingography,
      300–301
    laparoscopy, 301–302
    ovulation documentation,
      297–299, 298f
    postcoital test, 296
    semen analysis, 299–300,
      299t
  future of, 316–317
  prognostic factors
    of, 287–294, 288f, 290f,
      290f
    duration, 289, 290t, 292,
      291f
    lifestyle, 292–294
  treatment of, 302–316
    endometriosis, 303–304
    male factor, 309–310
    ovulatory factor, 303–306
      Clomid, 303–304
      gonadotropins, 305–306
      letrozole, 304
      metformin, 304–305
      ovarian drilling, 306
    tubal factor, 308–309
    unexplained, 311–316–311t
      clomiphene citrate, 312
      controlled ovarian
        hyperstimulation,
        312
      expectant management,
        311–312
      intracytoplasmic sperm
        injection, 315–316

Infertility (Continued)
treatment of (Continued)
unexplained (Continued)
in vitro fertilization,
312–315, 314f
uterine factor, 307–308
Inflammatory bowel disease,
614–616, 615b, 616f,
609b, 610f
Inheritance modes, family
history, cancer risk
assessment and, 46–47
autosomal dominant, 46
autosomal recessive, 46
chromosomal, 47
mitochondrial, 47
multifactorial, 47
x-linked dominant/recessive,
46–47
Inherited gene mutations, 52–53
Injectable contraceptives,
168–169
Instillation agents, second-
trimester pregnancy
termination and, 246–247
Internal iliac arteries, 77, 77f
Internal pudendal artery, 78, 78f
Interstitial cystitis
associated conditions of, 666
background of, 663
diagnosis of, 667–668, 668b
disease spectrum, 665–666,
666f
epidemiology of, 663–664
etiology of, 664–665, 665f
evaluation of, 668–673,
670t, 672f
pathology of, 672–673
symptoms of, 666–667, 667b
treatment of, 673–679, 673b
behavioral and self help,
673–674, 673b
bladder instillations, 673b,
676–677
nerve stimulation,
673b, 678
oral medications, 673b,
675–676
pain management, 673b,
677–678
surgical, 673b, 678–679

Interstitial ectopic pregnancy,
279–280, 280f
Interureteric ridge, 90
Intracytoplasmic sperm injection,
infertility and, 315–316
Intraepithelial lesions, of cervix,
treatment of, 451–455,
451f, 452f, 452t
cold-knife conization, 454
cryosurgery, 452–453
hysterectomy, 454–455
laser vaporization, 453
loop electrosurgical excision
procedure, 453–454,
454b, 454f
Intrauterine device (IUD),
170–176
abnormal bleeding and, 174
after abortion insertion of, 173
action mechanism of, 171–172
adolescence and, 173
adverse effects of, 174–176
cautionary conditions,
172–173
chronic medical problems and,
173–174
contraindications of, 172
expulsion and, 174
infection and, 175
nulliparous women, 173
pain and, 174
patient selection for, 172–174
perforation and, 175
postpartum insertion of, 173
pregnancy complications and,
175–176
prior ectopic pregnancy, 173
problem management and,
174–176
strings not visible on speculum
examination and, 174
types of, 170–171
Levonorgestrel, 171
Tcu-380 (Copper), 170–171
Intravenous conjugated equine
estrogen, for abnormal
uterine bleeding, 359
Invasive anal carcinoma, 636
Irritable bowel syndrome (IBS),
104, 105b
Ischium, 73, 74f

Isotonic solutions, hysteroscopy
and, 779
IUD. See Intrauterine device

J
Jacobaeus, 755

K
Kalk, Heinz, 755
Kallmann syndrome, 21

L
Labia, 81, 81f
fused, 220
Labia majora, 16, 17f, 18t
Labia minora, 15, 17f, 18t
anomalies of, 220
fused labia, 220
hypertrophy, 219
Labioscrotal, swelling of, 15
Labor, induction of, second-
trimester pregnancy
termination and, 246–250
instillation agents, 246–247
misoprostol, 247–248
oxytocin, 247
prostaglandins, 247
special considerations in,
248–250, 249t
Lactation, contraceptives and, 182
Lactational mastitis, 502
Lacunar ligament, 74f, 75
Langenbeck, Conrad Johann
Martin, 707
Laparoscopic hysterectomy,
727, 730–734, 729t,
728–729f
Laparoscopy
complication prevention,
769–772
contraindications, 769–770,
770b
indications, 769–770,
770b
intraoperative checklist,
770–771, 771f
electrosurgical
complications, 771
pneumoperitoneum
complications,
770–771, 772t

Laparoscopy (Continued)
  electrosurgery principles,
    756–760
    bipolar electrosurgery,
      759–760, 760f
    monopolar electrosurgery,
      759–760
    physics, 756–757, 756f
    waveforms, 757
      blended current, 757,
        758f, 758t, 759t
      modulated current, 757
      nonmodulated, 757
  endometriosis and, 327–329,
    328f, 329f
  equipment for, 762–763
    ancillary ports, 766
    classic entry, 763–768, 764f
    direct trocar insertion, 765
    initial entry, 763, 764f
    initial trocar placement, 763
    open laparoscopy, 765
    optical trocar technique,
      766
    radial expanding access
      cannulas, 766
    visualization, 762–763,
      762f
  history of, 755–756
  infertility and, 301–302
  laparotomy vs., ectopic
    pregnancy and, 271–272
  operative instrumentation for,
    271–272
  postoperative consideration in,
    273–274
    gastrointestinal
      complications,
      774–775
    general considerations,
      772–774
    genitourinary complications,
      775–776
    reproductive tract injury,
      777
    vascular complications, 776
  preoperative considerations,
    760–761
    checklist in, 760–761, 761f
  specimen removal, 768–769,
    768f

Laparoscopy (Continued)
  specimen removal (Continued)
    robotic laparoscopy,
      768–769, 769f
Laparotomy, laparoscopy vs.,
  ectopic pregnancy and,
  271–272
Laser vaporization, for cervical
  intraepithelial lesions, 453
Late phenotypic onset, 46
Lateral internal sphincterotomy,
  627
Lateral sacral artery, 73, 78f
LDLs. See Low-density
  lipoproteins
LeFort colpocleisis, pelvic organ
  prolapse and, 569–570,
  570f
Leiomyomas
  clinical manifestations of,
    460–461, 461b
  diagnosis of, 462–469
    diagnostic studies,
      463–469
      hysterosalpingography,
        466, 467f
      hysteroscopy, 466–469,
        468f
      magnetic resonance
        imaging, 465, 466f
      ultrasonography,
        463–464, 464–465f
    history, 462–463b
    physical examination,
      462–463
  reproductive function effects,
    461–462
  in reproductive-age women,
    492–493, 492–493f
  treatment of, 469–478
    future of, 477–478
    medical, 469–470
      gonadotropin-releasing
        hormone agonists,
        470
      nonsteroidal anti-
        inflammatory agents,
        469
      oral contraceptive pills,
        469
    surgical, 470–471

Leiomyomas (Continued)
  treatment of (Continued)
    surgical (Continued)
      abdominal myomectomy,
        472, 473f
      hysterectomy, 471–472
      hysteroscopic
        myomectomy,
        473–475, 475b
      uterine fibroid
        embolization,
        475–477, 475b,
        477b, 478b
  types of, 460f
  uterine, hysterectomy and,
    710–712
Letrozole, infertility and, 304
Levator ani muscles, 75–76, 75f,
  76f
Levonorgestrel intrauterine
  device, 171
  abnormal uterine bleeding and,
    360
LH. See Luteinizing hormone
Lichen planus, of vulva,
  418–419
Lichen sclerosus, of vulva,
  414–415
Lichen simplex chronicus (LSC),
  of vulva, 415–416
Li-Fraumeni Syndrome, 58
Ligaments, of pelvis,
  73–75, 74f
Liquid-based cytology, for
  cervical neoplasia,
  433–444
Longitudinal vaginal septum,
  216–217
Loop electrosurgical excision
  procedure, for cervical
  intraepithelial lesions,
  453–454, 454b, 454f
Low-density lipoproteins (LDLs),
  130–131, 133t
LSC. See Lichen simplex
  chronicus
Lumbar plexus, nerves of, 80–83,
  80–83f
Lung cancer
  risk factors for, 103b
  screening for, 146

Luteinizing hormone (LH), 24, 25, 26, 32–33, 34
Lymphatic/vascular metastasis theory, 323
Lymphogranuloma venereum, 527–528
Lynch, Henry, 64

M
Magnetic resonance imaging (MRI)
 of endometrium, 358
 of leiomyomas, 465, 466
Male pattern baldness, 391
Male pronucleus, 3
Males
 external genitalia of, 15, 18t
  penile urethra, 15, 17f, 18t
  penoscrotal hypospadias, 15, 17f, 18t
  phallus, 15, 17f, 18t
  scrotum, 15, 17f, 18t
 fertilization, pronucleus, 3
 genital ducts of appendix of the testis, 15
  ductus deferens, 15
  efferent ducts, 15
  ejaculatory duct, 15
  epididymis, 15
  prostatic utricle, 15
  seminal vesicle, 15
 infertility and, 310–311
 pattern baldness of, 391
 pronucleus, 3
 sterilization of, 181
Marshall-Marchetti-Krantz (MMK) procedure, 599–600
Masses, of pelvis
 in adolescence, 482–487, 482b
  adnexal masses, 485–487, 484f, 486f, 487b
  congenital obstructive lesions, 483
  functional ovarian cysts, 483–485, 484f
  ovarian masses, 483
  ovarian neoplasms, 485
 in children, 481–482, 482b
 in newborn, 481–482

Masses, of pelvis (Continued)
 in reproductive-age women, 487–494, 488b
  endometrioma, 491
  leiomyomas, 492–493, 492f
  ovarian neoplasms, 489–491, 489f, 490b
  ovarian remnant syndrome, 491–492
  peritoneal inclusion cysts, 493–494, 493f
Mastalgia, 499
Mastectomy, prophylactic, for hereditary breast cancer, 62
Matrix metalloproteinases inhibition, for endometriosis, 340
Mayer-Rokitansky-Küster-Hauser syndrome. *See* Müllerian agenesis
MCI. *See* Mild cognitive impairment
Median umbilical ligament, 19f, 20
Meiosis, 1, 2f
Melanoma, of vulva, 426, 426b
Membranous urethra, 19f, 20
Memory, menopause and, 392–393
Menometrorrhagia, 348
Menopausal bleeding, abnormal uterine bleeding and, 354–355, 355b
Menopause, 39–40
 cardiovascular disease and, 402–405, 404b, 403t
 definition of, 383–384
 diagnostic markers of, 384
 physical examination during, 405–406
  cancer screening, 405–406
  of thyroid, 406, 406t
 physiology of, 383–384
 skeletal changes, 394–402
  diagnosis of, 395–396, 395b, 397t
  osteoporosis, 394–395
  risk factors of, 395
  treatments for, 396, 398–402

Menopause (Continued)
 skeletal changes (Continued)
  treatments for (Continued)
   alcohol decrease, 402
   bisphosphonates, 399–400
   caffeine decrease, 402
   calcitonin-salmon, 401
   calcium supplements, 401
   hip protector pads, 402
   hormonal therapy, 396, 398–399
   muscle strengthening, 402
   parathyroid hormone, 400–401
   selective estrogen-receptor modulators, 400
   smoking decrease, 402
   vitamin D supplement, 401–402
 symptoms of, 385–394
  atrophic vaginitis, 388–389, 389b
  cognition, 392–393
  dementia, 392–393
  hair effects, 391–392
  headaches, 391
  hot flashes, 386b
  memory, 392–393
  menstrual irregularity, 385, 385b
  mood changes, 392
  nail effects, 391–392
  sexual function, 393–394
  skin effects, 391–392
  sleep changes, 392
  urinary incontinence, 389–391
  vasomotor, 385–387, 386, 387t, 388b, 388t
 terminology of, 383–384
Menorrhagia, 348
 in adolescence, 201–202, 202b, 203t
Menstrual cycle, 30–35, 367–369, 368t
 follicular phase, 30–32, 31f, 33f
 luteal phase, 34–35
 ovulation, 33–34

Menstrual cycle (Continued)
  physiology of, 367–369, 368f, 369t
Menstrual dysfunction. See Abnormal uterine bleeding
Menstrual irregularity, menopause and, 385, 385b
Mesoderm, 7, 7f, 10
  paraxial, 8
Mesonephric duct, 15
Mesonephros, 16, 17
Mesorectum, 609
Metanephric mesoderm, 17
Metanephros, 17
Metformin, infertility and, 304–305
Methotrexate, ectopic pregnancy and direct injection, 278
  multidose systemic, 274–275, 275t
  single-dose systemic, 275
Methotrexate/misoprostol, pregnancy termination, 253, 253t
Metrorrhagia, 348
Microbicides, contraceptives and, 177–178
Microsatellites, 56
Middle rectal artery, 78, 78f
Mild cognitive impairment (MCI), 150
Misoprostol, pregnancy termination, 247–248, 251–252
Missed abortion, 225
Mitochondrial, family history, cancer risk assessment and, 47
Mitosis, 2f
Modified McCall culdoplasty, for uterine/vaginal vault prolapse, 561–562, 562f
Mona pubis, 16, 17f, 18t
Mons veneris, 83, 84f
Mood changes, menopause and, 392
  symptoms of, 392
Morula, 3
MRI. See Magnetic resonance imaging

MUC. See Mucosal ulcerative colitis
Mucosal ulcerative colitis (MUC), 614–615, 615b, 615f
Müllerian agenesis, 208–212, 210t
Müllerian tubercle, 14
Multidose systemic methotrexate, ectopic pregnancy and, 274–275, 275t
  medical management of, 274–275, 275t
Multifactorial, family history, cancer risk assessment and, 47
Muscles, of pelvis, 75–76, 75f, 76f
Musculoskeletal system, well-woman exam and, 110–111
Mutated gene classes, 54–56
Myocardial infarction, risk factors for, 101b
Myomas. See Leiomyomas
Myomectomy, for abnormal uterine bleeding, 361

N
Nails, menopause and, 391–392
National Institute of Diabetes and Digestive and Kidney Diseases (NIDDK), 667, 668b
National Society of Genetic Counselors, 44
Neoplasia, cervical, screening for, 442–447
  cervical sampling, 443, 443b
  HPV DNA adjunct to, 444–445
  liquid-based cytology, 443–444
  modern recommendations, 445–447, 446f, 446t, 447b
  negative, 444–445
Neoplasms, ovarian
  in adolescence, 482–483
  in reproductive-age women, 487–489, 488f, 489b
Nephrons, 19, 19f

Nerves
  of anterior abdominal wall, 80–81, 80f, 81f
  of breasts, 492
  of lumbar plexus, 80–83, 80–83f
  of pelvis, 80–83, 80f–83f
  stimulation of, interstitial cystitis, 667b, 678
Neural folds, 8
Neural groove, 8
Neural plate, 8
Neurologic injury, gynecologic surgery and, 704
Newborns
  ambiguous genitalia in, 205–208, 206f, 206b, 207b
  pelvic mass of, 481–482
NIDDK. See National Institute of Diabetes and Digestive and Kidney Diseases
Nonlactational (subareolar) abscess, of breasts, 502–503
Nonpolyposis colorectal, hereditary cancer syndrome, 64–67
  chemoprevention in, 67
  clinical manifestations of, 64, 65b, 65f
  genetic testing in, 64–66
  management of, 66–67
  surgical strategies for, 67
  surveillance of, 66
Nonsteroidal anti-inflammatory drugs
  for abnormal uterine bleeding, 353
  for endometriosis, 329
Norplant, 169
Notochordal process, 8
Nuva Ring, 167

O
Obesity, 106
Obturator artery, 78, 78f
Obturator externus muscle, 76, 76f
Obturator internus muscle, 76, 76f

Oligomenorrhea, 347
One-cell embryo, 3, 4f
Oocytes, 1, 2
Oogonia, 1, 14, 14f
Oophorectomy, prophylactic
    hysterectomy and, 738–741
    for ovarian cancer, 63–64
Optical biopsy diagnosis, for
    cervical cancer, 448, 449f
Optical trocar technique, for
    laparoscopy, 766
Oral contraceptives
    for abnormal uterine bleeding,
      353
    combined, 162–167, 162b,
      163t, 164t, 166b
      action mechanisms of, 162
      contraindications of,
        162–163, 162b, 163t
      noncontraceptive benefits,
        165, 166b
      preparations for, 166–167
      prescription guidelines for,
        163–164t
      risks of, 163–165, 164t
      side effects of, 163–165
    for endometriosis, 332t, 334
    leiomyomas, 464
Ortho Evra, 168
Osteoporosis, 107, 108b,
    394–395
    prevention health care and,
      138–139, 138b, 140t
    prevention of, 140t
    risk factors for, 135b
    treatment of, 140t
Ovarian drilling, infertility and,
    306
Ovarian ectopic pregnancy, 281
Ovarian remnant syndrome, in
    reproductive-age women,
    487
Ovary, 27–30
    androgens, 27, 30
    cancer of, screening for, 141
    cysts of
      in adolescence, 198
      functional, 483–484,
        484f
      in prepuberty patients,
        188–189

Ovary (Continued)
    estrogen, 30, 30t
    hereditary cancer syndrome,
      58–64
      cancer screening, 61–62
      oophorectomy, prophylactic,
        62–63
      risk reduction of, 63
    masses of, in adolescence,
      482
    progestin, 27, 29t
    reproductive cycle androgens,
      29, 30
      estrogen, 29, 29t
      perhydrocyclopentano
        phenanthrene, 27, 27f
      progestin, 27, 29t
      steroid hormone
        biosynthesis, 27,
        28–28f
Ovulation, 39
Ovulatory factor, infertility and,
    303–306
    Clomid, 303–306
    gonadotropins, 305–306
    letrozole, 304
    metformin, 304–305
    ovarian drilling, 306
Oxytocin, pregnancy
    termination, 247
Oxytocin and vasopressin, 26

P
Paget's disease, 425, 636
Pain abdominal, causes of, 105,
    106b
    intrauterine device and, 170
    management of in first-
      trimester pregnancy
      termination, 230–232
    interstitial cystitis, 667b,
      671–672
    of pelvis, 210–211,
      206b, 679
    in adolescence, 198–199,
      199b
    diagnosis of, 683
    differential diagnosis of,
      680–683, 680b
    treatment of, 677–678
    of vulva, 416–423

Pain abdominal, causes of
    (Continued)
    of vulva (Continued)
      Behçet's disease, 419
      erosive diseases, 416–420
      herpes simplex virus,
        416–420, 418t
      lichen planus, 418–419
      syndromes, 420–423
      ulcerative diseases, 416–420
      vestibulitis, 420–423
      vestibulodynia, 420–423
      vulvodynia, 420–423
Palmer, Raol, 708
Pap smear. See Papanicolaou
    smear
Papanicolaou, George, 423–424
Papanicolaou (Pap) smear, 423
Paraovarian cysts, 15
Parathyroid hormone,
    menopause and, 400
Paravaginal defect repair, for
    anterior vaginal wall
    prolapse, 572, 575
Paraxial mesoderm, 8
Paroophoron, 15
Patch contraceptive, 168
PCOS. See Polycystic ovarian
    syndrome
Pectineal ligament, 74f, 75
Pelvic diaphragm, 75–76, 75f,
    76f
    anatomy of, 545–547, 546f
Pelvic floor
    anatomy of, 89–96, 545
      bladder, 90
      endopelvic fascia, 88–89,
        89f, 90f
      pelvic diaphragm, 93–95
      pelvic organ support, 92
      ureter, 87f, 90
      urethra, 90–92, 91f
      urethral support, 95–96, 96f
      vesical support, 95–96, 96f
    dysfunction pathophysiology
      of, 547–549
    risk factors for, 549–550
Pelvic inflammatory disease,
    533–535, 535b, 536b
Pelvic organ prolapse (POP)
    cost of, 543–544

Pelvic organ prolapse (POP)
(Continued)
diagnosis of, 550–551
physical examination,
551–552
staging, 552–553
symptoms of, 550–551
epidemiology of, 543
gynecologic assessment of, 116
hysterectomy and, 707,
745–746
natural history of, 544
nonsurgical management of,
557–560
behavior modification, 558
expectant, 557–558
pessary, 558–560, 55b,
559f, 560b
pathophysiology of, 547–549
risk factors for, 549–550, 549b
staging of, 552
diagnostic tests, 557
Pelvic organ prolapse
quantification, 552–557,
553–556f, 556b
surgical repair techniques, 561
anterior vaginal wall
prolapse anterior
colporrhaphy,
571–572, 573–574f
paravaginal defect repair,
572, 575
enterocele, 561
graft reconstructive, 579
obliterative operations,
569–571
colpectomy, 571
colpocleisis, 571
LeFort colpocleisis,
569–570, 570f
posterior vaginal wall
prolapse, 575
discrete rectovaginal
fascia defect repair,
576–579, 577f, 578f
posterior colporrhaphy,
575–576
posterior perineorrhaphy,
575–576
uterine/vaginal vault
prolapse, 561–569

Pelvic organ prolapse
quantification (Continued)
surgical repair techniques
(Continued)
uterine/vaginal vault
prolapse (Continued)
abdominal
sacrocolpopexy,
567–569, 568f
hysterectomy, 561
iliococcygeus fascia
suspension,
565–567, 566f
modified McCall
culdoplasty,
561–562, 562f
sacrospinous ligament
suspension, 565
uteropexy, 569
uterosacral ligament
vaginal vault
suspension,
563–564, 564f
vaginal enterocele repair,
564–565
terminology of, 544–545
anterior vaginal wall
prolapse, 544
apical prolapse, 544
enterocele, 544–545
posterior vaginal wall
prolapse, 544
uterovaginal prolapse, 544
Pelvic Organ Prolapse
Quantification (POPQ), 121,
552–556, 553–556f, 556f
Pelvis arteries of, 77–79,
77–79f
bones of, 73–75, 74f
ligaments of, 73–75, 74f
mass of
in adolescence, 482–487,
482b
adnexal masses, 485–487,
484f, 486f, 487b
congenital obstructive
lesions, 483
functional ovarian cysts,
483–485, 484f
ovarian masses, 483
ovarian neoplasms, 485

Pelvis arteries of (Continued)
mass of (Continued)
in children, 481–482, 482b
in newborn, 481–482
in reproductive-age women,
487–494, 488b
endometrioma, 491
leiomyomas, 492–493,
492f
ovarian neoplasms,
489–491, 489f, 490b
ovarian remnant
syndrome,
491–492
peritoneal inclusion cysts,
493–494, 493f
muscles of, 75–76, 75f, 76f
nerves of, 80–83, 80f, 81f
pain of, 198–199, 199b, 679,
747–748
in adolescence, 198–199,
199b
diagnosis of, 683
differential diagnosis of,
680–683, 680b
treatment of, 683–684
Penile urethra, 15, 17f, 18t,
19f, 20
Penoscrotal hypospadias, 15,
18f, 18t
PEP. See Persistent ectopic
pregnancy
Perhydrocyclop
entanophenanthrene,
ovaries and, 27, 27f
Perimenopause, 384
abnormal uterine bleeding in,
353–354
adnexal mass in, 494–495,
493f, 494f
contraceptives and, 183
Perineal body, gynecologic
assessment of,
119–120
Perineal membrane, anatomy
of, 547
Perineal space, muscles of, 85f
deep, 85, 84f
superficial, 84, 85f
Perineum, blood supply of,
86, 86f

Peritoneal inclusion cysts, in reproductive-age women, 493–494, 493f

Persistent ectopic pregnancy (PEP), surgical management of, 273–274, 274b

Peutz-Jeghers Syndrome, 58

Phallus, 15, 17f, 18t

Phenotypical sex, 11

Pinworms, 188–190

Piriformis muscle, 76, 76f

Pituitary, 25–27
  antidiuretic hormone, 26
  dysfunction of primary amenorrhea and, 369–370
    secondary amenorrhea and, 372–373
  gonadotropins, 25
  regulation of, 25–26
  oxytocin and vasopressin, 26
  posterior pituitary hormones, 26–27
  prolactin, 26

PMDD. See Premenstrual dysmorphic disorder

PMS. See Premenstrual syndrome

Polycystic ovarian syndrome (PCOS), 370, 375–376

Polymenorrhea, 347

POP. See Pelvic Organ Prolapse

POPQ. See Pelvic Organ Prolapse Quantification

Postcoital test, infertility and, 296

Posterior colporrhaphy, for posterior vaginal wall prolapse, 575–576

Posterior perineorrhaphy, for posterior vaginal wall prolapse, 575–576

Posterior vaginal wall prolapse, surgical repair techniques of, 576
  discrete rectovaginal fascia defect repair, 576–579, 577f, 578f
  posterior colporrhaphy, 575–576

Posterior vaginal wall prolapse, surgical repair techniques of (Continued)
  posterior perineorrhaphy, 575–576

Postmenopausal bleeding, 348

Postmenopause adnexal mass in, 494–495, 493f, 494f
  pelvic abscess in, 495

Pregnancy breast cancer and, 517–518
  hysteroscopy and, 780–781
  intrauterine device and, 170–172

Pregnancy, ectopic
  assisted reproduction and, 261
  clinical presentation of, 262–265
  diagnostic modalities in, 265–271
    culdocentesis, 269, 271
    laboratory tests, 265–266
    quantitative serum hCG, ultrasonography plus, 268–269, 269f
    ultrasonography, 266–268, 267f, 268t, 269f, 270t
      quantitative serum hCG plus, 268–269, 270f
    uterine curettage, 271
  epidemiology of, 257–259
    incidence of, 257, 258f
    mortality, 258–259, 258f
  failed contraception, 261
  functional factors in, 260–261
  infertility, 261
  location of, 262, 263f
  medical management of, 274–278
    direct injection methotrexate, 278
    multidose systemic methotrexate, 274–275, 275t
    patient counseling in, 277, 277b
    patient monitoring in, 276–277
    patient safety in, 277–278
    patient selection in, 276, 276b

Pregnancy, ectopic (Continued)
  medical management of (Continued)
    single-dose systemic methotrexate, 275
  natural history of, 262–265
  pathogenesis of, 259–262
  reproductive performance after, 283–284, 283b
  Rh sensitization, 279
  risk factors of, 259–262, 259t
  salpingitis, 259–260
  signs of, 264–265, 264t
  sterilization, 261
  surgical management of, 271–274
    conservative surgery, 272–273, 273f
    laparotomy vs. laparoscopy, 271–272
    persistent, 273–274, 274b
    radical surgery, 272
  symptoms of, 264–265, 264t
  treatment of, medical vs. surgical, 278–279
    efficacy, 278–279
    expectant management, 279
    safety, 278–279
  tubal abortion, 262–263
    tubal injury in, 259–260, 260f
    tubal rupture, 263, 264f
    tubal surgery, 261
  types of, uncommon, 279–280
    abdominal, 280–281
    cervical, 281–282
    heterotopic, 282
    interstitial, 279–280, 280f
    ovarian, 281

Pregnancy loss
  early, 225–227
    diagnosis of, 225–226
    epidemiology of, 225
    management of, 226–227
  recurrent, 227–228
    diagnosis of, 229–230, 230t, 231t
    etiologies of, 228–229
      anatomic, 228

Pregnancy loss *(Continued)*
  recurrent *(Continued)*
    etiologies of *(Continued)*
      behavioral, 229–230
      endocrinologic, 228
      environmental, 229–230
      genetic, 228
      immunologic, 229
      infectious, 228
      social, 229–230
      thrombophilic, 229
    management of, 226–227,
      230t
Pregnancy termination
  care after, 244–246, 245b
  counseling for, 232
  early medical, 250–254
    methotrexate/misoprostol,
      253, 253t
    mifepristone, 250–251
    mifepristone/misoprostol
      abortion provision,
      251–252, 251b, 252b
    complications of,
      252–253, 253t
    misoprostol, 253–254
  epidemiology of, 230–231
  first-trimester, 232–233,
    232–239, 233t, 234t
    complication incidence,
      238–239
    complication management,
      238–239
    gestational age
      determination,
      232–233, 233t, 234t
    pain management,
      236–238
    pregnancy diagnosis,
      232–233, 233t, 234t
    preoperative evaluation,
      234, 235t
    products of conception
      examination, 238
    surgical technique, 234–236
  long-term effects of,
    254–255
  second-trimester, 239–244,
    239t, 240–241t
    complication incidence, 244,
      244t

Pregnancy termination
  (Continued)
  second-trimester *(Continued)*
    complication management,
      244, 244t
    by labor induction
      246–250
      instillation agents,
        246–247
      misoprostol, 247–248
      oxytocin, 247
      prostaglandins, 247
      special considerations in,
        248–250, 249t
    preoperative cervical
      preparation, 242–243,
      242t
    special considerations,
      243–244
    surgical technique, 243
Premature ovarian failure,
  373
Premenarchal girls,
  abnormal uterine
  bleeding in, 353
Premenstrual dysmorphic
  disorder (PMDD), 378–380,
  379b
  evaluation of, 379–380
  pathophysiology of, 379
  treatment of, 379–380
Premenstrual syndrome (PMS),
  378–380, 379b
  evaluation of, 379–380
  pathophysiology of, 379
  treatment of, 379–380
Prepuberty patients
  conditions of, common,
    188–193
    ovarian cysts, 192–193
    pinworms, 188
    vaginal bleeding, 190–192,
      191b
    vulvovaginitis, 188, 190b,
      191b, 191f
  examination approach of,
    187–188
    Tanner Classification, 188,
      189f
Prevention health care
  cancer screening

Prevention health care
  (Continued)
  cancer screening *(Continued)*
    breast, 145, 141
    cervical, 145–146
    colorectal, 146, 147t
    lung, 146
    ovarian, 145
    skin, 146, 148
  for cardiovascular disease,
    126–138
    aspirin and, 137–138
    diabetes, 133–134, 134t,
      135b, 136t, 137t
    dyslipidemia, 130–133,
      132t, 133t
    exercise, 137
    HRT and, 137–138
    hypertension, 127–130,
      128t, 129t, 130t
    prevention of, 137–138
    risk factor assessment,
      126–127, 127b
    smoking, 135, 137
  dementia, 150, 151b
  depression, 148–149
  domestic violence, 150–152
  immunizations, 141,
    142–144t
  osteoporosis, 138–139, 138b,
    140t
  substance abuse, 152–154
  thyroid disease, 139
Primary villi, 5
Primitive heart tubes, 8
Primitive node, 7
Primitive sex cords, 13
Primitive streak, 6, 7f
Primordial germ cells, 30
Progesterone, for abnormal
  uterine bleeding, 359
Progestin
  for endometriosis, 332t
  ovaries and, 27, 30t
Progestin-only pill, 168
Prolactin, 26
Pronephros, 16
Prostaglandins, pregnancy
  termination, 247
Prostatic urethra, 19f, 20
Prostatic utricle, 15

Proteinuria
  differential diagnosis of, 11b
  evaluation of, 112b
Proto-oncogenes, mutations
  of, 54
Pruritus, of vulva, 412–416,
  414–416
  candidiasis, 413–414
  dermatitis, 412–413
  dermatologic conditions,
    414–416
    lichen sclerosus,
      414–415
    lichen simplex chronicus,
      415–416
    psoriasis, 416
  lichen sclerosus, 414–415
  lichen simplex chronicus,
    415–416
  psoriasis, 416
Psoriasis, of vulva, 416
Psychosocial assessment, well-
  woman exam and,
  114–115
  anxiety disorders,
    114–115
  eating disorders,
    114, 114b
  violence against woman,
    115–116
Puberty, 38–39 See also
  Adolescence; See also
  Prepuberty patients
  adrenarche, 38
  breasts and, 39, 39t
  delayed, in adolescence,
    193–194, 194b, 196,
    196f
  gonadarche, 38–39
  physical changes in, 39, 39t
  pubic hair and, 39, 39t
Pubic hair, puberty and,
  39, 39t
Pubis, 73, 74f
Pulmonary system, well-woman
  exam and, 102–103, 103b

Q
Quantitative serum hCG, ectopic
  pregnancy and, 268–269,
  269f

R
Radial expanding access
  cannulas, for laparoscopy,
  766
Radiation therapy, for breast
  cancer, 515–516
Rectal prolapse, 622–624, 623b,
  625b
Rectocele, 619–620
Reduced penetrance, 46
Renal system, well-woman exam
  and, 110
Reproductive cycle
  coordination of, 21, 22f
  endometrium, 35–38
    anatomy of, 35
    breakdown of, 37–38
    proliferative phase of,
      35–36, 36f
    secretory phase of, 36–37,
      37f
  hypothalamic axis, regulation
    of, 23–24
  hypothalamus, 21–25
    adrenocorticotropic
      hormone, 24
    catecholamines, 24
    corticotropin-releasing
      hormone, 24–25
    gonadotropin-releasing
      hormone, 21–23
    growth hormone-releasing
      factor, 24–25
    somatostatin, 24–25
    thyroid-stimulating
      hormone, 24–25
    thyrotropin-releasing
      hormone, 24–25
  menopause, 39–40
  menstrual cycle, 30–35
    follicular phase, 30–32, 31f,
      33f
    luteal phase, 34–35
    ovulation, 33–34
  ovary, 27–30
    androgens, 29
    estrogen, 29–30, 30t
    perhydrocyclo-
      pentanophenanthrene,
      27, 27f
    progestin, 27, 29t

Reproductive cycle (Continued)
  ovary (Continued)
    steroid hormone
      biosynthesis, 27,
      27–28f
  pituitary, 25–27
    antidiuretic hormone, 26
    gonadotropins, 25
      regulation of, 25–26
    oxytocin and vasopressin,
      26
    posterior pituitary
      hormones, 26–27
    prolactin, 26
  puberty, 38–39
    adrenarche, 38
    gonadarche, 38–39
    physical changes in, 39, 39t
Reproductive organs
  cervix, 87f, 88–89
  fallopian tubes, 87f, 88
  ovaries, 87–88, 87f
  uterus, 87f, 88–89, 89f
  vagina, 87f, 89
Reproductive-age women, pelvic
  masses in, 487–494, 488b
  endometrioma, 491
  leiomyomas, 492–493, 492f
  ovarian neoplasms, 489–491,
    489f, 490b
  ovarian remnant syndrome,
    491–492
  peritoneal inclusion cysts,
    493–494, 493f
Rete testis, 13, 13f
Retrograde menstruation theory,
  322
Retropubic procedures, for
  urinary incontinence,
  598–601
  Burch colosuspension, 599,
    600f
  complications of, 601
  Marshall-Marchetti-Krantz
    procedure, 599–600
  outcomes of, 601
  paravaginal defect repair,
    600–601
  patient selection for, 598–599
Rh sensitization, ectopic
  pregnancy and, 279

Richardson, E. H., 708
Rokitansky syndrome, 15

S

Sacrospinous ligament, 74f, 75
Sacrospinous ligament
    suspension, for uterine/
    vaginal vault prolapse, 565
Sacrotuberous ligament, 74f, 75
Sacrum, 73, 74f
Saline infusion sonography, of
    endometrium, 357, 357b
Salpingitis, 259–260
Sarah Lawrence College, 44
SCJ. *See* Squamocolumnar
    junction
Screening
    for cancer
        bowel disorder guidelines,
            612b
        of breasts, 145, 141
            hereditary, 58
        of cervix, 145–146
        colorectal, 146, 147t
        of lungs, 146
        of ovaries, 145
        of skin, 146, 148
    for cervical neoplasia, 442–447
        cervical sampling, 443, 443b
        HPV DNA adjunct to, 444
        liquid-based cytology,
            443–444
        modern recommendations,
            445–447, 446f, 446t,
            447b
        negative, 444–445
    hereditary cancer syndromes
        of breast, 61
        of ovaries, 61–62
    menopause and, physical
        examination during,
        405–406, 405t
    prevention health care
        breast, 145, 141
        cervical, 145–146
        colorectal, 146, 147t
        lung, 146
        ovarian, 145
        skin, 146, 148
    well-woman exam and,
        99–100

Scrotum, 15, 17f, 18t
Second-trimester pregnancy
    termination, 239–244,
    239t, 240–241t
    complication incidence,
        238–239, 239t
    complication management,
        238–239, 239t
    by labor induction, 246–250
        instillation agents, 246–247
        misoprostol, 247–248
        oxytocin, 247
        prostaglandins, 247
        special considerations in,
            248–250, 249t
    preoperative cervical
        preparation, 242–243,
        232t
    special considerations,
        248–249
    surgical technique, 243
Selective estrogen-receptor
    modulators, menopause
    and, 400
Semen, analysis of, infertility and,
    299–300
Seminal vesicle, 15
Septate uteri, 213–214, 214f
Serum markers, endometriosis
    and, 329
Sex-specific expression, 46
Sexual differentiation, 11
Sickle cell disease, contraceptives
    and, 184
Single-dose systemic
    methotrexate, ectopic
    pregnancy and, 275t
Sirenomelia, 10, 11f
Skeletal, changes, menopause
    and, 394–402
    diagnosis of, 395–396, 395b,
        397t
    osteoporosis, 394–395
    risk factors of, 395
    treatments for, 396, 399–402
        alcohol decrease, 402
        bisphosphonates, 399–400
        caffeine decrease, 402
        calcitonin-salmon, 401
        calcium supplements, 401
        hip protector pads, 402

Skeletal, changes, menopause
    and (*Continued*)
    treatments for (*Continued*)
        hormonal therapy, 396,
            398–399
        muscle strengthening, 402
        parathyroid hormone,
            400–401
        selective estrogen-receptor
            modulators, 400
        smoking decrease, 402
        vitamin D supplement, 401
Skin
    assessment of, well-woman
        exam and, 113–114
    cancer of, screening for, 146,
        148
    effects, menopause, symptoms
        of, 391–392
    menopause and, 391–392
Sleep, disordered, respiratory
    conditions associated with,
    103b
Smoking
    cardiovascular disease and,
        135, 137
    cervical cancer and,
        434–435
    decrease in, menopause and
Somatostatin, 24–25
Somites, 8
Spermicides, 177–178
Sponge, 177
Spontaneous abortion, 225
Squamocolumnar junction (SCJ),
    430
Sterility, 287
Sterilization, 178–181
    ectopic pregnancy
        and, 261
    hysteroscopic, 180–181
    laparoscopic techniques, 180
    of male, 181
    minilaparotomy, 179–180
Steroid hormone biosynthesis,
    27, 27–28f
Stratum compactum, 36
Stratum spongiosum, 36
Subfertility, 287
Substance abuse, 152–154
    gynecologic surgery and, 692

Suburethral sling procedure, for urinary incontinence, 601–604
  complications of, 604
  outcomes of, 604
  patient selection for, 602
  technique for, 602–603
Superior gluteal artery, 77, 78f
Superior vesical artery, 78, 78f
Surgery. *See* Gynecologic surgery
Surgical site infection prophylaxis, gynecologic surgery and, 694–695
Syncytiotrophoblast, 4
Syphilis, 525–527
Systemic hormonal contraceptives, 159, 162–170
  combined oral, 162–167, 162b, 163t, 164t, 166b
  contraceptive patch, 168
  implants, 169–170
  injectables, 168–169
  progestin-only pill, 168
  vaginal ring, 167t
Systemic therapy, for breast cancer, 512

T

Tanner Classification, 188, 189f
Tcu-380 (Copper) intrauterine device, 170–171
TDLU. *See* Terminal duct lobular unit
Terminal duct lobular unit (TDLU), 498
Therapeutic amenorrhea, 376–377
Threatened abortion, 225
Thrombosed hemorrhoid, 625
Thyroid, disease of, prevention health care and, 139
Thyroid disorders, 107b
Thyroid-stimulating hormone (TSH), 24
Thyrotropin-releasing hormone (TRH), 24–25
Tools
  for endometrium evaluation, 356–358
    biopsy, 356
    hysteroscopy, 358–359

Tools (*Continued*)
  for endometrium evaluation (*Continued*)
    magnetic resonance imaging, 358
    saline infusion sonography, 357, 357b
    transvaginal ultrasound, 356–357
  for vulva examination, 410
    biopsy, 411–412
    colposcopy, 412
    cultures, 411
    serologies, 411
    wet mount/potassium hydroxide preparation, 411
Total joint replacement, gynecologic surgery and, 691
Transvaginal needle suspension procedures, for urinary incontinence, 604–605
Transvaginal ultrasonography (TVUS), 458
Transvaginal ultrasound, of endometrium, 356–357
Transverse vaginal septum, 218–219
Treponema pallidum, 411
TRH. *See* Thyrotropin-releasing hormone
Trophectoderm, 3
Trophoblast, 4, 5, 6f
TSH. *See* Thyroid-stimulating hormone
Tuberculosis, 528–529
Tubo-ovarian abscess, 535–536
TVUS. *See* Transvaginal ultrasonography
2001 Bethesda System, 436–442
  adenocarcinoma, 441–442
  endometrial cells, 437
  glandular cell abnormalities, 440–441, 439b, 439f
  negative intraepithelial lesion, 437
  negative malignancy, 437
  specimen adequacy, 437
  squamous cell abnormalities, 437–440, 438–440b, 439f

U

UFE. *See* Uterine fibroid embolization
UI. *See* Urinary incontinence
Ultrasonography
  ectopic pregnancy and, 266–268, 267f, 268t, 269f, 270t
  quantitative serum hCG plus, 268–269, 269f
  of leiomyomas, 463–464, 464–465f
Unicornuate uterus, 214–215, 214f
Urachus, 19f, 20
Ureter, 19f, 20
Ureteric buds, 16–17, 19f
Urethra, 19f, 20
  gynecologic assessment of, 119
Urethral groove, 16, 17f, 18t
Urethral meatus, 73, 84f
Urinary incontinence (UI)
  anatomic structures related to 584–585
  behavioral approaches in, 594–595
  classification of, 587–588
    extra-urethral, 588
    mixed, 587–588
    overflow, 588
    stress, 587
    uncategorized, 588
    urge, 587
  medical management of, 598–606
    detrusor overactivity, 596–598
    stress, 596
  menopause and, 389–391
  neurophysiology of, 585–587, 586f
  patient history in, 589–591, 590t
  pelvic floor, physiotherapy of, 595–596
  physical examination of, 591–592
  predisposing factors of, 588–589
  surgical management of, 598–606

Urinary incontinence (UI)
(Continued)
surgical management of
(Continued)
bulk enhancing agent
injection, 605–606
complications of, 601
outcomes of, 601
periurethral technique,
605
transurethral technique,
605
retropubic procedures,
598–601
Burch colosuspension,
599, 600f
complications of, 601
Marshall-Marchetti-
Krantz procedure,
599–600
outcomes of, 601
paravaginal defect repair,
600–601
patient selection for,
598–599
suburethral sling procedure,
602–603
complications of, 604
outcomes of, 604
patient selection for, 602
technique for, 602–603
transvaginal needle
suspension procedures,
604–605
urodynamic testing in,
593–594, 593f
Urinary retention, gynecologic
surgery and, 687
Urinary system, in embryology,
16–20
allantois, 19f, 20
bladder, 19f, 20
collecting tubules, 19
ejaculatory ducts, 19f, 20
median umbilical ligament,
19f, 20
membranous urethra, 19f, 20
mesonephric duct, 17
mesonephros, 16, 17
metanephric mesoderm, 17
metanephros, 16
nephrons, 19, 19f

Urinary system, in embryology
(Continued)
penile urethra, 19f, 20
pronephros, 16
prostatic urethra, 19f, 20
urachus, 19f, 20
ureter, 19f, 20
ureteric buds, 16–17, 19f
urethra, 19f, 20
urogenital sinus, 19–20
vestibule of the vagina, 19f, 20
Urinary tract, injuries of,
631–651
bladder injury, 648–650
intraoperative management,
648–650, 649f
intraoperative recognition,
648–650, 649f
epidemiology of, 633–635,
639–640b
procedure types, 640–641,
640b
hysterectomy and, 742–743
postoperative management,
650
postoperative recognition of,
650–651
prevention of, 641–642
abdominal surgery,
643–644
anatomy, 642–643, 643f
laparoscopic surgery,
644–645, 645f
vaginal surgery,
644, 645f
ureteral injury, 646–648
intraoperative recognition,
646–647
surgical management,
647–648
urethral injury, 651
Urinary tract infections (UTIs),
537–541
cystitis, 538–539, 539b
pyelonephritis, 541
urethritis, 538
Urogenital fold, 15, 17f, 18t
Urogenital sinus, 19–20
Urogenital system, in
embryology, 10–20
external genitalia, 15
genetic sex, 11

Urogenital system, in embryology
(Continued)
genital ducts, 14–16
gonadal sex, 11
gonads, 12–14, 13f
phenotypical sex, 11
sexual differentiation, 11
urinary system, 16–20
allantois, 19f, 20
bladder, 19f, 20
collecting tubules, 19
ejaculatory ducts, 19f, 20
median umbilical ligament,
19f, 20
membranous urethra, 19f,
20
mesonephric duct, 16
mesonephros, 16, 17
metanephric mesoderm, 17
metanephros, 16
nephrons, 19, 19f
penile urethra, 19f, 20
pronephros, 16
prostatic urethra, 19f, 20
urachus, 19f, 20
ureter, 19f, 20
ureteric buds, 16–17, 19f
urethra, 19f, 20
urogenital sinus, 19–20
vestibule of the vagina, 19f,
20
Uterine anomalies, 208–219
classification of, 208–219,
209b, 210t, 212–217f
bicornuate uterus, 213, 214f
cervical agenesis, 217–218,
217f
didelphic uterus, 214–215,
215f
longitudinal vaginal septum,
216–217
Müllerian agenesis, 208,
212, 209t
septate uteri, 213–214, 215f
transverse vaginal septum,
218–219
unicornuate uterus, 214,
215, 215f
uterine didelphys, 215–216,
215f
uterine horns, 212–213,
212f

809

Uterine anomalies (*Continued*)
  incidence of, 208
Uterine artery, 78, 79f
Uterine bleeding, abnormal in
  adolescence, 201–202,
  202b, 203b, 353, 353b
  diagnosis of, 349–352, 350b,
    351b
  endometrial cancer,
    355, 356b
  endometrial hyperplasia,
    355–356b
  intrauterine device and, 170
  menopausal bleeding,
    354–355, 355b
  oral contraceptives for, 358
  outcomes of, 364
  pathophysiology of, 348–349,
    349b
  perimenopause, 353–354
  premenarchal girls, 353
  prevalence of, 348
  signs of, 353
  symptoms of, 349
  therapy for, 358
    medical, 358
      Danazol, 359
      gonadotropin-releasing
        hormone, 359–360
      intravenous conjugated
        equine estrogen, 359
      levonorgestrel intrauterine
        device, 360
      nonsteroidal anti-
        inflammatory drugs,
        358
      oral contraceptive pills,
        358
      progesterone, 359
    surgical, 360–361
      dilation and curettage,
        362
      endometrial ablation, 362,
        363t
      hysterectomy, 361
      management of,
        362–363
      myomectomy, 361
      operative hysteroscopy,
        360–361
      uterine fibroid
        embolization, 361

Uterine bleeding, abnormal in
  adolescence (*Continued*)
  von Willebrand's disease,
    352–353
Uterine curettage, ectopic
  pregnancy
  and, 271
Uterine didelphys, 215–216,
  215f, 216f
Uterine fibroid embolization
  (UFE), 475–477, 475b,
  475b, 477b
  for abnormal uterine bleeding,
    353
Uterine horns, 108f, 212–213,
  212f
Uterine leiomyomas,
  hysterectomy and,
  710–712
Uterine/vaginal vault prolapse,
  surgical repair techniques of,
  61–79
  abdominal sacrocolpopexy,
    567–569, 568f
  hysterectomy, 561
  iliococcygeus fascia
    suspension, 565–567,
    561b
  modified McCall culdoplasty,
    561–562, 552f
  sacrospinous ligament
    suspension, 565
  uteropexy, 569
  uterosacral ligament vaginal
    vault suspension,
    563–564, 563f
  vaginal enterocele repair,
    564–565
Uteropexy, for uterine/vaginal
  vault prolapse, 569
Uterosacral ligament vaginal
  vault suspension, for
  uterine/vaginal vault
  prolapse, 563–564, 564f
Uterovaginal anomalies,
  200–201
Uterus
  anomalies of, classification
    of bicornuate uterus,
    213–214, 214f
  didelphic uterus, 214–215,
    214f

Uterus (*Continued*)
  anomalies of, classification
    of bicornuate uterus
    (*Continued*)
    unicornuate uterus,
      214–215, 214f
  bicornuate, 213, 214f
  didelphic, 214–215, 214f
  dysfunction of, secondary
    amenorrhea and,
    372–375
  enlarged, removal of, vaginal
    hysterectomy, 722–725
  normal support mechanism,
    545–547, 546f
  reproductive organs, 86f, 87,
    87f
  unicornuate, 214–215, 214f
UTIs. *See* Urinary tract infections

V
Vagina
  bleeding of, 190–192, 191b
  gynecologic assessment of,
    116–118
  normal support mechanism,
    545, 547, 546f
Vaginal anomalies, 208–218
  classification of, 208–219,
    209b, 210t, 212–217f
    bicornuate uterus,
      213, 214f
    cervical agenesis,
      217, 217f
    didelphic uterus, 214–216,
      215f
    longitudinal vaginal septum,
      216–217
    Müllerian agenesis,
      208–212, 209t
    septate uteri, 213–214, 215f
    transverse vaginal septum,
      218–219
    unicornuate uterus,
      214–215, 214f
    uterine didelphys, 215–216,
      215f
    uterine horns, 108f,
      212–213, 212f
Vaginal enterocele repair, for
  uterine/vaginal vault
  prolapse, 564–565

Vaginal hysterectomy, 719–722, 728f
  enlarged uterus removal, 722–725
Vaginal plate, 14
Vaginal ring, 167
Vaginitis
  bacterial vaginosis, 529–530, 530b
  trichomoniasis, 530–531
  vulvovaginal candidiasis, 530, 531b
Vaginoscopy, hysterectomy, 783
Variable expressivity, 46–47
Vasomotor symptoms, menopause and, 385–388, 387, 387t, 388b, 388t
Vesicovaginal fistulas, hysterectomy and, 743–744
Vestibule, 83, 84f
  of vagina, 19f, 20
Vestibulitis, of vulva, 420–423
Vestibulodynia, of vulva, 420–423
Villi
  anchoring, 10
  free/terminal, 10
  primary, 8, 9f
  secondary, 8, 9f
  tertiary, 8, 9f
Violence
  domestic, 150–152
  against woman, 115–116
Viral hepatitis, 537
Viruses, DNA alterations, in cancer cells, 53–54
Vitamin D supplement, menopause and, 401
Von Willebrand's disease (VWD), 352–353
Vulva
  anatomy of, 409–410
  examination of, diagnostic tools for, 411–412
    biopsy, 411–412
    colposcopy, 412
    cultures, 411
    serologies, 411
    wet mount/potassium hydroxide preparation, 411

Vulva (Continued)
  gynecologic assessment of, 116–118
  history of, 410
  infections of, 523–524
    genital warts, 524, 524b
    parasitic, 523–524
  pain of, 416–418
    Behcet's disease, 419
    erosive diseases, 416–418
    herpes simplex virus, 418, 418t
    lichen planus, 418–419
    syndromes, 420–423
    ulcerative diseases, 416–418
    vestibulitis, 420–423
    vestibulodynia, 420–423
    vulvodynia, 420–423
  palpable masses of, 423–425
    Bartholin's abscess, 426–427
    Bartholin's gland carcinoma, 426, 426b
    basal cell carcinoma, 426, 426b
    hidradenitis suppurativa, 426–427
    human papillomavirus, 423–424, 424t
    melanoma, 426, 426b
    non-squamous cell malignancies, 426, 426b
    Paget's disease, 425
    VIN, 423–425, 424t
    vulvar condyloma, 423–425, 424t
  physical examination of, 410
  pruritus of, 412–413
    candidiasis, 413–414
    dermatitis, 412–413
    dermatologic conditions, 414–415
      lichen sclerosus, 414–415
      lichen simplex chronicus, 415–416
      psoriasis, 416
Vulvar condyloma, 423–425, 424t
Vulvodynia, of vulva, 420–423
Vulvovaginitis, 188, 190b, 191b, 191f

VWD. *See* von Willebrand's disease

W
Waveforms, laparoscopy, 755–756
  blended current, 755, 756f, 758t, 759t
  modulated current, 757
  nonmodulated, 757
Well-woman exam
  history and, 100–116, 100b
    breast assessment, 113
      breast cancer, 113
      fibroadenoma, 113
      fibrocystic changes, 113
    cardiovascular system, 101–102
    endocrine system, 106–109
    gastrointestinal system, 103–106
    musculoskeletal system, 110–112
    psychosocial assessment, 114
      anxiety disorders, 114–115
      eating disorders, 114, 114b
      violence against woman, 115–116
    pulmonary system, 102–103, 103b
    renal system, 100
    skin assessment, 113–114
  prevention and, 99–100
  screening for, 99–100
Wertheim, Ernst, 708
Wound care, gynecologic surgery and, 701–702

X
Xeroderma pigmentosum, 58
X-linked dominant/recessive, family history, cancer risk assessment and, 46–47

Y
Yolk sac, 5, 7f, 10

Z
Zona pellucida, 31
Zygote, 1, 3, 4f